Cognitive Functioning and Brain Plasticity

Cognitive Functioning and Brain Plasticity

Editor: Hudson Webb

MURPHY & MOORE
www.murphy-moorepublishing.com

www.murphy-moorepublishing.com

MURPHY & MOORE

Cataloging-in-Publication Data

Cognitive functioning and brain plasticity / edited by Hudson Webb.
p. cm.
Includes bibliographical references and index.
ISBN 978-1-63987-117-9
1. Cognitive neuroscience. 2. Neuroplasticity. 3. Cognition. 4. Neuropsychology. 5. Neurophysiology. I. Webb, Hudson.
QP360.5 .C64 2021
612.823 3--dc23

Murphy & Moore Publishing,
1 Rockefeller Plaza,
New York City, NY 10020, USA

ISBN 978-1-63987-117-9 (Hardback)

Contents

Preface

This book has been a concerted effort by a group of academicians, researchers and scientists, who have contributed their research works for the realization of the book. This book has materialized in the wake of emerging advancements and innovations in this field. Therefore, the need of the hour was to compile all the required researches and disseminate the knowledge to a broad spectrum of people comprising of students, researchers and specialists of the field.

The ability of the brain to structurally and functionally alter itself is called brain plasticity. Plasticity, or the ability to change, is one of the most important aspects of neural development and regular functioning. It is also observed as a response to a change in the environment or advancing age. The potential of a person to gain cognitive skills under certain situations or conditions is termed as cognitive plasticity. These cognitive skills can be enhanced through different methods such as observational learning and practice. The study of cognitive plasticity assumes a difference between a person's current cognitive performance and their untapped potential. This book presents the complex subject of cognitive functioning and brain plasticity in the most comprehensible and easy to understand language. From theories to research to practical applications, case studies related to all contemporary topics of relevance to this field have been included in it. This book will help the readers in keeping pace with the rapid changes in this field.

At the end of the preface, I would like to thank the authors for their brilliant chapters and the publisher for guiding us all-through the making of the book till its final stage. Also, I would like to thank my family for providing the support and encouragement throughout my academic career and research projects.

Editor

1

Plasticity of Brain Wave Network Interactions and Evolution across Physiologic States

Kang K. L. Liu[1, 2], *Ronny P. Bartsch*[3], *Aijing Lin*[1, 4], *Rosario N. Mantegna*[5, 6] *and Plamen Ch. Ivanov*[1, 7, 8*]

[1] *Laboratory for Network Physiology, Department of Physics, Boston University, Boston, MA, USA,* [2] *Department of Neurology, Beth Israel Deaconess Medical Center, Harvard Medical School, Boston, MA, USA,* [3] *Department of Physics, Bar-Ilan University, Ramat Gan, Israel,* [4] *Department of Mathematics, School of Science, Beijing Jiaotong University, Beijing, China,* [5] *Dipartimento di Fisica e Chimica, Viale delle Scienze, University of Palermo, Palermo, Italy,* [6] *Center for Network Science and Department of Economics, Central European University, Budapest, Hungary,* [7] *Division of Sleep Medicine, Brigham and Women's Hospital, Harvard Medical School, Boston, MA, USA,* [8] *Institute of Solid State Physics, Bulgarian Academy of Sciences, Sofia, Bulgaria*

Edited by:
Ido Kanter,
Bar Ilan University, Israel

Reviewed by:
Sebastiano Stramaglia,
Università degli Studi di Bari, Italy
Wolfgang Kinzel,
Universität Würzburg, Germany

***Correspondence:**
Plamen Ch. Ivanov
plamen@buphy.bu.edu

Neural plasticity transcends a range of spatio-temporal scales and serves as the basis of various brain activities and physiologic functions. At the microscopic level, it enables the emergence of brain waves with complex temporal dynamics. At the macroscopic level, presence and dominance of specific brain waves is associated with important brain functions. The role of neural plasticity at different levels in generating distinct brain rhythms and how brain rhythms communicate with each other across brain areas to generate physiologic states and functions remains not understood. Here we perform an empirical exploration of neural plasticity at the level of brain wave network interactions representing dynamical communications within and between different brain areas in the frequency domain. We introduce the concept of time delay stability (TDS) to quantify coordinated bursts in the activity of brain waves, and we employ a system-wide Network Physiology integrative approach to probe the network of coordinated brain wave activations and its evolution across physiologic states. We find an association between network structure and physiologic states. We uncover a hierarchical reorganization in the brain wave networks in response to changes in physiologic state, indicating new aspects of neural plasticity at the integrated level. Globally, we find that the entire brain network undergoes a pronounced transition from low connectivity in Deep Sleep and REM to high connectivity in Light Sleep and Wake. In contrast, we find that locally, different brain areas exhibit different network dynamics of brain wave interactions to achieve differentiation in function during different sleep stages. Moreover, our analyses indicate that plasticity also emerges in frequency-specific networks, which represent interactions across brain locations mediated through a specific frequency band. Comparing frequency-specific networks within the same physiologic state we find very different degree of network connectivity and link strength, while at the same time each frequency-specific network is characterized by a different signature pattern of sleep-stage stratification, reflecting a remarkable flexibility in response to change in physiologic state. These new aspects of neural plasticity demonstrate that in addition to dominant brain waves, the network of brain wave interactions is a previously unrecognized hallmark of physiologic state and function.

Keywords: neural plasticity, network physiology, brain wave interactions, time delay stability, sleep

1. INTRODUCTION

Physiological systems and organisms exhibit complex dynamics that continuously change with transitions across physiologic states and conditions by adapting neuronal regulatory mechanisms to optimize function and adequately respond to internal and external stimuli (Ivanov et al., 1999; Kantelhardt et al., 2002; Karasik et al., 2002; Ivanov et al., 2007; Schmitt et al., 2009; Schumann et al., 2010; Bartsch et al., 2012). The ability to perform variety of functions and to adapt to short-term and long-term changes in the environment results from high degree of plasticity in the nervous system. Neural plasticity occurs at multiple levels of organization and over a broad range of time scales (Destexhe and Marder, 2004). At the microscopic level, the ability of neurons to react to different inputs and in response to generate various output dynamics serves as a fundamental building block for a broad range of brain functions (Tononi and Cirelli, 2014). Neurons communicate with each other through chemical and electrical synapses, and the temporal firing patterns of presynaptic neurons, various neuropeptides, and neuromodulator neurons (Marder and Thirumalai, 2002) as well as the specific timing of activation of presynaptic and post-synaptic neuron activity modulate synaptic strength (Abbott and Nelson, 2000; Sjöström and Nelson, 2002) and induce synaptic plasticity that further empowers functional variation. Changes in the intrinsic firing properties of individual neurons (Marder et al., 1996) as well as modulation of synaptic strength (Kandel, 2001) play important role in the mechanisms underlying neuronal circuit plasticity (Abeles, 1991; Katz and Frost, 1996; Engel et al., 2001), which in turn affects the integrative properties of neurons leading to transitions in large network behavior. Thus, as a direct consequence of plasticity at the neuronal, synaptic, and circuitry level a variety of brain waves emerge with different dominant rhythms (Steriade et al., 1993; Traub et al., 2001; Steriade and Timofeev, 2003; Hill and Tononi, 2005; Millman et al., 2010; Olcese et al., 2010).

At the integrated system level, plasticity and neuromodulation have crucial roles in altering excitability in the brain and regulating physiological states such as sleep and wake (Gorgoni et al., 2013). Such modulation of excitatory and inhibitory brain activity during different physiologic states and conditions leads to specific brain waves with dominant frequencies—e.g., higher frequency α-wave associated with higher excitability and dis-synchronous cortical activation during quiet wake, and low frequency δ-wave associated with low excitability and global synchronous activation during deep sleep (Kryger et al., 1994; Massimini et al., 2005; Niedermeyer and da Silva, 2005; Siegel, 2005). In addition to dominant brain waves, physiological states are characterized by specific signatures in the temporal modulation of brain waves (Linkenkaer-Hansen et al., 2001; Poil et al., 2008) and their synchronization across different locations (White et al., 1998; Kopell et al., 2000).

The majority of studies in the field have focused on mechanisms of neural plasticity at the microscopic level of neurons, synapses (Jahnke et al., 2008; Deger et al., 2012; Helias et al., 2014) and neuronal circuits (Vardi et al., 2013, 2015), and on the role particular brain waves play in modulating neural plasticity (Diekelmann and Born, 2010). A fundamental question is how brain waves, which carry important information on physiologic function and result from complex mechanisms of neural plasticity, dynamically communicate with each other and collectively coordinate as a network to produce physiologic states. Here we investigate how neural plasticity is manifested through dynamic interactions of brain waves across different frequency bands and brain locations, and how these interactions facilitate physiologic functions. Since neural plasticity at the microscopic level can be modulated by physiologic states (Stefan et al., 2000; Wolters et al., 2005; Schmidt et al., 2006; Huber et al., 2007), thus leading to changes in physiologic function, we hypothesize that transitions across physiologic states would not only lead to changes in dominant brain waves and their temporal organization but will also modulate the coupling between different brain waves and the entire network of their interactions. Further, we hypothesize that the network dynamics of brain wave interactions and their evolution across physiologic states will provide (i) new information on functional plasticity and (ii) a new hallmark of physiological state derived from the network of brain wave interactions.

To address the fundamental question of how different brain waves dynamically communicate as a network, we develop a novel approach inspired by the new interdisciplinary field of Network Physiology (Bashan et al., 2012; Bartsch and Ivanov, 2014; Ivanov and Bartsch, 2014). This field focuses on understanding complex physiologic function as an emergent phenomenon from network interactions among diverse dynamical systems (network nodes). To identify and quantify networks of brain wave interactions, we introduce the concept of time delay stability (TDS) to analyze coordinated bursts in brain wave activity within different physiologically-relevant frequency bands and across different brain areas. Specifically, we investigate how networks of brain wave interactions evolve with different sleep stages (deep sleep, light sleep, rapid eye movement sleep, and wake) because: (i) sleep stages are well-defined physiologic states (Kryger et al., 1994) with external environmental inputs significantly reduced; (ii) sleep is essential for neural plasticity at the microscopic level (Huber et al., 2008); and (iii) disrupting sleep influences motor behaviors, vigilance, and cognitive functions at the integrated system level (Stickgold, 2005; Born et al., 2006; Rye et al., 2012).

Moreover, recent sleep investigations indicate a previously unknown non-homeostatic, non-equilibrium process that underlies the micro-architecture of sleep-stage and arousal transitions on time scales from seconds to hours, where inhibitory and excitatory brain activations appear to be coupled through a common self-organized criticality (SOC) type mechanism (Lo et al., 2002, 2004, 2013). Based on these observations we hypothesize that as a result of the underlying neuronal plasticity, brain waves coordinate their bursting activities across different frequency bands and brain locations to generate distinct physiologic functions. We further hypothesize that networks representing diverse brain wave interactions carry important information about the nature of physiologic function during specific physiologic states, and that the evolution of such brain wave networks across physiologic states reveals new aspects of functional plasticity.

The aim of this study is to bridge the gap between (i) investigations of neuronal and synaptic plasticity on the microscopic level and on mechanisms of vertical integration to generate specific brain waves in neuronal networks, and (ii) phenomenological studies of physiologic states and functions at the macroscopic system level. The Network Physiology approach we present here fills in this gap through investigations of the horizontal integration among brain waves with different physiologic function, and by probing how physiologic states modulate the network of brain wave interactions across physiologically-relevant frequency bands and brain areas. This study provides first insights on the collective network behavior of diverse brain waves, and how such networks undergo complex reorganization with transitions across distinct physiologic states (such as sleep stages) to facilitate advanced brain functions and physiologic regulation.

2. MATERIALS AND METHODS

2.1. Statement of Ethical Approval

The data we used in this work are pre-existing multi-channel physiologic recordings from EU SIESTA databases. The detailed protocol of the SIESTA database can be found in Klösch et al. (2001). All participants provided written informed consent.

The research protocol was approved by the Institutional Review Boards of Boston University (Boston, MA, USA) and was conducted according to the principles expressed in the Declaration of Helsinki.

2.2. Subject Data

We analyze continuously recorded multi-channel physiological data obtained from 36 healthy young subjects (18 female, 18 male, with ages between 20 and 40, average 29 years) during night-time sleep (average record duration is 7.8 h). We focus on physiological dynamics during sleep as sleep stages are well-defined physiological states, and external influences due to physical activity or sensory inputs are reduced during sleep. Sleep stages are scored in 30 s epochs by sleep lab technicians based on standard criteria (Rechtschaffen and Kales, 1968). Specifically, we analyze EEG data from six scalp locations (frontal left—Fp1, frontal right—Fp2, central left—C3, central right—C4, occipital left—O1, and occipital right—O2). In order to compare these very different signals with each other and to study interrelations between them, we extract the following time series from the raw EEG signals: the spectral power of seven frequency bands of the EEG in moving windows of 2 s with a 1 s overlap: δ (0–4 Hz), θ (4–8 Hz), α (8–12 Hz), σ (12–16 Hz), β (16–20 Hz), γ_1 (20–34 Hz), and γ_2 (34–100 Hz).

2.3. Time Delay Stability

One key aspect of neuronal plasticity and synaptic plasticity is the time-dependent behavior of single neurons and their synaptic connections (Buzsáki et al., 2012). Heterogeneous distribution in the response latency and characteristic times scales of various neurons and synapses generate complex temporal dynamics in electrophysiological signals including bursting oscillations and long-range correlated brain waves (Denker et al., 2004).

The complexity in the output EEG signals characterized by non-stationarity, continuous fluctuation poses a great challenge in identifying and quantifying dynamical interactions between EEG signals. This challenge is further compounded by the intrinsic time delay between neuronal activity that emerges at different brain locations, which makes traditional cross-correlation techniques inadequate. Here, we adapt a new framework from Network Physiology to analyze brain network interactions based on the concept of Time Delay Stability (TDS), a method tailor-made for quantifying interactions through the output signals of diverse systems (Bashan et al., 2012; Bartsch et al., 2014).

To probe the interaction between EEG spectral power in two frequency bands A and B, we consider their output signals $\{a\}$ and $\{b\}$ each of length N. We divide both signals $\{a\}$ and $\{b\}$ into N_L overlapping segments ν of equal length $L = 60$ s. We choose an overlap of $L/2 = 30$ s, which corresponds to the time resolution of conventional sleep-stage-scoring epochs, and thus $N_L = [2N/L] - 1$. Next, we calculate $C^{\nu}_{ab}(\tau) = \frac{1}{L}\sum_{i=1}^{L} a^{\nu}_{i+(\nu-1)L/2} b^{\nu}_{i+(\nu-1)L/2+\tau}$, which is the cross-correlation function within each segment $\nu \in [1, N_L]$ by applying periodic boundary conditions. For each segment ν, we define the time delay τ^{ν}_0 to correspond to the maximum in the absolute value of the cross-correlation function $C^{\nu}_{ab}(\tau)$ in this segment (**Figure 1**).

Time periods of stable interrelation between two signals are represented by segments of approximately constant τ_0 in the newly defined series of time delays, $\{\tau^{\nu}_0\}|_{\nu\in[1,N_L]}$. In contrast, absence of stable coupling between the signals corresponds to large fluctuations in τ_0. We identify two systems as linked if their corresponding signals exhibit a time delay that does not change by more than ±1 for several consecutive segments ν. We track the values of τ_0 along the series $\{\tau^{\nu}_0\}$: when for at least four out of five consecutive segments ν (corresponding to a window of 5×30 s) the time delay remains in the interval $[\tau_0 - 1, \tau_0 + 1]$, these segments are labeled as stable. This procedure is repeated for a sliding window with a step size one along the entire series $\{\tau^{\nu}_0\}$. The % TDS is finally calculated as the fraction of stable points in the time series $\{\tau^{\nu}_0\}$ (**Figure 1**). We have tested several different values for the window size L, i.e., $L = 30$, 60, 120, and 180 s with non-overlapping windows as well as window overlaps $L/2$ and $L/4$. The overall TDS results were not significantly different for the different combinations of L and overlap, however, there was a tendency to noisier τ_0 vs. t signals for shorter windows and less overlap. On the other hand larger windows reduce the time resolution of the TDS. We chose $L = 60$ s with an overlap of 30 s because this choice was most sensitive to sleep-stage transitions that are scored in 30 s epochs (**Figure 1**), consistent with the traditional sleep research time scales.

2.4. Visualization Approach and TDS Brain-networks

To visually inspect and dissect the complex communications between one brain area and others that are mediated through

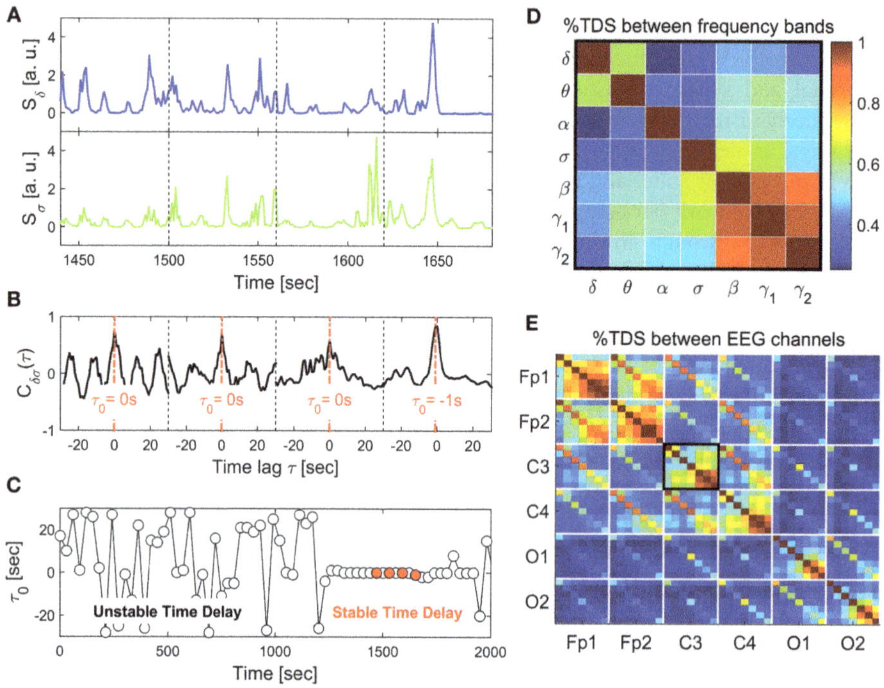

FIGURE 1 | Schematic presentation of the Time Delay Stability (TDS) method and TDS matrix representing the degree of coupling between different frequency bands across brain locations. (A) Segments of brain EEG power spectra S_δ and S_σ for the δ- and σ-band shown for four consecutive 60 s time windows. **(B)** Coordinated bursts in S_δ and S_σ lead to pronounced cross-correlation $C_{\delta\sigma}$ within each time window. The time lag τ_0 that corresponds to the peak in the cross-correlation function $C_{\delta\sigma}(\tau)$ represents the time delay between the two signals. **(C)** Time delay τ_0 between S_δ and S_σ plotted as a function of time for consecutive 60 s windows moving with a step of 30 s. Four red dots represent τ_0 for the four windows shown in the above panels. Note the transition at $\sim$ 1200 s from a segment with strongly fluctuating τ_0 to a stable time delay regime with $\tau_0 \approx$ constant. Such regime of time delay stability (TDS) indicates the onset of physiological coupling. The fraction of time when TDS is observed in the EEG recording, i.e., % TDS, quantifies the degree of coupling strength. Longer periods of TDS between S_δ and S_σ reflect stronger coupling. **(D)** TDS matrix representing the degree of coupling between different physiologically relevant EEG frequency bands ($\delta, \theta, \alpha, \sigma, \beta, \gamma_1, \gamma_2$) derived from the C3 channel. Matrix elements represent % TDS, where the color code is shown in the vertical bar. **(E)** Block-matrix representing the degree of TDS coupling between EEG channels (Fp1, Fp2, C3, C4, O1, O2) and between EEG frequency bands. Each off-diagonal block element corresponds to a specific pair of EEG channels and each diagonal block element represents the coupling between different frequency bands within the same EEG channel, as shown in **(D)**.

various frequency bands, these interactions are mapped onto a network where group averaged TDS links strength are scaled with the line thickness of the corresponding network links.

Network nodes with different colors represent seven different frequency bands ($\delta, \theta, \alpha, \sigma, \beta, \gamma_1, \gamma_2$). Each set of seven nodes ordered as a heptagon forms a vertex on the hexagon representing six EEG channels from particular brain locations: 2 Frontal areas (Fp1 and Fp2), 2 Central areas (C3 and C4), and 2 Occipital areas (O1 and O2).

These networks consists of intra-channel links at a chosen channel/location and inter-channel links between the chosen channel location and other brain areas. The intra-channel links for a given channel location are plotted using a gray color code where the darkness and the width of the line are scaled with the link strength. The inter-channel links are plotted with the color representing the frequency band located at the chosen channel (C3, Fp1, or O1) and the line thickness is scaled with the link strength.

If an inter-channel link ends at a node with the same color as the link itself, this link represents interactions between spectral power of the same frequency bands at different locations. We define these links as same-frequency links. Otherwise, links whose color do not match with the node color represent communications between two different frequency bands, and thus are defined as cross-frequency links.

3. RESULTS

3.1. Plasticity in Brain Wave Interactions Across the Entire Brain

Utilizing our TDS method and network approach, we identify and quantify coupling between brain waves defined by physiologically-relevant EEG frequency bands. We build a network of brain wave interactions, where network nodes represent diverse brain waves at different brain locations and network links represent the strength of TDS coupling between brain waves across the entire brain.

We find that brain-wave network links exhibit complex patterns in the coupling strength between frequency bands across different brain locations as represented by the TDS block-matrix elements (**Figure 2**). Moreover, we find that during distinct

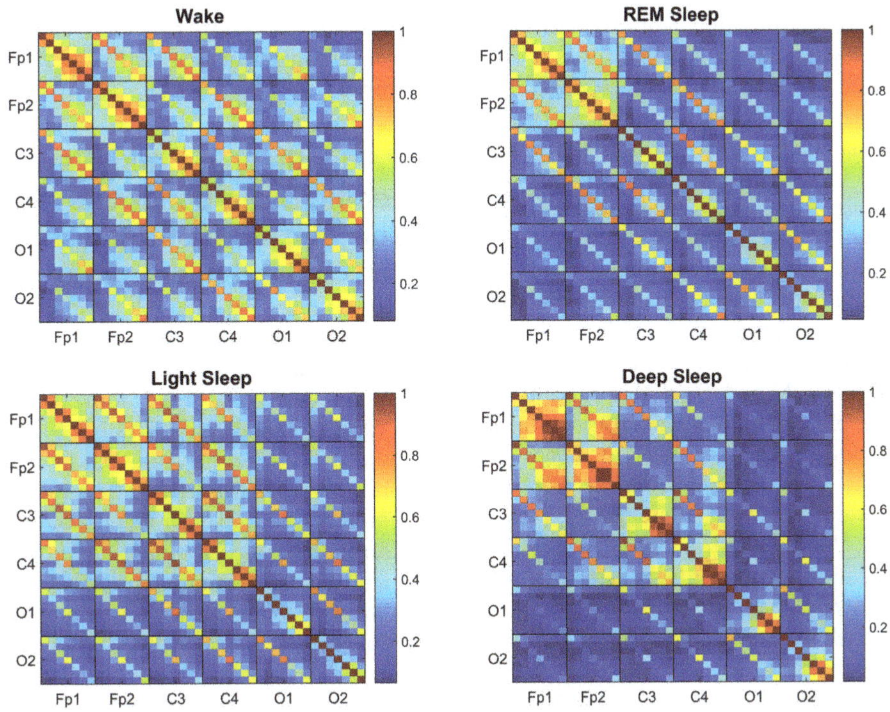

FIGURE 2 | Transitions in the Time Delay Stability (TDS) matrix across physiologic states indicate neural response and plasticity in brain wave interactions at the integrated level. Group-averaged Time Delay Stability (TDS) block-matrices during distinct physiologic states (sleep stages) obtained from continuous 8-h EEG recordings during sleep from 36 healthy subjects. Color code represents the average strength of TDS coupling between brain waves (distinct EEG frequency bands) across different brain locations as quantified by % TDS—i.e., the fraction of time out of the total duration of a given sleep stage throughout the night when TDS is observed. Parallel diagonal lines across each off-diagonal matrix block indicate strong coupling between the same EEG frequency band derived from different EEG-channel locations (e.g., coupling of δ_{C3}–δ_{C4}, α_{O1}–α_{O2} etc.). This behavior is consistently observed for all sleep stages indicating that a significant part of the brain-brain interactions across different brain areas are mediated through coupling between the same frequency bands. Transitions in the TDS matrix across different sleep stages are associated with reorganization in brain-network connectivity as reflected by (i) different configurations in the strength of the off-diagonal matrix elements that represent coupling between different EEG frequency bands in both the diagonal and off-diagonal matrix blocks, and (ii) the overall strength of coupling (% TDS, shown by color code)—lower connectivity during Deep Sleep and REM, higher during Light Sleep and highest brain-network connectivity in Wake. Such complex reorganization in the strength of brain interactions (represented by network links in the following figures) across different frequency bands and brain locations demonstrates remarkable plasticity of the brain-network in response to change of physiologic state and function.

physiologic states (sleep stages) the entire brain adjusts the configuration and strength of network connections between brain waves leading to a hierarchical network re-organization with transitions across physiologic states. This demonstrates a remarkable neural plasticity in the way brain waves coordinate their bursting activity at the integrated system level to produce physiologic functions associated with each physiologic state. Specifically, the network of brain wave interactions undergoes a pronounced transition from less connected state during Deep Sleep and REM to a highly connected state in Light Sleep and Wake (**Figure 2**).

Generally, the strongest links in the network structure of brain wave interactions are those links between brain waves of different frequencies at the same EEG-channel location (i.e., intra-channel interactions) as represented by the diagonal matrix blocks in the TDS matrix. In contrast, interactions among brain waves from different EEG-channel locations (i.e., inter-channel links) are weaker as represented by the off-diagonal matrix blocks (**Figure 2**). Further, considering all inter-channel links that represent interactions between the same brain waves exhibit strongest coupling, as shown by the dominant diagonal elements in each off-diagonal matrix block (**Figure 2**). These network features are consistently observed for all sleep stages, indicating a universal and robust structure in brain wave interactions independent of physiologic states. Moreover, our results show that a significant part of the brain wave interactions across different brain areas is mediated through the coupling between brain waves in the same frequency bands.

Comparing the TDS matrix for different sleep stages, we find that in each matrix block the most significant change in the network of brain wave interactions occurs for the off-diagonal matrix elements, which represent interactions between brain waves of different frequencies (**Figure 2**). Such dramatic re-organization in network connectivity and link strength between different brain waves (from either the same or from different brain locations) indicates high degree of neural plasticity and modulation of global cooperative behavior of brain wave interactions to accommodate physiologic function during different physiologic states. Notably, the underlying mechanism of such neural plasticity influences predominantly the interactions between pairs of different brain waves (as demonstrated by the large color variation in off-diagonal matrix elements across sleep stages, **Figure 2**). Our analyses show that neural plasticity also affects the generally stronger links between same brain waves, although to a smaller degree (smaller color variation of diagonal matrix elements across sleep stages, **Figure 2**).

To further assess plasticity in the network of brain wave interactions we compare the rank distribution of the coupling strength of brain-network links connecting brain waves from different EEG-channel locations (inter-channel links). We find that there is a pronounced stratification in the rank distributions with lowest values for most of the brain wave interactions during Deep Sleep, higher during REM and Light Sleep and highest during Wake (**Figure 3**). Moreover, these rank distributions fall into two separate categories—fast decay for REM and Deep Sleep, and slow decay for Light Sleep and Wake. The separation in two categories is most pronounced for link strength interactions above 45% TDS, where the rank distributions for REM and Deep Sleep as well as the distributions for Light Sleep and Wake practically coincide (**Figure 3**).

Generally, intra-channel interactions are stronger compared to inter-channel links. In particular, Links associated with Frontal areas have higher strength compared to Central and Occipital areas (**Figure 2**). Links that represent interactions between the same frequency band have higher strength in general compared to those interactions between different frequency bands, as evidenced by the color code of the diagonal vs. off-diagonal elements in each matrix block for different sleep stages (**Figure 2**).

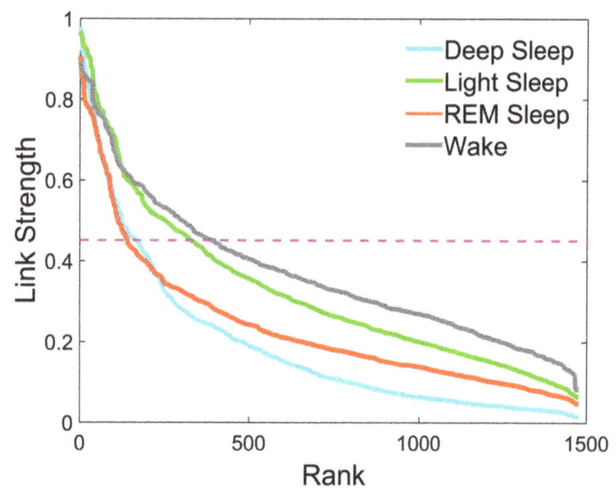

FIGURE 3 | Rank distribution of the strength of network links connecting different brain waves across brain areas. Group averaged coupling strength of inter-channel network links between different brain areas represented by the matrix elements in the off-diagonal matrix blocks of the TDS matrix shown in **Figure 2** is ranked separately for different sleep stages. Rank 1 corresponds to the strongest link in the network with highest degree of Time Delay Stability (TDS) between a pair of brain waves. The rank distributions for different sleep stages are characterized by different strength of the network links measured in % TDS—consistently lower values for most links during Deep Sleep, higher values during REM and highest during Light Sleep and Wake. Magenta dashed line represents a threshold of 45% TDS. Notably, links above the 45% TDS threshold exhibit two distinct forms of rank distributions—fast decay for Deep Sleep and REM vs. much slower decay for Light Sleep and Wake.

3.2. Plasticity in Brain Wave Interactions at Specific Brain Locations—Hierarchical Reorganization of Intra-channel and Inter-channel Interactions

To better understand the role of individual brain areas in the network of brain wave interactions, we consider subnetworks associated with specific brain locations. Specifically, we consider six subnetworks associated with the six EEG channels in the experimental setup (Section 2), where each subnetwork represents the set of network links between different frequency bands (network nodes) derived from a given EEG frequency band and brain waves at all other brain areas (EEG locations).

Our results show a strong and robust symmetry between the left and right hemisphere in both network topology and link strength configurations. For example, we find that for each physiologic state, the subnetwork associated with the C3 channel is almost identical to the one associated with the C4 channel. Thus, we only present and discuss the results obtained for the channels located in the left hemisphere (C3, Fp1, and O1).

3.2.1. Central Channel C3

3.2.1.1. Intra-channel network at C3

The intra-channel network represents flow of communication (as measured by % TDS, Section 2.3) carried by the spectral power of different frequency bands of the EEG signal recorded at one specific channel location. We find that the connectivity of the intra-channel network at C3 channel changes significantly across distinct physiologic states—we observe a lowest connectivity in REM, a higher one in Wake and Light Sleep and the highest connectivity during Deep Sleep. Notably, in Deep Sleep we observe that most links are associated with high frequency β, γ_1, γ_2 bands, which form a dark triangle in **Figure 4**.

3.2.1.2. Inter-channel network associated with C3

The inter-channel network represents interactions between one channel location and all other brain areas. By investigating the inter-channel network associated with C3, we find that the network undergoes a very pronounced reorganization with transition across sleep stages. This network reorganization, both in network structure and link strength, is more pronounced compared to the reorganization of we observe in the intra-channel network of C3 (**Figure 4**).

Central-Central interaction. Our analyses show that inter-channel links that connect same frequency bands (i.e., same-frequency links) at different central channel locations remain strong (> 45% TDS) during all sleep stages. In contrast, inter-channel links that connect different frequency bands (i.e., cross-frequency links) at the two Central channels C3 and C4 change significantly across different sleep stages. Central-Central cross-frequency links are weak with < 45% TDS during REM (not visible on the network graph), stronger during Deep Sleep

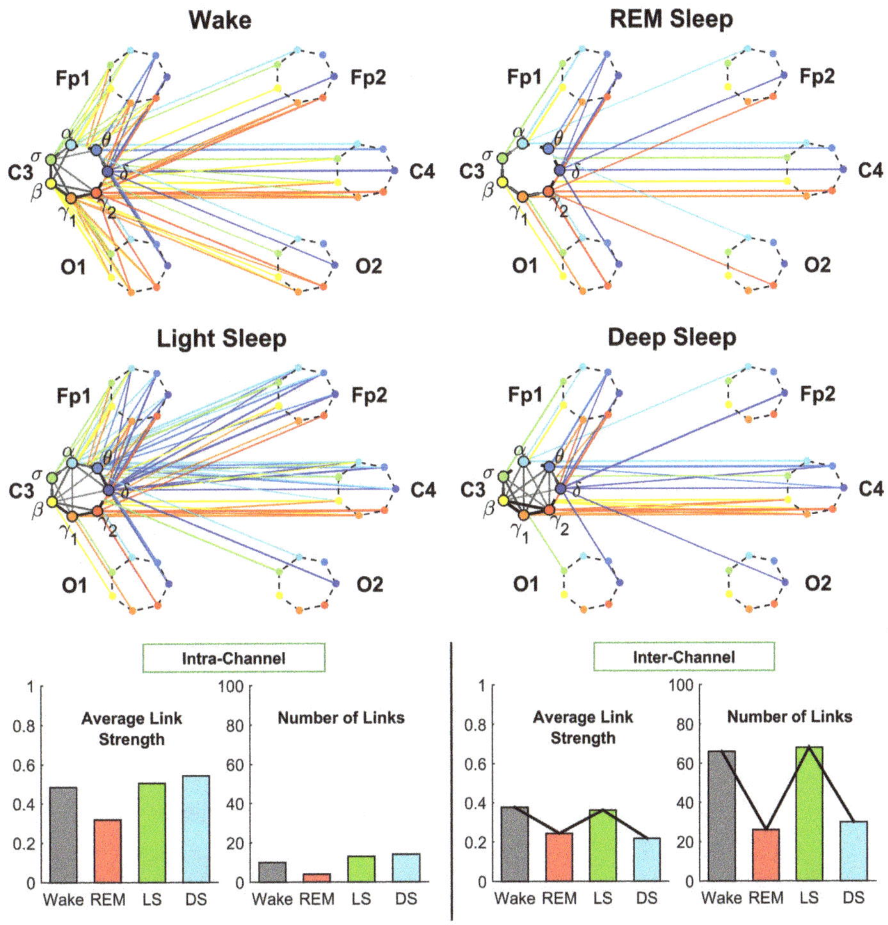

FIGURE 4 | Neural plasticity represented by transitions in the sub-networks of brain wave interactions centered at the Central C3 channel. Network nodes with different colors represent seven different frequency bands (δ, θ, α, σ, β, γ_1, γ_2) derived from EEG signals. Each set of seven nodes ordered as a heptagon forms a vertex on the hexagon representing six EEG channels from particular brain locations: Two Frontal areas (Fp1 and Fp2), two Central areas (C3 and C4), and two Occipital areas (O1 and O2). Interactions between frequency bands derived from the C3 channel (intra-channel links) are color-coded in gray scale. Interactions between frequency bands derived from the C3 channel and network nodes in all other EEG channels are represented by inter-channel links shown with the same color as the corresponding frequency band (network node) at C3. Line thickness represents the group-averaged link strength as measured by % TDS, and only links with % TDS $\geq$ 45% are shown (threshold in **Figure 3**). Both the intra-channel networks (involving links between the frequency nodes at C3) and inter-channel networks (colored links between nodes at C3 and nodes at all other channels) undergo complex hierarchical reorganization across sleep stages, indicating pronounced plasticity in the way frequency bands communicate locally within the C3 Central area and with frequency bands at other brain areas. The intra-channel subnetwork at C3 exhibits low connectivity during REM, medium connectivity during Wake and Light Sleep, and becomes highly connected during Deep Sleep. A similar sleep-stage pattern is also observed for the intra-channel links strength. In contrast, the inter-channel subnetwork between C3 and other brain areas undergoes a very different transition in network connectivity and link strength—from low connectivity in REM and Deep Sleep to high connectivity in Light Sleep and Wake. Note that an identical network structure and reorganization across sleep stages is observed for the Central C4 channel (not shown), indicating a robust symmetry between the left and right hemisphere.

and Wake, and reach their maximum strength during Light Sleep as shown in **Figure 4**.

Central-Frontal interaction. We find that inter-channel links representing connections observed between brain waves at the Central and Frontal channels have lower connectivity in REM and Deep Sleep, higher connectivity in Wake and become highly connected during Light Sleep. In general, we find that inter-channel links within the same hemisphere (C3-Fp1) are stronger than cross-hemisphere links (C3-Fp2) in all sleep stages.

Central-Occipital interaction. Further we observe that Central-Occipital brain wave interactions are much weaker (lower network connectivity) compared to Central-Central or Central-Frontal brain wave interactions, a behavior which is consistent for all sleep stages (**Figure 4**). Nonetheless, the connectivity of Central-Occipital subnetwork follows a similar sleep-stage stratification pattern as all other inter-channel subnetworks associated with C3—lower connectivity during Deep Sleep and REM, and higher connectivity during Light Sleep and Wake (**Figure 4**).

3.2.2. Frontal Channel Fp1

Next we consider the intra- and inter-channel subnetworks associated with the Frontal Channel Fp1. We observe that these subnetworks also exhibit pronounced plasticity, however, undergo a very different reorganization with sleep stage transitions as shown in **Figure 5**.

3.2.2.1. Intra-channel network at Fp1

Our analyses show that in contrast to the intra-channel network observed for the C3 channel (**Figure 5**), the intra-channel network at Fp1 remains highly connected across all sleep stages. However, the overall connectivity of the intra-channel networks at Fp1 exhibits a specific sleep-stage stratification pattern with network connectivity and average link strength similar for all sleep stages, which is different from the pattern observed at C3 where network connectivity and link strength are lower during REM and Wake and higher during Light and Deep Sleep.

3.2.2.2. Inter-channel network associated with Fp1

We find that inter-channel network of brain wave interactions associated with Fp1 location exhibits a pronounced pattern with lower connectivity during REM and Deep Sleep and much higher connectivity dying Wake and Light Sleep as shown in **Figure 5**. Notably, this sleep-stage stratification pattern is very similar to the one we find for the C3 location (**Figure 5**). Further, we find a similar stratification pattern for the average link strength though it is less pronounced compared to network connectivity (**Figure 5**).

Frontal-Frontal interaction. In contrast to the pronounced sleep-stage stratification pattern in link strength of Central-Central interactions (**Figure 4**), we find that Frontal-Frontal inter-channel interactions remain strong across all sleep stages

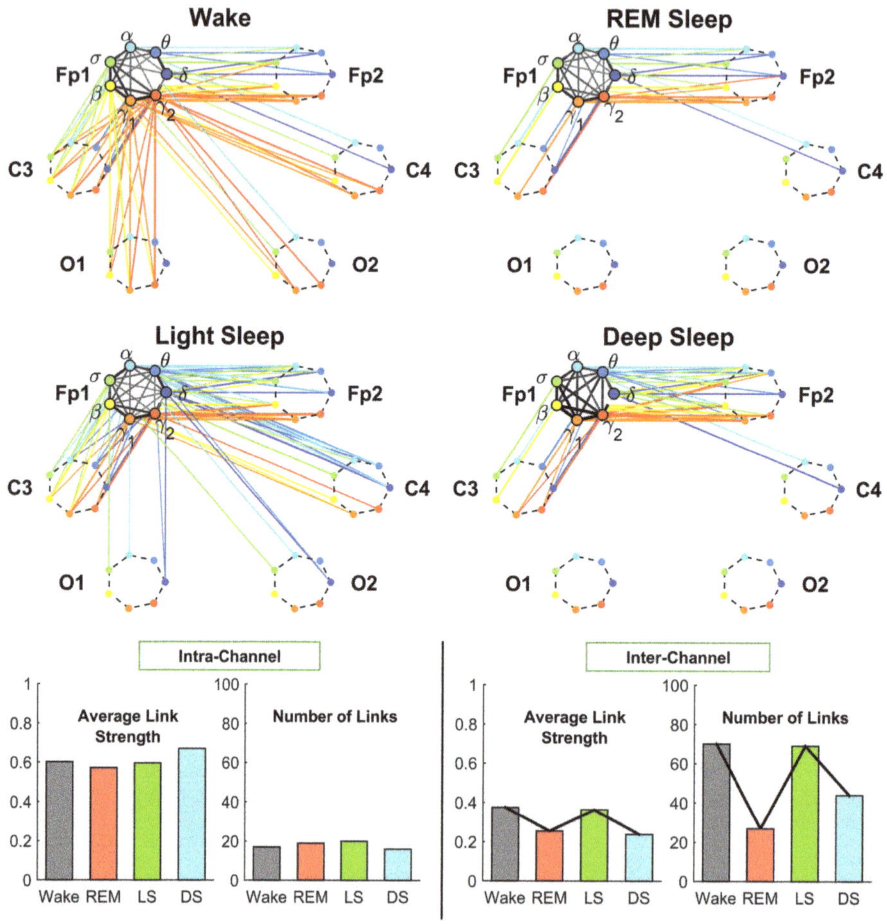

FIGURE 5 | Neural plasticity represented by transitions in the sub-networks of brain interactions centered at the Frontal Fp1 channel. Network nodes and network links are illustrated in the same way as described in **Figure 4**. Line thickness represents the group-averaged link strength as measured by % TDS, and only links with % TDS $\geq$ 45% are shown. Intra-channel sub-networks (links in gray scale) between different frequency nodes at the Fp1 channel exhibit high connectivity and link strength in all sleep stages. This is in contrast to the pronounced stratification in connectivity and average link strength observed for the C3 intra-channel sub-networks shown in **Figure 4**, and indicates a reduced plasticity in the intra-channel communications within the Frontal Fp1 area. A very different behavior is exhibited by the inter-channel sub-network representing interactions between frequency nodes at the Fp1 location and frequency nodes at other brain areas, which is characterized by a pronounced reorganization in both global connectivity and link strength configurations: Deep Sleep and REM are characterized by low global connectivity of the inter-channel sub-network and dominant links between Fp1 and the neighboring Frontal and Central areas; in contrast, global connectivity is high during Wake and Light Sleep with emerging Frontal-Occipital links that are predominantly mediated through the high frequency bands during Wake (red color links) and mainly through the low frequency bands during Light Sleep (blue color links). Note that an identical network structure and reorganization across sleep stages is observed for the Frontal Fp2 channel (not shown), indicating a robust symmetry between the left and right hemisphere.

for both same-frequency and cross-frequency links (**Figure 5**). This observation indicates that the frontal area exhibit very different plasticity and functional role in response to sleep stage transitions.

Frontal-Occipital interaction. In contrast to Frontal-Frontal, and Frontal-Central brain wave interactions, we find that Frontal-Occipital subnetworks (Fp1-O1 and Fp1-O2) are relatively sparse during Wake and Light Sleep and with practically no connections during REM and Deep Sleep (**Figure 5**).

Further, we find that during Light Sleep, Frontal-Occipital brain wave interactions are mainly mediated through the relatively low frequency δ , α , σ bands, while in contrast, during Wake, these interactions are mediated through the high frequency bands (β , γ_1 , γ_2).

3.2.3. Occipital Channel O1

3.2.3.1. Intra-channel network at O1

We find that intra-channel network of brain wave interactions at the Occipital O1 location is characterized by low connectivity during Light Sleep and REM, intermediate during Deep Sleep and high connectivity during Wake. We also observe a similar pattern for the average link strength of the O1 intra-channel network (**Figure 6**).

We note that sleep-stage transitions in the intra-channel network connectivity and average link strength at the O1 location exhibit a very different pattern (**Figure 6**) compared to the intra-channel networks observed at the C3 and Fp1 location (**Figures 4, 5**). Moreover, both network connectivity and average link strength at O1 are significantly lower compared to the C3 and Fp1 location.

These observations indicate a remarkable plasticity in brain wave network interactions, where brain wave activations modulate the neural signal at each brain location by varying the interrelation between different frequency bands in response to change in physiologic state. Further, the different level of network connectivity and average links strength, as well as the different patterns of reorganization in brain wave intra-channel interactions we discovered at different brain locations indicate a complex hierarchically structured mechanism of plasticity in brain dynamics to facilitate distinct physiologic functions.

3.2.3.2. Inter-channel network associated with O1

Occipital-Occipital interaction. Investigating the inter-channel network of brain wave interactions associated with the O1 brain location, we find that Occipital-Occipital interactions are predominantly mediated through same-frequency inter-channel links in all sleep stages.

In contrast, cross-frequency inter-channel links undergo transitions in links strength across sleep stages—weak links during REM, Deep Sleep and Light Sleep (not shown in **Figure 6**) and strong links during Wake (above the threshold of 45% TDS, **Figure 6**) that involve high frequency β , γ_1 , γ_2 bands. Notably, emergence of strong cross-frequency links between the high frequency bands is consistently observed with transition to Wake for the inter-channel subnetworks associated with Central (**Figure 4**), Frontal (**Figure 5**), and Occipital areas (**Figure 6**).

Occipital-Central and Occipital-Frontal inter-channel brain wave interactions are discussed in the Sections 3.2.1 and 3.2.2 above.

3.2.4. Dominant Frequency of Inter-channel Communications

Our investigations of the subnetworks of inter-channel brain wave interactions associated with the Central (**Figure 4**), Frontal (**Figure 5**), and Occipital areas (**Figure 6**) reveal a consistent pattern, where network connectivity and average link strength are high during Wake and Light Sleep, and lower during REM and Deep Sleep. This stratification pattern represents a previously unknown basic rule of neural plasticity underlying brain wave dynamics. Moreover, this pattern contrasts with the traditional classification of sleep stages where Deep Sleep and Light Sleep are considered similar and are categorized as Non-REM Sleep.

While network connectivity and average link strength of the inter-channel subnetworks show a similarity between Wake and Light Sleep, a closer inspection reveals that during Wake brain wave interactions are predominantly mediated through high frequency β , γ_1 , γ_2 bands, whereas during Light Sleep most links correspond to interactions between lower frequency δ , θ , α bands.

In summary, our results show that each brain area follows its own rule with respect to the intra-channel communications between different frequency bands. In contrast, brain wave interactions across different locations exhibit a robust sleep-stage stratification pattern in network connectivity and average link strength. These observations suggest the possible presence of two distinct mechanisms of plasticity that regulate the network communications across different physiologic states.

3.3. Plasticity of Individual Brain Rhythms and Complex Transitions in Frequency-specific Networks Across Physiologic States

Our investigations show that brain wave interactions between different frequency bands at different brain locations exhibit strong sleep-stage specificity—as represented by dramatic change in the off-diagonal elements of the TDS block matrices (**Figure 2**) and by cross-frequency links in the Central, Frontal, and Occipital subnetwork during different sleep stages (**Figures 4–6**). In contrast, brain wave interaction mediated through the same frequency band (e.g., parallel diagonal lines in the TDS block matrices **Figure 2**) are stronger in all sleep stages compared to the cross-frequency links, indicating an important role of same-frequency links in facilitating communications between different brain locations.

To better understand the role of same-frequency interactions across brain areas and how these interactions respond to change in physiologic states, we obtain frequency-specific networks (**Figure 7**) as the ensemble of inter-channel links connecting a specific frequency band at different brain locations (network nodes). We find that brain interactions mediated through specific frequency bands are (i) associated with very different network

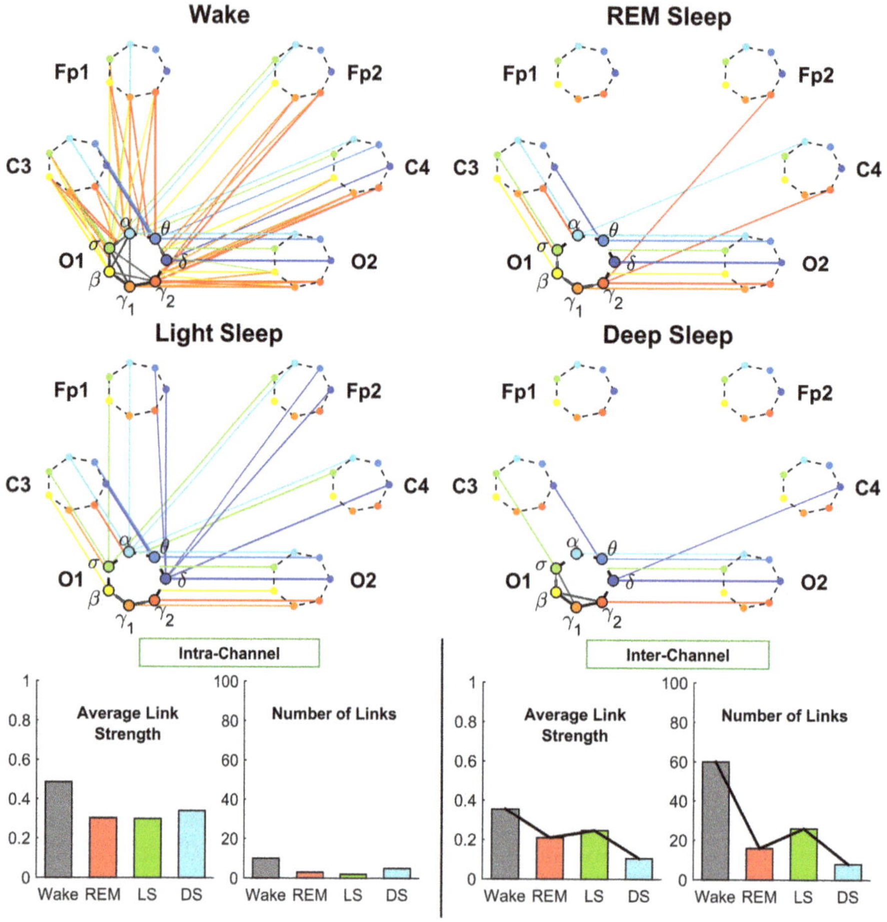

FIGURE 6 | Neural plasticity represented by transitions in the sub-networks of brain interactions centered at the Occipital O1 channel. Network nodes and network links are illustrated in the same way as described in **Figures 4, 5**. Line thickness represents the group-averaged link strength as measured by % TDS, and only links with % TDS ≥ 45% are shown. In contrast to the intra-channel sub-networks of brain interactions across frequency bands within the Central C3 area (**Figure 4**) and within the Frontal Fp1 area (**Figure 5**), the intra-channel sub-networks at the Occipital O1 channel have weak links and are generally less connected for all sleep stages—very low connectivity during REM and Light Sleep, slightly higher during Deep Sleep and highest during Wake. In contrast to the intra-channel sub-networks at the Occipital O1 location, the inter-channel sub-networks associated with the O1 channel exhibit pronounced sleep-stage stratification in global connectivity and average link strength—low connectivity during Deep Sleep and REM, and higher connectivity during Light Sleep and Wake, where brain interactions are predominantly mediated through low frequency bands during Light Sleep (blue color links) and through the high frequency bands during Wake (red color links). A similar sleep-stage stratification pattern in the overall connectivity and average link strength of the inter-channel sub-network is consistently observed for the Central C3 and Frontal Fp1 channels (**Figures 4, 5**) indicating a general rule of network reorganization underlying neural plasticity in brain interactions between frequency bands across brain areas. Note that an identical network structure and reorganization across sleep stages is observed for both O1 and O2 channels, indicating a robust symmetry between the left and right hemisphere that is also observed for the frontal and central channels (**Figures 4, 5**).

structure within a given physiologic state, and (ii) exhibit distinct patterns of hierarchical reorganization with transition across physiologic states (**Figure 7**).

Specifically, the network of brain wave interactions across different locations mediated through the δ band is highly connected in Light and Deep Sleep, indicating a strong coordination of bursting activity in the δ band across different brain locations. This is consistent with early reports of global synchronous slow wave brain activity during Non-REM Sleep (Gorgoni et al., 2013). In contrast, the network of the σ band is highly connected during Light Sleep, indicating a strong coordination of spindles at different brain locations. Networks for high frequency β, γ_1, γ_2 bands show similar sleep-stage stratification—i.e., highly connected in Wake, and much less connected in REM, Light and Deep Sleep. Notably, there is a general pattern in network connectivity and links strength where networks of all frequency bands are weakly connected during Deep Sleep and REM, and strongly connected during Light Sleep and Wake (**Figures 7, 8A**). This appears to be a robust sleep-stage stratification pattern, as we also observe it for the inter-channel subnetworks associated with the Central, Frontal and Occipital locations that involve interactions between all frequency bands (**Figures 4–6**).

Comparing frequency-specific networks within the same physiologic state, we find very different degree of network connectivity and link strength for the different bands. During

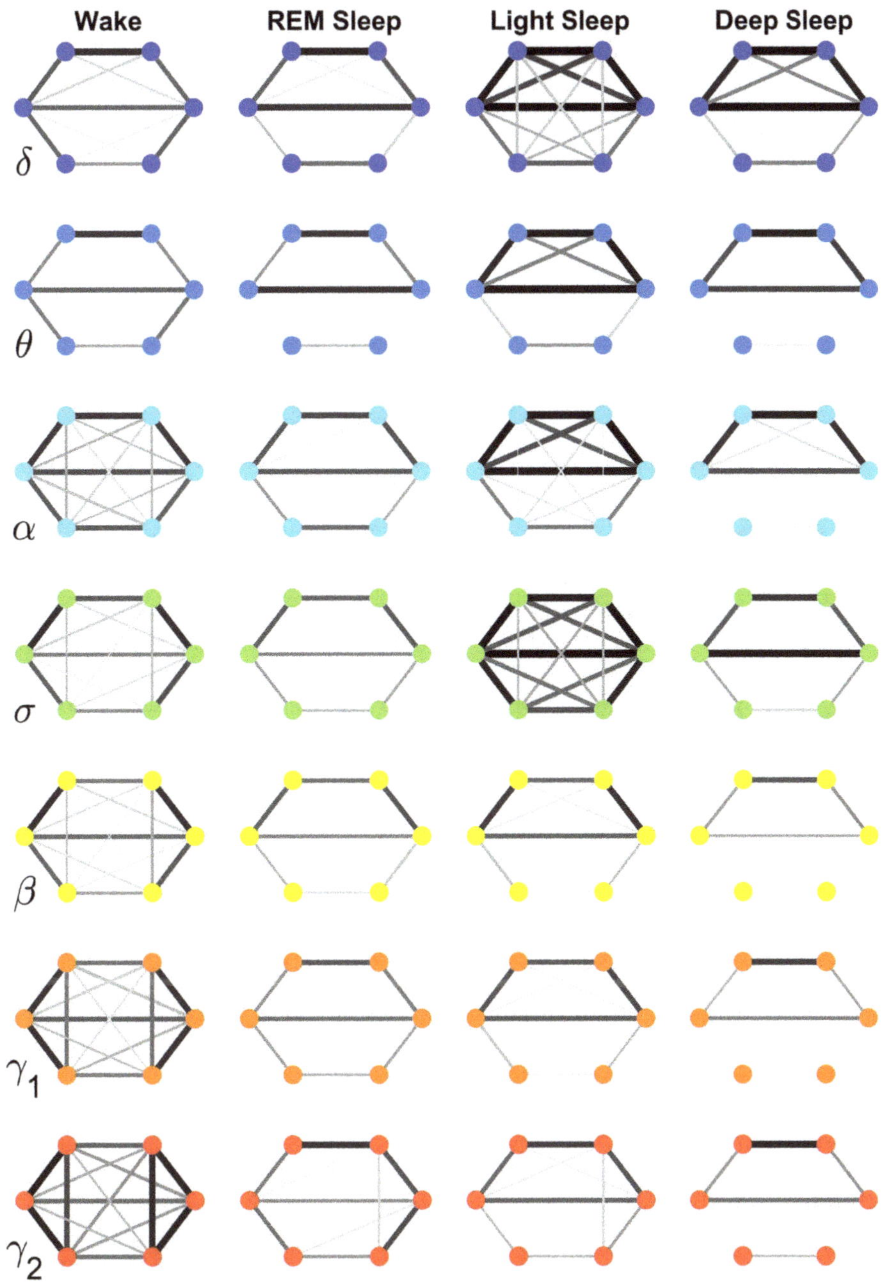

FIGURE 7 | Neural plasticity in the frequency domain represented by reorganization of network interactions across brain areas mediated through a specific frequency band across physiologic states. Network nodes represent six different brain areas: Frontal Fp1 and Fp2 (top vertices of the hexagon), Central C3 and C4 (middle vertices), and Occipital O1 and O2 (bottom vertices). Node colors indicate different frequency bands through which the inter-channel brain interactions are mediated. Group-averaged TDS links strength is represented by line thickness and by different color on gray scale. Only links with % TDS $\geq$ 45% are shown. Brain interactions mediated through specific frequency bands are associated with very different network structure within a given physiologic state, and exhibit distinct patterns of hierarchical reorganization with transition across physiologic states. Specifically, networks representing brain interactions in the δ and σ band are highly connected and with stronger links in Light Sleep, whereas networks representing brain interactions in the α, γ_1, and γ_2 band are highly connected and with stronger links during Wake. Notably, network characteristics during Deep Sleep and REM are similar for almost all frequency bands.

Deep and Light Sleep, the inter-channel interactions are mainly mediated through the δ and σ band. However, during Deep Sleep the network of δ band is dominant where as during Light Sleep the network of σ band is dominant (**Figure 8A**). Further, during REM we find that networks of all frequency bands have comparable contributions to the inter-channel brain wave communications, with slight prevalence of network interactions in the α and γ bands (**Figure 8A**). In contrast, the high-frequency γ_1 and γ_2 bands dominates the inter-channel interactions during Wake.

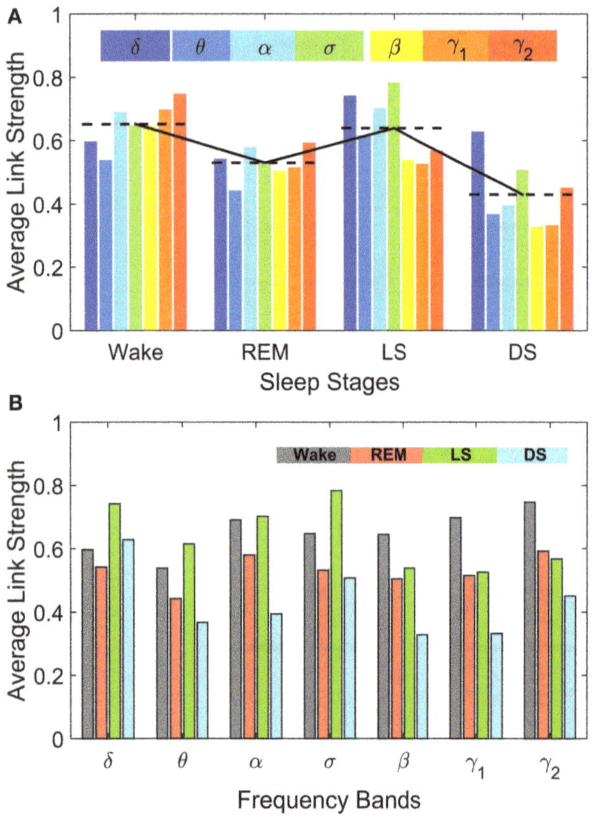

FIGURE 8 | Sleep-stage stratification patterns in the average strength of inter-channel brain interactions mediated through specific frequency bands. Average link strength in the frequency-specific networks of inter-channel interactions shown in **Figure 7** are grouped by sleep stages **(A)** and by frequency bands **(B)**, respectively. **(A)** demonstrates the degree of involvement of different frequency bands in inter-channel brain communications in each physiologic state (sleep stage). In Deep Sleep inter-channel interactions are mainly mediated through the lowest frequency δ band, while in Light Sleep both the δ band and the mid-frequency σ band associated with sleep spindle activity dominate the interactions between different brain areas. For REM sleep, the average link strength of inter-channel brain networks is similar for all frequency bands. In contrast, during Wake the α band and the high-frequency γ_1 and γ_2 bands dominate the inter-channel brain interactions. **(B)** Average link strength of brain network interactions mediated through different frequency bands exhibit distinct sleep-stage stratification patterns. For brain network interactions in the high-frequency $\beta, \gamma_1, \gamma_2$ bands, the average link strength is high during Wake, lower during REM and Light Sleep, and lowest during Deep Sleep. In contrast, the interactions in the mid- and low-frequency bands are characterized by different sleep-stage stratification in the average link strength—indicating pronounced plasticity of brain network interactions in the frequency domain.

Our investigation reveals that each frequency-specific network is characterized by a different signature pattern of sleep-stage stratification in average link strength, reflecting different neural plasticity of brain activation in different frequency bands. Specifically, we uncover two distinct categories of sleep-stage stratification. For high frequency networks corresponding to $\beta, \gamma_1, \gamma_2$ bands, the average link strength is high during Wake, intermediate (with similar values) during REM and Light Sleep and low during Deep Sleep (**Figure 8B**). In contrast, for the low and intermediate frequency $\delta, \theta, \alpha, \sigma$ bands, the frequency-specific networks are characterized by a different pattern of sleep-stage stratification—higher connectivity and stronger links during Wake and Light Sleep and lower connectivity during REM and Deep Sleep (**Figure 8B**).

4. SUMMARY AND DISCUSSION

Recent developments in the new field of Network Physiology indicate that complex physiologic functions could be understood through investigating networked communications between diverse dynamical components (Bashan et al., 2012; Bartsch and Ivanov, 2014; Ivanov and Bartsch, 2014). Adapting this integrative approach to multi-channel EEG signals, our investigation reveals a wealth of information about the dynamical interactions between various brain rhythms at different brain locations.

We find that complex network communications between brain waves that encompass not only the coordinated activation across different brain locations within the same frequency band but also previously unexplored interactions across different frequency bands that have been traditionally associated with distinct physiologic states and functions. Our results demonstrate that both network connectivity and strength of brain wave interactions significantly change with transition from one physiologic state to another. This finding indicates that in addition to the traditional view defining physiologic state and function through the prism of a distinct or dominant brain rhythm, networks of interactions across different brain waves and locations are a fundamental signature of physiologic states.

Our observations that brain wave network interactions evolve with transition from one physiologic state to another following a particular pattern of reorganization indicate a new aspect of neural plasticity reflected in the coordinated activation of different brain rhythms across brain areas. Specifically, the plasticity of brain wave network interaction is manifested at three levels of brain dynamics:

(1) *Globally:* the entire network of brain interactions across all brain locations and frequency bands undergoes a pronounced transition from a less connected state during Deep Sleep and REM to a highly connected state in Light Sleep and Wake.
(2) *Locally:* each brain area has its own characteristics pattern of network interactions between brain waves for a given physiologic state. Further, network interactions associated with a particular brain location exhibit specific pattern of reorganization with transitions across physiologic states.
(3) *In the frequency domain:* networks of interactions across brain areas that are mediated through the same frequency band are characterized by different structure and link strength, and exhibit different reorganization patterns across sleep stages.

These observations indicate a complex and hierarchical organization in brain wave interactions that changes in response to different physiologic states. Specifically, we find that intra-channel networks representing interactions between different brain rhythms at the same location exhibit location-specific patterns of reorganization across physiologic states. In contrast, the inter-channel networks exhibit a universal pattern of sleep-stage stratification for the Central, Frontal and Occipital areas that is characterized by high connectivity and link strength during Wake and Light Sleep, and low connectivity and link strength during REM and Deep Sleep.

Compared to other kinds of dynamical and functional brain maps constructed from fMRI, MEG, or BOLD signals (Bullmore and Sporns, 2009), and recent investigations on the structural-functional relationship at the neural circuits level (Bonifazi et al., 2009) as well as at the integrated brain level (Diez et al., 2015), our approach based on the TDS method focuses on the coordinated bursting activity of brain waves in different frequency domains. Generally, this integrative approach allows us to investigate how multi-component dynamical systems self-organize as a result of network interactions among components in order to generate complex functions, and to elucidate the mechanism underlying the evolution of system dynamics across states and conditions. The presented here approach provides a new kind of detailed brain maps allowing us to track the evolution and dynamics of brain functional states in real time, and can be broadly applied to quantify brain wave network interactions under different neuropathological conditions to derive novel biomarkers based on the brain network characteristics. Indeed, our new observations of similarity in network structure between REM and Deep Sleep, and between Wake and Light Sleep provide new insight to traditional sleep research, where Light Sleep and Deep Sleep are often considered similar and classified together as a Non-REM state. Further, in contrast to traditional interpretation of α rhythms as being irregular, localized, and desynchronized, and associated with arousals and quiet wake (Kryger et al., 1994; Siegel, 2005; Born et al., 2006), our findings demonstrate a robust network representing coordinated bursts of α waves activation across different brain locations, as well as a distinct pattern in the evolution of α wave network interactions with transition across sleep stages.

Our observations trigger new questions about the role of neural plasticity not only in generating specific brain rhythms but also in facilitating brain wave communications globally and locally, as well as across different frequency bands. Since networks of local and global brain wave interactions exhibit distinct characteristics, our findings raise the hypothesis that different mechanisms of neural plasticity may be responsible for the local or global aspect of brain rhythms communications. Our work demonstrates the utility of the Network Physiology approach in understanding physiologic state and function in the context of network communications between different brain waves.

The reported here findings of plasticity in brain wave network interactions will facilitate further efforts to bridge microscopic mechanisms of neuronal plasticity with emergent brain dynamics at the system level. Current investigations focus on understanding the role of neuronal and synaptic plasticity in generating particular brain rhythms associated with a specific physiologic state and function. Our empirical observations may guide further efforts in exploring mechanisms of neuronal and synaptic plasticity that also account for the complex hierarchical organization of network interactions between brain rhythms.

AUTHOR CONTRIBUTIONS

RB wrote the algorithm. KL, RB, and AL analyzed the data. KL, AL, PI, and RM participated in the development of the network analysis of TDS matrices. KL, RB, AL, and PI prepared the manuscript. PI initiated the investigation and supervised all aspects of the work. All authors discussed the results and commented on the manuscript.

ACKNOWLEDGMENTS

We acknowledge support from the W M Keck Foundation, National Institutes of Health (NIH Grant 1R01- HL098437), the Office of Naval Research (ONR Grant 000141010078), the US-Israel Binational Science Foundation (BSF Grant 2012219). RB acknowledges support from EC- FP7 Marie Curie Fellowship (IIF 628159). AL acknowledges support from the National Natural Science Foundation of China (Grant no. 61304145) and the Fundamental Research Funds for the Central Universities (Grant no. 2014RC014).

REFERENCES

Abbott, L. F., and Nelson, S. B. (2000). Synaptic plasticity: taming the beast. *Nat. Neurosci.* 3(Suppl.), 1178–1183. doi: 10.1038/81453

Abeles, M. (1991). *Corticonics: Neural Circuits of the Cerebral Cortex*. Cambridge, UK: Cambridge University Press.

Bartsch, R. P., and Ivanov, P. Ch. (2014). Coexisting forms of coupling and phase-transitions in physiological networks. *Commun. Comput. Inform. Sci.* 438, 270–287. doi: 10.1007/978-3-319-08672-9_33

Bartsch, R. P., Liu, K. K. L., Ma, Q. D. Y., and Ivanov, P. Ch. (2014). Three independent forms of cardio-respiratory coupling: transitions across sleep stages. *Comput. Cardiol.* 41, 781–784.

Bartsch, R. P., Schumann, A. Y., Kantelhardt, J. W., Penzel, T., and Ivanov, P. Ch. (2012). Phase transitions in physiologic coupling. *Proc. Natl. Acad. Sci. U.S.A.* 109, 10181–10186. doi: 10.1073/pnas.1204568109

Bashan, A., Bartsch, R. P., Kantelhardt, J. W., Havlin, S., and Ivanov, P. Ch. (2012). Network physiology reveals relations between network topology and physiological function. *Nat. Commun.* 3, 702. doi: 10.1038/ncomms1705

Bonifazi, P., Goldin, M., Picardo, M. A., Jorquera, I., and Cattani, A. (2009). GABAergic hub neurons orchestrate synchrony in developing hippocampal networks. *Science* 326, 1419–1424. doi: 10.1126/science.1175509

Born, J., Rasch, B., and Gais, S. (2006). Sleep to remember. *Neuroscientist* 12, 410–424. doi: 10.1177/1073858406292647

Bullmore, E., and Sporns, O. (2009). Complex brain networks: graph theoretical analysis of structural and functional systems. *Nat. Rev. Neurosci.* 10, 186–198. doi: 10.1038/nrn2575

Buzsáki, G., Anastassiou, C. A., and Koch, C. (2012). The origin of extracellular fields and currents—EEG, ECoG, LFP and spikes. *Nat. Rev. Neurosci.* 13, 407–420. doi: 10.1038/nrn3241

Deger, M., Helias, M., Rotter, S., and Diesmann, M. (2012). Spike-timing dependence of structural plasticity explains cooperative synapse formation in the neocortex. *PLoS Comput. Biol.* 8:e1002689. doi: 10.1371/journal.pcbi.1002689

Denker, M., Timme, M., Diesmann, M., Wolf, F., and Geisel, T. (2004). Breaking synchrony by heterogeneity in complex networks. *Phys. Rev. Lett.* 92:074103. doi: 10.1103/PhysRevLett.92.074103

Destexhe, A., and Marder, E. (2004). Plasticity in single neuron and circuit computations. *Nature* 431, 789–795. doi: 10.1038/nature03011

Diekelmann, S., and Born, J. (2010). The memory function of sleep. *Nat. Rev. Neurosci.* 11, 114–126. doi: 10.1038/nrn2762

Diez, I., Bonifazi, P., Escudero, I., Mateos, B., Muñoz, M. A., Stramaglia, S., et al. (2015). A novel brain partition highlightsthe modular skeleton shared bystructure and function. *Sci. Rep.* 5:10532. doi: 10.1038/srep10532

Engel, A. K., Fries, P., and Singer, W. (2001). Dynamic predictions: oscillations and synchrony in top-down processing. *Nat. Rev. Neurosci.* 2, 704–716. doi: 10.1038/35094565

Gorgoni, M., D'Atri, A., Lauri, G., Rossini, P. M., Ferlazzo, F., and De Gennaro, L. (2013). Is sleep essential for neural plasticity in humans, and how does it affect motor and cognitive recovery? *Neural Plast.* 2013, 1–13. doi: 10.1155/2013/103949

Helias, M., Tetzlaff, T., and Diesmann, M. (2014). The correlation structure of local neuronal networks intrinsically results from recurrent dynamics. *PLoS Comput. Biol.* 10:e1003428. doi: 10.1371/journal.pcbi.1003428

Hill, S., and Tononi, G. (2005). Modeling sleep and wakefulness in the thalamocortical system. *J. Neurophysiol.* 93, 1671–1698. doi: 10.1152/jn.00915.2004

Huber, R., Esser, S. K., Ferrarelli, F., Massimini, M., Peterson, M. J., and Tononi, G. (2007). TMS-induced cortical potentiation during wakefulness locally increases slow wave activity during sleep. *PLoS ONE* 2:e276. doi: 10.1371/journal.pone.0000276

Huber, R., Määttä, S., Esser, S. K., Sarasso, S., Ferrarelli, F., Watson, A., et al. (2008). Measures of cortical plasticity after transcranial paired associative stimulation predict changes in electroencephalogram slow-wave activity during subsequent sleep. *J. Neurosci.* 28, 7911–7918. doi: 10.1523/JNEUROSCI.1636-08.2008

Ivanov, P. Ch., and Bartsch, R. P. (2014). *Network Physiology: Mapping Interactions Between Networks of Physiologic Networks, Chapter 10.* Cham: Springer International Publishing.

Ivanov, P. Ch., Bunde, A., Amaral, L. A. N., Havlin, S., Fritsch-Yelle, J., Baevsky, R. M., et al. (1999). Sleep-wake differences in scaling behavior of the human heartbeat: analysis of terrestrial and long-term space flight data. *Europhys. Lett.* 48, 594–600.

Ivanov, P. Ch., Hu, K., Hilton, M. F., Shea, S. A., and Stanley, H. E. (2007). Endogenous circadian rhythm in human motor activity uncoupled from circadian influences on cardiac dynamics. *Proc. Natl. Acad. Sci. U.S.A.* 104, 20702–20707. doi: 10.1073/pnas.0709957104

Jahnke, S., Memmesheimer, R.-M., and Timme, M. (2008). Stable irregular dynamics in complex neural networks. *Phys. Rev. Lett.* 100:048102. doi: 10.1103/PhysRevLett.100.048102

Kandel, E. R. (2001). The molecular biology of memory storage: a dialogue between genes and synapses. *Science* 294, 1030–1038. doi: 10.1126/science.10 67020

Kantelhardt, J. W., Ashkenazy, Y., Ivanov, P. Ch., Bunde, A., Havlin, S., Penzel, T., et al. (2002). Characterization of sleep stages by correlations in the magnitude and sign of heartbeat increments. *Phys. Rev. E* 65:051908. doi: 10.1103/PhysRevE.65.051908

Karasik, R., Sapir, N., Ashkenazy, Y., Ivanov, P. Ch., Dvir, I., Lavie, P., et al. (2002). Correlation differences in heartbeat fluctuations during rest and exercise. *Phys. Rev. E* 66:062902. doi: 10.1103/PhysRevE.66.062902

Katz, P. S., and Frost, W. N. (1996). Intrinsic neuromodulation: altering neuronal circuits from within. *Trends Neurosci.* 19, 54–61.

Klösch, G., Kemp, B., Penzel, T., Schlögl, A., Rappelsberger, P., Trenker, E., et al. (2001). The SIESTA project polygraphic and clinical database. *IEEE Eng. Med. Biol. Mag.* 20, 51–57. doi: 10.1109/51.932725

Kopell, N., Ermentrout, G. B., Whittington, M. A., and Traub, R. D. (2000). Gamma rhythms and beta rhythms have different synchronization properties. *Proc. Natl. Acad. Sci. U.S.A.* 97, 1867–1872. doi: 10.1073/pnas.97.4.1867

Kryger, M. H., Roth, T., and Dement, W. C., (eds.). (1994). *Principles and Practice of Sleep Medicine.* Philadelphia, PA: Elsevier Saunders.

Linkenkaer-Hansen, K., Nikouline, V. V., Palva, J. M., and Ilmoniemi, R. J. (2001). Long-range temporal correlations and scaling behavior in human brain oscillations. *J. Neurosci.* 21, 1370–1377.

Lo, C.-C., Amaral, L. A. N., Havlin, S., Ivanov, P. Ch., Penzel, T., Peter, J.-H., et al. (2002). Dynamics of sleep-wake transitions during sleep. *Europhys. Lett.* 57, 625–631. doi: 10.1209/epl/i2002-00508-7

Lo, C.-C., Bartsch, R. P., and Ivanov, P. Ch. (2013). Asymmetry and basic pathways in sleep-stage transitions. *Europhys. Lett.* 102:10008. doi: 10.1209/0295-5075/102/10008

Lo, C.-C., Chou, T., Penzel, T., Scammell, T. E., Strecker, R. E., Stanley, H. E., et al. (2004). Common scale-invariant patterns of sleep-wake transitions across mammalian species. *Proc. Natl. Acad. Sci. U.S.A.* 101, 17545–17548. doi: 10.1073/pnas.0408242101

Marder, E., Abbott, L. F., and Turrigiano, G. G. (1996). Memory from the dynamics of intrinsic membrane currents. *Proc. Natl. Acad. Sci. U.S.A.* 93, 13481–13486.

Marder, E., and Thirumalai, V. (2002). Cellular, synaptic and network effects of neuromodulation. *Neural Netw.* 15, 479–493. doi: 10.1016/S0893-6080(02)00043-6

Massimini, M., Ferrarelli, F., Huber, R., Esser, S. K., Singh, H., and Tononi, G. (2005). Breakdown of cortical effective connectivity during sleep. *Science* 309, 2228–2232. doi: 10.1126/science.1117256

Millman, D., Mihalas, S., Kirkwood, A., and Niebur, E. (2010). Self-organized criticality occurs in non-conservative neuronal networks during/up/'states. *Nat. Phys.* 6, 801–805. doi: 10.1038/nphys1757

Niedermeyer, E., and da Silva, F., (eds.) (2005). *Electroencephalography: Basic Principles, Clinical Applications, and Related Fields.* Philadelphia, PA: LWW.

Olcese, U., Esser, S. K., and Tononi, G. (2010). Sleep and synaptic renormalization: a cocomputation study. *J. Neurophysiol.* 104, 3476–3493. doi: 10.1152/jn.00593.2010

Poil, S.-S., van Ooyen, A., and Linkenkaer-Hansen, K. (2008). Avalanche dynamics of human brain oscillations: relation to critical branching processes and temporal correlations. *Hum. Brain Mapp.* 29, 770–777. doi: 10.1002/hbm.20590

Rechtschaffen, A., and Kales, A. (1968). *A Manual of Standardized Terminology, Techniques and Scoring System for Sleep Stages of Human Subjects.* Bethesda, MD: U.S. Dept. of Health, Education, and Welfare.

Rye, D. B., Bliwise, D. L., Parker, K., Trotti, L. M., Saini, P., Fairley, J., et al. (2012). Modulation of vigilance in the primary hypersomnias by endogenous enhancement of gaba-a receptors. *Sci. Transl. Med.* 4, 161–151. doi: 10.1126/scitranslmed.3004685

Schmidt, C., Peigneux, P., Muto, V., Schenkel, M., Knoblauch, V., Muench, M., et al. (2006). Encoding difficulty promotes postlearning changes in sleep spindle activity during napping. *J. Neurosci.* 26, 8976–8982. doi: 10.1523/JNEUROSCI.2464-06.2006

Schmitt, D. T., Stein, P. K., and Ivanov, P. Ch. (2009). Stratification pattern of static and scale-invariant dynamic measures of heartbeat fluctuations across sleep stages in young and elderly. *IEEE Trans. Biomed. Eng.* 56, 1564–1573. doi: 10.1109/TBME.2009.2014819

Schumann, A. Y., Bartsch, R. P., Penzel, T., Ivanov, P. Ch., and Kantelhardt, J. W. (2010). Aging effects on cardiac and respiratory dynamics in healthy subjects across sleep stages. *Sleep* 33, 943–955.

Siegel, J. M. (2005). Clues to the functions of mammalian sleep. *Nature* 437, 1264–1271. doi: 10.1038/nature04285

Sjöström, P. J., and Nelson, S. B. (2002). Spike timing, calcium signals and synaptic plasticity. *Curr. Opin. Neurobiol.* 12, 305–314. doi: 10.1016/S0959-4388(02)00325-2

Stefan, K., Kunesch, E., Cohen, L. G., Benecke, R., and Classen, J. (2000). Induction of plasticity in the human motor cortex by paired associative stimulation. *Brain* 123, 572–584. doi: 10.1093/brain/123.3.572

Steriade, M., McCormick, D. A., and Sejnowski, T. J. (1993). Thalamocortical oscillations in the sleeping and aroused brain. *Science* 262, 679–685.

Steriade, M., and Timofeev, I. (2003). Neuronal plasticity in thalamocortical networks during sleep and waking oscillations. *Neuron* 37, 563–576. doi: 10.1016/S0896-6273(03)00065-5

Stickgold, R. (2005). Sleep-dependent memory consolidation. *Nature* 437, 1272–1278. doi: 10.1038/nature04286

Tononi, G., and Cirelli, C. (2014). Sleep and the price of plasticity: from synaptic and cellular homeostasis to memory consolidation and integration. *Neuron* 81, 12–34. doi: 10.1016/j.neuron.2013.12.025

Traub, R. D., Kopell, N., Bibbig, A., Buhl, E. H., LeBeau, F., and Whittington, M. A. (2001). Gap junctions between interneuron dendrites can enhance synchrony of gamma oscillations in distributed networks. *J. Neurosci.* 21, 9478–9486.

Vardi, R., Goldental, A., Marmari, H., Brama, H., Stern, E. A., Sardi, S., et al. (2015). Neuronal response impedance mechanism implementing cooperative networks with low firing rates and μs precision. *Front. Neural Circuits* 9:29. doi: 10.3389/fncir.2015.00029

Vardi, R., Timor, R., Marom, S., Abeles, M., and Kanter, I. (2013). Synchronization by elastic neuronal latencies. *Phys. Rev. E* 87:012724. doi: 10.1103/PhysRevE.87.012724

White, J. A., Chow, C. C., Ritt, J., Soto-Treviño, C., and Kopell, N. (1998). Synchronization and oscillatory dynamics in heterogeneous, mutually inhibited neurons. *J. Comput. Neurosci.* 5, 5–16.

Wolters, A., Schmidt, A., Schramm, A., Zeller, D., Naumann, M., Kunesch, E., et al. (2005). Timing-dependent plasticity in human primary somatosensory cortex. *J. Physiol.* 565, 1039–1052. doi: 10.1113/jphysiol.2005.084954

2

Does Combined Physical and Cognitive Training Improve Dual-Task Balance and Gait Outcomes in Sedentary Older Adults?

Sarah A. Fraser[1], Karen Z.-H. Li[2], Nicolas Berryman[3,4], Laurence Desjardins-Crépeau[4,5], Maxime Lussier[4], Kiran Vadaga[2], Lora Lehr[4,5], Thien Tuong Minh Vu[4,6], Laurent Bosquet[7] and Louis Bherer[4,6]*

[1]Interdisciplinary School of Health Sciences, University of Ottawa, Ottawa, ON, Canada, [2]Department of Psychology, Concordia University, Montréal, QC, Canada, [3]Sports Studies, Bishop's University, Sherbrooke, QC, Canada, [4]Centre de Recherche de l'Institut Universitaire de Gériatrie de Montréal, Montréal, QC, Canada, [5]Department of Psychology, Université du Québec à Montréal, Montréal, QC, Canada, [6]Medecine, Université de Montréal, Montréal, QC, Canada, [7]Laboratoire MOVE (EA6314), Faculté des Sciences du Sport, Université de Poitiers, Poitiers, France

Edited by:
Claudia Voelcker-Rehage, Chemnitz University of Technology, Germany

Reviewed by:
Sean Commins, Maynooth University, Ireland
Wei Peng Teo, Deakin University, Australia

***Correspondence:**
Sarah A. Fraser
sarah.fraser@uottawa.ca

Everyday activities like walking and talking can put an older adult at risk for a fall if they have difficulty dividing their attention between motor and cognitive tasks. Training studies have demonstrated that both cognitive and physical training regimens can improve motor and cognitive task performance. Few studies have examined the benefits of combined training (cognitive and physical) and whether or not this type of combined training would transfer to walking or balancing dual-tasks. This study examines the dual-task benefits of combined training in a sample of sedentary older adults. Seventy-two older adults (≥60 years) were randomly assigned to one of four training groups: Aerobic + Cognitive training (CT), Aerobic + Computer lessons (CL), Stretch + CT and Stretch + CL. It was expected that the Aerobic + CT group would demonstrate the largest benefits and that the active placebo control (Stretch + CL) would show the least benefits after training. Walking and standing balance were paired with an auditory n-back with two levels of difficulty (0- and 1-back). Dual-task walking and balance were assessed with: walk speed (m/s), cognitive accuracy (% correct) and several mediolateral sway measures for pre- to post-test improvements. All groups demonstrated improvements in walk speed from pre- (M = 1.33 m/s) to post-test (M = 1.42 m/s, $p < 0.001$) and in accuracy from pre- (M = 97.57%) to post-test (M = 98.57%, p = 0.005).They also increased their walk speed in the more difficult 1-back (M = 1.38 m/s) in comparison to the 0-back (M = 1.36 m/s, $p < 0.001$) but reduced their accuracy in the 1-back (M = 96.39%) in comparison to the 0-back (M = 99.92%, $p < 0.001$). Three out of the five mediolateral sway variables (Peak, SD, RMS) demonstrated significant reductions in sway from pre to post test (p-values < 0.05). With the exception of a group difference between Aerobic + CT and Stretch + CT in accuracy, there were no significant group differences after training.

Results suggest that there can be dual-task benefits from training but that in this sedentary sample Aerobic + CT training was not more beneficial than other types of combined training.

Keywords: dual-task gait, dual-task balance, combined training (physical and cognitive dual-task training), transfer effects

INTRODUCTION

Standing balance and walking are two motor activities that are assumed to be automatic in nature and not requiring a great degree of conscious thought. However, in real life situations, it is rare that we are simply standing still or walking without attending to some secondary task (i.e., walking and talking). Research that examines the ability to attend to two tasks simultaneously during gait and balance suggests that both younger and older adults involve some executive processes (planning, inhibiting, and switching/coordinating) in order to manage these dual-task situations (Woollacott and Shumway-Cook, 2002; Allali et al., 2008; Hausdorff et al., 2008). A large literature associates these executive processes with the prefrontal cortex (PFC; Miyake et al., 2000; Stuss and Alexander, 2000; Gunning-Dixon and Raz, 2003). The PFC has been shown to be an area that is sensitive to age-associated declines with aging (Buckner, 2004; Hedden and Gabrieli, 2004). Moreover, studies suggest that cognitive functions largely subserved by the PFC can be improved through physical exercise and cognitive training interventions (Colcombe and Kramer, 2003; Erickson et al., 2007; Kramer and Erickson, 2007; Braver et al., 2009; Klingberg, 2010; Bherer et al., 2013). Given the potential plasticity of the PFC and its association with executive functions, the goal of the current study was to assess the benefits of combined physical and cognitive training on dual-task gait and balance in a sample of sedentary older adults.

Although both younger and older adults may involve executive function processes to manage dual-task gait and balance, the literature suggests that the ability of older adults to manage such situations is reduced in comparison to younger adults (Woollacott and Shumway-Cook, 2002; Fraser et al., 2007; Li et al., 2012; Fraser and Bherer, 2013). Further, when active and sedentary older adults are compared, sedentary older adults demonstrate a greater risk of cognitive and physical declines that can influence executive functions and ultimately increase fall risk (Thibaud et al., 2011). This risk increases in dual-task situations (Montero-Odasso et al., 2012). In addition, certain types of dual-task combinations can increase the dual-task interference (Fraser and Bherer, 2013). In particular cognitive tasks that are more executive in nature seem to interfere more with gait (Al-Yahya et al., 2011; Buracchio et al., 2011; Walshe et al., 2015). A systematic review and meta-analysis found that cognitive tasks with "mental tracking" (pg. 725) increased the interference during walking to a greater degree than simple reaction time tasks (Al-Yahya et al., 2011). The literature on motor-cognitive dual-tasks has certainly demonstrated that both cognitive and motor factors might be contributing to these age differences in dual-task abilities (Woollacott and Shumway-Cook, 2002; Hausdorff et al., 2008; Schaefer and Schumacher, 2010). In general, older adults with mild cognitive impairment or dementia tend to walk more slowly than healthy older adults (Montero-Odasso et al., 2012). In addition, the measurement of gait during dual-task has also revealed differences in gait parameters between healthy and cognitively impaired seniors (Sheridan et al., 2003; Springer et al., 2006; Muir et al., 2012) and fallers and non-fallers (Springer et al., 2006; Montero-Odasso et al., 2012). Such findings suggest that dual-task gait might be an important clinical marker of cognitive decline and falls risk (Montero-Odasso et al., 2012).

Similarly, maintaining standing balance is considered a complex skill that requires several elements and cognitive processing has been identified as one of them (Horak, 2006). In comparison to the gait literature, the literature on dual-task balance assessments demonstrates that this approach has been successful in differentiating fallers from non-fallers (Brauer et al., 2001; Condron et al., 2002; Hauer et al., 2003) and somewhat successful in differentiating healthy older adults from those with cognitive impairment (Zijlstra et al., 2008; Muir-Hunter et al., 2014). More research using static balance dual-tasks is required to determine if this type of assessment can identify different forms of cognitive impairment. Despite this, gait and balance are both postural control tasks and common to both is the association with executive functions (van Iersel et al., 2008) and the potential for cognitive plasticity.

Cognitive plasticity and enhanced motor function have been targeted with intervention studies. Several intervention studies have demonstrated that exercise training can improve cognitive outcomes (Predovan et al., 2012; Bherer et al., 2013; Langlois et al., 2013; Berryman et al., 2014; Bherer, 2015) and physical outcomes (Shumway-Cook et al., 1997; Cadore et al., 2013; de Labra et al., 2015). Regarding specific types of exercise training, aerobic training in particular has been associated with enhanced executive functions (Kramer et al., 1999; Hall et al., 2001; Colcombe and Kramer, 2003) and increased activations in the frontal and parietal cortices (Colcombe et al., 2004, 2006). However, most review and meta-analyses tend to suggest that exercise intervention combining aerobic and strength training components lead to greater improvement in cognition (Colcombe and Kramer, 2003). Cognitive training (CT) can also lead to improvement (Segev-Jacubovski et al., 2011; Belleville and Bherer, 2012) in several cognitive domains including working memory, attention, and executive functions (Li et al., 2008; Kueider et al., 2012; Leung et al., 2015). There is however, some debate about the transfer of cognitive training to untrained tasks or everyday activities (Lee et al., 2012; Lussier et al., 2015). Despite this, some cognitive training interventions have shown transfer demonstrating improved motor outcomes in older adults in balance (Li et al., 2010), gait (Verghese et al., 2010), balance and gait (Smith-Ray et al., 2013) and activities of daily living (Willis et al., 2006). More specifically, in the first three studies mentioned, participants received a computerized cognitive training (seated at a computer) and outcome measures such as mediolateral sway (Li et al., 2010), gait speed in single and dual-task walking (Verghese et al., 2010) and timed-up-and go and distracted walking (Smith-Ray et al., 2013) improved in comparison to control groups that did not receive this training.

When exploring training specific to motor-cognitive dual-task situations, a systematic review specific to dual-task outcomes, revealed that motor-cognitive dual-task training was beneficial to standing balance performance and that walking outcomes were improved by both single-task and dual-task training (Wollesen and Voelcker-Rehage, 2013). It is important to note that a majority of the studies contained in the review trained the component tasks either separately (cognitive task alone or motor task alone) or concurrently (dual-task condition in which cognitive and motor task were trained simultaneously), then assessed single- and dual-task performances with the same combination of tasks. None of the studies looked specifically at combined cognitive and physical training and transfer to untrained dual-task balance and gait tasks.

A recent systematic review of combined cognitive and physical training interventions in older adults with or without cognitive impairment demonstrated that this type of combined training was beneficial in two of the three studies on older adults without cognitive impairment and four out of the five studies examining individuals with cognitive impairment (Law et al., 2014). Only one of the studies contained in the review examined dual-task walking as an outcome measure and included an active placebo control group that received low intensity exercise training (Schwenk et al., 2010). This study found that training older individuals with cognitive impairment in dual-task walking, at an adaptive level of difficulty (challenging the patients), led to improvements in dual-task walk outcomes in comparison to the placebo control. While this study is explicitly highlighted as a well-designed randomized control trial in the review, there were a few critiques. Specifically, components of the dual-task assessed at pre-and post-intervention were similar to the tasks being trained and the placebo control did not have the same hours of training.

Taken together, there are few studies that have explicitly examined transfer from a combined cognitive and physical training program to dual-task gait and balance outcomes in a sample of sedentary older adults. There were several outcome measures included in this large mobility study (see Desjardins-Crépeau et al., 2016). Only the results specific to balance and gait dual-task outcomes are reported here. The goal of the current study was to assess whether or not combined cognitive and physical training benefits transferred to dual-task walk and balance outcomes and whether or not there would be synergistic effects when combining cognitive dual-task training and aerobic training which have demonstrated specific benefits to executive function. In the present study, there were four training groups including either aerobic, cognitive or active control conditions. The first three groups all contained components designed to improve executive function and the last group was considered our active placebo-placebo control. All groups were expected to benefit to some degree from training but we expected the Aerobic + CT group to demonstrate greater improvements in dual-task walking and balance outcomes than the other three groups after training. Further, we expected that the placebo-placebo control would demonstrate the least amount of benefits to dual-task walking and balance outcomes in comparison to the three other groups which all included conditions designed to improve executive function.

MATERIALS AND METHODS

Participants

Sedentary older adults (≥60 years old) who performed less than 150 min of physical activity per week were recruited from public advertisements (flyers, newspapers) and from the research center's participant pool. One hundred and thirty six individuals passed our phone screening, which had the following exclusion criteria: history of neurological disease or major surgery in the year preceding the study, uncorrected auditory or visual impairments, smoking, severe mobility limitations or any other physical activity contraindications, and being currently engaged in any structured physical activity. The 136 were randomly assigned to one of the four training groups (Aerobic + Cognitive Training (CT); Aerobic + Computer lessons (CL); Stretch + CT, Stretch + CL). Our Aerobic + CT group contained both physical and cognitive components to improve executive function and our placebo-placebo control containing no aerobic or cognitive dual-task training was the Stretch + CL group. Of those 136, 11 abandoned the study before beginning any training (for personal reasons, time constraints, or recent injuries that restricted their ability to participate). Of the 125 who entered into the study and provided written and informed consent that conformed to the Montreal Geriatric Institute ethics committee and the Declaration of Helsinki, 22 abandoned during training and 31 were excluded, at post-test, for the following reasons: wearing a hearing aid (affected performance on auditory task with headset), having a Geriatric Depression Score greater than 11 (which is suggestive of mild/moderate depression), and insufficient training (less than 75% of training sessions completed). Reasons for abandoning typically related to: injury outside the lab that impeded participation; death in the family; and other commitments. Those who abandoned were equally distributed across the training groups. This study was carried out in accordance with the recommendations of human research by the ethics committee of the Montreal Geriatric Institute. The protocol was approved by this ethics committee.

Descriptive characteristics (i.e., age, education, etc.) of the participants included in the final sample (n = 72; 51 women/21 men) are presented in **Table 1** at the beginning of the "Results" Section. It is important to note that we began balance assessments in the third cohort recruited for this study, as such, there are fewer participants in each of the training groups that completed the dual-task balance assessments. For

TABLE 1 | Descriptive characteristics of the participants by training group.

	Aerobic + CT	Aerobic + CL	Stretch + CT	Stretch + CL	Group differences? *p*-value
Participants	21	17	18	16	
Age (years)	71.90 (6.84)	70.53 (7.34)	72.22 (5.93)	71.13 (5.40)	0.86
Education (years)	13.81 (2.62)	16.06 (2.19)	13.89 (4.39)	15.00 (2.73)	0.11
6MWT (meters)	508.45 (75.49)	538.53 (76.39)	511.50 (80.81)	513.06 (62.68)	0.61
PPT (score)	32.40 (2.42)	32.18 (3.52)	31.83 (1.92)	33.00 (1.83)	0.59
ABC (score)	82.68 (2.9)	83.82 (2.9)	85.03 (2.9)	89.08 (3.2)	0.49
MMSE	28.48 (1.25)	28.88 (1.05)	29.39 (0.70)	28.50 (1.37)	0.06
GDS	4.57 (3.34)	4.18 (2.68)	3.11 (3.31)	2.44 (2.37)	0.14

Note: 6MWT, 6 min walk test (total meters completed in 6 mins); PPT, modified Physical Performance Test (max score 36); ABC balance questionnaire (max score 100% confidence in balance abilities); MMSE, Mini Mental State Exam (a global measure of cognition, max score 30); GDS, Geriatric Depression Scale (scores equal to or above 11 are indicative of mild/moderate depression).

dual-task balance, $n = 15$ (Aerobic + CT); $n = 12$ (Aerobic + CL); $n = 16$ (Stretch + CT); and $n = 11$ (Stretch + CL).

Protocol

All participants underwent pre-testing across 3 days. On Day 1, pre-testing involved: a comprehensive medical exam with a geriatrician. On Day 2, participants completed a full neuropsychological battery and a dual-task cognitive training baseline on the computer (see Desjardins-Crépeau et al., 2016 for a detailed description of the protocol). Finally on Day 3, participants completed a battery of physical tests (including the 6 min walk test, the timed-up-and-go, and the short physical performance battery) and dual-task walking and balance assessments. Upon completion of the pre-testing groups of 4–8 individuals began their respective training protocol, which involved 12 weeks of training 3 times a week. All participants had two 60 min sessions of physical exercise (aerobic or stretch) and one 60 min session of cognitive stimulation (dual-task training or computer lessons). The mixed aerobic training involved a 5 min warm up, 15 min of lower body resistance training, 30 min of cardiovascular exercise on a treadmill and a cool down. Intensity of the exercise increased over the sessions based on each individuals' ratings of perceived exertion on the Borg (1998) scale. The Stretching and toning group also had a 5 min warm-up and cool down but spent the majority of the training time (50 min) performing whole body stretching exercises mainly in a seated position. The computer dual-task training involved two visual discrimination tasks (number and shape discrimination) that were based on previous cognitive training paradigms (Bherer et al., 2005, 2006, 2008). Participants were encouraged to be as accurate and rapid as possible at responding to the tasks alone (single-task) and simultaneously (dual-task). Participants were provided continuous feedback on their response time (during the session) and provided feedback for both response time and accuracy at the end of each session. In contrast to the dual-task training, those who received computer lessons had demonstrations and trials with different computer applications (i.e., word and excel) and learned how to search the internet. At the end of the 12 weeks, all participants returned for 2 days of post-testing. The first day of post-testing involved completing the same neuropsychological assessments completed at pre-test and the second day of post-testing involved completing the same battery of physical tests and dual-task walk and balance assessments.

Main Outcome Measures

Cognitive Accuracy: N-back Task (With and Without Concurrent Walking/Balance)

The n-back task is a working memory task that can be parametrically manipulated to increase the memory load during testing (Jaeggi et al., 2003; Doumas et al., 2008). Typically during an n-back task, a series of stimuli are presented and the participant is asked to remember and respond to the stimuli that they heard "n" items-back (0-back, 1-back, etc.). In the lowest load version (0-back), individuals simply have to remember and report the stimuli they just heard. As the number of items back increases, the working memory load increases placing greater attentional demands on the individual (Jaeggi et al., 2003; Doumas et al., 2008). The auditory n-back used in this study involves working memory and mental tracking as the participant has to remember the numbers that are continuously being presented and as a new number is presented say out-loud the number they heard one item back. During the balance task, in order to minimize muscle fatigue from repeated balance assessments (Helbostad et al., 2010), we chose to complete the dual-task balance with the 1-back only. During the walk portion, we used two levels of difficulty the 0-back and the 1-back version of the task (with and without concurrent walking). In all conditions (single (n-back only) and dual-task (n-back + motor task)), a mean accuracy score was computed (percent correct of total possible responses (%)).

The n-back task in the current study has already successfully demonstrated differences in cognitive performances during walking in sample of older women who completed a combined training intervention (Fraser et al., 2014). In this auditory n-back, the to-be-remembered stimuli were numbers (0–9). A visual depiction of the 0-back and 1-back conditions is presented in **Figure 1**. The numbers were recorded in a female voice and soundfiles (wavfiles) of each number were used in pseudo-randomly ordered lists of numbers that were presented

0-back

Stimuli	9	1	7	2	0	3	...
	↓	↓	↓	↓	↓	↓	
Response	9	1	7	2	0	3	...

1-back

Stimuli	9	1	7	2	0	3 ...	
		↓	↓	↓	↓	↓	↓
Response	None	9	1	7	2	0	3 ...

FIGURE 1 | An example of the stimuli presented and vocal response expected from the participant for the 0-back and 1-back conditions. *Note*: In the 0-back condition the participant hears a number "9" and immediately responds "9". In the 1-back condition the participant hears the first stimuli "9" and has to keep it in mind until they hear the second stimuli "1" and at this point they respond with the first item they heard "9", then they have to keep in mind the "1" until presented with the next stimuli, and so on.

using E-prime2 software (Psychology Software Tools Inc., Sharpsburg, PA, USA). The numbers were pseudo-randomly ordered to ensure that there were no repeats (9-9) and no ordered series (1-2-3). The numbers were presented through wireless headphones (Sennheiser Canada, Pointe-Claire, QC, Canada). For DT-balance, six lists of eight numbers were created; two were used for practice and the remaining for the test phase. For DT-walk, 10 lists of 12 numbers were created; two lists were used for practice and the remaining for the test phase. Since there were two levels of n-back in the DT-walk these lists were used twice.

Mobility Measures: Posture and Gait

In both balance and the walk portions of the physical assessment after instructions were provided, the participants wore headphones for both the practice and test phases. Prior to any testing, the dominant leg of the participant was assessed by having the participant begin walking from a standing position three times (Fraser et al., 2007). The leg most often used for gait initiation was considered the dominant leg. For the balance portion participants had to maintain balance with their eyes open, arms at their sides, on their dominant leg for 20 s with and without the 1-back task. Postural control was assessed with a Matscan floor mat that captures the plantar pressures and forces of the foot (Tekscan, Boston, MA, USA). The Matscan raw data was converted to center of pressure measures. In the current study, we measured area (cm^2), velocity, peak to peak dispersion, and standard deviation of sway values specific to the mediolateral (ML) and anterior-posterior (AP) directions. Based on the training benefits reported in ML sway in the study by Li et al. (2010), we have focused on area and ML sway variables measured during single- and dual-task balance (Peak ML (cm), SD ML (cm), RMS ML (cm^2), Velocity ML (cm/s)). Mean scores for each of the ML sway values were computed. In addition, at the end of the pre- and post-test sessions, we asked each participant to complete the Activities-Specific Balance Confidence (ABC) scale (Powell and Myers, 1995) in order to have a standardized questionnaire of balance confidence in everyday activities. The scale has 16 items which are rated on a 0%–100% scale of confidence, higher scores (closer to 100%) indicate that the individual is completely confident in their balance ability during the activity in question. A mean confidence value from all 16-items was calculated for Pre- and Post-test.

For the walk portion, participants had to walk down a 37-m hallway at a comfortable self-selected pace for 30 s with and without the n-back task. Each meter in the hallway was marked on the floor and an experimenter remained with the participant during walk trial and recorded the number of steps taken. The participant was cued to stop and remain still at the end of each trial by a beep in the head set and the experimenter measured from the dominant heel to the nearest meter marked on the floor to obtain accurate measures of distance. Each walk trial had a fixed time (30 s), therefore meters per second (walk speed) was calculated for each participant. Mean walk speed values (m/s) were calculated for each participant for single and dual-task walking.

Procedure: Pre-Test and Post-Test Dual-Task Assessments

Each participant included in the final sample completed pre- and post-training physical assessments. At the beginning of each physical assessment session, participants were weighed (kg) and their height (cm) and abdominal circumference (cm) measurements recorded. In a seated position the participants were explained the n-back task and told that they would complete this task while seated and while balancing on one foot. They then completed single-task cognitive (SC; 1-back only) practice. Once their dominant leg was determined, the participant then practiced single balance (SB; balancing only) and practiced dual-task balancing (DTBal; balance and 1-back). All trials SC, SB, DT-bal were 20 s in duration and started with three warning beeps and finished with a single beep. After practice, the participants completed the test phase, in which the condition order was (ABCCBA): SC, SB, DTBal, DTBal, SB, SC. This ABCCBA order allowed the different conditions to be distributed throughout the test phase and fatigue in any one condition minimized.

Once the balance portion of the physical assessment was complete, the experimenter explained the walk portion of the experiment. Similar to the balance portion the condition order for the walk portion had practice on each condition (SC, single walk (SW), and DT-walk) followed by a similar ABCCBA order to the balance test. All conditions were 30 s in duration and began with three beeps and finished with one beep. In comparison to the balance portion, the walk portion had additional conditions such that each participant had the following test order (SC, SC, SW, DT-walk, DT-walk, DT-walk, DT-walk, SW, SC, SC). Each participant completed this order with the 0-back task and then with the 1-back task.

Statistical Analyses

Training Effects

Prior to presenting any transfer from training to our single and dual-task walk outcomes, it is important to state whether or not the four groups improved after training. With respect to physical training, we expected groups who received aerobic training would have greater physical benefits than our groups who received stretch training. Improvements in physical training were assessed with Pre-Post 6 min walk test (6MWT). A one way ANOVA on mean post-test scores for this variable was conducted to assess group differences. With respects to cognitive dual-task computer training, we examined if groups who received cognitive training were able to diminish their dual-task costs on a visual dual-task to a greater extent to those who did not receive cognitive dual-training. Change scores were computed ((dual-task costs (PRE)-dual-task costs (POST))/dual-task costs (POST)). Groups with higher change scores demonstrate diminished dual-task costs after training. These change scores were also subjected to a one way ANOVA to test group differences in training effects.

Single and Dual-Task Walk Data

A full model was conducted to test within and between main effects and interactions for our variable of interest (walk speed). In order to assess difficulty effects, tasks effects, time effects and training group differences in walk speed, we conducted a $2 \times 2 \times 2 \times 4$ ANOVA on mean walk speed with the following within-subjects factors: Task (Single vs. Dual), Time (Pre vs. Post-test), and Difficulty (0-back vs. 1-back) and the between-subjects factor was Group (Aerobic + CT, Aerobic + CL, Stretch + CT, Stretch + CL). The same ANOVA was used to test any mean differences in accuracy (% correct).

Single and Dual-Task Balance Data

The analysis of the dual-task balance data differed from the walk data in that it involved only one level of the n-back task (1-back). For each ML-sway variable and cognitive accuracy score (means only), $2 \times 2 \times 4$ ANOVAs were conducted with the within-subjects factors of Time (Pre vs. Post), Task (single vs. dual) and the between-subjects factor of Group (Aerobic + CT, Aerobic + CL, Stretch + CT, Stretch + CL). For all statistical analyses, IBM SPSS Statistical package version 21 was used, the alpha was set at (0.05) for significance and all *post hoc* comparisons were Bonferroni corrected.

RESULTS

Training Effects

The one way ANOVAs on physical improvements after training revealed that all our groups improved on their 6MWT and there were no significant differences between the groups ($p = 0.21$). The ANOVA on the dual-task cost change scores revealed significant differences between the groups, $F_{(1,67)} = 4.63$, $p = 0.005$, $\eta^2 = 0.17$. The groups that received cognitive training had higher change scores than those that did not receive cognitive training and there were no differences in the two groups that received cognitive training (Aerobic + CT and Stretch + CT; $p = 0.22$). Stretch + CT dual-task cost change ($M = 1.19$) was greater than Aerobic + CL ($M = 0.02$; $p = 0.002$) and Stretch + CL ($M = 0.05$; $p = 0.005$). Aerobic + CT dual-task cost change ($M = 0.74$) was greater than Aerobic + CL ($M = 0.02$; $p = 0.04$) and marginally greater than Stretch + CL ($M = 0.05$; $p = 0.07$).

Single and Dual-Task Walk Data

The walk speed means were subjected to a $2 \times 2 \times 2 \times 4$ ANOVA in order to assess within-subjects effects of difficulty, task and time and between-subjects effects of group. The ANOVA revealed a main effect of time, $F_{(1,68)} = 27.83$, $p < 0.001$, $\eta^2 = 0.29$, in which walk speed means were greater at post-test ($M = 1.42$ m/s, $SE = 0.03$ m/s) than at pre-test ($M = 1.33$ m/s, $SE = 0.03$ m/s). The ANOVA also revealed a main effect of task, $F_{(1,68)} = 193.92$, $p < 0.001$, $\eta^2 = 0.74$, in which participants walk speeds were greater in single-task ($M = 1.39$ m/s, $SE = 0.02$ m/s) than in dual-task ($M = 1.35$ m/s, $SE = 0.02$ m/s). With respects to difficulty, there was also a main effect, $F_{(1,68)} = 37.80$, $p < 0.001$, $\eta^2 = 0.36$, in which participants walked faster in the more difficult 1-back condition ($M = 1.38$ m/s, $SE = 0.02$ m/s) than in the 0-back condition ($M = 1.36$ m/s, $SE = 0.02$ m/s).

The ANOVA also revealed two significant interactions. The first, a task by difficulty interaction $F_{(1,68)} = 4.56$, $p = 0.036$, $\eta^2 = 0.06$, supported the main effect findings such that single-task (ST) walk speed was greater than dual-task (DT) walk speed in both 0-back ($M_{ST} = 1.38$ m/s, $SE_{ST} = 0.02$ m/s $> M_{DT} = 1.34$ m/s, $SE_{DT} = 0.02$ m/s) and 1-back ($M_{ST} = 1.41$ m/s, $SE_{ST} = 0.02$ m/s $> M_{DT} = 1.36$ m/s, $SE_{DT} = 0.02$ m/s). Further, although in both difficulty levels there were significant differences in ST and DT, the mean difference was higher in the 1-back contrast (0.05 m/s) than in the 0-back contrast (0.04 m/s). In addition, a time by task by difficulty interaction, $F_{(1,68)} = 5.83$, $p = 0.02$, $\eta^2 = 0.08$, demonstrated that there were differences between single-task and dual-task at each difficulty level, such that walk speed was greater in single-task vs. dual-task and greater in 1-back vs. 0-back, but that these differences were less at post-test (p-values for contrasts < 0.02) compared to pre-test (p-values for contrasts <0.003; see **Figure 2** for mean single and dual-task values across time and difficulty level). Please see **Table 2** for the mean dual-task walk speed values across time, difficulty level and group.

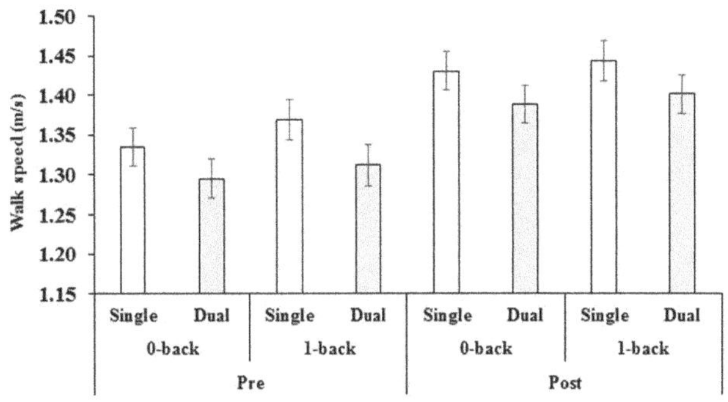

FIGURE 2 | Mean pre- and post-test values for single and dual-task walk speed for both difficulty levels. *Note*: Error bars = standard error of the mean.

TABLE 2 | Dual task mean values for walk speed and accuracy for each group, time and difficulty level.

	Aerobic + CT				Aerobic + CL			
Time	**Pre**		**Post**		**Pre**		**Post**	
Difficulty	**0-back**	**1-back**	**0-back**	**1-back**	**0-back**	**1-back**	**0-back**	**1-back**
Walk speed (m/s)	1.27 (0.05)	1.28 (0.05)	1.36 (0.04)	1.37 (0.05)	1.28 (0.05)	1.31 (0.05)	1.42 (0.05)	1.43 (0.05)
Accuracy (%)	99.89 (0.30)	91.74 (1.47)	100 (0.18)	94.16 (1.24)	99.33 (0.33)	97.59 (1.64)	100 (0.20)	96.52 (1.38)
	Stretch + CT				**Stretch + CL**			
Time	**Pre**		**Post**		**Pre**		**Post**	
Difficulty	**0-back**	**1-back**	**0-back**	**1-back**	**0-back**	**1-back**	**0-back**	**1-back**
Walk speed (m/s)	1.27 (0.05)	1.29 (0.05)	1.39 (0.05)	1.39 (0.05)	1.36 (0.05)	1.37 (0.06)	1.38 (0.05)	1.41 (0.05)
Accuracy (%)	100 (0.32)	96.59 (1.59)	99.62 (0.19)	96.97 (1.34)	100 (0.06)	93.18 (1.69)	100 (0.20)	97.87 (1.42)

Note: Standard error of the mean (SE) reported in the brackets beside the mean value.

Single and Dual-Task Accuracy Data (% Correct)

Similar to the walk speed data, the mean accuracy scores (% correct) were subjected to a 2 × 2 × 2 × 4 ANOVA in order to assess within-subjects effects of difficulty, task, and time and between-subjects effects of group. There were four significant main effects and three interactions with difficulty. There was a main effect of time, $F_{(1,68)} = 8.38$, $p = 0.005$, $\eta^2 = 0.11$, in which accuracy was higher at post-test ($M = 98.57\%$, $SE = 0.20\%$) than at pre-test ($M = 97.57\%$, $SE = 0.36\%$). There was also a main effect of task, $F_{(1,68)} = 7.80$, $p = 0.007$, $\eta^2 = 0.10$, in which accuracy was higher in single-task ($M = 98.60\%$, $SE = 0.25\%$) than in dual-task ($M = 97.72\%$, $SE = 0.27\%$). The main effect of difficulty, $F_{(1,68)} = 72.64$, $p < 0.001$, $\eta^2 = 0.52$, went in the expected direction with participants providing more accurate responses in the easier 0-back ($M = 99.92\%$, $SE = 0.05\%$) in comparison to the more difficult 1-back condition ($M = 96.39\%$, $SE = 0.41\%$). There was also a main effect of group, $F_{(1,68)} = 2.96$, $p = 0.038$, $\eta^2 = 0.12$, in which the Aerobic + CT group had lower accuracy scores ($M = 97.18\%$, $SE = 0.38\%$) than the three other groups (Aerobic + CL ($M = 98.29\%$, $SE = 0.42\%$); Stretch + CT ($M = 98.70\%$, $SE = 0.41\%$); and Stretch + CL ($M = 98.46\%$, $SE = 0.44\%$)). This group effect was further qualified by a significant difficulty by group interaction, $F_{(1,68)} = 3.24$, $p = 0.027$, $\eta^2 = 0.13$, in which the Aerobic + CT group had lower 1-back accuracy scores ($M = 94.38\%$, $SE = 0.76\%$) than the Stretch + CT group ($M = 97.50\%$, $SE = 0.82\%$) only. In addition to this interaction, there was a difficulty by time interaction, $F_{(1,68)} = 7.08$, $p = 0.01$, $\eta^2 = 0.09$, which demonstrated that there were no differences pre to post-test ($p = 0.49$) in the 0-back condition, but there were significant improvements from pre ($M = 95.25\%$, $SE = 0.71\%$) to post-test ($M = 97.54\%$, $SE = 0.41\%$) in the 1-back condition. Finally, there was a difficulty by task interaction, $F_{(1,68)} = 6.27$, $p = 0.015$, $\eta^2 = 0.08$, in which there were only significant differences in single ($M = 97.21\%$, $SE = 0.50\%$) and dual-task ($M = 95.58\%$, $SE = 0.53\%$) in the 1-back condition. Please see **Table 2** for the mean dual-task accuracy values across time, difficulty level and group. Please see **Figure 3** for mean single- and dual-task accuracy across time and difficulty level.

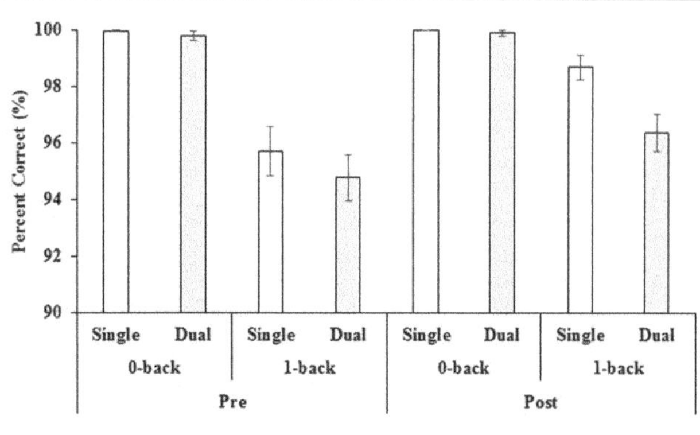

FIGURE 3 | Mean pre- and post-test values for single and dual-task accuracy for both difficulty levels. *Note*: Error bars = standard error of the mean.

Single and Dual-Task Mediolateral Balance Data

The balance dual-task involved only one level of difficulty, the 1-back. We conducted 2 × 2 × 4 mixed ANOVAs (time by task by group) on each sway variable and mean accuracy (% correct). For velocity there were no significant effects. For Peak sway, there was a main effect of time $F_{(1,50)} = 3.99$, $p = 0.05$, $\eta^2 = 0.07$, in which Peak sway was higher at Pre-test ($M = 11.68$ cm, $SE = 1.02$ cm/s) than at Post-test ($M = 9.80$ cm, $SE = 0.95$ cm). The standard deviation (SD) sway variable also demonstrated a significant main effect of time $F_{(1,50)} = 5.73$, $p = 0.02$, $\eta^2 = 0.10$, in which SD sway was higher at Pre-test ($M = 2.31$ cm, $SE = 0.22$ cm) than at Post-test ($M = 1.84$ cm, $SE = 0.21$ cm). A significant time by task by group interaction $F_{(1,50)} = 3.40$, $p = 0.025$, $\eta^2 = 0.17$ was also found for the SD variable. *Post hoc* analyses revealed that the Stretch + CL group had a significant difference ($p = 0.001$) in SD single-task (balancing alone) from Pre ($M = 2.86$, $SE = 0.49$) to Post ($M = 1.42$, $SE = 0.48$) while all other groups did not demonstrate any significant differences. The root mean squared (RMS) variable also demonstrated a main effect of time $F_{(1,50)} = 4.26$, $p = 0.04$, $\eta^2 = 0.08$, in which RMS was higher at Pre-test ($M = 25.40$ cm^2, $SE = 0.89$ cm^2) than at Post-test ($M = 23.47$ cm^2, $SE = 0.92$ cm^2). In addition, there was a significant time by task interaction $F_{(1,50)} = 7.55$, $p = 0.008$, $\eta^2 = 0.13$, in which single-task RMS was not significantly different from Pre- to Post-test ($p = 0.14$) but that dual-task RMS was higher at Pre-test ($M = 25.50$ cm^2, $SE = 0.90$ cm^2) than at Post-test ($M = 23.04$ cm^2, $SE = 0.91$ cm^2; $p = 0.015$). For the 1-back mean accuracy during balancing, the 2 × 2 × 4 mixed ANOVA revealed a main effect of time $F_{(1,50)} = 16.61$, $p < 0.001$, $\eta^2 = 0.24$, in which Post-test accuracy was higher ($M = 95.97\%$, $SE = 0.75\%$) than Pre-test accuracy ($M = 91.72\%$, $SE = 1.09\%$). There was also a main effect of task $F_{(1,50)} = 4.36$, $p = 0.042$, $\eta^2 = 0.08$, in which the single-task 1-back accuracy ($M = 95.10\%$, $SE = 0.89\%$) was higher than the dual-task 1-back accuracy ($M = 92.59\%$, $SE = 1.07\%$). There were no other significant effects or interactions. **Table 3** presents the mean dual-task mediolateral sway values for each group pre- and post-test.

DISCUSSION

In the current study, age-associated changes in physical and cognitive function were targeted with a combined training (physical and cognitive) protocol. Participants were randomly assigned to one of four different training protocols (Aerobic + CT, Aerobic + CL, Stretch + CT, Stretch + CL). The goal of the study was to assess whether or not the benefits of a combined training protocol would transfer to untrained gait and balance dual-tasks. Based on the literature, it was hypothesized that the Aerobic + CT group would demonstrate the greatest improvements in dual-task gait and balance in comparison to other groups. In addition, we predicted that the Stretch + CL group, our active control, would demonstrate the least improvements in dual-task gait and balance after training. Our findings only partially support our hypotheses, as we did find improvements in dual-task walk and balance outcomes from pre to post-test, but we did not find that our Aerobic + CT group improved to a greater degree than the other groups, or that our placebo-placebo control (Stretch + CL) improved the least.

Training Effects

All groups demonstrated improvements in our outcome measures for physical (6MWT) and cognitive dual-task training (dual-task cost change scores). In terms of physical training, the 6MWT did not reveal any differences between our groups in performance gains, such that the groups containing aerobic training did not benefit to a greater degree than the groups containing stretch training. For the cognitive training, a majority of the group contrasts suggest that the cognitive dual-task training was beneficial in reducing dual-task costs post-test for the groups that received this specific type of training compared to the other groups who had computer lessons.

Single and Dual-Task Walk Findings

Consistent across all groups, and confirming the dual-task effect, walk speed and accuracy were higher in single-task conditions vs. dual-task conditions. Interestingly, when examining main effects of difficulty, all groups walked faster in the harder difficulty level (1-back) when compared to the easier difficulty level (0-back) but all were less accurate in the 1-back compared to the 0-back. Increasing the speed of the motor response to dual-task conditions is similar to the facilitation findings we have found in dual-task treadmill walking (Fraser et al., 2007). When the walk speed was fixed, participants responded more rapidly to the cognitive task during walking when compared to responding in a seated position. Perhaps the ability to speed up ones response cognitively or in the present study increase walk speed in a more challenging dual-task allows for better management of the walking dual-task. The task by difficulty effect in walk speed does support that the 1-back difficulty level was more difficult than the 0-back difficulty level as the difference between single and dual-task walk speed were greatest in the 1-back condition. Further, accuracy levels overall were high, but 1-back accuracy levels are clearly poorer than 0-back accuracy levels which also support the manipulation of difficulty.

The full model also revealed that all the participants in our sample benefited from training. Post-test walk speed and accuracy values were greater than pre-test values and the differences between single and dual-task walk speeds were diminished at post-test. With the exception of a slight accuracy difference between our Aerobic + CT group and our Stretch + CT group, our walk results do not reveal specific group differences but rather demonstrate that all groups improved in their accuracy and walk speed from pre to post-test. Despite the lack of significant differences found in the full statistical model, from a clinical standpoint 0.05 m/s increase in walk speed represents a small meaningful change and 0.10 m/s represents substantial meaningful change (Perera et al., 2006; Kwon et al., 2009). In the current study, the only group that did not demonstrate a clinically significant change in walk speed from pre to post-test

TABLE 3 | Mean dual-task mediolateral (ML) sway values for each group and time.

	Aerobic + CT		Aerobic + CL		Stretch + CT		Stretch + CL	
Time	Pre	Post	Pre	Post	Pre	Post	Pre	Post
Velocity (cm/s)	4.87 (0.70)	3.69 (0.56)	4.40 (0.79)	3.47 (0.63)	5.07 (0.68)	5.13 (0.54)	4.22 (0.82)	4.05 (0.65)
Peak (cm)	11.72 (2.16)	8.83 (1.68)	11.28 (2.41)	6.96 (1.88)	12.64 (2.09)	10.92 (1.63)	10.27 (2.52)	11.36 (1.96)
SD (cm)	2.24 (0.47)	1.64 (0.47)	2.13 (0.52)	1.45 (0.53)	2.40 (0.45)	2.16 (0.46)	2.12 (0.55)	2.37 (0.55)
RMS (cm^2)	23.57 (1.68)	21.94 (1.71)	26.78 (1.88)	22.27 (1.92)	24.76 (1.63)	23.32 (1.66)	26.88 (1.97)	24.64 (2.00)
Accuracy (%)	87.16 (3.43)	97.14 (1.81)	93.39 (3.56)	98.98 (1.87)	87.14 (3.43)	92.86 (1.81)	90.08 (3.68)	93.97 (1.94)

Note: Standard error of the mean (SE) reported in the brackets beside the mean value.

was our active placebo control. Groups with an aerobic and/or cognitive training component demonstrated 0.09 m/s increase in walk speed or greater. As such, from a clinical point of view, it may be more beneficial to have an aerobic and/or a cognitive training component in a combined training protocol.

The results of the full model differ from the study by Schwenk et al. (2010) that targeted dual-task walk speed as a primary outcome and found significant group differences in their most difficult dual-task gait condition.

There are several possible reasons for these contrasting findings. First, Schwenk et al. (2010) chose a type of exercise training that was very close to their outcome measure, as such they successfully demonstrated near transfer (training effects in a task similar to the trained task). Our training protocol did not explicitly train dual-task walking abilities but rather focused on aerobic exercise and cognitive dual-task training at a computer. As such, our training was distinct from our outcome measure and we were assessing far transfer effects to dual-task walking. Our results suggest that any type of active intervention in a sample of sedentary older adults can improve dual-task gait. In addition, while both studies included a 12-week training protocol, in Schwenk et al.'s (2010) study the groups did not have the same number of intervention hours (control group had half the time of the experimental group), whereas all participants in our 12-week intervention were exposed to the same number of intervention hours and always trained in groups. It is unknown how this influences the differences in our findings but it is possible that the differences between our groups were reduced as they all had the same number of intervention hours. Another important difference between the studies, is that Schwenk et al. (2010) trained older adults with cognitive impairment (dementia) and we trained individuals without cognitive impairment. A meta-analysis examining the effects of aerobic exercise on cognitive performance suggests that greater improvements in memory may be seen in those with cognitive impairment compared to those without cognitive impairment (Smith et al., 2010). Although sedentary, our sample was relatively healthy, did not have cognitive impairment or functional limitations and this may have minimized the gains seen after training. One interesting similarity between the two studies is that the most consistent findings emerge in the more difficult condition. In our study, although we found robust differences in v and 1-back performances supporting a difficulty effect, it is possible that if we challenged our groups with an additional difficulty level (for example a 2-back) we would see differences between our training groups on a more challenging dual-task walk situation. Also, in the current study, we chose to focus on walk speed, in a relatively high functioning sample, other gait parameters (e.g., stride time variability) might have been more sensitive to training induced changes (Lamoth et al., 2011.

While it was important in the current study to control for the number of visits and interactions with training groups by including active control groups, another possible reason for improvements across all the groups may have been our alternate choice in physical training (stretch training). Although the stretch training in the current study did not target aerobic capacity it did have a resistance training component and the goal of improving lower body strength. The improvement in lower body strength may have transferred to improvements in walk speed. Indeed, there is some evidence that certain types of stretching/resistance training exercises can influence gait speed (Stanziano et al., 2009; van Abbema et al., 2015).

Single and Dual-Task Balance Findings

The main findings from the mediolateral sway measures were that all participants improved from pre to post-test in Peak sway, SD, RMS. In the SD variable, there was a time by task by group interaction in which the active placebo-placebo (Stretch + CL) had a significant improvement in single-task performance from pre-to post and the other groups did not demonstrate this effect. This finding should be interpreted with caution, as direct comparisons of the groups on the single-task sway measures by means of a one-way ANOVA did not find any significant differences between the groups. The RMS sway value also demonstrated a task by time interaction in which there were no improvements pre to post in single-task performances but there were improvements in dual-task performances (reduced sway). It is important to note also that our standardized paper and pencil measure of balance confidence, the ABC scale did not reveal any differences between our groups and all groups had high scores suggesting that our findings are not influenced by a lack of confidence in balance abilities.

In terms of accuracy on the 1-back task, all groups demonstrated the typical task effect in which single-task cognitive performance (seated in a chair) was more accurate than dual-task cognitive performance (while balancing). In addition, all groups improved their accuracy significantly from pre- to post-test. Similar to the dual-task gait findings, all participants improved in several (but not all) mediolateral postural sway variables and in their cognitive accuracy during balance. Our results also suggest that sedentary adults can demonstrate reduced sway (improved balance) after an active intervention protocol. There were limited task effects in the balance data, one interaction effect with time, task, and group in which there was single-task SD sway improvement in the Stretch + CL group that wasn't apparent in the other groups. This finding is difficult to explain, as the groups did not differ in single-task SD when the one-way ANOVA comparing groups was conducted. It may be the case that the limited sample size in the balance data influenced the outcome of the larger 2 × 2 × 4 mixed ANOVA. The RMS variable seems to be sensitive to task effects demonstrating dual-task balance improvements over time across groups, but additional research with larger sample sizes is needed to truly evaluate the importance of these variables for outcome measures of dual-task balance.

Limitations

Limitations specific to our training protocols and active control groups are discussed elsewhere (see Desjardins-Crépeau et al., 2016). Specific limitations for this portion of the study relate to the small sample size in the balance outcome measures, limiting our potential interpretation and the generalizability of results. Nonetheless, there is a very limited literature on dual-task static balance as an outcome measure for combined cognitive and physical training programs that do not train the components of the outcome measure being assessed (i.e., single and dual-task balance training). The results of this study can be used to inform selection of variables of interest in future combined intervention studies with static sway variables as outcomes. Regarding the dual-task gait outcomes, the sample size is larger and the changes in dual-task 1-back walk speed (see **Table 1**) argue against simple test re-test effects, as the three groups that had cognitive and/or aerobic training have higher gains in walk speed pre-post (Aerobic + CT: 0.09 m/s, Aerobic + CL:.12 m/s, and Stretch + CT: 0.10 m/s) than the placebo-placebo group (Stretch + CT: 0.04 m/s). Despite this, it is unclear given the findings what specifically led to improved dual-task gait performances. Given that we solicited sedentary older adults, who may have fewer outings and less social contact, it is possible that the social interaction produced by the regular group meetings contributed to improved outcomes in the current study and this not a factor that was measured in this study. It would be important in future combined cognitive and physical training studies to control for social factors of regular group sessions.

Further, it is important to note that our methodological choice of having a combined training protocol limited the number of training sessions we were able to provide to our participants on a weekly basis. Although our group has demonstrated cognitive improvements from a 12-week training protocol (Predovan et al., 2012) and balance benefits from cognitive training (Li et al., 2010) these training protocols were able to devote all the weekly sessions to a specific training type (either aerobic or cognitive) and as such might have boosted the benefits of training. In our protocol, we had to reduce the amount of cognitive training to once per week and physical training to twice per week in order to provide both cognitive and physical training in the same protocol. Wollesen and Voelcker-Rehage (2013), indicated in their review that not only did the type of training influence dual-task outcomes but the amount of training could also influence outcomes. As such, the combined protocol might have reduced the training effects as the amount of cognitive and physical training per week might not have been sufficient to demonstrate the potential synergistic effects of combined training.

CONCLUSION

Given the clinical importance of dual-task gait and balance assessments in identifying individuals at risk for falls and cognitive decline and the potential for training to improve dual-task balance and gait, future combined training studies should include dual-task outcome measures in order to tease out what kind of training (perhaps adaptive), how often, at what intensity, would be most beneficial to improve dual-task balance and gait. Future studies, utilizing portable imaging technologies such as functional near infra-red spectroscopy will complement the behavioral findings of this study and provide more clarity on cognitive plasticity in the PFC. Certainly, the training gains seen across all groups in walk and certain balance measures in the current study suggest that encouraging sedentary older adults to actively participate in a training protocol may have transferrable benefits to dual-task gait and balance that could potentially reduce fall risk and cognitive decline in this population.

AUTHOR CONTRIBUTIONS

SAF: design, protocol, training of graduate students, data analysis, manuscript write-up. KZ-HL: design, principal investigator, secured funding for the project, trained graduate student for balance data analysis, provided feedback. NB: design for physical assessments (6MWT, etc.) training of all trainers for the physical portion of study and data analysis of the physical data. LD-C: responsible for all the testing, data entry, and analysis of the neuropsychological data. ML: responsible for the cognitive training and computer lesson component, and all the data related to this component. KV: responsible for converting the raw balance data to center of pressure scores, provided feedback on preliminary version of manuscript. LL: responsible for the physcial training with participants, data entry for physical and neuropsychological data. TTMV: medical doctor responsible for all the clinical assessments of participants, provided feedback on preliminary version of manuscript. LBosquet: design, physical assessment, one of the principle investigators who secured funding for the project. LBherer: design, cognitive training component, principle investigator who secured funding for the project—provided feedback on several versions of the manuscript.

ACKNOWLEDGMENTS

This study was supported by a Canadian Institutes of Health Research grant (#187596) to LBherer, LBosquet and KZ-HL. SAF was supported by a "Fonds Québec Recherche en Nature et Technologies" Postdoctoral Fellowship and LBherer was supported by the Canadian Research Chair Program. We would like to thank all the research assistants, two study co-ordinators (Mélanie Renaud and Chantal Mongeau) and all the participants. The authors would like to thank the Canadian Institutes of Health Research that supported this large mobility in aging trial.

REFERENCES

van Abbema, R., De Greef, M., Crajé, C., Krijnen, W., Hobbelen, H., and Van Der Schans, C. (2015). What type, or combination of exercise can improve preferred gait speed in older adults? A meta-analysis. *BMC Geriatr.* 15:72. doi: 10.1186/s12877-015-0061-9

Allali, G., Assal, F., Kressig, R. W., Dubost, V., Herrmann, F. R., and Beauchet, O. (2008). Impact of impaired executive function on gait stability. *Dement. Geriatr. Cogn. Disord.* 26, 364–369. doi: 10.1159/000162358

Al-Yahya, E., Dawes, H., Smith, L., Dennis, A., Howells, K., and Cockburn, J. (2011). Cognitive motor interference while walking: a systematic review and meta-analysis. *Neurosci. Biobehav. Rev.* 35, 715–728. doi: 10.1016/j.neubiorev.2010.08.008

Bherer, L. (2015). Cognitive plasticity in older adults: effects of cognitive training and physical exercise. *Ann. N Y Acad. Sci.* 1337, 1–6. doi: 10.1111/nyas.12682

Bherer, L., Erickson, K. I., and Liu-Ambrose, T. (2013). A review of the effects of physical activity and exercise on cognitive and brain functions in older adults. *J. Aging Res.* 2013:657508. doi: 10.1155/2013/657508

Bherer, L., Kramer, A. F., Peterson, M. S., Colcombe, S., Erickson, K., and Becic, E. (2005). Training effects on dual-task performance: are there age-related differences in plasticity of attentional control? *Psychol. Aging* 20, 695–709. doi: 10.1037/0882-7974.20.4.695

Bherer, L., Kramer, A. F., Peterson, M. S., Colcombe, S., Erickson, K., and Becic, E. (2006). Testing the limits of cognitive plasticity in older adults: application to attentional control. *Acta Psychol. (Amst)* 123, 261–278. doi: 10.1016/j.actpsy.2006.01.005

Bherer, L., Kramer, A. F., Peterson, M. S., Colcombe, S., Erickson, K., and Becic, E. (2008). Transfer effects in task-set cost and dual-task cost after dual-task training in older and younger adults: further evidence for cognitive plasticity in attentional control in late adulthood. *Exp. Aging Res.* 34, 188–219. doi: 10.1080/03610730802070068

Belleville, S., and Bherer, L. (2012). Biomarkers of cognitive training effects in aging. *Curr. Transl. Geriatr. Exp. Gerontol. Rep.* 1, 104–110. doi: 10.1007/s13670-012-0014-5

Berryman, N., Bherer, L., Nadeau, S., Lauzière, S., Lehr, L., Bobeuf, F., et al. (2014). Multiple roads lead to Rome: combined high-intensity aerobic and strength training vs. gross motor activities leads to equivalent improvement in executive functions in a cohort of healthy older adults. *Age (Dordr)* 36:9710. doi: 10.1007/s11357-014-9710-8

Borg, G. (1998). *Borg's Perceived Exertion and Pain Scales.* Champaign, IL: Human Kinetics.

Brauer, S. G., Woollacott, M., and Shumway-Cook, A. (2001). The interacting effects of cognitive demand recovery of postural stability in balance-impaired elderly persons. *J. Gerontol. A Biol. Sci. Med. Sci.* 56, M489–M496. doi: 10.1093/gerona/56.8.m489

Braver, T. S., Paxton, J. L., Locke, H. S., and Barch, D. M. (2009). Flexible neural mechanisms of cognitive control within human prefrontal cortex. *Proc. Natl. Acad. Sci. U S A* 106, 7351–7356. doi: 10.1073/pnas.0808187106

Buckner, R. L. (2004). Memory and executive function in aging and AD: multiple factors that cause decline and reserve factors that compensate. *Neuron* 44, 195–208. doi: 10.1016/j.neuron.2004.09.006

Buracchio, T. J., Mattek, N. C., Dodge, H. H., Hayes, T. L., Pavel, M., Howieson, D. B., et al. (2011). Executive function predicts risk of falls in older adults without balance impairment. *BMC Geriatr.* 11:74. doi: 10.1186/1471-2318-11-74

Cadore, E. L., Rodríguez-Mañas, L., Sinclair, A., and Izquierdo, M. (2013). Effects of different exercise interventions on risk of falls, gait ability, and balance in physically frail older adults: a systematic review. *Rejuvenation Res.* 16, 105–114. doi: 10.1089/rej.2012.1397

Condron, J. E., Hill, K. D., and Dip, G. (2002). Reliability and validity of a dual-task force platform assessment of balance performance: effect of age, balance impairment, and cognitive task. *J. Am. Geriatr. Soc.* 50, 157–162. doi: 10.1046/j.1532-5415.2002.50022.x

Colcombe, S. J., Erickson, K. I., Scalf, P. E., Kim, J. S., Prakash, R., McAuley, E., et al. (2006). Aerobic exercise training increases brain volume in aging humans. *J. Gerontol. A Biol. Sci. Med. Sci.* 61, 1166–1170. doi: 10.1093/gerona/61.11.1166

Colcombe, S., and Kramer, A. F. (2003). Fitness effects on the cognitive function of older adults: a meta-analytic study. *Psychol. Sci.* 14, 125–130. doi: 10.1111/1467-9280.t01-1-01430

Colcombe, S. J., Kramer, A. F., Erickson, K. I., Scalf, P., McAuley, E., Cohen, N. J., et al. (2004). Cardiovascular fitness, cortical plasticity, and aging. *Proc. Natl. Acad. Sci. U S A* 101, 3316–3321. doi: 10.1073/pnas.0400266101

de Labra, C., Guimaraes-Pinheiro, C., Maseda, A., Lorenzo, T., and Millán-Calenti, J. C. (2015). Effects of physical exercise interventions in frail older adults: a systematic review of randomized controlled trials. *BMC Geriatr.* 15:154. doi: 10.1186/s12877-015-0155-4

Desjardins-Crépeau, L., Berryman, N., Fraser, S. A., Vu, T. T. M., Kergoat, M.-J., Li, K. Z. H., et al. (2016). Effects of combined physical and cognitive training on fitness and neuropsychological outcomes in healthy older adults. *Clin. Interv. Aging*, 11, 1287–1299. doi: 10.2147/cia.s115711

Doumas, M., Smolders, C., and Krampe, R. T. (2008). Task prioritization in aging: effects of sensory information on concurrent posture and memory performance. *Exp. Brain Res.* 187, 275–281. doi: 10.1007/s00221-008-1302-3

Erickson, K. I., Colcombe, S. J., Wadhwa, R., Bherer, L., Peterson, M. S., Scalf, P. E., et al. (2007). Training-induced functional activation changes in dual-task processing: an fMRI study. *Cereb. Cortex* 17, 192–204. doi: 10.1093/cercor/bhj137

Fraser, S. A., and Bherer, L. (2013). Age-related decline in divided attention: from theoretical lab research to practical real life situations. *Wiley Interdiscip. Re. Cogn. Sci.* 4, 623–640. doi: 10.1002/wcs.1252

Fraser, S. A., Elliott, V., de Bruin, E. D., Bherer, L., and Dumoulin, C. (2014). The effects of combined pelvic floor muscle training and virtual-reality dance rehabilitation on dual-task gait and cognition in women with mixed urinary incontinence. *Games Health J.* 3, 172–178. doi: 10.1089/g4h.2013.0095

Fraser, S. A., Li, K. Z. H., DeMont, R. G., and Penhune, V. B. (2007). The effects of balance status and age on muscle activation during walking under divided attention. *J. Gerontol. B Psychol. Sci. Soc. Sci.* 62B, P171–P178. doi: 10.1093/geronb/62.3.p171

Gunning-Dixon, F. M., and Raz, N. (2003). Neuroanatomical correlates of selected executive functions in middle-aged and older adults: a prospective MRI study. *Neuropsychologia* 41, 1929–1941. doi: 10.1016/s0028-3932(03)00129-5

Hall, C. D., Smith, A. L., and Keele, S. W. (2001). The impact of aerobic activity on cognitive function in older adults: a new synthesis based on the concept of executive control. *Eur. J. Cogn. Psychol.* 13, 279–300. doi: 10.1080/09541440126012

Hauer, K., Pfisterer, M., Weber, C., Wezler, N., Kliegel, M., and Oster, P. (2003). Cognitive impairment decreases postural control during dual-tasks in geriatric patients with a history of severe falls. *J. Am. Geriatr. Soc.* 51, 1638–1644. doi: 10.1046/j.1532-5415.2003.51517.x

Hausdorff, J. M., Schweiger, A., Herman, T., Yogev-Seligmann, G., and Giladi, N. (2008). Dual-task decrements in gait: contributing factors among healthy older adults. *J. Gerontol. A Biol. Sci. Med. Sci.* 63, 1335–1343. doi: 10.1093/gerona/63.12.1335

Hedden, T., and Gabrieli, J. D. (2004). Insights into the ageing mind: a view from cognitive neuroscience. *Nat. Rev. Neurosci.* 5, 87–96. doi: 10.1038/nrn1323

Helbostad, J. L., Sturnieks, D. L., Menant, J., Delbaere, K., Lord, S. R., and Pijnappels, M. (2010). Consequences of lower extremity and trunk muscle fatigue on balance and functional tasks in older people: a systematic literature review. *BMC Geriatr.* 10:56. doi: 10.1186/1471-2318-10-56

Horak, F. (2006). Postural orientation and equilibrium: what do we need to know about neural control of balance to prevent falls? *Age Ageing* 35, II7–II11. doi: 10.1093/ageing/afl077

van Iersel, M. B., Kessels, R. P. C., Bloem, B. R., Verbeek, A. L. M., and Olde Rikkert, M. G. M. (2008). Executive functions are associated with gait and balance in community-living elderly people. *J. Gerontol. A Biol. Sci. Med. Sci.* 63, 1344–1349. doi: 10.1093/gerona/63.12.1344

Jaeggi, S. M., Seewer, R., Nirkko, A. C., Eckstein, D., Schroth, G., Groner, R., et al. (2003). Does excessive memory load attenuate activation in the prefrontal cortex? Load-dependent processing in single and dual tasks: functional magnetic resonance imaging study. *NeuroImage* 19, 210–225. doi: 10.1016/s1053-8119(03)00098-3

Klingberg, T. (2010). Training and plasticity of working memory. *Trends Cogn. Sci.* 14, 317–324. doi: 10.1016/j.tics.2010.05.002

Kramer, A. F., and Erickson, K. I. (2007). Capitalizing on cortical plasticity: influence of physical activity on cognition and brain function. *Trends Cogn. Sci.* 11, 342–348. doi: 10.1016/j.tics.2007.06.009

Kramer, A. F., Hahn, S., Cohen, N. J., Banich, M. T., McAuley, E., Harrison, C. R., et al. (1999). Ageing, fitness and neurocognitive function. *Nature* 400, 418–419. doi: 10.1038/22682

Kueider, A. M., Parisi, J. M., Gross, A. L., and Rebok, G. W. (2012). Computerized cognitive training with older adults: a systematic review. *PLoS One* 7:e40588. doi: 10.1371/journal.pone.0040588

Kwon, S., Perera, S., Pahor, M., Katula, J. A., King, A. C., Groessl, E. J., et al. (2009). What is a meaningful change in physical performance? Findings from a clinical trial in older adults (the LIFE-P study). *J. Nutr. Health Aging* 13, 538–544. doi: 10.1007/s12603-009-0104-z

Lamoth, C. J., van Deudekom, F. J., van Campen, J. P., Appels, B. A., de Vries, O. J., and Pijnappels, M. (2011). Gait stability and variability measures show effects of impaired cognition and dual-tasking in frail people. *J. Neuroeng. Rehabil.* 8:2. doi: 10.1186/1743-0003-8-2

Langlois, F., Vu, T. T. M., Chassé, K., Dupuis, G., Kergoat, M.-J., and Bherer, L. (2013). Benefits of physical exercise training on cognition and quality of life in frail older adults. *J. Gerontol. B Psychol. Sci. Soc. Sci.* 68, 400–404. doi: 10.1093/geronb/gbs069

Law, L. L., Barnett, F., Yau, M. K., and Gray, M. A. (2014). Effects of combined cognitive and exercise interventions on cognition in older adults with and without cognitive impairment: a systematic review. *Ageing Res. Rev.* 15, 61–75. doi: 10.1016/j.arr.2014.02.008

Lee, H., Boot, W. R., Basak, C., Voss, M. W., Prakash, R. S., Neider, M., et al. (2012). Performance gains from directed training do not transfer to untrained tasks. *Acta Psychol.* 139, 146–158. doi: 10.1016/j.actpsy.2011.11.003

Leung, N. T., Tam, H. M., Chu, L. W., Kwok, T. C., Chan, F., Lam, L. C., et al. (2015). Neural plastic effects of cognitive training on aging brain. *Neural Plast.* 2015:535618. doi: 10.1155/2015/535618

Li, S. C., Schmiedek, F., Huxhold, O., Röcke, C., Smith, J., and Lindenberger, U. (2008). Working memory plasticity in old age: practice gain, transfer and maintenance. *Psychol. Aging* 23, 731–742. doi: 10.1037/a0014343

Li, K. Z. H., Abbud, G. A., Fraser, S. A., and DeMont, R. G. (2012). Successful adaptation of gait in healthy older adults during dual-task treadmill walking. *Neuropsychol. Dev. Cogn. B Aging Neuropsychol. Cogn.* 19, 150–167. doi: 10.1080/13825585.2011.628375

Li, K. Z. H., Roudaia, E., Lussier, M., Bherer, L., Leroux, A., and McKinley, P. A. (2010). Benefits of cognitive dual-task training on balance performance in healthy older adults. *J. Gerontol. A Biol. Sci. Med. Sci.* 65, 1344–1352. doi: 10.1093/gerona/glq151

Lussier, M., Brouillard, P., and Bherer, L. (2015). Limited benefits of heterogeneous dual-task training on transfer effects in older adults. *J. Gerontol. B Psychol. Sci. Soc. Sci.* doi: 10.1093/geronb/gbv105 [Epub ahead of print].

Miyake, A., Friedman, N. P., Emerson, M. J., Witzki, A. H., Howerter, A., and Wager, T. D. (2000). The unity and diversity of executive functions and their contributions to complex "frontal lobe" tasks: A latent variable analysis. *Cogn. Psychol.* 41, 49–100. doi: 10.1006/cogp.1999.0734

Muir, S. W., Speechley, M., Wells, J., Borrie, M., Gopaul, K., and Montero-Odasso, M. (2012). Gait assessment in mild cognitive impairment and Alzheimer's disease: the effect of dual-task challenges across the cognitive spectrum. *Gait Posture* 35, 96–100. doi: 10.1016/j.gaitpost.2011.08.014

Muir-Hunter, S. W., Clark, J., McLean, S., Pedlow, S., Van Hemmen, A., Montero-Odasso, M., et al. (2014). Identifying balance and fall risk in community-dwelling older women: the effect of executive function on postural control. *Physiother. Can.* 66, 179–186. doi: 10.3138/ptc.2013-16

Montero-Odasso, M., Verghese, J., Beauchet, O., and Hausdorff, J. M. (2012). Gait and cognition: a complementary approach to understanding brain function and the risk of falling. *J. Am. Geriatr. Soc.* 60, 2127–2136. doi: 10.1111/j.1532-5415.2012.04209.x

Perera, S., Mody, S. H., Woodman, R. C., and Studenski, S. A. (2006). Meaningful change and responsiveness in common physical performance measures in older adults. *J. Am. Geriatr. Soc.* 54, 743–749. doi: 10.1111/j.1532-5415.2006.00701.x

Powell, L. E., and Myers, A. M. (1995). The activities-specific balance confidence (ABC) scale. *J. Gerontol. A Biol. Sci. Med. Sci.* 50, M28–M34. doi: 10.1093/gerona/50A.1.M28

Predovan, D., Fraser, S. A., Renaud, M., and Bherer, L. (2012). The effect of three months of aerobic training on stroop performance in older adults. *J. Aging Res.* 2012:269815. doi: 10.1155/2012/269815

Schaefer, S., and Schumacher, V. (2010). The interplay between cognitive and motor functioning in healthy older adults: findings from dual-task studies and suggestions for intervention. *Gerontology* 57, 239–246. doi: 10.1159/000322197

Schwenk, M., Zieschang, T., Oster, P., and Hauer, K. (2010). Dual-task performances can be improved in patients with dementia A randomized controlled trial. *Neurology* 74, 1961–1968. doi: 10.1212/WNL.0b013e3181e39696

Segev-Jacubovski, O., Herman, T., Yogev-Seligmann, G., Mirelman, A., Giladi, N., and Hausdorff, J. M. (2011). The interplay between gait, falls and cognition: can cognitive therapy reduce fall risk? *Expert Rev. Neurother.* 11, 1057–1075. doi: 10.1586/ern.11.69

Sheridan, P. L., Solomont, J., Kowall, N., and Hausdorff, J. M. (2003). Influence of executive function on locomotor function: divided attention increases gait variability in Alzheimer's disease. *J. Am. Geriatr. Soc.* 51, 1633–1637. doi: 10.1046/j.1532-5415.2003.51516.x

Shumway-Cook, A., Gruber, W., Baldwin, M., and Liao, S. (1997). The effect of multidimensional exercises on balance, mobility, and fall risk in community-dwelling older adults. *Phys. Ther.* 77, 46–57.

Smith, P. J., Blumenthal, J. A., Hoffman, B. M., Cooper, H., Strauman, T. A., Welsh-Bohmer, K., et al. (2010). Aerobic exercise and neurocognitive performance: a meta-analytic review of randomized controlled trials. *Psychosom. Med.* 72, 239–252. doi: 10.1097/PSY.0b013e3181d14633

Smith-Ray, R. L., Hughes, S. L., Prohaska, T. R., Little, D. M., Jurivich, D. A., and Hedeker, D. (2013). Impact of cognitive training on balance and gait in older adults. *J. Gerontol. B Psychol. Sci. Soc. Sci.* 70, 357–366. doi: 10.1093/geronb/gbt097

Springer, S., Giladi, N., Peretz, C., Yogev, G., Simon, E. S., and Hausdorff, J. M. (2006). Dual-tasking effects on gait variability: the role of aging, falls and executive function. *Mov. Disord* 21, 950–957. doi: 10.1002/mds.20848

Stanziano, D. C., Roos, B. A., Perry, A. C., Lai, S., and Signorile, J. F. (2009). The effects of an active-assisted stretching program on functional performance in elderly persons: a pilot study. *Clin. Interv. Aging* 4, 115–120. doi: 10.2147/cia.s4152

Stuss, D. T., and Alexander, M. P. (2000). Executive functions and the frontal lobes: A conceptual view. *Psychol. Res.* 63, 289–298. doi: 10.1007/s004269900007

Thibaud, M., Bloch, F., Tournoux-Facon, C., Brèque, C., Rigaud, A. S., Dugué, B., et al. (2011). Impact of physical activity and sedentary behaviour on fall risks in older people: a systematic review and meta-analysis of observational studies. *Eur. Rev. Aging Phys. Act.* 9, 5–15. doi: 10.1007/s11556-011-0081-1

Verghese, J., Mahoney, J., Ambrose, A. F., Wang, C., and Holtzer, R. (2010). Effect of cognitive remediation on gait in sedentary seniors. *J. Gerontol. A Biol. Sci. Med. Sci.* 65, 1338–1343. doi: 10.1093/gerona/glq127

Walshe, E. A., Patterson, M. R., Commins, S., and Roche, R. A. (2015). Dual-task and electrophysiological markers of executive cognitive processing in older adult gait and fall-risk. *Front. Hum. Neurosci.* 9:200. doi: 10.3389/fnhum.2015.00200

Willis, S. L., Tennstedt, S. L., Marsiske, M., Ball, K., Elias, J., Koepke, K. M., et al. (2006). Long-term effects of cognitive training on everyday functional outcomes in older adults. *JAMA* 296, 2805–2814. doi: 10.1001/jama.296.23.2805

Wollesen, B., and Voelcker-Rehage, C. (2013). Training effects on motor-cognitive dual-task performance in older adults. *Eur. Rev. Aging Phys. Act.* 11, 5–24. doi: 10.1007/s11556-013-0122-z

Woollacott, M., and Shumway-Cook, A. (2002). Attention and the control of posture and gait: a review of an emerging area of research. *Gait Posture* 16, 1–14. doi: 10.1016/s0966-6362(01)00156-4

Zijlstra, A., Ufkes, T., Skelton, D. A., Lundin-Olsson, L., and Zijlstra, W. (2008). Do dual-tasks have an added value over single-tasks for balance assessment in fall prevention programs? A mini-review. *Gerontology* 54, 40–49. doi: 10.1159/000117808

3

Cognitive Flexibility Training: A Large-Scale Multimodal Adaptive Active-Control Intervention Study in Healthy Older Adults

Jessika I. V. Buitenweg[1*], *Renate M. van de Ven*[1], *Sam Prinssen*[1], *Jaap M. J. Murre*[1] and *K. Richard Ridderinkhof*[1,2]

[1] Department of Psychology, University of Amsterdam, Amsterdam, Netherlands, [2] Amsterdam Brain and Cognition, University of Amsterdam, Amsterdam, Netherlands

Edited by:
Soledad Ballesteros,
Universidad Nacional de Educación a Distancia, Spain

Reviewed by:
Ana M. Daugherty,
University of Illinois at Urbana–Champaign, United States
Julia Karbach,
Goethe University Frankfurt, Germany

***Correspondence:**
Jessika I. V. Buitenweg
j.i.v.buitenweg@uva.nl

As aging is associated with cognitive decline, particularly in the executive functions, it is essential to effectively improve cognition in older adults. Online cognitive training is currently a popular, though controversial method. Although some changes seem possible in older adults through training, far transfer, and longitudinal maintenance are rarely seen. Based on previous literature we created a unique, state-of-the-art intervention study by incorporating frequent sessions and flexible, novel, adaptive training tasks, along with an active control group. We created a program called TAPASS (Training Project Amsterdam Seniors and Stroke), a randomized controlled trial. Healthy older adults (60–80 y.o.) were assigned to a frequent- (FS) or infrequent switching (IS) experimental condition or to the active control group and performed 58 half-hour sessions over the course of 12 weeks. Effects on executive functioning, processing- and psychomotor speed, planning, verbal long term memory, verbal fluency, and reasoning were measured on four time points before, during and after the training. Additionally, we examined the explorative question which individual aspects added to training benefit. Besides improvements on the training, we found significant time effects on multiple transfer tasks in all three groups that likely reflected retest effects. No training-specific improvements were detected, and we did not find evidence of additional benefits of individual characteristics. Judging from these results, the therapeutic value of using commercially available training games to train the aging brain is modest, though any apparent effects should be ascribed more to expectancy and motivation than to the elements in our training protocol. Our results emphasize the importance of using parallel tests as outcome measures for transfer and including both active and passive control conditions. Further investigation into different training methods is advised, including stimulating social interaction and the use of more variable, novel, group-based yet individual-adjusted exercises.

Keywords: aging, cognitive training, executive functions, cognitive flexibility, videogames

INTRODUCTION

We live in a time of great societal changes in the Western world. Due in part to dramatic improvements in medical science, our aging population is expanding rapidly. As aging is associated with decreased cognitive functioning, the prevalence of age-related cognitive decline is an increasingly important issue. Decline of cognitive control, memory, and decision-making, among other functions, leads to greater dependence on family members and society. With recent increments of the retirement age in many countries, increasing numbers of older workers are expected to contribute to the workforce, but may cognitively fall behind. In order to ensure that older adults can live and work independently for as long as possible, research into possibilities of reducing this age-related decline of functioning is a pressing matter.

Enhancing cognitive functions or limiting their decline using cognitive training is currently a popular topic. Effectiveness of such trainings has been investigated with numerous intervention studies, for instance working memory training (Buschkuehl et al., 2008; Richmond et al., 2011; Rose et al., 2015), virtual reality training (Optale et al., 2010; Lövdén et al., 2012), and game training (Basak et al., 2008; Nouchi et al., 2012; van Muijden et al., 2012; Baniqued et al., 2013; Toril et al., 2016). Benefits of using at-home computer-based training programs are evident: they require no face-to-face contact, are easy to administer, and do not require traveling, which is especially advantageous when catering to more physically impaired individuals. Furthermore, they are cost efficient, and can be customized to a personal level in order to keep motivation optimal. In addition to the possible benefits for cognition, young and older adults also enjoy playing computer games in order to challenge themselves and for reasons of entertainment and—for certain games—social rewards (Allaire et al., 2013; Whitbourne et al., 2013). The gaming industry has conveniently caught on to this trend. As a result, countless commercial training websites and stand-alone applications offer a whole range of games that promise to contribute to cognitive reserve and slowed decline.

Research indicates, however, that not all types of games are enjoyed equally by the older population. Realistic first-person shooter games, though cognitively challenging, are perceived negatively by many older adults (Nap et al., 2009; McKay and Maki, 2010). Generally, casual games or games comprised of short mathematical- or memory activities are rated as most enjoyable and lead to higher compliance and beliefs about enhancement (Nap et al., 2009; Boot et al., 2013a).

Despite its popularity and market potential, the effectiveness of brain training remains a controversial topic. Results are inconsistent (Au et al., 2015; Dougherty et al., 2016) with some producing no transfer effects at all (Ackerman et al., 2010; Lee et al., 2012). Near transfer is often reported, especially after multitasking or task-switching designs (Karbach and Kray, 2009; Wang et al., 2011; Anguera et al., 2013) though far transfer is scarcely found (Green and Bavelier, 2008; Park and Bischof, 2013). Furthermore, a large variability in the degree of individual response to cognitive training is often observed (Langbaum et al., 2009; Melby-Lervag et al., 2016). For instance, general training benefit is often found to be dependent on higher age and lower baseline cognitive abilities, and in some cases on training gain and education (Verhaeghen et al., 1992; Bissig and Lustig, 2007; Langbaum et al., 2009; Zinke et al., 2014) although there is some evidence of increasing benefit after lower baseline scores (Ball et al., 2007; Whitlock et al., 2012).

We and others (e.g., Buitenweg et al., 2012; Slagter, 2012; van de Ven et al., 2016) raised a number of problematic issues often encountered in the training research literature. Among them were brief training periods (limited numbers of session/days/weeks), small sample sizes, absence of active control conditions, inapt competitive motivational incentives, and use of unimodal training tasks (incurring task-specific and even stimulus-specific rather than process-specific training benefits). On the basis of our review of optimal study design, training efficacy, and neurocognitive profiles of successful aging (Buitenweg et al., 2012), we suggested adding the elements of flexibility, novelty (Noice and Noice, 2008) and adaptiveness (Kelly et al., 2014) to training protocols to increase the chances of finding positive effects on cognitive functioning.

Due to the encountered issues in the literature, the current situation in the training field is inconclusive on training generalizability. We therefore created a unique, state-of-the-art, 12-week intervention study incorporating multimodal, novel, adaptive training games and frequent sessions. To induce flexibility, we transformed the idea of task switching training, which has lead to far transfer in Karbach and Kray (2009). We integrated switching between training games to create a more ecologically valid intervention, while using a number of switching tasks as our transfer measures. Besides this, we employed a number of measures with alternate (parallel) forms in order to minimize retest effects. In addition to including a number of essential elements, we are the first study adding flexibility as a key ingredient to training. We were especially interested in the question whether shifting attention between multiple functions during the training would transfer to decreasing switch costs. For this purpose, we required a task in which to present both alternating and repeating cues, which was possible using the switching paradigm previously used by Rogers and Monsell (1995). However, to evaluate effects on the entire construct of task switching, we combined additional measures in our secondary analysis. We included the clinically validated Delis-Kaplan Executive Function System—Trail Making Test and the online version of this task, in which (unlike in our main switch task) every response requires a switch, but participants still access basic knowledge of number- and letter systems. To incorporate a more ecologically valid measure of task switching, we also added the switch condition of the semantic fluency test, in which switching between activations of more covert representations is required.

We investigated whether an online training incorporating these crucial components can lead to transfer in an elderly population. Our training program consisted of two experimental conditions and an active control condition in a program called TAPASS (Training Project Amsterdam Seniors and Stroke). The TAPASS program has been used to determine the effects of cognitive flexibility training in stroke survivors by adding to the usual rehabilitation care (van de Ven et al., 2015).

Here, we focus on effectiveness of this program in the healthy aging population. Experimental groups differed in flexibility, novelty, and adaptiveness. Higher flexibility was created by having the subject switch more often in a session between cognitive domains from game to game. High novelty implied exposure to more different cognitive domains within one session. Adaptiveness refers to the extent to which game difficulty can be adapted dynamically to an individual's performance. The frequent switching (FS) group scored high on flexibility, novelty, and adaptiveness. The infrequent switching (IS) group contained high novelty and adaptiveness but low flexibility, and the mock training (MT) scored low on all three features. We investigated whether there are benefits of the experimental training on cognitive functioning, and if so, whether the switching component adds extra value to these effects. In addition, we explored the question whether training efficacy is modulated by individual characteristics, such as age, baseline functioning, or education.

As the current intervention is especially focused on inducing flexibility, we expected transfer to occur in functions of executive control (Buchler et al., 2008; Karbach and Kray, 2009; Buitenweg et al., 2012). Based on a classification model by Miyake et al. (2000) these are often separated into updating, inhibition, and shifting (dual tasking and task switching). Therefore, our main analysis was centered around measures of these constructs. For reasons of equal comparison, for the primary analysis we selected tasks that were all administered by computer at the lab.

In our secondary analysis, we included additional assessments of working memory and task switching as well as tasks from other domains. Due to their dependence on the frontal lobe, planning and verbal fluency are often counted among the executive functions as well (Fisk and Sharp, 2004; Phillips et al., 2006; Lewis and Miller, 2007) and can be subject to decline in older adults (Auriacombe et al., 2001; Sullivan et al., 2009; Kim et al., 2013). For this reason, we chose to include measures within these domains. In addition to the executive functions, processing speed often declines in later life (Salthouse, 2000), though training with a similar intervention has been seen to lead to improvements in this domain (Nouchi et al., 2012). As most of our training tasks included fast paced, timed games, we were interested to see whether the training would generalize to measures of processing speed. Additionally, as using the computer mouse was an important part in this study in completing the training tasks as well as the transfer measures, we also decided to include tasks of psychomotor speed. Finally, two more functions often found to diminish in older adults are reasoning ability and verbal long term memory (Davis et al., 2003; Harada et al., 2013), which have also seen improvements after similar interventions (Au et al., 2015; Barban et al., 2015). Measures of these constructs have been added to our battery of transfer tasks.

The purpose of this study was to test the hypothesis that a 12-week cognitive flexibility training would improve cognitive functions in healthy older adults. We expected to see the largest transfer effects on executive control performance after the frequent switch training, smaller effects after the infrequent switch training, and little to no effects after the MT. We expected differences between conditions to be smaller, yet in the same direction, on performance of other domains.

METHODS

Subjects

Our study entailed a randomized controlled double-blind design. Participants were recruited via media campaigns (pitch talks on regional radio stations and articles in local newspapers) and from a database of healthy older adults interested in participation in psychological research (www.seniorlab.nl). A total of 249 healthy participants signed up online on www.tapass.nl and were assessed for eligibility. Inclusion criteria included age above 60, willingness and cognitive ability to finish the 12-week training program, and daily access to a computer with internet connection. Exclusion criteria were a history of neuropsychiatric disorders, TIA or stroke, strongly impairing visual deficits, and colorblindness. Additionally, mental condition was estimated with the Telephone Interview Cognitive Status (TICS; Brandt et al., 1988): individuals scoring below 26 on this test were excluded. Eleven individuals did not fit the inclusion criteria and were excluded. Twenty-nine individuals withdrew before randomization, and another 51 before the first test session, due to health- and technical issues, or lack of time. The remaining 158 subjects were included in the final sample.

Subjects were randomly assigned to one of three conditions, with the exception of partners/spouses, who were always assigned to the same group. We minimized asymmetry in our three conditions using a minimization program (Minimpy; Saghaei and Saghaei, 2011) over the factors age, computer experience, TICS score, gender, and education. The minimization procedure was carried out by the principal investigators only. All subjects were given the same information regarding the intention of the experiment. They were told they would be placed in one of three different conditions, without explicit mention of a control condition. A schematic overview of the study design can be found in **Figure 1**.

Participants were compensated for travel costs and received free unlimited access to all games on www.braingymmer.com. Full written informed consent was given by all subjects prior to participation. The study was approved by the local Ethics Committee of the University of Amsterdam and registered under number 2012-BC-2566. All procedures were conducted in compliance with the Declaration of Helsinki, relevant laws, and institutional guidelines.

Study Protocol

A battery of online tests (Neurotask BV, 2012) was devised to measure effects of the training at four points in time: at baseline (T0), after 6 weeks of training (T1), after 12 weeks of training (T2), and 4 weeks post-training (T3). On T0 and T2, subjects also visited the university for a series of neuropsychological tests and computer tasks, and a small set of cognitive tests was administered via a link in the email. Additionally, subjective effects were measured using a series of questionnaires at all time points, and a subgroup of participants underwent Magnetic Resonance Imaging (MRI) scanning at T0 and T2. Results of

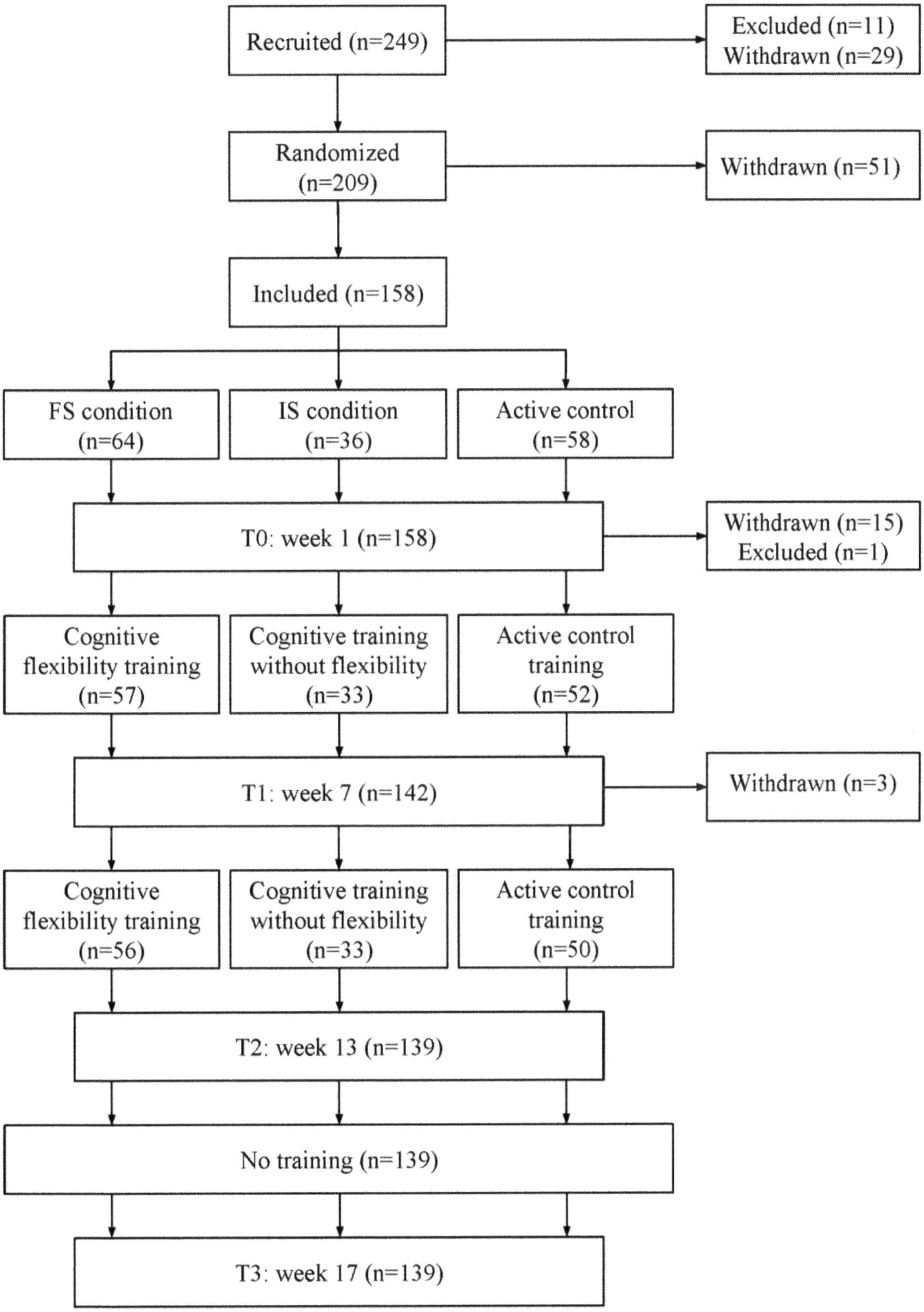

FIGURE 1 | Flow chart of the study design. FS, frequent switching; IS, infrequent switching.

these subjective and MRI measures will be reported separately. Testing on T0 and T2 was spread out over three different days, and on T1 and T3 over 2 days. Both the order of the test days for T0 and T2 and order of testing within the neuropsychological test battery were counterbalanced between subjects.

Neuropsychological assessments were conducted by a trained junior psychologist, who was blind to the training condition. As a check, neuropsychological assessors were asked to guess the condition of the subject. A separate test assessor administered four computer tasks, and introduced the training to subjects using instruction videos and a demonstration of the training platform and games. After their first visit to the university, subjects received a personalized instruction booklet with illustrations reminding them how to log on to the testing and training platforms, how to play each game, and how to report technical problems. It also gave useful information beyond the training, for example, how to download a new browser, and the importance of good posture during computer use. Subjects were assigned to a member of the research team who called them weekly to biweekly with standardized questions, would offer motivation and feedback and who could solve (technical) problems. Subjects were encouraged to email or call their contact with more urgent problems.

Subjects were requested to train five times a week for a half hour, on days and times of their choosing. Training activity was monitored. If no login was encountered for 2 days, an automatic email was sent to the subject. Subjects were encouraged to finish the training in 12 consecutive weeks. If training had to be interrupted for a period of more than 2 days, such as during a holiday, the missed trainings were added to the end of the 12 weeks.

After T3, participants filled out an exit questionnaire in which they were asked to rate the training and their own motivation. To verify blindness, we asked subjects to guess in which condition they had been included, in the case that one condition was less effective than the other. Subsequently, all subjects received login information for a lifetime account on the training website.

Intervention

All three training programs were based on the brain training website www.braingymmer.com. Games were originally programmed for the general population, but after running a pilot study, we altered the ones selected for our programs to fit the need of older participants. For example, many games commenced at too high speed and difficulty levels. This was adjusted in the research-dedicated "dashboard" version of the platform. In this platform, game presentation order was fully preprogrammed in order to prevent individuals from selecting their own tasks. Subjects had some extra time to finish after the time-period set aside for playing a certain game had been reached (e.g., 3 or 10 min) to prevent too abruptly ending a game.

All groups received the same amount and type of feedback after finishing a game or training session (see Supplementary Material 1). Additionally, all participants received standardized weekly to bi-weekly feedback and support from research team members who supervised them from baseline until 4 weeks post-training.

Cognitive Training

We designed a cognitive training based on nine games in three domains: reasoning, working memory, and attention (see Supplementary Material 2). In designing our intervention, we chose not to include training games which too closely resembled any of our transfer tasks. Each game consisted of 20 levels, increasing in difficulty. The order of games was selected in such a way that two games following one another were never from the same domain, to optimize variability and flexibility.

Subject performance was rated with up to three stars at the end of each game block. Adaptiveness was implemented by asking subjects to continue to the next difficulty level when reaching two or three stars. In case a subject reached the highest level (20), he or she was asked to improve performance on previous levels with two stars.

Within the cognitive training we created two groups: frequent switching (FS) and infrequent switching (IS). In the FS group, one training session consisted of 10 games of 3 min each, thus requiring subjects to frequently switch to a task aimed to train a different cognitive function than the one before. In the IS group, three games of 10 min each were played so that switching between game domains occurred less frequently. In the first week only, in order for subjects to become familiar with the games, both groups played the games for 10 min each. By the end of the intervention, the time spent on each game was similar across participants in the FS and IS groups.

Mock Training

For the MT, we selected games that provided equal visual stimulation and feedback and put equal demands on computer ability, but that were reduced in variability, flexibility, and adaptiveness, compared with the experimental conditions (see Supplementary Material 3). We selected four games that all put minimal demands on executive functions. Per session, subjects played three games of 10 min each, thus minimizing the need for flexibility. Unlike the FS and IS conditions, the MT was not adaptive. Although higher levels could be unlocked in the same manner, participants in the MT were instructed to remain on the same level for a week before continuing to the next level, regardless of the number of stars they received on a game.

Assessment Tasks

The effects of the flexibility training were estimated using pre- and post-measures on an extensive battery of computer tasks, neuropsychological paper-and-pen tests and computerized versions of these tests. For detailed task descriptions, see van de Ven et al. (2015).

Principal Analysis

For the principal analysis we used the executive functions as distinguished by Miyake et al. (2000): shifting (task switching and dual tasking), updating, and response inhibition. These were assessed with four computerized tasks. Task switching and dual tasking performances were measured using modified versions of a commonly used switch task (Rogers and Monsell, 1995) and dual task (Stablum et al., 2007). The two tasks were combined to save time. Switch cost was calculated as the difference between reaction time on switch trials and no-switch trials in milliseconds, with higher switch cost signifying lower cognitive flexibility (Rogers and Monsell, 1995). Dual task performance was assessed by the reaction time on speeded responses of the dual trials (Stablum et al., 2007). Updating performance was measured using the N-back task as used by de Vries and Geurts (2014) including 0-back, 1-back, and 2-back blocks. Performance on this task was calculated by the difference between the percentage correct on 2-back and percentage correct on 0-back items (Kirchner, 1958). The stop-signal task (Logan et al., 1984) was used to measure inhibition. Stop-signal reaction time (SSRT) was calculated by sorting all correct Go-trial reaction times, taking the time corresponding to the percentage of correct stop trials, and subtracting the mean stop-signal delay (SSD) from this number (Logan et al., 1984).

Secondary Analysis

Effectiveness of the training on a larger scale was assessed by using neuropsychological tests from eight cognitive domains: task switching, psychomotor speed, processing speed, planning, reasoning, working memory, long term memory, and verbal fluency. In most domains we included multiple tests. For the RAVLT, letter fluency, category fluency with- and without switch condition, and Raven Progressive Matrices, we used alternate assessment forms. Where necessary, raw scores were recoded such that higher scores always represent better performance.

In the domain of task switching, we included the Delis-Kaplan Executive Function System—Trail Making Test (D-KEFS TMT; Condition 4), the Trail Making Test-B (TMT-B), and a separate switch condition of the semantic fluency task. The D-KEFS TMT concerned the number-letter switching subtask, with the performance score calculated as the total time in seconds to complete connecting letters and numbers in alternating order (i.e., 1, A, 2, B, etc.; (Delis et al., 2001). The TMT-B pertained to the online version of this task, with performance assessed by the total time in seconds to complete connecting letters and numbers in alternating order (NeuroTask BV). The switch condition of the semantic fluency task consisted of alternating listing as many words as possible from two separate categories (male names and supermarket items, or female names and cities, counterbalanced over participants) in 1 min. Outcome measure is the number of correct words in the switch condition, subtracted from the average number of correct words produced in the same categories without switching (Troyer et al., 1997).

For psychomotor speed, we used five tasks, four of which were assessed online. In the drag-and-drop task, participants were required to use their computer mouse to drag round or square shapes into an empty border. Outcome measure is the total time in milliseconds to complete the task (Neurotask BV). In the drag-to-grid task, participants dragged 25 squares into a 5 × 5 grid using the mouse. Performance was assessed by the total time in milliseconds to complete the task (Neurotask BV). The click task required participants to click a spiral of circles of decreasing sizes using the mouse, with total time in milliseconds to complete the task signifying the outcome measure (Neurotask BV). The D-KEFS TMT (Condition 5) concerned the motor speed condition, with the performance score calculated as the total time in seconds to complete tracing a dotted line between a number of circles (Delis et al., 2001). The TMT-A pertained to the online version of this task, with performance assessed by the total time in seconds to complete connecting numbers (NeuroTask BV).

Processing speed was measured using the Digit Symbol Coding test (DSC; Wechsler, 2000) and an online version of this task (Neurotask BV). In this task, participants are required to pair a series of numbers to the correct symbol according to a given rule. Outcome measure on this task is the correct number of items completed in 2 min.

In planning, we used the Tower of London (ToL). This concerned the online version (Neurotask BV) based on the original task by Culbertson and Zillmer (2005), in which participants move colored beads from a starting position into the required position using a minimum amount of possible steps. Performance was assessed by the sum of the number of additional moves to solve the ToL, using a maximum score of 20.

In the reasoning domain, we included Raven's Progressive Matrices (Raven et al., 1998) as well as the Shipley Institute of living scale-2 (Zachary, 1991). For both reasoning tasks, the outcome measure we used was the total number correct on 20 items.

Working memory was assessed using two online tasks and three face-to-face tasks. A modified version of the Corsi block tapping task (Milner, 1971) was constructed for online assessment. Outcome measure was the longest correctly reproduced array of blocks (Neurotask BV). In the Paced Auditory Serial Addition Task (PASAT), participants needed to update the addition of numbers presented auditively. We administered two versions, in which numbers were delivered at a rate of, respectively, 3.4 and 2.8 s. As an outcome measure, we calculated the mean percentage correct of both versions (Gronwall, 1977). The Operation Span consisted of a series of letters presented sequentially that needed to be remembered while solving mathematical equations (Unsworth et al., 2005). Outcome measure for the Operation Span was the total number of correctly remembered letters. In Rey's Auditory Verbal Learning Test (RAVLT)-direct, participants were presented with a series of words auditively for five trials and recalled as many words as possible after each trial. We used the total number of words remembered after five trials as an outcome measure (Saan and Deelman, 1986). Lastly, in Letter Number Sequencing (LNS), participants were required to recall a series of numbers and letters in increasing or alphabetical order (Wechsler, 2000). For this measure, we used the total number of correct items.

In verbal long term memory, the delayed item of the RAVLT was used, in which the outcome measure was the total number of words recalled after a delay of 20 min (Saan and Deelman, 1986).

In the domain of verbal fluency, we used a semantic fluency task and a letter fluency task. In the semantic fluency task, participants produced as many words as possible in two different categories (male names and supermarket items, or female names and cities, counterbalanced over participants), each in 1 min (Thurstone, 1938). In the letter fluency task, participants produced as many words as possible starting with one of three different letters (P, G, and R on one time point, K, O, and M on the other time point, counterbalanced over participants), each in

1 min (Benton et al., 1989). For both tests, the outcome measure was the mean number of correct words.

To control for possible differences in fatigue and depression, we also examined baseline scores of the Checklist Individual Strength—Fatigue subscale (CIS-F) and the Hospital Anxiety Depression Scale—Depression subscale (HADS-D). The HADS-D (Zigmond and Snaith, 1983) measures subjective severity of depression and includes seven items on a four-point scale, with a maximum score of 21. The CIS-F (Vercoulen et al., 1997) measures subjective fatigue and the behavioral characteristics related to this concept. The scale consists of eight items, with scores ranging from 8 to 56. A score of 35 is regularly used as a cut-off to denote severe fatigue (Worm-Smeitink et al., 2017).

We designed an exit scale with four separate questions assessing perceived difficulty and enjoyment of the games, self-rated general cognitive enhancement, and whether participants would continue using the training. Although the scale is not validated, it serves as a necessary tool to judge participants' present and future view of the training. Participants rated these questions on T2 and T3, on a five-point Likert scale.

Training Performance

Training performance in all three groups was measured using a mean training z-score as well as a mean gain score between T0 and T2. Level high scores were calculated as a percentage of the maximal score on that level. Next, all were added up to a total game score for each training game. For the experimental conditions, domain scores were also made by averaging the three total scores within each domain, and a final score by averaging all three domain scores. For the MT, a final score was calculated by averaging over the four games. Subsequently, we computed a mean training score for all three training groups separately and transformed these to Z-scores to be able to compare MT and experimental training groups relative to each other. The gain score was calculated by subtracting the mean score attained after the first 10 min of playing from the mean score attained at the end of training.

Statistical Analysis

A first set of repeated-measures ANOVAs focused on the executive functions in the principal analysis, using time points T0 (baseline) and T2 (post-training). Scores on task switching and dual tasking, updating, and inhibition were used as dependent variables, with group (FS, IS or MT) as the independent variable. A second set of repeated-measures ANOVAs was carried out for the secondary measures. PASAT, ToL, TMT-A, and TMT-B were transformed due to non-normality. PASAT scores were raised to the 3rd power, a square root transformation was used on ToL data, and TMT-A and TMT-B scores were transformed using the formula $1/x^{0.14}$. When necessary, outcome measures were rescored so that a positive value indicated improvement. We computed correlations between significant transfer tasks and age, TICS score, and workouts completed to determine whether to add them as covariates to the primary and secondary ANOVAs. Education level required non-parametric correlation analysis (Spearman's Rho); all other measures used Pearson's correlation coefficient. To explore the extent to which individual characteristics influenced training benefits, significantly correlated covariates were added to a repeated-measures ANCOVA of the primary and secondary measures.

When a significant improvement was detected at T2 on one of the dependent variables also measured at T1 (after 6 weeks of training) and T3 (post-training follow up after 4 weeks), these were additionally added to the model to establish whether training effects were visible after 6 weeks of training, and whether they remained after training had ceased.

Grubbs' Extreme Studentized Deviation test was used to detect outliers (Grubbs, 1950). We ran analyses with- and without outliers. All reported results are without outliers, unless otherwise specified. IBM SPSS Statistics for Windows, version 22 (IBM Corp., Armonk, N.Y., USA) was used for all statistical analyses. Normality was checked using Shapiro-Wilk's test and by evaluating skewness and kurtosis. A *p*-value of 0.05 (two-tailed if not mentioned otherwise) was considered significant. For all analyses, Bonferroni corrections for multiple testing were used. Greenhouse-Geisser corrected degrees of freedom were used whenever sphericity was violated, though for the purpose of legibility the original degrees of freedom are reported.

RESULTS

Of the 158 subjects we tested on baseline, 1 person was excluded before starting the training due to difficulty understanding the transfer tasks, 5 experienced substantial health problems, 3 reported lack of time, 5 did not enjoy the training, and another 5 experienced technical issues. There was no difference in gender, TICS score, education level, or training group between the final sample and dropouts (all p's > 0.19) though there was a significant difference in age [sustainers $M = 67.77$, SD 5.0; dropouts $M = 72.3$, $SD = 7.8$, $t_{(20, 134)} = -2{,}454$, $p = 0.023$]. The subsequent results are based on the remaining 139 subjects (age 60–80, $M = 67.8$, 60.4% female, mean years of education 13.7).

Because participants receiving MRI scans were only assigned to either the frequent switch training or the MT, these groups contain a higher number of participants than the infrequent switch condition. Fifty-six subjects were allocated to the frequent switch training, 33 subjects to the infrequent switch training, and 50 subjects to the MT. Before training, the three training groups did not differ in gender, level of education, TICS score, age, or computer experience (all p's > 0.26), as expected after minimization (see **Table 1**). There was also no difference in fatigue or depression (all p's > 0.48). Of the 14 participants whose fatigue scores exceeded the cut-off of 35, 5 were in the frequent switch condition, 5 in the active control and 4 in the infrequent switch condition. On the exit questionnaire, an equal number of people in each group reported having started new activities or training other than ours [$\chi^2_{(2, N = 139)} = 0.561$, $p = 0.77$].

Intervention

Average number of completed training sessions was 57.1 (28.6 h) and this did not differ between training groups [$F_{(2, 135)} = 0.438$, $p = 0.65$]. All three groups improved equally on all training tasks, judging from the z-scores [$F_{(2, 135)} = 0.192$, $p = 0.826$], though in terms of total gain, the experimental conditions improved

TABLE 1 | Subject demographics.

	FS ($n = 56$)	IS ($n = 33$)	MT ($n = 50$)	p
Age	67.8 ± 5.0	67.9 ± 5.4	67.6 ± 5.1	0.97
Gender (% female)	64.3	63.6	54	0.51[a]
Level of education	5.9 ± 0.9	5.8 ± 0.7	5.9 ± 0.9	0.76
TICS score	35.6 ± 2.5	35.7 ± 2.3	35.2 ± 1.8	0.51
Prior computer use	5.6 ± 0.8	5.4 ± 1.6	5.8 ± 0.8	0.11
CIS-F	20.0 ± 11.5	21.1 ± 11.5	18.1 ± 11.80	0.48
HADS-D	2.2 ± 2.6	2.5 ± 2.6	2.1 ± 2.1	0.73

Values are Mean ± SD; p-values are based on ANOVA unless otherwise specified; Prior computer use based on seven-point scale (from 1= less than once a month to 7= more than 4 h a day); Level of education based on seven-point scale (from 1= unfinished primary school to 7= university); FS, frequent switching experimental group; IS, infrequent switching experimental group; MT, mock training group; TICS, Telephone Interview for Cognitive Status; CIS-F, Checklist Individual Strength–Fatigue subscale; HADS-D, Hospital Anxiety Depression Scale-Depression subscale.

[a]*p-value based on χ^2.*

significantly more than did the active control [$F_{(2,\,135)} = 6.698$, $p = 0.002$].

Although the active control condition was asked to maintain a single game level for a set week, we discovered that many active control participants continued playing beyond this level, thus diminishing differences in adaptiveness between our training groups. It appeared that 42% of control participants played more than 10% of their training time beyond the highest allowed level (level 9), and 26% played more than 30% of their time beyond this level. Besides this, 25 subjects (39% of IS subjects, 21% of FS subjects) scored a maximal number of points at the highest possible level on one or two of the nine games, thereby compromising adaptiveness among both experimental groups. Although many of these cases occurred only in the last few weeks of the training period, these events may have led to suboptimal differences between the MT and the experimental conditions.

Subjects were told after participation that we had made use of two conditions: one of which we expected would be less effective than the other. When asked whether they believed they had been in the more effective or less effective condition, participants were more likely to assume they had been in the experimental condition: 71% of FS and IS and 59% of MT expected they had received our more effective training. Neuropsychological assessors did not guess subjects' training group above chance level, both before training [39%; $\chi^2_{(4,\,N=105)} = 2.73$, $p = 0.60$] and after training [33%; $\chi^2_{(4,\,N=105)} = 4.07$, $p = 0.39$]. We can therefore assume that both neuropsychological assessors and participants themselves remained blind to the training conditions.

Besides this, there was no difference between the three conditions in the perceived difficulty or enjoyment of the games, self-rated cognitive enhancement, number of completed training sessions, or the degree to which they would like to continue playing the games (all p's > 0.28), showing that all interventions were enjoyed equally.

Transfer Effects

The statistics of the primary and secondary analyses reported below are detailed in **Table 2**. Main effects of Group were absent throughout and will not be discussed further. ANCOVA outcomes are reported where appropriate.

Principle Analysis: Executive Functions

On task switching, all three groups significantly improved their scores over Time, but a Time * Group interaction did not reach significance. A similar pattern was seen on the dual task, with a main effect of Time that was not modulated by Group. This time effect disappeared when correcting for the number of workouts [$F_{(1,\,128)} = 0.721, p = 0.397, \eta^2_p = 0.006$]. Time effects for N-back and Stop-signal task did not survive Bonferroni correction, and no modulation by Group was found. Equivalent results appeared when outliers were included.

Secondary Analysis

Most of the secondary measures were subject to improvement with Time, as described below, but none of these effects were modulated by Group. Performance on 2 out of 3 cognitive flexibility tasks improved over time for all three groups. Both the DKEFS TMT and the online version of the TMT-B showed decreased switching latency. No significant effects were found for performance on the switch condition of the semantic fluency task. Psychomotor speed improved on the online TMT-A and the three mouse ability tasks (Click, Drag-and-drop, and Drag-to-grid). The motor speed condition of the DKEFS TMT did not show a significant Time effect. Processing speed improved in both the original DSC as the online version of the task. A significant Time effect was found for the ToL. In the reasoning domain, a significant Time effect was observed for the SILS. The score on the RPM did not change significantly. On tasks of working memory, both PASAT and RAVLT-direct improved over Time, whereas no change appeared on the online Corsi or the Operation Span. The score on the LNS was not significant after Bonferroni correction. No Time effect was found on long term memory measured with the RAVLT-delay. Finally, both semantic and letter fluency did not improve over Time for any of the groups. With outliers included in the data, the results showed the same pattern.

All Time effects disappeared when correcting for age, baseline TICS score, number of completed training sessions, or education level, regardless of whether one or multiple covariates were used.

Follow-Up Effects

As specific training effects were lacking, T1 measurements were not examined. An explorative repeated-measures ANOVA was run for tasks which did exhibit a significant Time effect and had also been administered at T3. All of these measures improved even further on T3, revealing higher effect sizes for all tasks [Switch task: $F_{(1,\,125)} = 59.167, p < 0.001, \eta^2_p = 0.32$; ToL: $F_{(1,\,115)} = 37.237$, $p < 0.001$, $\eta^2_p = 0.25$; online DSC: $F_{(1,\,100)} = 101.421$, $p < 0.001$, $\eta^2_p = 0.50$; TMT-A: $F_{(1,\,112)} = 43.755$, $p < 0.001$, $\eta^2_p = 0.28$; TMT-B: $F_{(1,\,112)} = 53.234$, $p < 0.001$, $\eta^2_p = 0.32$; Click task: $F_{(1,\,112)} = 16.933$, $p < 0.001$, $\eta^2_p = 0.13$; Drag-and-drop: $F_{(1,\,109)} = 39.465$, $p < 0.001$, $\eta^2_p = 0.27$; Drag-to-grid: $F_{(1,\,113)} = 60.085$, $p < 0.001$, $\eta^2_p = 0.35$]. However, these Time effects did not interact with Group for any of these measures, and no

TABLE 2 | Transfer results.

Measure	Group												Comparison											
	FS ($n = 56$)				IS($n = 33$)				MT ($n = 50$)				Time				Group				Time*Group			
	Pre-training		Post-training		Pre-training		Post-training		Pre-training		Post-training		*df*	*F*	*P*	η_P^2	*df*	*F*	*P*	η_P^2	*df*	*F*	*P*	η_P^2
	M	*s.d.*	*M*	*s.d.*	*M*	*s.d.*	*M*	*s.d.*	*M*	*s.d.*	*M*	*s.d.*												
PRINCIPAL																								
Switch task	−348	175	−276	155	−368	266	−298	143	−367	225	−321	172	1;130	16.13	**<0.001**	0.11	2;130	0.238	0.79	0.004	2;130	0.535	0.59	0.01
Dual task	−1,215	274	−1,122	264	−1,241	302	−1,141	223	−1,290	300	−1,210	328	1;130	40.96	**<0.001**	0.24	2;130	0.702	0.5	0.01	2;130	0.078	0.93	0.001
SSRT	−258	48	−243	61	−269	56	−251	63	−265	61	−259	59	1;120	4.277	0.04	0.03	2;120	0.782	0.46	0.01	2;120	0.304	0.74	0.01
N-back	−10.2	7.4	−8.3	4.9	−9.2	4.5	−8.3	8.0	−11.4	7.8	−9.1	6.2	1;125	4.955	0.03	0.04	2;125	0.865	0.42	0.01	2;125	0.218	0.8	0.003
SECONDARY																								
D-KEFS TMT-4	−86.0	27.8	−80.7	31.0	−87.1	30.1	−71.1	22.1	−88	34	−77.8	31.7	1;133	16.796	**<0.001**	0.11	2;133	0.299	0.74	0.004	2;133	1.387	0.25	0.02
TMT-B	−71.7	29.3	−61.8	20.0	−72.6	31.7	−64.1	20.4	−71.3	21.0	−63.4	17.1	1;120	31.211	**<0.001**	0.21	2;120	0.312	0.73	0.01	2;120	0.519	0.6	0.01
Sem. fluency switch	−3.2	4.1	−3.6	4.2	−2.9	3.5	−5.3	4.5	−4.8	5.2	−4.8	4.1	1;129	3.653	0.06	0.03	2;129	2.362	0.1	0.04	2;129	1.66	0.19	0.03
Drag-and-drop	−37.3	9.7	−34.8	9.2	−39.2	8.5	−33.7	6.3	−42.6	17.1	−36.1	7.9	1;119	17.399	**<0.001**	0.13	2;119	1.877	0.16	0.03	2;119	1.289	0.28	0.02
Drag-to-grid	−62.8	13.5	−57.8	11.8	−66.4	13.1	−59.3	9.1	−65.3	12.2	−58.6	10.6	1;120	58.206	**<0.001**	0.33	2;120	0.535	0.59	0.01	2;120	0.706	0.5	0.01
Click task	−30.7	12.6	−27.3	8.2	−29.9	13.5	−26.0	6.0	−30.0	12.8	−25.2	7.1	1;118	12.549	**0.001**	0.1	2;118	0.333	0.72	0.01	2;118	0.159	0.85	0.003
TMT-A	40.6	11.3	37.4	7.0	42.9	10.4	36.7	8.6	43.9	15.2	37.4	7.7	1;119	27.518	**<0.001**	0.19	2;119	0.713	0.49	0.01	2;119	2.137	0.12	0.04
D-KEFS TMT-5	−28.1	9.6	−27.3	10.3	−26.2	7.9	−25.8	9.8	−27.8	9.5	−26.8	8.5	1;136	2.135	0.15	0.02	2;136	0.405	0.67	0.01	2;136	0.093	0.91	0.00
DSC	66.4	12.8	69.6	14.0	66.4	13.6	68.5	12.5	65.8	13.0	68.6	13.8	1;136	20.666	**<0.001**	0.13	2;136	0.054	0.95	0.001	2;136	0.255	0.78	0.00
DSC online	37.9	5.3	40.0	6.3	37.5	4.7	40.0	4.5	37.2	4.9	39.9	4.9	1;108	66.755	**<0.001**	0.38	2;108	0.082	0.92	0.002	2;108	0.498	0.61	0.01
ToL	33.5	23.3	27.1	17.9	33.4	21.4	22.4	15.9	37.0	24.4	22.3	19.1	1;123	24.059	**<0.001**	0.16	2;123	0.302	0.74	0.01	2;123	1.392	0.25	0.02
RPM	18.3	1.6	17.8	1.8	18.2	1.7	18.8	1.4	18.2	1.5	18.3	1.5	1;129	0.05	0.82	0	2;129	0.929	0.4	0.01	2;129	3.378	0.04	0.05
Shipley	15.3	2.8	15.9	3.0	15.8	2.7	17.1	2.5	15.8	2.7	16.5	2.7	1;130	23.496	**<0.001**	0.15	2;130	1.193	0.31	0.02	2;130	1.001	0.37	0.02
Corsi online	5.8	1.2	5.9	0.9	5.9	1.5	5.9	1.2	5.6	1.2	5.9	1.0	1;122	0.573	0.45	0.01	2;122	0.290	0.75	0.01	2;122	0.297	0.74	0.01
PASAT	96.7	16.5	103.5	16.2	96.6	14.6	103.6	11.2	93.8	16.5	101.2	13.5	1;133	67.008	**<0.001**	0.34	2;133	0.683	0.51	0.01	2;133	0.13	0.88	0.00
OSPAN	52.5	13.8	54.3	13.1	51.9	12.2	54.3	15.9	53.4	10.8	56.9	10.6	1;89	3.69	0.06	0.04	2;89	0.324	0.72	0.01	2;89	0.188	0.83	0.00
LNS	10.3	2.2	10.4	2.5	9.9	2.4	10.5	2.6	10.2	2.4	10.6	2.4	1;136	4.663	0.03	0.03	2;136	0.081	0.92	0.001	2;136	0.478	0.62	0.01
RAVLT	47.6	9.5	49.2	10.2	45.5	9.1	48.1	9.8	46.1	9.4	48.1	8.8	1;131	11.854	**<0.001**	0.08	2;131	0.435	0.65	0.01	2;131	0.219	0.8	0.00
RAVLT delay	10.6	3.1	11.1	3.0	9.3	2.9	10.0	3.2	10.4	2.8	10.6	2.8	1;131	5.744	0.02	0.04	2;131	1.853	0.16	0.03	2;131	0.599	0.55	0.01
Sem. fluency	23.4	4.8	23.4	5.7	22.6	4.6	24.1	5.3	23.8	5.1	23.2	5.2	1;129	0.487	0.49	0	2;129	0.014	0.99	0.001	2;129	2.146	0.12	0.03
Letter fluency	47.4	13.1	47.8	13.1	43.8	12.2	43.9	11.4	44.4	10.9	44.6	10.9	1;130	0.13	0.72	0	2;130	1.408	0.25	0.02	2;130	0.011	0.99	0.00

p-values are based on repeated-measures ANOVA; Bonferroni-corrected significant values in bold; η_p^2 = partial eta squared (effect size); FS, frequent switching experimental group ; IS, infrequent switching experimental group; MT, mock training; SSRT, stop-signal reaction time; D-KEFS, Delis-Kaplan Executive Function System; TMT, Trail Making Test; sem, semantic; DSC, Digit Symbol Coding; ToL, Tower of London; RPM, Raven's Progressive Matrices; PASAT, Paced Auditory Serial Addition Test; LNS, Letter Number Sequencing; RAVLT, Rey Auditory Verbal Learning Test. TM T A and B, DKEFS 4 and 5, Drag-and-drop , Drag-to-grid and Click task in sec.; switchtask, dual task, SSRT in msec.; N-back in % correct.

Time effects remained when correcting for age, education level, baseline TICS score, and number of completed training sessions, regardless of whether one or multiple covariates were used.

Extra Analyses

We added an extra analysis, examining a possible interaction between Time, Group, and switch task trial type (switch- and non-switch trials). This three-way interaction was not significant [$F_{(6, 360)} = 0.233, p = 0.943, \eta_p^2 = 0.004$].

To examine whether there was a significant difference in training benefit of Group after adjusting for baseline performance, we ran a separate number of ANCOVA's using difference scores on all measures, including baseline scores as a covariate. There was a difference in score on the Raven's Progressive Matrices [$F_{(2,128)} = 4.111, p < 0.019, \eta_p^2 = 0.060$] between the frequent- and infrequent switch conditions, when adjusting for baseline RPM score. However, this value did not survive Bonferroni correction.

DISCUSSION

We investigated the possibility to train cognitive functioning in older adults using a computerized cognitive training. For this purpose, we designed an intervention with multimodal, novel, adaptive training tasks, a built-in element of flexibility, and frequent training sessions to optimize transfer, and selected a number of transfer tests with parallel forms to minimize retest effects. Based on previous literature (Mahncke et al., 2006; Karbach and Kray, 2009; Düzel et al., 2010) we expected far transfer to several executive functions. Improvement over time was found on training tasks as well as on multiple transfer tasks covering all domains. Our primary analyses showed that older adults benefited from training across the main domains of executive function (updating, shifting, inhibition; Miyake et al., 2000). Our secondary analyses partially confirmed these findings: improvements were seen in planning, reasoning, two out of three cognitive flexibility tests, two out of five working memory tests, and two out of three psychomotor speed tests; while no improvement was observed for IQ, long-term memory, and fluency. Improvements were further amplified 4 weeks after training completion.

Most importantly, however, the experimental training that capitalized on flexibility, novelty, and adaptiveness as central features did not lead to more progress than the trainings without these elements. This suggests that there was no additional advantage of these key ingredients in training tasks, and that improvements were induced mainly by other causes.

On outcome measures where a covariate was included, all time effects disappeared. Although covariates were added only if a significant correlation with a measure occurred, on plotting the covariate data it appeared that different values of each covariate affected the various measures differently. This suggests that the covariation effects were not systematic across covariates, and therefore did not add to the model to explain training effects.

Our study had a number of limitations, some of which it shares with similar studies in the literature.

Generic Factors: Motivation, Expectation, and Placebo Effects

The effects on training benefits from training-non-specific factors such as attention, motivation, expectancy, and placebo may have played a larger role than anticipated. Long-term intensive training interventions are accompanied by degrees of personal attention as well as motivation that in themselves may suffice to enhance cognitive performance. Moreover, such programs may induce an expectancy to improve, which has proven to generate powerful placebo effects across a wide range of domains and paradigms (Boot et al., 2013b; Dougherty et al., 2016; Foroughi et al., 2016).

Thus, one explanation also for the present set of findings is that of a placebo or subject-expectancy effect. In the information booklet that aspirant participants received at the beginning of the study, we informed them about our intention to investigate whether benefit from training was a possibility, and stated our hope to find positive effects on cognitive functioning. Although it also explained that we were not sure whether this would be the case, we might have inadvertently given subjects the notion that we expected benefit, thus leading them to put extra effort in post-training performance. The finding that a majority of our participants had assumed to be in the experimental condition, may support this notion. A similar pattern has been observed in Foroughi et al. (2016), in which subjects who had responded to a suggestive flyer displayed more improvement on cognitive functions, compared to a control group responding to a non-suggestive flyer. Elsewhere, we will report on how participants perceived their progress subjectively. If a subject-expectancy or placebo effect has indeed influenced the current results, these improvements might appear in their subjective reports, shedding more light on the question of overall time-based improvement.

A similar, but slightly different interpretation is that of the Hawthorne effect (Green and Bavelier, 2008), referring to subjects' tendency to perform better on tasks when they are working toward a common goal or when a need for attention is satisfied by participating in research. In our case, as all three conditions received a certain amount of social stimulation, this might have led to increased motivation to perform well on the post-training measurements.

Potential Limitations: Challenge Levels, Group Composition, and Social Cohesion

Based on previous studies using computerized training (Basak et al., 2008; van Muijden et al., 2012; Ballesteros et al., 2014; Kühn et al., 2014), we assumed that using the current set of nine games—with 20 levels each—would provide ample variation and challenge for 12 weeks. Nonetheless, some evidence suggests this challenge was not always met in our experiment. First, a considerable number of participants found themselves reaching the maximum score for at least one of the games within a number of weeks before the end of the training, diminishing adaptiveness in these groups. In addition, on the exit questionnaire, some participants in the frequent switch training commented that the training was too simple or repetitive, or specifically criticized adaptiveness, reflecting that learning in the first half of levels was too gradual and in the second half too steep; we did not answer to all personal needs for challenge. An improvement for future studies is to implement more variable and novel activities tailored to individual demands to further optimize performance increases. Yet, by and large, most participants experienced the tasks as aptly challenging, with the levels of variability and adaptiveness contributing to that experience.

Training in our active control group, on the other hand, might have been too challenging. We had meant to generate novelty only in the frequent- and in FS conditions, and assumed that by selecting only four, less multimodal, games in the active control condition, novelty would be minimal. However, for many participants (across groups) playing games seemed in itself to be a sufficiently novel activity to incur small cognitive effects. Many participants had not previously used a mouse in the relatively fast manner that was necessary in our games and computer tasks. The strong transfer effects to mouse ability tasks in all three groups supports this assumption. Another point to consider is that the limitation on adaptiveness in the control condition was compromised by the fact that many participants continued past the maximally allowed weekly game level, causing the control condition to be more challenging than intended. Thus, our control condition may have unintentionally targeted similar functions as in the experimental conditions. This is especially evident when comparing our design to those of other studies. Overall, many training studies that find more evident transfer than the current study have employed active control conditions that appear distinctly less active than the experimental conditions, spending fewer hours on assigned tasks and having markedly less interaction with the researchers. Some only use a passive control condition, or none at all. Our results stress the value of including an active control condition that receives equal attention and training time, yet creates no overlap in the engagement of functions.

Furthermore, for many of our subjects, participating in the training involved more than just playing the games and may have included aspects such as following a link in an email to get to the online test batteries, downloading a new browser, (later) starting up the correct browser, and navigating to the right page. Although all of our subjects used their computer regularly and knew about basic internet use, such actions beyond the training itself often exceeded those of their usual activities and, thus, may have constituted a type of unintended cognitive training.

However, results from our stroke sample, described elsewhere (van de Ven et al., 2017), suggest that this has had only a minor effect. In this sample, we investigated effects of the TAPASS training in recovering stroke patients, including a no-contact waiting list condition. This group showed equal improvements to the experimental intervention and active control, including mouse ability tasks. This suggests that playing games or increased use of a mouse could not have been the main factor behind the transfer effects that we found. Instead, the improvements in this study, appearing in all three training groups, are more likely to have been caused by retest effects. Almost all tests with parallel forms did not reach significance in any of the groups. Also, there was no indication that improvement was limited to specific cognitive processes, as transfer effects were not exclusive to specific domains. Testing frequency thus seems to be the most important factor underlying these time effects. Although we included parallel tests where available, future studies might benefit from using parallel tests only, to minimize these retest-effects. Furthermore, using the statistical analysis used at present, we have not fully been able to uncover further knowledge of the individual differences in training benefit. More thorough analyses are necessary to provide additional insight into the individual learning processes and contribute to future interventions.

Our design largely lacked social interaction with other participants, which might have provided additional stimulation (Ybarra et al., 2008; Charles and Carstensen, 2010). Also, although the focus for this project was on the effectiveness of the popular home-based training tasks, some recent evidence reveals that for non-impaired older adults, individual at-home training might not be as effective as group training (Kelly et al., 2014; Lampit et al., 2014) or training sessions provided in the lab (Basak et al., 2008; Lövdén et al., 2012; Ballesteros et al., 2014). Among reasons given are optimization of adherence and compliance, as well as providing motivation to master more difficult training tasks. Possibly, participants in these studies may have benefited more from the training due to this procedure, producing more conspicuous results than the home-based training method presented here. Yet, as we contacted participants frequently with motivational telephone calls, it is unclear whether increased transfer in the experimental conditions would have occurred, if subjects had received face-to-face support from a trainer instead.

In our current study, we used a set of commercially available games targeted at the general population to train their cognitive functions. Naturally, commercial- and scientific games are created with different intentions in mind, yet in this case, we expect this to be less of a concern, as we took care to adapt each game, as well as the design of the intervention, to fit our scientific objectives, with the additional benefit of generalizing more to other functions than the frequently used commercial games.

A potential methodological limitation of this study was the homogeneity of our elderly sample, with a high educational level and relatively few cognitive complaints. This is characteristic of participants interested in volunteering in research experiments, increased further by the inevitable self-selection due to our inclusion criteria, such as the requirement to own a modern computer and to be willing to spend 12 weeks on our training. This raises the question to what degree cognitive improvement could have been attained in a sample with ample daily cognitive stimulation and minimal need to improve functions. A sample of older, less fit individuals might be more representative in displaying the benefit for the population. However, logistically it is difficult to encourage lower-educated, more cognitively impaired individuals to participate in research, let alone spend a sufficient amount of time on such an intervention. Despite subjects' demographic homogeneity, we noticed a large test score variability within groups, overshadowing any differences between them.

CONCLUSION

Our cognitive flexibility training, using elements based on previously effective cognitive interventions, did not produce the expected near- and far transfer. Although training benefits were observed almost across the board, equal effects appeared in the active control group. Taken at face value, our results with commercially available training games suggest that this type of training may yield cognitive benefits among older adults. In our experimental design, however, we could not disentangle training effects from those attributable to test practice, expectancy, and motivation. Our parallel study with recovering stroke patients (van de Ven et al., 2017), which included a wait list condition, suggests that such factors may well have overshadowed the beneficial effect of the training itself and that training effects on cognition could be rather small. Additional investigation into different training methods is advised, including stimulation of social interaction and the use of more variable, novel, group-based yet individual-adjusted activities. Our results further emphasize the importance of using parallel forms as outcome measures for transfer and including both passive and active control conditions.

As a future direction, we may observe that a thus far underexplored territory pertains to individual differences in "trainability" or the susceptibility to benefits from particular aspects of a training. For instance, it may prove fruitful to explore which cognitive or neural connectivity profiles are predictive of who will improve in what domain. If brain training is to be successful in a meaningful way, we first have to learn more about which determinants are key in tailor-made interventions to maximize far transfer.

ETHICS STATEMENT

This study was carried out in accordance with the recommendations of the guidelines formulated by the Ethics Review Board of the Faculty of Social and Behavioral Sciences, University of Amsterdam, The Netherlands, with written informed consent from all subjects. All subjects gave written informed consent in accordance with the Declaration of Helsinki. The protocol was approved by the aforementioned Ethics Review Board of the University of Amsterdam.

AUTHOR CONTRIBUTIONS

JB and RvdV contributed to conception and design of the study and were responsible for data collection. JB and SP analyzed the data. JB interpreted the data and wrote the manuscript. JB, RvdV, SP, JM, and KR critically revised the article and approved this version to be published.

FUNDING

This project is part of the research program "Evidence-based adaptive brain training in seniors: Effects of brain structure and dopaminergic system on individual differences in trainability" funded by the Netherlands Initiative Brain and Cognition (NIHC), a part of the Netherlands Organization for Scientific Research (NWO) under grant number 056-12-010. This quick-results project is embedded in the pillar "Healthy cognitive aging."

ACKNOWLEDGMENTS

The authors would like to thank all participants and their relatives for participating in the study; all students for assisting in recruitment, testing and coaching of participants, and Dezzel media for making Braingymmer available for our study.

REFERENCES

Ackerman, P. L., Kanfer, R., and Calderwood, C. (2010). Use it or lose it? Wii brain exercise practice and reading for domain knowledge. *Psychol. Aging* 25, 753. doi: 10.1037/a0019277

Allaire, J. C., McLaughlin, A. C., Trujillo, A., Whitlock, L. A., LaPorte, L., and Gandy, M. (2013). Successful aging through digital games: socioemotional differences between older adult gamers and non-gamers. *Comput. Hum. Behav.* 29, 1302–1306. doi: 10.1016/j.chb.2013.01.014

Anguera, J. A., Boccanfuso, J., Rintoul, J. L., Al-Hashimi, O., Faraji, F., Janowich, J., et al. (2013). Video game training enhances cognitive control in older adults. *Nature* 501, 97–101. doi: 10.1038/nature12486

Au, J., Sheehan, E., Tsai, N., Duncan, G. J., Buschkuehl, M., and Jaeggi, S. M. (2015). Improving fluid intelligence with training on working memory: a meta-analysis. *Psychon. Bull. Rev.* 22, 366–377. doi: 10.3758/s13423-014-0699-x

Auriacombe, S., Fabrigoule, C., Lafont, S., Jacqmin-Gadda, H., and Dartigues, J. (2001). Letter and category fluency in normal elderly participants: a population-based study. *Aging Neuropsychol. Cogn.* 8, 98–108. doi: 10.1076/anec.8.2.98.841

Ball, K., Edwards, J. D., and Ross, L. A. (2007). The impact of speed of processing training on cognitive and everyday functions. *J. Gerontol. Ser. B* 62, 19–31. doi: 10.1093/geronb/62.special_issue_1.19

Ballesteros, S., Prieto, A., Mayas, J., Toril, P., Pita, C., Ponce de León, L., et al. (2014). Brain training with non-action video games enhances aspects of cognition in older adults: a randomized controlled trial. *Front. Aging Neurosci.* 6:277. doi: 10.3389/fnagi.2014.00277

Baniqued, P. L., Lee, H., Voss, M. W., Basak, C., Cosman, J. D., Desouza, S., et al. (2013). Selling points: What cognitive abilities are tapped by casual video games? *Acta Psychol.* 142, 74–86. doi: 10.1016/j.actpsy.2012.11.009

Barban, F., Annicchiarico, R., Pantelopoulos, S., Federici, A., Perri, R., Fadda, L., et al. (2015). Protecting cognition from aging and Alzheimer's disease: a computerized cognitive training combined with reminiscence therapy. *Int. J. Geriatric Psychiatry* 31, 340–348. doi: 10.1002/gps.4328

Basak, C., Boot, W. R., Voss, M. W., and Kramer, A. F. (2008). Can training in a real-time strategy video game attenuate cognitive decline in older adults? *Psychol. Aging* 23, 765. doi: 10.1037/a0013494

Benton, A., Hamsher, K. D., and Sivan, A. (1989). *Multilingual Aphasia Examination*. Iowa, IA: AJA Associates.

Bissig, D., and Lustig, C. (2007). Who benefits from memory training? *Psychol. Sci.* 18, 720–726. doi: 10.1111/j.1467-9280.2007.01966.x

Boot, W. R., Champion, M., Blakely, D. P., Wright, T., Souders, D. J., and Charness, N. (2013a). Video games as a means to reduce age-related cognitive decline: attitudes, compliance, and effectiveness. *Front. Psychol.* 4:31. doi: 10.3389/fpsyg.2013.00031

Boot, W. R., Simons, D. J., Stothart, C., and Stutts, C. (2013b). The pervasive problem with placebos in psychology: why active control groups are not sufficient to rule out placebo effects. *Perspect. Psychol. Sci.* 8, 445–454. doi: 10.1177/1745691613491271

Brandt, J., Spencer, M., and Folstein, M. (1988). The telephone interview for cognitive status. *Cogn. Behav. Neurol.* 1, 111–118.

Buchler, N. G., Hoyer, W. J., and Cerella, J. (2008). Rules and more rules: The effects of multiple tasks, extensive training, and aging on task-switching performance. *Mem. Cogn.* 36, 735–748. doi: 10.3758/MC.36.4.735

Buitenweg, J. I., Murre, J. M., and Ridderinkhof, K. R. (2012). Brain training in progress: a review of trainability in healthy seniors. *Front. Hum. Neurosci.* 6:183. doi: 10.3389/fnhum.2012.00183

Buschkuehl, M., Jaeggi, S. M., Hutchison, S., Perrig-Chiello, P., Däpp, C., Müller, M., et al. (2008). Impact of working memory training on memory performance in old-old adults. *Psychol. Aging* 23, 743. doi: 10.1037/a0014342

Charles, S. T., and Carstensen, L. L. (2010). Social and emotional aging. *Ann. Rev. Psychol.* 61, 383–409. doi: 10.1146/annurev.psych.093008.100448

Culbertson, W., and Zillmer, E. (2005). *Tower of London Drexel University: Technical Manual.* Toronto, ON: Multi-Health Systems.

Davis, H. P., Small, S. A., Stern, Y., Mayeux, R., Feldstein, S. N., and Keller, F. R. (2003). Acquisition, recall, and forgetting of verbal information in long-term memory by young, middle-aged, and elderly individuals. *Cortex* 39, 1063–1091. doi: 10.1016/S0010-9452(08)70878-5

de Vries, M., and Geurts, H. M. (2014). Beyond individual differences: are working memory and inhibition informative specifiers within ASD? *J. Neural Trans.* 121, 1183–1198. doi: 10.1007/s00702-014-1225-z

Delis, D. C., Kaplan, E., and Kramer, J. (2001). *Delis-Kaplan Executive Function System.* San Antonio, TX: Psychological Corporation.

Dougherty, M. R., Hamovitz, T., and Tidwell, J. W. (2016). Reevaluating the effectiveness of n-back training on transfer through the bayesian lens: support for the null. *Psychon. Bull. Rev.* 23, 306–316. doi: 10.3758/s13423-015-0865-9

Düzel, E., Bunzeck, N., Guitart-Masip, M., and Düzel, S. (2010). NOvelty-related motivation of anticipation and exploration by dopamine (NOMAD): implications for healthy aging. *Neurosci. Biobehav. Rev.* 34, 660–669. doi: 10.1016/j.neubiorev.2009.08.006

Fisk, J. E., and Sharp, C. A. (2004). Age-related impairment in executive functioning: updating, inhibition, shifting, and access. *J. Clin. Exp. Neuropsychol.* 26, 874–890. doi: 10.1080/13803390490510680

Foroughi, C. K., Monfort, S. S., Paczynski, M., McKnight, P. E., and Greenwood, P. M. (2016). Placebo effects in cognitive training. *Proc. Natl. Acad. Sci. U.S.A.* 113, 7470–7474. doi: 10.1073/pnas.1601243113

Green, C. S., and Bavelier, D. (2008). Exercising your brain: a review of human brain plasticity and training-induced learning. *Psychol. Aging* 23, 692. doi: 10.1037/a0014345

Gronwall, D. M. (1977). Paced auditory serial-addition task: a measure of recovery from concussion. *Percept. Mot. Skills* 44, 367–373. doi: 10.2466/pms.1977.44.2.367

Grubbs, F. E. (1950). Sample criteria for testing outlying observations. *Ann. Mathemat. Stat.* 21, 27–58. doi: 10.1214/aoms/1177729885

Harada, C. N., Love, M. C. N., and Triebel, K. L. (2013). Normal cognitive aging. *Clin. Geriatr. Med.* 29, 737–752. doi: 10.1016/j.cger.2013.07.002

Karbach, J., and Kray, J. (2009). How useful is executive control training? Age differences in near and far transfer of task-switching training. *Dev. Sci.* 12, 978–990. doi: 10.1111/j.1467-7687.2009.00846.x

Kelly, M. E., Loughrey, D., Lawlor, B. A., Robertson, I. H., Walsh, C., and Brennan, S. (2014). The impact of cognitive training and mental stimulation on cognitive and everyday functioning of healthy older adults: a systematic review and meta-analysis. *Ageing Res. Rev.* 15, 28–43. doi: 10.1016/j.arr.2014.02.004

Kim, B. J., Lee, C. S., Oh, B. H., Hong, C. H., Lee, K. S., Son, S. J., et al. (2013). A normative study of lexical verbal fluency in an educationally-diverse elderly population. *Psychiatry Investigat.* 10, 346–351. doi: 10.4306/pi.2013.10.4.346

Kirchner, W. K. (1958). Age differences in short-term retention of rapidly changing information. *J. Exp. Psychol.* 55, 352. doi: 10.1037/h0043688

Kühn, S., Gleich, T., Lorenz, R. C., Lindenberger, U., and Gallinat, J. (2014). Playing super mario induces structural brain plasticity: gray matter changes resulting from training with a commercial video game. *Mol. Psychiatry* 19, 265–271. doi: 10.1038/mp.2013.120

Lampit, A., Hallock, H., and Valenzuela, M. (2014). Computerized cognitive training in cognitively healthy older adults: a systematic review and meta-analysis of effect modifiers. *PLoS Med.* 11:e1001756. doi: 10.1371/journal.pmed.1001756

Langbaum, J. B., Rebok, G. W., Bandeen-Roche, K., and Carlson, M. C. (2009). Predicting memory training response patterns: results from ACTIVE. *J. Gerontol. Ser. B* 64, 14–23. doi: 10.1093/geronb/gbn026

Lee, H., Boot, W. R., Basak, C., Voss, M. W., Prakash, R. S., Neider, M., et al. (2012). Performance gains from directed training do not transfer to untrained tasks. *Acta Psychol.* 139, 146–158. doi: 10.1016/j.actpsy.2011.11.003

Lewis, M. S., and Miller, L. S. (2007). Executive control functioning and functional ability in older adults. *Clin. Neuropsychol.* 21, 274–285. doi: 10.1080/13854040500519752

Logan, G. D., Cowan, W. B., and Davis, K. A. (1984). On the ability to inhibit simple and choice reaction time responses: a model and a method. *J. Exp. Psychol.* 10:276.

Lövdén, M., Schaefer, S., Noack, H., Bodammer, N. C., Kühn, S., Heinze, H., et al. (2012). Spatial navigation training protects the hippocampus against age-related changes during early and late adulthood. *Neurobiol. Aging* 33:e22. doi: 10.1016/j.neurobiolaging.2011.02.013

Mahncke, H. W., Connor, B. B., Appelman, J., Ahsanuddin, O. N., Hardy, J. L., Wood, R. A., et al. (2006). Memory enhancement in healthy older adults using a brain plasticity-based training program: a randomized, controlled study. *Proc. Natl. Acad. Sci. U.S.A.* 103, 12523–12528. doi: 10.1073/pnas.0605194103

McKay, S. M., and Maki, B. E. (2010). Attitudes of older adults toward shooter video games: an initial study to select an acceptable game for training visual processing. *Gerontechnology* 9, 5–17. doi: 10.4017/gt.2010.09.01.001.00

Melby-Lervag, M., Redick, T. S., and Hulme, C. (2016). Working memory training does not improve performance on measures of intelligence or other measures of far transfer: evidence from a meta-analytic review. *Perspect. Psychol. Sci.* 11, 512–534. doi: 10.1177/1745691616635612

Milner, B. (1971). Interhemispheric differences in the localization of psychological processes in man. *Br. Med. Bull.* 27, 272–277. doi: 10.1093/oxfordjournals.bmb.a070866

Miyake, A., Friedman, N. P., Emerson, M. J., Witzki, A. H., Howerter, A., and Wager, T. D. (2000). The unity and diversity of executive functions and their contributions to complex frontal lobe tasks: a latent variable analysis. *Cogn. Psychol.* 41, 49–100. doi: 10.1006/cogp.1999.0734

Nap, H., De Kort, Y., and IJsselsteijn, W. (2009). Senior gamers: preferences, motivations and needs. *Gerontechnology* 8, 247–262. doi: 10.4017/gt.2009.08.04.003.00

Noice, H., and Noice, T. (2008). An arts intervention for older adults living in subsidized retirement homes. *Aging Neuropsychol. Cogn.* 16, 56–79. doi: 10.1080/13825580802233400

Nouchi, R., Taki, Y., Takeuchi, H., Hashizume, H., Akitsuki, Y., Shigemune, Y., et al. (2012). Brain training game improves executive functions and processing speed in the elderly: a randomized controlled trial. *PLoS ONE* 7:e29676. doi: 10.1371/journal.pone.0029676

Optale, G., Urgesi, C., Busato, V., Marin, S., Piron, L., Priftis, K., et al. (2010). Controlling memory impairment in elderly adults using virtual reality memory training: a randomized controlled pilot study. *Neurorehabil. Neural Repair* 24, 348–357. doi: 10.1177/1545968309353328

Park, D. C., and Bischof, G. N. (2013). The aging mind: neuroplasticity in response to cognitive training. *Dialog. Clin. Neurosci.* 15, 109–119.

Phillips, L. H., Kliegel, M., and Martin, M. (2006). Age and planning tasks: the influence of ecological validity. *Internat. J. Aging Hum. Devel.* 62, 175–184. doi: 10.2190/EM1W-HAYC-TMLM-WW8X

Raven, J., Raven, J. C., and Court, J. H. (1998). *Manual for Raven's Progressive Matrices and Vocabulary Scales—Section 3: Standard Progressive Matrices.* Oxford: Oxford Psychologists Press.

Richmond, L. L., Morrison, A. B., Chein, J. M., and Olson, I. R. (2011). Working memory training and transfer in older adults. *Psychol. Aging* 26, 813. doi: 10.1037/a0023631

Rogers, R. D., and Monsell, S. (1995). Costs of a predictible switch between simple cognitive tasks. *J. Exp. Psychol.* 124, 207.

Rose, N. S., Rendell, P. G., Hering, A., Kliegel, M., Bidelman, G. M., and Craik, F. I. (2015). Cognitive and neural plasticity in older adults' prospective memory following training with the virtual week computer game. *Front. Hum. Neurosci.* 9:592. doi: 10.3389/fnhum.2015.00592

Saan, R., and Deelman, B. (1986). *De 15-Woordentest a en b Een Voorlopige Handleiding*. Groningen: Afdeling Neuropsychologie.

Saghaei, M., and Saghaei, S. (2011). Implementation of an open-source customizable minimization program for allocation of patients to parallel groups in clinical trials. *J. Biomed. Sci. Eng.* 4, 734. doi: 10.4236/jbise.2011.411090

Salthouse, T. A. (2000). Aging and measures of processing speed. *Biol. Psychol.* 54, 35–54. doi: 10.1016/S0301-0511(00)00052-1

Slagter, H. A. (2012). Conventional working memory training may not improve intelligence. *Trends Cogn. Sci.* 16, 582–583. doi: 10.1016/j.tics.2012.10.001

Stablum, F., Umiltà, C., Mazzoldi, M., Pastore, N., and Magon, S. (2007). Rehabilitation of endogenous task shift processes in closed head injury patients. *Neuropsychol. Rehabil.* 17, 1–33. doi: 10.1080/13506280500411111

Sullivan, J. R., Riccio, C. A., and Castillo, C. L. (2009). Concurrent validity of the tower tasks as measures of executive function in adults: a meta-analysis. *Appl. Neuropsychol.* 16, 62–75. doi: 10.1080/09084280802644243

Thurstone, L. L. (1938). *Primary Mental Abilities*. Chicago, IL: University of Chicago Press.

Toril, P., Reales, J. M., Mayas, J., and Ballesteros, S. (2016). Video game training enhances visuospatial working memory and episodic memory in older adults. *Front. Hum. Neurosci.* 10:206. doi: 10.3389/fnhum.2016.00206

Troyer, A. K., Moscovitch, M., and Winocur, G. (1997). Clustering and switching as two components of verbal fluency: evidence from younger and older healthy adults. *Neuropsychology* 11:138. doi: 10.1037/0894-4105.11.1.138

Unsworth, N., Heitz, R. P., Schrock, J. C., and Engle, R. W. (2005). An automated version of the operation span task. *Behav. Res. Methods* 37, 498–505. doi: 10.3758/BF03192720

van de Ven, R. M., Buitenweg, J. I., Schmand, B., Veltman, D. J., Aaronson, J. A., Nijboer, T. C., et al. (2017). Brain training improves recovery after stroke but waiting list improves equally: a multicenter randomized controlled trial of a computer-based cognitive flexibility training. *PLoS ONE* 12:e0172993. doi: 10.1371/journal.pone.0172993

van de Ven, R. M., Murre, J. M., Veltman, D. J., and Schmand, B. A. (2016). Computer-based cognitive training for executive functions after stroke: a systematic review. *Front. Hum. Neurosci.* 10:150. doi: 10.3389/fnhum.2016.00150

van de Ven, R. M., Schmand, B., Groet, E., Veltman, D. J., and Murre, J. M. (2015). The effect of computer-based cognitive flexibility training on recovery of executive function after stroke: rationale, design and methods of the TAPASS study. *BMC Neurol.* 15:144. doi: 10.1186/s12883-015-0397-y

van Muijden, J., Band, G. P., and Hommel, B. (2012). Online games training aging brains: Limited transfer to cognitive control functions. *Front. Hum. Neurosci.* 6:221. doi: 10.3389/fnhum.2012.00221

Vercoulen, J. H. M. M., Bazelmans, E., Swanink, C. M. A., Fennis, J. F. M., Galama, J. M. D., Jongen, P. J. H., et al. (1997). Physical activity in chronic fatigue syndrome: assessment and its role in fatigue. *J. Psychiatr. Res.* 31, 661–673.

Verhaeghen, P., Marcoen, A., and Goossens, L. (1992). Improving memory performance in the aged through mnemonic training: a meta-analytic study. *Psychol. Aging* 7, 242–251. doi: 10.1037/0882-7974.7.2.242

Wang, M. Y., Chang, C. Y., and Su, S. Y. (2011). What's cooking? - cognitive training of executive function in the elderly. *Front. Psychol.* 2:228. doi: 10.3389/fpsyg.2011.00228

Wechsler, V. D. (2000). *Wechsler Adult Intelligence Scale (WAIS-III) Nederlandstalige Bewerking. Technische Handleiding.* Lisse: Swets and Zeitlinger.

Whitbourne, S. K., Ellenberg, S., and Akimoto, K. (2013). Reasons for playing casual video games and perceived benefits among adults 18 to 80 years old. *Cyberpsychol. Behav. Soc. Netw.* 16, 892–897. doi: 10.1089/cyber.2012.0705

Whitlock, L. A., McLaughlin, A. C., and Allaire, J. C. (2012). Individual differences in response to cognitive training: using a multi-modal, attentionally demanding game-based intervention for older adults. *Comput. Hum. Behav.* 28, 1091–1096. doi: 10.1016/j.chb.2012.01.012

Worm-Smeitink, M., Gielissen, M., Bloot, L., van Laarhoven, H. W. M., van Engelen, B., van Riel, P., et al. (2017). The assessment of fatigue: psychometric qualities and norms for the checklist individual strength. *J. Psychosomat. Res.* 98, 40–46. doi: 10.1016/j.jpsychores.2017.05.007

Ybarra, O., Burnstein, E., Winkielman, P., Keller, M. C., Manis, M., Chan, E., et al. (2008). Mental exercising through simple socializing: social interaction promotes general cognitive functioning. *Pers. Soc. Psychol. Bull.* 34, 248–259. doi: 10.1177/0146167207310454

Zachary, R. (1991). *The Manual of the Shipley Institute of Living Scale*. Los Angeles, CA: Western Psychological Services.

Zigmond, A. S., and Snaith, R. P. (1983). The hospital anxiety and depression scale. *Acta Psychiatr. Scand.* 67, 361–370.

Zinke, K., Zeintl, M., Rose, N. S., Putzmann, J., Pydde, A., and Kliegel, M. (2014). Working memory training and transfer in older adults: effects of age, baseline performance, and training gains. *Dev. Psychol.* 50, 304–315. doi: 10.1037/a0032982

4

Acute Exercise Improves Motor Memory Consolidation in Preadolescent Children

Jesper Lundbye-Jensen[1,2,3]*, *Kasper Skriver*[1,2,3], *Jens B. Nielsen*[2] *and Marc Roig*[4,5]

[1]*Department of Nutrition, Exercise and Sports, University of Copenhagen, Copenhagen, Denmark,* [2]*Department of Neuroscience and Pharmacology, University of Copenhagen, Copenhagen, Denmark,* [3]*Copenhagen Centre for Team Sport and Health, University of Copenhagen, Copenhagen, Denmark,* [4]*Memory and Motor Rehabilitation Laboratory (MEMORY-LAB), Feil and Oberfeld Research Centre, Jewish Rehabilitation Hospital, Montreal Center for Interdisciplinary Research in Rehabilitation (CRIR), Laval, QC, Canada,* [5]*School of Physical and Occupational Therapy, Faculty of Medicine, McGill University, Montreal, QC, Canada*

Edited by:
Claudia Voelcker-Rehage, Technische Universität Chemnitz, Germany

Reviewed by:
Keita Kamijo, Waseda University, Japan
David L. Wright, Texas A&M University, USA
Darla M. Castelli, University of Texas at Austin, USA

***Correspondence:**
Jesper Lundbye-Jensen
jlundbye@nexs.ku.dk

Objective: The ability to acquire new motor skills is essential both during childhood and later in life. Recent studies have demonstrated that an acute bout of exercise can improve motor memory consolidation in adults. The objective of the present study was to investigate whether acute exercise protocols following motor skill practice in a school setting can also improve long-term retention of motor memory in preadolescent children.

Methods: Seventy-seven pre-adolescent children (age 10.5 ± 0.75 (SD)) participated in the study. Prior to the main experiment age, BMI, fitness status and general physical activity level was assessed in all children and they were then randomly allocated to three groups. All children practiced a visuomotor tracking task followed by 20 min of rest (CON), high intensity intermittent floorball (FLB) or running (RUN) with comparable exercise intensity and duration for exercise groups. Delayed retention of motor memory was assessed 1 h, 24 h and 7 days after motor skill acquisition.

Results: During skill acquisition, motor performance improved significantly to the immediate retention test with no differences between groups. One hour following skill acquisition, motor performance decreased significantly for RUN. Twenty-four hours following skill acquisition there was a tendency towards improved performance for FLB but no significant effects. Seven days after motor practice however, both FLB and RUN performed better when compared to their immediate retention test indicating significant offline gains. This effect was not observed for CON. In contrast, 7 days after motor practice, retention of motor memory was significantly better for FLB and RUN compared to CON. No differences were observed when comparing FLB and RUN.

Conclusions: Acute intense intermittent exercise performed immediately after motor skill acquisition facilitates long-term motor memory in pre-adolescent children, presumably by promoting memory consolidation. The results also demonstrate that the effects can be accomplished in a school setting. The positive effect of both a team game (i.e., FLB) and running indicates that the observed memory improvements are determined to a larger extent by physiological factors rather than the types of movements performed during the exercise protocol.

Keywords: motor memory, consolidation, retention, exercise, learning, children

INTRODUCTION

During the recent years, there has been an increasing focus on the potential effects of exercise on health, cognitive functions and also learning. The quality of public education has rarely been more debated than it is currently, with the discussion focusing on measures that can optimize academic performance of school children (Danish Ministry of Education, 2014). One of the means by which authorities are presently looking to facilitate academic performance in school children, is by incorporating more physical activity in and outside physical education (PE; Alvang, 2010). This initiative is supported by research indicating that there is a positive relation between high levels of aerobic fitness (Åberg et al., 2009; Lambourne et al., 2013), participation in vigorous physical activity (Coe et al., 2006) and academic achievements, even when time is taken from the normal curriculum and dedicated to exercise (Sallis et al., 1999; Ahamed et al., 2007).

These findings are part of a larger body of research showing that exercise can be beneficial for a variety of brain functions (for reviews see Hillman et al., 2008; Taubert et al., 2015). Both chronic and acute exercise can have beneficial effects on cognitive functions (Hillman et al., 2009, 2014) and facilitate the formation and retention of several types of memory (Roig et al., 2013). In children, chronic exercise is associated with significant memory-related benefits such as better academic performance (Coe et al., 2006; Singh et al., 2012; Booth et al., 2014) and cognitive functions (Sibley and Etnier, 2003; Hillman et al., 2014). Similarly, studies investigating the effects of an acute bout of exercise on memory have documented positive effects on cognitive functions including memory in adults (Winter et al., 2007; Kamijo et al., 2009; Labban and Etnier, 2011) and children (Hillman et al., 2009; Pesce et al., 2009; Ellemberg and St-Louis-Deschênes, 2010). Additionally, a meta-analysis found acute exercise to have small but consistent effects on simultaneous or subsequent performance of a memory-related task (Chang et al., 2012). While both chronic and acute exercise can benefit memory functions and effects may be interrelated, the distinction is important since the underlying mechanisms may differ and effects may relate to different aspects of memory.

Memory can crudely be divided into declarative and nondeclarative memory, and a major emphasis is placed on formation and retention of declarative memory in the educational system, e.g., geographical knowledge or recall of names (Squire, 1992). Declarative memory has also been a main focus for the majority of studies mentioned in the previous paragraph. Acquisition and retention of skills does however also play a major role both in the educational curriculum and in the lives of children and adults in general and skill learning requires the formation and retention of procedural or motor memory. It is thus also relevant to investigate how exercise may influence motor memory functions.

Recent studies have demonstrated that motor skills in preadolescent children are related to objective measures of cognitive functions, academic performance (Geertsen et al., 2016) and to academic achievement in adolescence (Kantomaa et al., 2013), and that daily PE and increased focus on motor skill training during compulsory school years can improve both motor skills and academic performance in adolescence (Ericsson and Karlsson, 2014). Finally, since motor (or procedural) memory is both associated with motor skills, but also supports language (Ullman, 2004) and certain social skills (Lieberman, 2000), motor skills may additionally subserve academic learning. Since motor skills are important in everyday life, and we need to acquire and retain a multitude of skills throughout life, these findings justify an increased focus on the principles and mechanisms involved in motor skill learning and motor memory in children.

Considering the effects of acute exercise on skill learning and motor memory, Roig et al. (2012) demonstrated in adults that an acute bout of intense exercise can facilitate long-term memory of a novel motor skill, when performed either before or after initial motor practice (Roig et al., 2012). The study also revealed that the effect was larger when exercise was performed after learning, indicating that exercise benefits the consolidation processes subserving retention of motor memory. Recently, it has been demonstrated also in adults, that consolidation and motor memory is influenced by the timing and intensity of exercise following skill learning (Thomas et al., 2016a,c). Thus, an acute bout of high intensity exercise performed in close temporal proximity to the skill acquisition and thus in the early consolidation phase is preferable for influencing motor memory consolidation positively. However, since these studies were conducted in a lab setting with able-bodied adult male subjects, it remains unknown whether acute exercise can benefit motor memory consolidation in preadolescent children. This question is important to elucidate given the potential for promoting skill learning in children, and in order to elucidate neuroplastic mechanisms underlying memory functions in children. Furthermore, it remains unknown whether the type of the employed exercise protocol plays a role for eliciting positive effects of exercise on motor memory.

The aim of this study was therefore to investigate if a single bout of intense exercise performed after motor skill learning, promotes long-term motor memory in preadolescent children since this has not been investigated in previous studies. Our main hypothesis was that long-term motor memory would be improved in children performing an intense physical activity after skill acquisition, compared to a passive control group. Additionally, we wanted to elucidate whether different types of intense exercise may affect long-term memory differentially.

MATERIALS AND METHODS

Participating Children

Seventy-eight ethnically diverse children from 3rd and 4th grade were recruited to participate in the study (see **Table 1**). They were all naïve to the visuomotor accuracy-tracking task (MT) used to assess skill learning and retention of motor memory. Exclusion criteria for participation were: history of neurological or psychiatric diseases as well as current intake of medications

TABLE 1 | Characteristics of the children in the control (CON), floorball (FLB) and running (RUN) groups.

	CON	FLB	RUN
Participants (*n*)	26	26	25
Boys/Girls	13/13	16/10	15/10
Age (Years)	10.3 ± 0.6	10.4 ± 0.7	10.8 ± 0.8*
BMI (Weight/Height^2)	18.3 ± 2.6	17.1 ± 2.0	17.7 ± 2.9
Cardiovascular fitness (VO_{2peak} mlO2/kg/min)	42.4 ± 3.4	42.5 ± 3.6	41.1 ± 1.9
Physical Activity (PAQ-C, METS)	3.43 ± 0.6	3.41 ± 0.5	3.3 ± 0.7
HR_{avg} during exercise	NA	197 ± 7$^+$	191 ± 8
HR_{peak} during exercise	NA	199 ± 6	201 ± 10

*Data are reported as mean ± SD. BMI = Body mass index, Cardiovascular fitness is estimated peak VO_2 consumption using the yoyo-test, PAQ-C, General Physical activity level questionnaire for children; METs, Metabolic Equivalents; HR, Heart rate). *Denotes significantly different from other groups (p < 0.05). $^+$Denotes significantly different from RUN (p < 0.05).*

affecting the central nervous system. The legal guardians of all participating children gave informed written consent on behalf of their child prior to participation. One child withdrew consent before completing the experiment. Blocked-randomization was used to assign children to either running (RUN), floorball (FLB) or control (CON) groups. The groups were matched on gender, age, BMI and fitness level since these factors may influence the effect of acute exercise on performance in cognitive tests, and possibly motor performance (Kamijo et al., 2009; Stroth et al., 2009). The study was performed in accordance with the Declaration of Helsinki II. The ethics committee for the Greater Copenhagen area approved the study (protocol: H-2-2012-169).

Study Design

Design Overview

The experiment was designed as a randomized controlled trial and included four separate sessions (**Figure 1**). The pre-examination consisted of an aerobic fitness test to assess fitness level. The following session was the main experiment during which the children practiced the motor task. After motor practice the children rested (CON), played FLB or ran (RUN) for 20 min. Retention tests were performed 1 h, 24 h and 7 days after initial practice of the motor task.

Pre-Examination

At least 1 week prior to the main experiment, all children completed a Yo-Yo Interval Restitution Children's test to assess their aerobic fitness. This test provides an estimate of the maximal oxygen consumption ($VO_{2\text{-peak}}$; Bendiksen et al., 2013). During the test, heart rate was monitored (Polar Team System, Kempele, Finland).

Main Experiment and Retention Tests

Children were tested in groups of four, with all four being assigned to the same experimental group. They were seated at independent workstations along with an experimenter that followed them throughout the experiment. Initially children were given a brief description of the experiment. Afterwards, the weight, height and body composition (Innerscan, Tanita, Tokyo, Japan) of each child was measured. Additionally, the children completed an Edinburgh Handedness Questionnaire to assess handedness and Physical Activity Questionnaire for Children (PAQ_C) to estimate daily physical activity level (Kowalski et al., 2004).

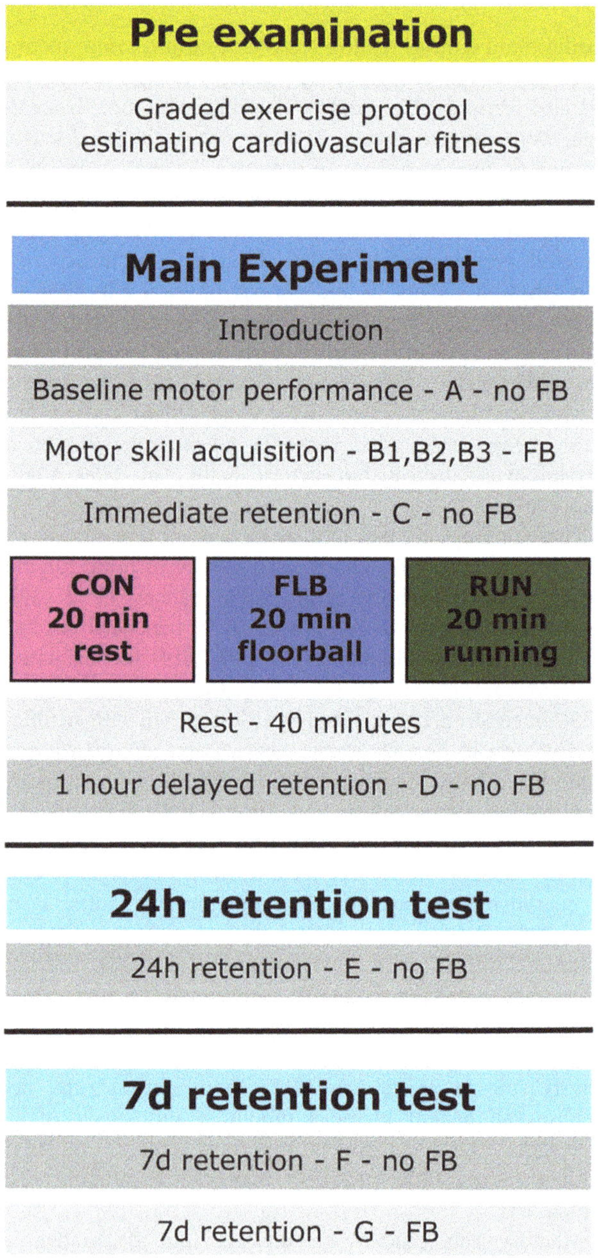

FIGURE 1 | Schematic overview of the experimental design. FB, Augmented Feedback; CON, control group; FLB, floorball group; RUN, running group.

Following this, the children practiced MT (see detailed information below). Immediately after motor practice, the children engaged in 20 min of rest (CON), FLB or running (RUN). After the interventions, all children rested 40 min during which they were allowed to read magazines or watch cartoons.

The motor task employed in this study was a modified version of the visuomotor accuracy tracking task previously applied in other experiments (Roig et al., 2012; Thomas et al., 2016a,b,c). In short, the children were comfortably seated at a table, with their forearm resting on the table. Immediately in front of the child was a computer screen. The children were instructed to control a computer mouse with their preferred hand.

The motor task setup was established using a customized software application (Matlab®, R2013b, Mathworks), allowing the child to control the vertical position (y-axis) of a cursor that moved left to right across the screen in 8 s i.e., with a constant speed. Based on the cursor's automatic movement along x-axis and the child's movement of the cursor on the y-axis, a trajectory was created, representing the trace drawn by the cursor's movement during the respective trial.

Children were allowed 1 min of familiarization, during which they could freely move the cursor on an empty screen i.e., without a target. Following familiarization, actual motor practice (acquisition) was initiated. For each trial, the child was required to match the cursor as accurately as possible to a preset target (Roig et al., 2012). Eight different targets with different, but predictable trajectories were displayed in a random order (see Thomas et al., 2016b). All eight target trajectories started and ended at target mean positioned in the middle of the visual display, and all targets required the child to move the cursor both upwards and downwards from target mean.

For each trial, motor performance was calculated based on the root mean square error (RMSE) between the preset target and the trace produced by the child. In order to provide intuitive augmented feedback on motor performance to the children, motor performance was transformed to a 0–100 score. The score was defined as the mean of absolute vertical errors between the cursor and target in relation to target mean. If the error exceeded two times the distance from target to target mean, the score for this data point was set to zero. An RMSE of 0 equaled a score of 100 (see Thomas et al., 2016b).

The motor task was performed in blocks of 24 trials arranged so that each block contained three rounds of the eight different targets. Following each trial there was a 2 s pause during which augmented feedback on motor performance could be provided. To promote learning, the following feedback was provided: (1) knowledge of result (KR) was presented as the score ranging 0–100; (2) knowledge of performance was represented by a picture displaying the target with the trace produced by the child superimposed; (3) since the difficulty and thereby scores of individual traces varied, the child was provided with an average of KR for every full eight-targets cycle completed as a measure of average performance.

Augmented feedback was omitted from baseline and retention blocks to test memory and minimize the effect of feedback dependency and (re)learning (Salmoni et al., 1984). The children performed one block of baseline MT performance (A), followed by three blocks of acquisition (B_1–B_3). A 1-min break was allowed between adjoining blocks. Subsequently the children completed four blocks of MT to assess retention: immediately after (C), 1 h (D), 24 h (E) and 7 days (F) after motor practice, respectively (see **Figure 1**). One additional block of motor practice (block G) with augmented feedback was performed after the retention test on day seven to elucidate potential ceiling effects in motor performance.

Intervention Protocols

The intermittent exercise protocol used in both RUN and FLB was based on the exercise intervention applied in Roig et al. (2012). The intensity of the physical activity was relatively high, since some studies, including our own data (Thomas et al., 2016c), have indicated that high work intensity during consolidation leads to larger effect of the intervention (Angevaren et al., 2007; Winter et al., 2007).

Both FLB and RUN represent activities, which are frequently employed in school-settings. The activities were thus chosen based on ecological validity. While the physiological requirements of running in some aspects can be matched to those of FLB (e.g., average heart rate), FLB additionally involves more complex motor skills, decision making, teamwork and competition. The aim of the three group design was thus to include a passive control and if the results demonstrated differential effects of FLB and RUN, the design would suggest that differences would likely be related to the additional requirements of FLB in the aforementioned domains.

FLB played indoor FLB on a court measuring 6.6 × 14 m. The two teams each consisted of two children and one adult experimenter. The experimenters participated in the game to ensure that the flow and intensity of the game was maintained throughout the activity. The intensity of the game varied in a similar intermittent pattern for all children in FLB: 2 min instructions—in 3 min low intensity warm up—3 min of high intensity—2 min low intensity—3 min high intensity—2 min low intensity—3 min high intensity—2 min low intensity. Consequently the children performed a total of 9 min high intensity exercise. The running exercise took place at an indoor square track measuring 6.6 × 14 m. The children in RUN were required to exercise following an intermittent protocol as described for FLB thus totaling 9 min of high intensity running.

While performing high intensity exercise, the childrens' heart rate was monitored online and results stored for offline analysis (Polar Team 2 System, Polar, Finland). This was also the case for three pilot experiments preceding the main experiment. The purpose of these pilot experiments was to determine the heart rates for children following the exercise protocol by playing FLB. During the main experiment, the aim was to reach similar heart rates as in the pilot experiments. This was ensured by experimenters monitoring heart rates online and verbally encouraging the children in both exercise groups. The children in the CON group were resting seated comfortably with the opportunity to watch cartoons for 20 min.

Data Analysis

Children's Characteristics and Exercise Data

Average heart rate (HR_{avg}) and peak heart rate (HR_{peak}) data were determined for each of the three intervals of high intensity exercise. Peak heart rate (HR_{peak}) represented the highest heart rate observed during the exercise protocol and HR_{avg} the average of the peak heart rate observed in the three high intensity intervals. Differences in children's characteristics between experimental groups were compared using one-way analysis of variance (ANOVA). A significant difference between groups was assumed if $p < 0.05$.

Motor Learning and Memory

Motor performance scores obtained in each 24-trial block were averaged, providing a total of nine data points for each child (block A to G). Motor learning and memory was assessed by measuring acquisition (block A to C) and retention (block C to G) separately. A one-way ANOVA was applied to investigate differences between groups at baseline (block A). This test was needed to rule out the possibility of differences in baseline motor skill performance. Motor learning was analyzed with two-way repeated measures (RM) ANOVA with TIME (block A to C) and GROUP as factors. Motor memory was analyzed with a two-way RM ANOVA with TIME (block C to G) and GROUP as factors.

In the second ANOVA model the motor performance scores in the delayed retention tests (i.e., retention at 1 h, 24 h and 7 days) were normalized to scores at immediate retention (block C). This was done to ensure that the analysis of motor memory factorized differences among groups in skill performance at the end of acquisition.

If sphericity was violated when applying an ANOVA (as determined using Mauchly's test) the Greenhouse-Geisser correction was used. Furthermore, if a significant main or interaction effect was established in any ANOVA model, *post hoc* pairwise comparisons were performed using student's *t*-test. To reduce the risk of type I errors, the α-level was adjusted to $p \leq 0.017$ thus applying a modified Bonferroni's correction procedure for the *post hoc* tests (0.05/3—0.05 divided by the number of comparisons within blocks; Roig et al., 2012). In addition, to elucidate if any statistical significant offline effects of memory could be documented within each experimental group, paired *t*-tests were carried out, comparing block C with blocks D, E, F and G, respectively. To reduce the risk of type I errors the α-level was adjusted to $p \leq 0.0125$ (i.e., 0.05 divided by the number of comparisons within groups; Roig et al., 2012). To further investigate the time course of potential offline effects on motor skill retention, time-weighed regression analysis was performed within single subjects over the follow-up period including data from the immediate retention test and delayed retention at 24 h and 7 days (block C, E, F). A time-weighed slope measure was extracted for each individual, and entered into a one-way ANOVA to test for differences in offline mechanisms between groups. This procedure has previously been applied by Reis et al. (2009) to assess retention effects.

All statistical analyses were performed using IBM SPSS Statistics 22 for PC employing two-tailed probability tests. All *p*-values for *t*-tests are reported uncorrected. The results are provided as mean ± SEM unless otherwise reported.

RESULTS

Description of Children and Groups

The baseline characteristics of the children participating in the three groups are summarized in **Table 1**. There were no significant differences between groups with regards to $VO_{2\text{-peak}}$ ($F_{(2,69)} = 1.33$; $p = 0.272$), BMI ($F_{(2,74)} = 1.56$; $p = 0.218$), body fat percentage ($F_{(2,74)} = 0.34$; $p = 0.717$), PAQ_C score ($F_{(2,74)} = 0.33$; $p = 0.743$). There was a difference in age ($F_{(2,74)} = 3.46$; $p = 0.037$) with RUN being older compared to CON ($t = 2.33$; $p = 0.024$) and FLB ($t = 2.02$; $p = 0.048$). For heart rate measurements obtained during exercise, HR_{peak} was not different between exercise groups ($F_{(1,49)} = 0.37$; $p = 0.374$). In contrast, HR_{avg} was significantly higher during FLB compared to RUN ($t = 2.86$; $p = 0.006$).

Motor Skill Acquisition

There were no differences in baseline motor performance between groups ($F_{(2,72)} = 0.61$; $p = 0.549$; see **Figure 2**). A two-way RM ANOVA assessing the effect of motor skill acquisition revealed no effect of either GROUP ($F_{(2,72)} = 0.43$; $p = 0.654$) or a GROUP-TIME interaction ($F_{(2,72)} = 1.15$; $p = 0.322$). Conversely there was an effect of TIME on motor performance baseline to immediate retention ($F_{(1,72)} = 314$; $p < 0.001$) across groups. These finding suggest similar baseline motor performance and skill acquisition for all groups (see **Figure 2**). The average motor performance score obtained at the immediate retention test following motor practice (59.61 ± 0.92) was significantly improved compared to average performance at baseline (43.67 ± 1.11; $t = 18.42$; $p < 0.001$).

Delayed Retention

Motor performance scores obtained in delayed retention tests were normalized to immediate retention for the experimental groups to depict relative changes (**Figure 3**). Visual inspection of

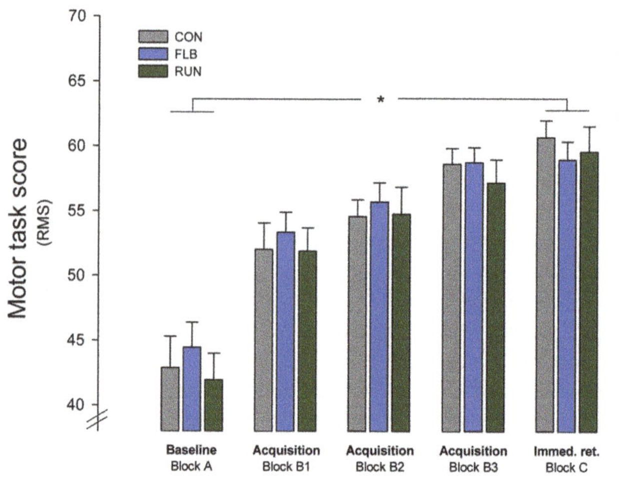

FIGURE 2 | Motor skill acquisition. Group mean scores in the motor task at baseline (block A), during motor practice (blocks B1, B2, B3) and in the immediate retention test (block C; group mean ± SEM) (Immed. ret.: immediate retention test). *Significantly different ($p < 0.05$).

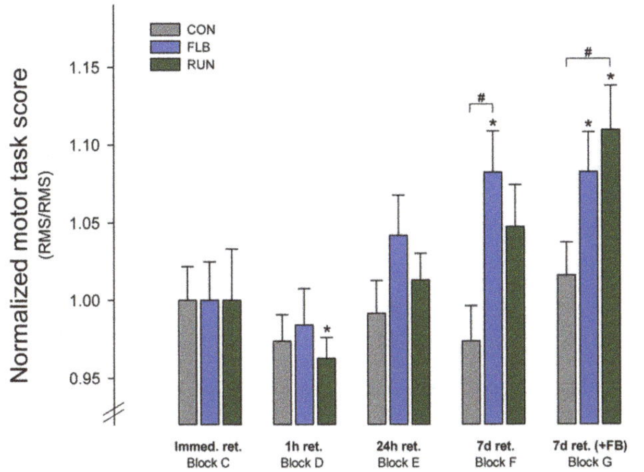

FIGURE 3 | Retention of motor skill. Group mean scores in the motor task at block C to G for the three experimental groups (group mean ± SEM). The retention scores are normalized to performance in the immediate retention test (block C). Immed. ret.: immediate retention test; 1 h ret.: 1 h retention test; 24 h ret.: 24 h retention test; 7 d ret. −FB: 7 days retention without augmented feedback (KR); 7 d ret. +FB: 7 days retention with augmented feedback (KR); #significantly different from control group ($p < 0.017$); *significantly different from immediate retention ($p < 0.0125$).

these results indicated that the exercise groups performed better in the delayed retention tests compared to CON, and the two-way RM ANOVA showed a statistically significant GROUP-TIME interaction ($F_{(5.972,215)} = 3.30$; $p = 0.004$). In addition, there was a main effect of TIME on retention ($F_{(2.986,215)} = 15.83$; $p < 0.001$), thus suggesting offline effects. *Post hoc* tests revealed that FLB performed significantly better than CON in block F (no augmented feedback on task performance) 7 days after motor practice ($t = 3.12$; $p = 0.003$). RUN also tended to perform better than CON ($t = 2.09$; $p = 0.041$, α-level adjusted $p \leq 0.017$). There was no difference between FLB and RUN ($t = 1.22$; $p = 0.228$).

In block G however also 7 days after motor practice, the task was performed with augmented feedback on motor performance to investigate effects of continued practice. Within-block comparisons of motor performance for block G showed that RUN performed significantly better compared to CON, ($t = 2.54$; $p = 0.014$), and FLB still tended to perform better than CON ($t = 1.97$; $p = 0.05$, α-level adjusted $p \leq 0.017$). There were no differences between FLB and RUN ($t = 0.513$; $p = 0.611$). The findings thus demonstrate that 7 days after initial motor practice, both FLB and RUN performed better compared to CON. Visual inspection of **Figure 3** confirms that there was no ceiling effect for motor performance in the tracking task.

Offline Effects within and between Intervention Groups

The assessment of offline effects in the three intervention groups revealed that children in RUN displayed a significant drop in motor performance from the immediate retention test (C) to block D, 1 h after the end of practice and 40 min after exercise ($t = 2.76$; $p = 0.011$). This decrease in motor performance was not observed for FLB or CON.

Assessment of offline effects across 24 h and 7 days showed that children in the FLB group displayed an offline gain in motor performance from the immediate retention test (block C) to block F ($t = 3.11$; $p = 0.003$) and block G ($t = 3.23$; $p = 0.002$) 7 days later. RUN also performed significantly better in block G after 7 days compared to block C ($t = 4.0$; $p = 0.001$), while there were no offline gains in motor performance for children in the CON group.

Offline changes in motor skill were also assessed by means of time-weighed slope measure calculated within single subjects for changes in motor performance between the immediate retention test and delayed retention at 24 h and 7 days (blocks C, E, F; **Figure 4**). The one-way ANOVA revealed a significant effect of GROUP ($F_{(2,75)} = 5.0$; $p = 0.009$) and *post hoc* comparisons revealed that the slope parameter was significantly higher in FLB ($t = 3.32$; $p = 0.0017$) compared to CON (**Figure 4B**). The slope parameter also tended to be higher for RUN compared to CON ($t = 2.23$; $p = 0.032$, α–level adjusted $p \leq 0.017$). There was no difference between FLB and RUN ($t = 0.863$; $p = 0.39$). These findings indicate offline gains in motor memory for both exercise groups compared to the control group.

DISCUSSION

The present study is to our knowledge the first to investigate: (1) whether a single bout of acute intense intermittent exercise following skill acquisition can improve motor memory consolidation in preadolescent children; and (2) whether different types of acute exercise employed in a school setting are accompanied by differential effects on motor memory and skill learning.

The results demonstrate that an acute bout of intense exercise performed after practicing a novel motor task improves long-term motor memory. In accordance with Roig et al. (2012) we have thus demonstrated that exercise can facilitate retention following skill learning through an effect on motor memory consolidation also in pre-adolescent children. Furthermore, we investigated the effects of different exercise interventions including running and FLB, which represents a team-oriented exercise intervention, demonstrating that team-sports can be effective in reinforcing the consolidation and retention of long-term motor memory. The finding that long-term motor memory was enhanced in both exercise groups indicates that the type of exercise does not seem to be essential to achieve a memory-facilitating effect. Most likely, timing, intensity and duration of exercise are more important parameters for facilitating memory consolidation processes (Angevaren et al., 2007; Chang et al., 2012; Roig et al., 2013; Thomas et al., 2016a,c).

While no study to our knowledge assessed effects of acute exercise on motor memory consolidation in preadolescents, Pesce et al. (2009) previously demonstrated a positive effect of acute exercise on declarative memory in this group, when submaximal exercise preceded the memory encoding and

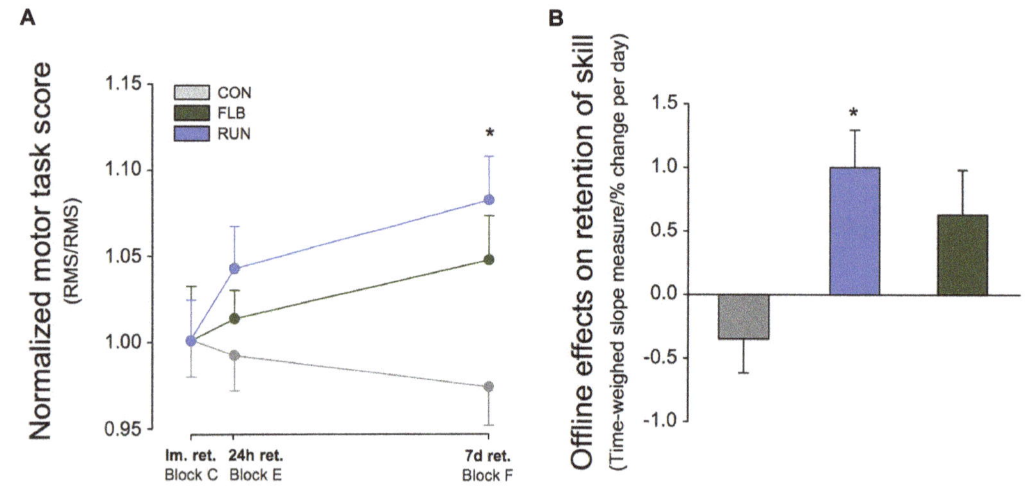

FIGURE 4 | Offline Effects. (A) Changes in motor performance between the immediate retention test and the delayed retention tests without feedback (KR) at 24 h and 7 days (Block C, E, F). *Significantly different from control group ($p < 0.017$) and immediate retention ($p < 0.0125$). **(B)** Time-weighed slope measure for offline changes in motor performance between immediate retention, 24 h and 7 days retention (C,E,F), calculated within single subjects. *Significantly different from control group ($p < 0.05$).

retrieval. In this case, exercise may have influenced both declarative memory formation and storage. Furthermore, Pesce et al. (2009) did not assess long-term retention thereby potentially missing further offline effects of the exercise. Delayed retention tests are highly important in order to assess interventional effects on consolidation (Kantak and Winstein, 2012), since the formation of both long-term declarative (McGaugh, 2000) and motor memory as in the present study (Brashers-Krug et al., 1996) can persist for many hours after acquisition. In the present study, skill acquisition preceded exercise, and this design including delayed retention tests enable us to demonstrate that the acute bout of exercise, enhanced memory through an effect on consolidation processes.

The timing of both the exercise relative to skill acquisition and the delayed retention tests are important in order to elucidate the effects of exercise on motor memory (Statton et al., 2015; Roig et al., 2016; Thomas et al., 2016a). In the current study, exercise followed motor practice with a short delay, which may be important for the positive effect on consolidation (Roig et al., 2016; Thomas et al., 2016a). Indeed, Thomas et al. (2016a) recently demonstrated that the temporal proximity between the exercise bout and motor practice has a positive influence on motor memory consolidation. This may relate to the potential temporal gradient of the consolidation processes following motor practice.

It is noteworthy that significant effects of exercise on motor memory improvements may appear long after the performance of the exercise bout and not immediately after. Indeed in the present study, memory and thus motor performance was significantly enhanced in the exercise groups 7 days after encoding, even though there was a detrimental effect in the running group 1 h after motor practice. Other studies have found non-significant or even detrimental effects of acute exercise on memory when retention tests were employed during or shortly after a moderate to high intensity exercise bout (Roig et al., 2013). This approach is not appropriate to assess effects on memory because the proximity of the retention test to the exercise stimulus can easily mask potential gains in memory due to exercise-induced fatigue and/or arousal, particularly when exercise is performed at a high intensity (Roig et al., 2016). Thus although intense running was accompanied by an acute detrimental effect on motor performance, this did not preclude delayed gains in the RUN group.

The finding of improved motor memory for the exercise groups 7 days after motor practice is consistent with previous studies (Roig et al., 2012; Skriver et al., 2014; Thomas et al., 2016a,c). While previous studies have also found significant effects of exercise 24 h after motor practice, this was only a tendency for FLB in the current study. Both groups did however display offline improvements from immediate retention to the 7-day retention test (see **Figures 3, 4**). It is possible that the effects of exercise evolve long after synaptic consolidation processes (Dudai, 2012) and that several days are required to see the effects of exercise on memory consolidation. Sleep-dependent processes may also be involved in the exercise-induced improvements in motor memory consolidation and this could contribute to the delayed effects (Dudai, 2012). In addition, the retrieval and motor practice inherent in the 24 h retention test and the following reconsolidation may contribute to the effects on delayed motor memory observed at 7 days.

Although there were no significant differences between the two exercise groups and both groups displayed different degrees of offline gains in motor performance, it is also noteworthy that there seemed to be apparent differential effects. Whereas FLB demonstrated significant offline improvements from immediate retention to 7 days retention and performed better compared to the control group, this effect was less pronounced for RUN. The running group however displayed a marked gain in performance with continued motor practice on day 7. In line with this, Rhee et al. (2016) also recently noted a latent effect of exercise on the development of motor performance with continued practice, and this may represent an alternative way in which exercise-mediated consolidation effects can influence motor memory and development of motor skills. Thus, acute exercise may both promote both consolidation processes, reconsolidation and facilitate learning with continued motor practice differentially. In essence however, both FLB and RUN ultimately led to improvements in motor memory in the current study.

Moderate to vigorous acute exercise preceding encoding has previously been demonstrated to promote declarative memory in children (Pesce et al., 2009) and adults (Winter et al., 2007) as well as motor skill acquisition (Statton et al., 2015). In a recent study by Thomas et al. (2016c) it was found that higher intensity exercise following skill acquisition was accompanied by more pronounced effects on motor memory compared to moderate intensity exercise. In agreement with previous studies in adults (Roig et al., 2012; Skriver et al., 2014) the present results demonstrate that high-intensity exercise following skill learning can promote consolidation of memory in children.

Indeed children in both exercise groups displayed high heart rates and thus performed exercise at a high intensity during the intermittent intervention. The groups displayed small differences concerning age and heart rate during exercise. The difference in age for RUN occurred due to an unexpected delay due to national labor disputes, causing a relatively larger part of children in RUN to participate in the main experiment 2 months later than planned. Since the groups were matched prior to initiation of the main experiment, this led to the observed small but significant difference for RUN. However, since neither age nor HR_{avg} were related to acquisition (age: $r = -0.111$; $p = 0.338$; HR_{avg}: $r = 0.171$; $p = 0.229$) or retention (age: $r = 0.109$; $p = 0.348$; HR_{avg}: $r = 0.003$; $p = 0.99$) these differences were considered to be of minor importance to the interpretation and validity of the results.

While mean HR was high and comparable between exercise groups, FLB and running are naturally different in several aspects. While running is a continuous activity, FLB naturally is a more intermittent activity and although exercise-protocols were also matched on time, the inherent intermittent nature of FLB may have influenced the anaerobic metabolism compared to running. FLB also involves decision making, varied movements also for the upper body in addition to a team element and competition. It is based on the design of the present study not possible to say to which extent these differences may have influenced the results, but further studies may elucidate whether these factors could influence motor memory processes.

The finding in the present study that motor memory consolidation and long-term motor memory can be enhanced by both FLB and running is consistent with the findings of Thomas et al. (2016b) in adults. This does however not mean that it is not relevant to consider exercise type. The finding that team sport in addition to running can boost long-term memory in children is important, since the classic experimental exercise regimes on treadmills or bike ergometers, are far from the regular activities that pre-adolescent children experience in school settings, e.g., playing during recess or PE. The applicability of team sports allows flexibility in selecting a more motivating and manageable activity depending on individual and group preferences.

A recent study has documented that the fitness levels of the younger population are declining (Tomkinson and Olds, 2007) making any effort that stimulates participation in regular physical activity ever more relevant. Furthermore, the level of fundamental movement skills in childhood is correlated to level of physical activity and obesity (Morgan et al., 2013) and physical activity can mediate the association between childhood motor functions and adolescents' academic achievements (Kantomaa et al., 2013). Since increased focus on motor skills combined with incorporation of exercise in education institutions can benefit both skill learning and academic achievements as demonstrated by Ericsson and Karlsson (2014), this underlines the importance of early-life motor skill training.

Skill learning is important and the mechanisms subserving formation and retention of declarative and nondeclarative memory (Censor et al., 2012) are to a large degree similar. Although memory systems are distinct, recent studies have made it conceivable that declarative and procedural memories can and do indeed interact (Robertson, 2012), and memories are not necessarily confined to independent systems. The functional connection between memory processes may contribute to the observed long-term effects of motor skill training on academic performance (Ericsson and Karlsson, 2014), and it suggests that consolidation of declarative memory might also benefit from acute exercise (Kandel et al., 2014). Caution should however be taken when extrapolating the current results to other types of memory or exercise, and studies assessing the long-term effects of acute exercise on declarative and nondeclarative memory are needed to conclusively document such effects.

The present results demonstrate that acute exercise in temporal proximity to a skill learning session can facilitate memory consolidation following acquisition and thus retention of motor memory. Based on the obtained measurements, it is difficult to infer in detail, which mechanisms could be involved in the observed effects of exercise on motor memory. Given that exercise was placed immediately following motor practice, long-term motor memory is most likely influenced by positive influences of the exercise on consolidation processes involving neuroplastic changes in the central nervous system (Brashers-Krug et al., 1996; Lundbye-Jensen et al., 2011; Taubert et al., 2015). We have in a previous study in adults found relations between exercise-induced effects on motor memory and changes in concentrations of specific biomarkers in peripheral blood samples (Skriver et al., 2014). This analysis demonstrated that higher concentrations of brain derived neurotrophic factor (BDNF), norepinephrine and lactate correlated with better retention of motor memory. Recently, a similar relationship was found between delayed motor memory and changes in corticospinal excitability following exercise (Ostadan et al., 2016).

Whether these associations may also be found for preadolescent children remains to be elucidated. Future studies could thus focus on investigating the mechanisms underlying the observed effects through application of e.g., electrophysiological or neuroimaging techniques in children.

In addition to investigating the mechanisms underlying the behavioral effects observed in the current study, future studies could investigate the potential effects of strategically implementing acute exercise in longer interventions thus combining acute and chronic exercise with the aim of influencing e.g., skill learning and motor memory. In addition to the direct transferability of the behavioral findings to school settings, the results of the present study could also be relevant for rehabilitation training with the purpose of improving long-term outcome of the rehabilitative treatment (Vaynman and Gomez-Pinilla, 2005), with acquisition and retention of motor skills being particularly important for physical rehabilitation. However, studies targeting clinical populations with mobility impairments are required before finally making such recommendations.

CONCLUSION

The present study is to our knowledge the first to demonstrate that acute intense intermittent exercise performed immediately after motor skill acquisition facilitates long-term motor memory in pre-adolescent children, presumably by promoting memory consolidation. The results also demonstrate that the effects can be accomplished in a school setting. The positive effect of exercise both as a team game (i.e., FLB) and running indicates that the observed memory improvements are determined to a larger extent by physiological factors such as intensity and timing of exercise, rather than the types of movements performed.

AUTHOR CONTRIBUTIONS

JL-J, KS, JBN and MR designed the experiment. JL-J and KS collected the data. JL-J, KS and MR conducted the required data analysis. All authors contributed to drafting the manuscript, and approved the final version of the manuscript.

ACKNOWLEDGMENTS

We would like to thank Lene Norbert Henriksen, Alexander Mogensen, Jonas Roland Knudsen, Caroline Borup Andersen, Cecilie Karlsson, Camilla Linde and Sidse Nikoline Stavad for their assistance with data collection. We would like to thank the school, teachers, and most importantly the children for participating in the study.

REFERENCES

Åberg, M. A. I., Pedersen, N. L., Toren, K., Svartengren, M., Bäckstrand, B., Johnsson, T., et al. (2009). Cardiovascular fitness is associated with cognition in young adulthood. *Proc. Natl. Acad. Sci. U S A* 106, 20906–20911. doi: 10.1073/pnas.0905307106

Ahamed, Y., Macdonald, H., Reed, K., Naylor, P. J., Liu-Ambrose, T., and McKay, H. (2007). School-based physical activity does not compromise children's academic performance. *Med. Sci. Sports Exerc.* 39, 371–376. doi: 10.1249/01.mss.0000241654.45500.8e

Alvang, D. (2010). Fysisk aktivitet og motion i folkeskolen. *Danish Ministry of Education.* Available online at: https://www.uvm.dk/publikationer/folkeskolen/2010-fysisk-aktivitet-og-motion-i-folkeskolen

Angevaren, M., Vanhees, L., Wendel-Vos, W., Verhaar, H. J., Aufdemkampe, G., Aleman, A., et al. (2007). Intensity, but not duration, of physical activities is related to cognitive function. *Eur. J. Cardiovasc. Prev. Rehabil.* 14, 825–830. doi: 10.1097/HJR.0b013e3282ef995b

Bendiksen, M., Ahler, T., Clause, H., Wedderkopp, N., and Krustrup, P. (2013). The use of Yo-Yo intermittent recovery level 1 and Andersen testing for fitness and maximal heart rate assessments of 6- to 10-year-old school children. *J. Strength Cond. Res.* 27, 1583–1590. doi: 10.1519/JSC.0b013e318270fd0b

Booth, J. N., Leary, S. D., Joinson, C., Ness, A. R., Tomporowski, P. D., Boyle, J. M., et al. (2014). Associations between objectively measured physical activity and academic attainment in adolescents from a UK cohort. *Br. J. Sports Med.* 48, 265–270. doi: 10.1136/bjsports-2013-092334

Brashers-Krug, T., Shadmehr, R., and Bizzi, E. (1996). Consolidation in human motor memory. *Nature* 382, 252–255. doi: 10.1038/382252a0

Censor, N., Sagi, D., and Cohen, L. G. (2012). Common mechanisms of human perceptual and motor learning. *Nat. Rev. Neurosci.* 13, 658–664. doi: 10.1038/nrn3315

Chang, Y. K., Labban, J. D., Gapin, J. I., and Etnier, J. L. (2012). The effects of acute exercise on cognitive performance: a meta-analysis. *Brain Res.* 1453, 87–101. doi: 10.1016/j.brainres.2012.02.068

Coe, D. P., Pivarnik, J. M., Womack, C. J., Reeves, M. J., and Malina, R. M. (2006). Effect of physical education and activity levels on academic achievement in children. *Med. Sci. Sports Exerc.* 38, 1515–1519. doi: 10.1249/01.mss.0000227537.13175.1b

Danish Ministry of Education. (2014). Improving the Public School—overview of reform of standards in the Danish public school (primary and lower secondary education). Available online at: https://www.uvm.dk/publikationer/engelsksprogede/2014-improving-the-public-school

Dudai, Y. (2012). The restless engram: consolidations never end. *Annu. Rev. Neurosci.* 35, 227–247. doi: 10.1146/annurev-neuro-062111-150500

Ellemberg, D., and St-Louis-Deschênes, M. (2010). The effect of acute physical exercise on cognitive function during development. *Psychol. Sport. Exerc.* 11, 122–126. doi: 10.1016/j.psychsport.2009.09.006

Ericsson, I., and Karlsson, M. K. (2014). Motor skills and school performance in children with daily physical education in school—a 9-year intervention study. *Scand. J. Med. Sci. Sports* 24, 273–278. doi: 10.1111/j.1600-0838.2012.01458.x

Geertsen, S. S., Thomas, R., Larsen, M. N., Dahn, I. M., Andersen, J. N., Krause-Jensen, M., et al. (2016). Motor skills and exercise capacity are associated with objective measures of cognitive functions and academic performance in preadolescent children. *PLoS One* 11:e0161960. doi: 10.1371/journal.pone.0161960

Hillman, C. H., Erickson, K. I., and Kramer, A. F. (2008). Be smart, exercise your heart: exercise effects on brain and cognition. *Nat. Rev. Neurosci.* 9, 58–65. doi: 10.1038/nrn2298

Hillman, C. H., Pontifex, M. B., Castelli, D. M., Khan, N. A., Raine, L. B., Scudder, M. R., et al. (2014). Effects of the FITKids randomized controlled trial on executive control and brain function. *Pediatrics* 134, e1063–e1071. doi: 10.1542/peds.2013-3219

Hillman, C. H., Pontifex, M. B., Raine, L. B., Castelli, D. M., Hall, E. E., and Kramer, A. F. (2009). The effect of acute treadmill walking on cognitive control and academic achievement in preadolescent children. *Neuroscience* 159, 1044–1054. doi: 10.1016/j.neuroscience.2009.01.057

Kamijo, K., Hayashi, Y., Sakai, T., Yahiro, T., Tanaka, K., and Nishihira, Y. (2009). Acute effects of aerobic exercise on cognitive function in older adults. *J. Gerontol. B Psychol. Sci. Soc. Sci.* 64B, 356–363. doi: 10.1093/geronb/gbp030

Kandel, E. R., Dudai, Y., and Mayford, M. R. (2014). The molecular and systems biology of memory. *Cell* 157, 163–186. doi: 10.1016/j.cell.2014.03.001

Kantak, S. S., and Winstein, C. J. (2012). Learning-performance distinction and memory processes for motor skills: a focused review and perspective. *Behav. Brain Res.* 228, 219–231. doi: 10.1016/j.bbr.2011.11.028

Kantomaa, M. T., Stamatakis, E., Kankaanpää, A., Kaakinen, M., Rodriguez, A., Taanila, A., et al. (2013). Physical activity and obesity mediate the association between childhood motor function and adolescents' academic achievement. *Proc. Natl. Acad. Sci. U S A* 110, 1917–1922. doi: 10.1073/pnas.1214574110

Kowalski, K. C., Crocker, P. R. E., and Donen, R. M. (2004). *The Physical Activity Questionnaire for Older Children (PAQ-C) and Adolescents (PAQ-A) Manual.* Saskatoon: Universtiy of Saskatchewan.

Labban, J. D., and Etnier, J. L. (2011). Effects of acute exercise on long-term memory. *Res. Q. Exerc. Sport* 82, 712–721. doi: 10.5641/027013611x13275192111943

Lambourne, K., Hansen, D. M., Szabo, A. N., Lee, J., Herrmann, S. D., and Donnelly, J. E. (2013). Indirect and direct relations between aerobic fitness, physical activity and academic achievement in elementary school students. *Ment. Health Phys. Act.* 6, 165–171. doi: 10.1016/j.mhpa.2013.06.002

Lieberman, M. D. (2000). Intuition: a social cognitive neuroscience approach. *Psychol. Bull.* 126, 109–137. doi: 10.1037/0033-2909.126.1.109

Lundbye-Jensen, J., Petersen, T. H., Rothwell, J. C., and Nielsen, J. B. (2011). Interference in ballistic motor learning: specificity and role of sensory error signals. *PLoS One* 6:e17451. doi: 10.1371/journal.pone.0017451

McGaugh, J. L. (2000). Memory—a century of consolidation. *Science* 287, 248–251. doi: 10.1126/science.287.5451.248

Morgan, P. J., Barnett, L. M., Cliff, D. P., Okely, A. D., Scott, H. A., Cohen, K. E., et al. (2013). Fundamental movement skill interventions in youth: a systematic review and meta-analysis. *Pediatrics* 132, e1361–e1383. doi: 10.1542/peds.2013-1167

Ostadan, F., Centeno, C., Daloze, J. F., Frenn, M., Lundbye-Jensen, J., and Roig, M. (2016). Changes in corticospinal excitability during consolidation predict acute exercise-induced off-line gains in procedural memory. *Neurobiol. Learn. Mem.* 136, 196–203. doi: 10.1016/j.nlm.2016.10.009

Pesce, C., Crova, C., Cereatti, L., Casella, R., and Bellucci, M. (2009). Physical activity and mental performance in preadolescents: effects of acute exercise on free-recall memory. *Ment. Health Phys. Act.* 2, 16–22. doi: 10.1016/j.mhpa.2009.02.001

Reis, J., Schambra, H. M., Cohen, L. G., Buch, E. R., Fritsch, B., Zarahn, E., et al. (2009). Noninvasive cortical stimulation enhances motor skill acquisition over multiple days through an effect on consolidation. *Proc. Natl. Acad. Sci. U S A* 106, 1590–1595. doi: 10.1073/pnas.0805413106

Rhee, J., Chen, J., Riechman, S. M., Handa, A., Bhatia, S., and Wright, D. L. (2016). An acute bout of aerobic exercise can protect immediate offline motor sequence gains. *Psychol. Res.* 80, 518–531. doi: 10.1007/s00426-015-0682-9

Robertson, E. M. (2012). New insights in human memory interference and consolidation. *Curr. Biol.* 22, R66–R71. doi: 10.1016/j.cub.2011.11.051

Roig, M., Nordbrandt, S., Geertsen, S. S., and Nielsen, J. B. (2013). The effects of cardiovascular exercise on human memory: a review with meta-analysis. *Neurosci. Biobehav. Rev.* 37, 1645–1666. doi: 10.1016/j.neubiorev.2013.06.012

Roig, M., Skriver, K., Lundbye-Jensen, J., Kiens, B., and Nielsen, J. B. (2012). A single bout of exercise improves motor memory. *PLoS One* 7:e44594. doi: 10.1371/journal.pone.0044594

Roig, M., Thomas, R., Mang, C. S., Snow, N. J., Ostadan, F., Boyd, L. A., et al. (2016). Time-dependent effects of cardiovascular exercise on memory. *Exerc. Sport Sci. Rev.* 44, 81–88. doi: 10.1249/JES.0000000000000078

Sallis, J. F., McKenzie, T. L., Kolody, B., Lewis, M., Marshall, S., and Rosengard, P. (1999). Effects of health-related physical education on academic achievement: project SPARK. *Res. Q. Exerc. Sport* 70, 127–134. doi: 10.1080/02701367.1999.10608030

Salmoni, A. W., Schmidt, R. A., and Walter, C. B. (1984). Knowledge of results and motor learning: a review and critical reappraisal. *Psychol. Bull.* 95, 355–386. doi: 10.1037/0033-2909.95.3.355

Sibley, B. A., and Etnier, J. L. (2003). The relationship between physical activity and cognition in children: a meta-analysis. *Pediatr. Exerc. Sci.* 15, 243–256. doi: 10.1123/pes.15.3.243

Singh, A., Uijtdewilligen, L., Twisk, J. W. R., van Mechelen, W., and Chinapaw, M. J. M. (2012). Physical activity and performance in school. *Arch. Pediatr. Adolesc. Med.* 166, 49–55. doi: 10.1001/archpediatrics.2011.716

Skriver, K., Roig, M., Lundbye-Jensen, J., Pingel, J., Kiens, B., and Nielsen, J. B. (2014). Acute exercise improves motor memory: exploring potential biomarkers. *Neurobiol. Learn. Mem.* 116, 46–58. doi: 10.1016/j.nlm.2014.08.004

Squire, L. R. (1992). Declarative and nondeclarative memory: multiple brain systems supporting learning and memory. *J. Cogn. Neurosci.* 4, 232–243. doi: 10.1162/jocn.1992.4.3.232

Statton, M. A., Encarnacion, M., Celnik, P., and Bastian, A. J. (2015). A single bout of moderate aerobic exercise improves motor skill acquisition. *PLoS One* 10:e0141393. doi: 10.1371/journal.pone.0141393

Stroth, S., Hille, K., Spitzer, M., and Reinhardt, R. K. (2009). Aerobic endurance exercise benefits memory and affect in young adults. *Neuropsychol. Rehabil.* 19, 223–243. doi: 10.1080/09602010802091183

Taubert, M., Villringer, A., and Lehmann, N. (2015). Endurance exercise as an "endogenous" neuro-enhancement strategy to facilitate motor learning. *Front. Hum. Neurosci.* 9:692. doi: 10.3389/fnhum.2015.00692

Thomas, R., Beck, M. M., Lind, R. R., Korsgaard Johnsen, L. K., Geertsen, S. S., Christiansen, L., et al. (2016a). Acute exercise and motor memory consolidation: the role of exercise timing. *Neural Plast.* 2016:6205452. doi: 10.1155/2016/6205452

Thomas, R., Flindtgaard, M., Skriver, K., Geertsen, S. S., Christiansen, L., Johnsen, L. K., et al. (2016b). Acute exercise and motor memory consolidation: does exercise type play a role? *Scand. J. Med. Sci. Sports* doi: 10.1111/sms.12791 [Epub ahead of print].

Thomas, R., Johnsen, L. K., Geertsen, S. S., Christiansen, L., Ritz, C., Roig, M., et al. (2016c). Acute exercise and motor memory consolidation: the role of exercise intensity. *PLoS One* 11:e0159589. doi: 10.1371/journal.pone.0159589

Tomkinson, G. R., and Olds, T. S. (2007). Secular changes in aerobic fitness test performance of Australasian children and adolescents. *Med. Sport Sci.* 50, 168–182. doi: 10.1159/000101361

Ullman, M. T. (2004). Contributions of memory circuits to language: the declarative/procedural model. *Cognition* 92, 231–270. doi: 10.1016/j.cognition.2003.10.008

Vaynman, S., and Gomez-Pinilla, F. (2005). License to run: exercise impacts functional plasticity in the intact and injured central nervous system by using neurotrophins. *Neurorehabil. Neural Repair* 19, 283–295. doi: 10.1177/1545968305280753

Winter, B., Breitenstein, C., Mooren, F., Voelker, K., Fobker, M., Lechtermann, A., et al. (2007). High impact running improves learning. *Neurobiol. Learn. Mem.* 87, 597–609. doi: 10.1016/j.nlm.2006.11.003

5

Older Adults with Mild Cognitive Impairments Show Less Driving Errors after a Multiple Sessions Simulator Training Program but Do Not Exhibit Long Term Retention

Normand Teasdale[1,2]*, *Martin Simoneau*[1,2], *Lisa Hudon*[1], *Mathieu Germain Robitaille*[1], *Thierry Moszkowicz*[3], *Denis Laurendeau*[3], *Louis Bherer*[4,5], *Simon Duchesne*[6,7] *and Carol Hudon*[6,8]

[1] Department of Kinesiology, Faculty of Medicine, Université Laval, Quebec City, QC, Canada, [2] Centre intégré universitaire de santé et de services sociaux de la Capitale-Nationale et Centre d'excellence sur le vieillissement de Québec, Quebec City, QC, Canada, [3] Computer Vision and Systems Laboratory, Department of Electrical Engineering, Université Laval, Quebec City, QC, Canada, [4] PERFORM Centre, Concordia University, Montreal, QC, Canada, [5] Department of Medicine, University of Montreal and Montreal Heart Institute, Montreal, QC, Canada, [6] Centre de recherche de l'Institut universitaire en santé mentale de Québec, Quebec City, QC, Canada, [7] Département de Radiologie, Faculté de Médecine, Université Laval, Quebec City, QC, Canada, [8] École de psychologie, Université Laval, Quebec City, QC, Canada

Edited by:
Stephane Perrey,
University of Montpellier, France

Reviewed by:
Arun Bokde,
Trinity College, Dublin, Ireland
Anouk Vermeij,
Radboud University Nijmegen,
Netherlands

***Correspondence:**
Normand Teasdale
normand.teasdale@kin.ulaval.ca

The driving performance of individuals with mild cognitive impairment (MCI) is suboptimal when compared to healthy older adults. It is expected that the driving will worsen with the progression of the cognitive decline and thus, whether or not these individuals should continue to drive is a matter of debate. The aim of the study was to provide support to the claim that individuals with MCI can benefit from a training program and improve their overall driving performance in a driving simulator. Fifteen older drivers with MCI participated in five training sessions in a simulator (over a 21-day period) and in a 6-month recall session. During training, they received automated auditory feedback on their performance when an error was noted about various maneuvers known to be suboptimal in MCI individuals (for instance, weaving, omitting to indicate a lane change, to verify a blind spot, or to engage in a visual search before crossing an intersection). The number of errors was compiled for eight different maneuvers for all sessions. For the initial five sessions, a gradual and significant decrease in the number of errors was observed, indicating learning and safer driving. The level of performance, however, was not maintained at the 6-month recall session. Nevertheless, the initial learning observed opens up possibilities to undertake more regular interventions to maintain driving skills and safe driving in MCI individuals.

Keywords: MCI, driving, learning, training, retention

INTRODUCTION

Mild cognitive impairment (MCI) is characterized by objective memory impairments with or without other cognitive deficits such as language, attention or executive function disorders (Petersen, 2004). The autonomy of many MCI individuals is relatively preserved, but a gradual functional decline can be observed when the cause of this syndrome is a neurodegenerative disease.

One of the most frequent causes of MCI is Alzheimer's disease (AD; Elias et al., 2000; Albert et al., 2011). Although there is some variability between studies regarding its prevalence, MCI could affect between 3% to 32% of the elderly population (65 years and older; Ward et al., 2012).

Compared to older adults with normal cognition, individuals with MCI and those with clinical mild dementia show similar rates of driving cessation and frequency (O'Connor et al., 2010). Also, there are several questionnaire studies showing that a significant proportion of older individuals with a diagnosis of MCI or dementia are active drivers and will continue to drive for several years after having received their clinical diagnosis (Silverstein, 2008; Betz and Lowenstein, 2010; Turcotte, 2012; O'Connor et al., 2013). Although it is well known that older drivers tend to underestimate the number of trips they take and provide inaccurate estimates of their traveled distance (Blanchard et al., 2010; Porter et al., 2015), these data are important because they suggest that older individuals with MCI are active drivers.

So far, all studies that have examined driving among MCI individuals reported that most of these persons can drive safely (Wadley et al., 2009; Frittelli et al., 2009). However, maneuvers involving executive functions, such as left turns (i.e., crossing a lane with traffic going the opposite direction), changing lanes and maintaining the vehicle in the center of the lane, are considered suboptimal in participants with MCI (Grace et al., 2005; Dawson et al., 2009; Wadley et al., 2009). In some driving simulation studies, drivers with MCI have shown poor control of speed (driving at slow speed and greater variability of speed than healthy individuals) and lateral position (weaving, driving off the road), and improper distance with a lead vehicle (Freund et al., 2002; Pavlou et al., 2016).

As cognitive function declines and dementia progresses, driving can become a serious traffic safety problem (Hunt et al., 1993, 1997; Dubinsky et al., 2000; Rizzo et al., 2001; Uc et al., 2005). Because the driving abilities of individuals with MCI are expected to worsen with the decline of cognitive capabilities, there is currently a debate about whether or not individuals diagnosed with MCI should also be allowed to continue to drive (Olsen et al., 2014). However, a recent Cochrane review (Martin et al., 2013) clearly highlights the lack of construct validity of current approaches to assess driving performance and the identification of at-risk drivers. Using data from a large-scale prospective cohort study, the Maryland Prospective Older Driver Study (Staplin et al., 2003), the authors have estimated that the cognitive test that most strongly predicted future crashes would, if used as a screening tool, potentially prevent six crashes per 1000 people over 65 years of age screened. This, however, would be achieved at the price of stopping the driving of 121 people who would not have had a crash. Martin et al. (2013) suggested that, although declining driving skills raise understandable concerns about crash risk, these data suggest that screening currently discriminates unfairly against older drivers. A similar suggestion arises from the work of Jeong et al. (2012) who showed no differences in the history of crashes and traffic citations for a period of 3 years between healthy elderly drivers and older drivers with MCI.

Clearly, the identification of at-risk drivers is problematic (Bédard et al., 2008; Gamache et al., 2010; Bédard and Dickerson, 2014). For older drivers with MCI, transitioning to alternative transportations is an option that needs to be considered as driving cessation will occur in the future (Carr and Ott, 2010; Wheatley et al., 2014). Before this potential transition occurs, one approach could be to examine whether or not these individuals can be retrained to maintain or even improve their actual level of driving performance. An interesting observation is that procedural memory (implicit learning) is preserved in individuals with MCI, as well as in people having clinically probable AD (McEvoy and Patterson, 1986; van Halteren-van Tilborg et al., 2007; Gobel et al., 2013). Implicit learning, contrary to explicit learning, takes place without awareness, often by repetition, and without reference to explicit knowledge learned previously (Vinter and Perruchet, 2002; van Halteren-van Tilborg et al., 2007). According to Willingham (1998) and Willingham and Goedert-Eschmann (1999), there could be an interaction effect between implicit and explicit learning, and implicit motor-skill learning could take place in parallel during explicit learning when a movement response is done. Complex sequence of actions can be learned implicitly (Witt and Willingham, 2006). With driving, knowledge of road safety rules is explicit knowledge, but several of the maneuvers involve implicit learning. For example, people explicitly know they should brake at an intersection with a stop sign, but releasing the accelerator and dosing the pressure on the brake pedal when braking is an implicit learning task that takes place while practicing. With healthy individuals, several studies have reported the maintenance of the acquired skills several months after implicit learning (Albouy et al., 2008; Gheysen et al., 2010; Doyon et al., 2011; Rose et al., 2011; Simon et al., 2012). Furthermore, two recent studies have demonstrated that this type of intervention brings measurable functional changes in the brain in healthy adults (Oosterman et al., 2008; Gheysen et al., 2010).

There is currently a lack of evidence as to whether or not MCI patients can benefit from a driving training program. In a recent pilot study (Teasdale et al., 2016), we examined if individuals with MCI could benefit from a training program in a driving simulator (five sessions over a 3-week period). None of these individuals participated in the current study. For several maneuvers (speeding, not using the turn signal, verification of the blind spot, tailgating), a gradual and significant decrease in the number of errors was noted. Individuals with MCI also showed implicit learning, with their braking showing a shorter and more uniform deceleration with training. These data are important as they suggest that individuals with MCI can be trained to drive more safely. In this new research project, we wanted to replicate these initial results. As well, we had a particular interest in testing if this initial learning decays when there is no rehearsal. To test this hypothesis, we recruited a group of drivers with MCI. They first participated in a 5-session training program within a 21-day period. Then, a 6-month recall session without any feedback was given. This last session was a transfer test serving the purpose to examine if the participants were able to transfer the improved performance observed within the first 21 days

(5 sessions) to a new context approximating what is needed in a real-world setting (i.e., driving alone without any additional verbal feedback on the performance; Lee, 1988; Schmidt and Bjork, 1992).

MATERIALS AND METHODS

Participants

Fifteen elderly individuals with amnestic MCI (eight single-domain; seven multiple-domain) were recruited from memory clinics. Participants had a valid driving license, normal or corrected to normal vision (6/15 or better on the Snellen test) and declared driving regularly (>3 times a week). This experimental group included 13 men and 2 women (age range: 60–89, mean age (±SD): 72.0 ± 8.8 years, education (years ± SD): 14.6 ± 2.7). None of the participants had a significant decrease in functional autonomy, but all were showing objective cognitive problems, including at least memory impairment. This decline in cognitive functioning was first detected through participants' complaints, which in turn were confirmed by a close relative. To confirm the presence of MCI, procedures similar to those adopted by Gaudreau et al. (2015) were followed. Briefly, the MCI was confirmed based on a battery of clinical and neuropsychological tests that was administered. As well, each case was discussed by a team of clinicians in order to reach a consensus regarding the status of participants. All participants met the core clinical criteria for MCI as defined by Albert et al. (2011). On their first visit to the laboratory, participants were briefed about the requirements of the experiment and invited to read and sign an informed consent declaration approved by the Ethics Committee of the *Institut Universitaire en Santé Mentale de Québec*.

Questionnaire and General Driving Assessment

All participants completed a general verbal questionnaire (driving habit questionnaire, DHQ) that included items on driving (frequency of driving and average km/week, presence of an accident during the last years; Owsley et al., 1999). This information regarding self-reports of driving exposure was only used to verify if participants were active drivers. As well, the DHQ includes several questions about avoidance behaviors during the past 3 months (driving outside the immediate neighborhood, left turns (crossing a lane with traffic going the opposite direction), night driving, bad weather, rush hours, highways). For each of these questions, there was also a secondary question regarding the confidence in their driving ability (5-point scale from 0 = no difficulty to 5 = great difficulty). A summary of the responses is provided in **Table 1**.

Before each session, participants were asked if they were in their usual state of fitness (that is, not suffering from a cold or flu or hangover) and were made aware the simulator could make them feel uncomfortable (nausea, dizziness, general discomfort and headache). They were instructed to inform the experimenter if this happened and were told to stop the simulation session before they felt discomfort or illness that could lead to emetic responses. They were told the experiment would stop immediately without any prejudice for them. To prevent simulation sickness situations to occur, the temperature within the room was maintained around 19°C with proper airflow using a ceiling vent positioned just above the driver.

Simulator

A fixed-based open-cab simulator powered by STISIM Drive 3.0 (System Technology Inc., Hawthorne, CA, USA) was used for training purposes. Images were projected on a screen (1.45 m high × 2.0 m wide) located 2.2 m from the steering wheel using a projector (Hitachi CPX8) displaying a 40° horizontal by 30° vertical field-of-view with the center of the screen located at eye-level through the mid-line of the subject. The simulator has an automatic transmission. Steering movements and displacements of the accelerator and brake pedals were also recorded (Computer Measurement PCI DAS08, 12-bit A/D) during driving. The simulator included a digital input/output board (Computer Measurement PCI-DIO24) allowing to record activation and deactivation of the turn signals. The cabin had genuine vehicle parts, and a fully instrumented dashboard (Tessier et al., 2009) leaving the entire screen for presenting the road environment. Audio feedback of the engine noise was provided through two speakers positioned in front of the vehicle. Two USB video cameras (Webcam C905, Logitech, Silicon Valley, CA, USA) were used, one was mounted on the cab facing the subject and zoomed to capture head and eye movements while the other one captured the scenario displayed on the screen. A magnetic tracker (Flock of Birds, Ascension Technology Corporation, Burlington, VT, USA) secured on the driver's head recorded head movements while driving. To comply with the 40° field of view of our simulator, there was no right or left-turn maneuver at intersections (i.e., crossing a lane at a right angle with traffic going the opposite direction), and moderate curves were presented (smallest radius of curvature of 120 m).

To detect driving errors, custom-made software was developed using STISIM 3 open module. The open module fed all information about the scenario and the simulation to a second computer through an Ethernet TCP/IP connection. This information was processed in real-time to evaluate the driving performance. The software also included a module to determine head and eye movements when a lane change was performed (Metari et al., 2013). A description of the driving feedback that were provided is presented below.

Procedure

At the first driving session, participants were explained the study, completed the DHQ, and were familiarized with the simulator. Then, they were given five simulator sessions on five different days within a 21-day period. A 6-month recall session was then held without any feedback. At each session, the participants drove a 6 km practice run (with less graphical information than the experimental scenario) to familiarize themselves with the

TABLE 1 | Summary of the self-reported driving habits.

	Mean (standard deviation)	
Driving days per week	5.6 (1.3)	
Average km/week	216 (191)	
Presence of accident during the last years	1 MCI with two accidents, and 1 MCI with one accident	
During the last 3 months, did you avoid... (number of drivers)		
Driving outside immediate neighborhood		0
Left turns (i.e., crossing a lane with traffic going the opposite direction		1
Night driving		4
Bad weather (rain)		0
Rush hours		1
Highways		0

simulator and recorded instructions. They were asked to comply with local traffic regulations throughout the experiment. The width and markings of the lanes were implemented according to governmental rules and speed limits, and advisory signs appeared throughout the scenario. Intersections with a stop sign or a traffic light were presented. No emergency braking response was necessary unless a driving error was made. During the familiarization run (for the first session as well as for all training sessions), general explanations were provided whenever a driver requested specific information regarding the auditory feedback that were provided, and the experimenter made sure that drivers understood the message relevant to each feedback and responded with appropriate corrective responses. The feedback provided were developed based on previous reports of typical errors reported for drivers having cognitive problems (Grace et al., 2005; Dawson et al., 2009; Wadley et al., 2009; Pavlou et al., 2016; Teasdale et al., 2016). They included maneuvers involving executive functions, such as changing lanes (indicating the intent to change lanes and verifying the blind spot) and proper control of the vehicle (speed, variability of the lateral position, and control of the vehicle at intersections). After the familiarization, participants rested for 5 min before they were given a continuous 27.48-km long scenario with urban and semi-urban two-way and four-way roads with minor grade changes. The scenario included recorded instructions to inform the driver about requested maneuvers (for example, instructions to overtake securely a slower-moving vehicle ahead of them) and conditional feedback about specific maneuvers when a driving error was detected by the simulator. No additional information was provided. For the 6-month recall session, the participants drove the familiarization session followed by the 27.48-km long scenario. As mentioned above, no feedback was given during this recall session. A brief description of the feedback provided is now presented.

Speeding

The scenario included urban and semi-urban sections with speed limits set at 35 km/h, 50 km/h and 70 km/h. The distance traveled within each of these zones was 650 m, 12,570 m and 14,260 m, respectively. Subsections were arranged within the scenario to represent naturalistic driving conditions. Throughout the drive, a threshold of 10-km/h above the speed limit was accepted (the actual speed was always available through an analog speedometer located within the simulator dashboard). Consequently, for each speed zone, exceeding the speed limit by more than 10 km/h triggered an immediate auditory feedback ("Your current speed exceeds the speed limit. You should slow down"). The driver had to reduce their speed below the 10 km/h threshold within the following 10 s to avoid an additional warning for the same speeding event.

Tailgating

This consists of driving too close to a frontward vehicle at a distance which does not guarantee avoiding a collision if stopping is required. The threshold was adapted to the speed of the driver using a time to contact measure. The threshold was set at 2 s. For example, at 50 km/h the minimum distance from the frontward vehicle needed to be greater than 27.7 m. A shorter distance would trigger a feedback ("Keep a safe distance from the vehicle preceding you"). Reducing the speed and/or increasing the distance from the frontward vehicle to increase the time to contact above the 2-s threshold within the next 10 s prevented the driver from receiving an additional feedback for the same tailgating event.

Weaving

Failure to control the lateral position of the vehicle is defined as weaving. In this study, we identified difficulties of drivers in maintaining the vehicle within the center of the road. A lateral positioning error was defined as maintaining the vehicle farther than 17.5% of the lane width from the center of the lane for 10 s. In other words, if the tires were less than 15 cm from the nearest road line for more than 10 s, a feedback was given ("You should maintain your vehicle in the center of the road").

Lane Changing

Fifteen lane change maneuvers were included within the scenario. Some of those were requested through a recorded command indicating to overtake a slower vehicle safely and to move back into the rightmost lane. Others were integrated within the scenario through the road design (for instance, lanes that were merging). A few additional lane change maneuvers could occur as a function of the driver's strategies. Whenever a lane change occurred, the system would verify the driver had signaled their intention to change lane before changing lanes (i.e., activation of the correct turn signal) and that a blind spot verification had occurred prior to initiating the lane change. When this was not the case, a feedback ("Verify your blind spot before changing lanes", "Activate your turn signal before changing lanes" or "Activate your turn signal and verify your blind spot before changing lanes") was provided as soon as the mid-line of the vehicle crossed the line separating two roadway lanes.

Vehicle Control at Intersections with a Stop Sign

Failure to stop completely at an intersection (speed <1 km/h for at least 1 s) or stopping beyond the stop line triggered a feedback as soon as drivers crossed the intersection ("You should stop your vehicle properly at the intersection").

Visual Search at Intersections with a Stop Sign

Drivers were instructed to look ahead and on their left and their right side to verify clearance before they entered the intersection. Ignoring this visual search triggered a feedback as soon as drivers crossed the intersection ("Just before entering the intersection, look left, ahead and right to check that the way is clear").

Vehicle Control at Red-Light Intersections

A permissive yellow-rule was adopted. Specifically, the driver could enter the intersection during the entire yellow interval, but a feedback was provided if the light turned red before the vehicle crossed the midpoint of the intersection ("You should stop at the intersection whenever the light is red"). As well, stopping beyond the stop line triggered a feedback as soon as drivers crossed the line ("You should stop your vehicle properly at the intersection").

Whenever a feedback was provided, an automatic 7 s delay was imposed before any other feedback could be given. A driving error occurring within this period would not trigger a delayed feedback but the error was recorded. This prevented consecutive feedback that could potentially overload the driver. No other feedback was provided. As well, no account of the driver's performance was given at the end of a session or before any given session. For the 6-month recall session, feedback was turned off and participants were simply asked to drive the same 27.48-km long scenario as safely as they would normally drive.

Data Analysis

For each session, we first analyzed the duration for driving the scenario. The results were submitted to a one-way ANOVA (first five sessions). We then compiled the number of errors made by each driver for each of the eight different types of driving errors (speeding, tailgating, weaving, omitting to indicate lane change, omitting to verify a blind spot, failure to stop properly at an intersection with a stop sign, failure to engage a visual search before entering an intersection with a stop sign, failure to stop properly at an intersection with a traffic light).

Because of the small number of subjects included in this study and the distribution of the error data, nonparametric statistical tests were adopted. First, we tested for each variable if learning occurred across the five training sessions using a non-parametric Friedman one-way analysis of variance (ANOVA). Significant differences were further examined using a Wilcoxon rank-sum test to examine more specifically if an improvement in the driving performance occurred between sessions 1 and 5. Further comparisons between two sessions were also made using the Wilcoxon rank-sum test (comparisons between sessions 6 and 5 or between sessions 6 and 1). All analyses were conducted using Statistica 13.0 (Dell Statsoft). The level of significance was set at 0.05.

RESULTS

Characteristics of the Participants

Overall, four participants (two men and two women) elected to stop their participation due to simulator sickness during the first session. Data for these individuals are not included in the 15 participants included in this study. The 6-month transfer session included 13 participants as 2 participants declined to come back for personal reasons. **Table 2** shows the sociodemographic and clinical/cognitive characteristics of the 15 participants. The sample included 2 women and 13 men. The mean age was 71 years and the mean education level was 14 years. No participant had clinical depression, but all had mild episodic memory impairment. The other cognitive functions were preserved at the group level, but as indicated in the "Materials and Methods" Section, some amnestic MCI subjects had additionally non-memory impairment. The most frequent non-memory impairment included language (i.e., naming or fluency) and/or executive deficits (i.e., inhibition). We compared participants with executive deficits with those without such deficits on the total number of errors observed at each session (Kolmogorov-Smirnov Two-Sample Tests). All comparisons were not significant and data for the 15 participants are presented thereafter.

Sessions 1 to 5: Training

The time for driving the scenario did not vary across sessions. On average, driving the 27.48-km long scenario took 43 min, 10 s ($F_{(4,56)} = 0.33$, $p = 0.855$). The number of errors compiled for each session for each dependent variable is presented in **Figure 1**. Across the first five sessions, there is a general decrease in the number of errors for nearly all variables. The main effect of session was significant for speeding ($\chi_{(15,4)} = 16.56$, $p = 0.002$), weaving ($\chi_{(15,4)} = 18.11$, $p = 0.001$), omitting to verify a blind spot ($\chi_{(15,4)} = 19.03$, $p = 0.0007$), visual search at intersections with a stop sign ($\chi_{(15,4)} = 24.39$, $p = 0.0000$), and vehicle control at intersections with a stop sign ($\chi_{(15,4)} = 10.16$, $p = 0.037$). For this latter condition, we did not observe an intersection for which the driver did not stop. All errors were failure to stop completely at the intersection, or stopping too far from or beyond the stop line. The number of omissions to indicate a lane change was small (on average, 1.7 omissions per session for the five sessions), and the small decrease that

TABLE 2 | Mean (standard deviation) sociodemographic and clinical characteristics of the participants.

	Raw score (SD)	*Z* score (SD)	Percentile (SD)
Sociodemographic characteristics			
Age (years)	71.7 (9.0)	–	–
Sex (Male/Female)	13/2	–	–
Education (years)	14.3 (2.5)	–	–
General cognitive functioning			
MoCA (/30)	24.3 (2.5)	−0.7 (1.0)	–
DRS (/144)	136.1 (4.9)	−0.1 (0.9)	–
Depressive symptoms			
GDS (/30)	4.8 (3.8)	–	–
Episodic memory			
RL/RI mean free recall 1, 2 and 3 (/16)	6.3 (1.8)	−1.7 (0.5)	–
RL/RI mean delayed free recall (/16)	7.2 (2.5)	−2.5 (1.5)	–
RL/RI mean total recall 1, 2 and 3 (/16)	37.0 (7.3)	–	6 (5.6)
RL/RI mean total delayed recall (/16)	13.4 (2.3)	–	6 (5.0)
3-min recall ROCFT (/36)	12.9 (6.1)	−0.5 (2.5)	–
Visuo-perception and visuo-construction			
Copy score ROCFT (/36)	29.4 (5.1)	−1.2 (2.0)	–
Size-match subtest (BORB) (/30)	27.1 (2.2)	−0.1 (0.9)	–
Information processing speed			
Coding subtest (WAIS-III)	52.1 (14.1)	0.1 (0.9)	–
Language and semantic memory			
BNT total (/15)	12.9 (1.9)	−0.1 (1.3)	–
Phonemic fluency (T-N-P)	31.6 (7.3)	−0.8 (0.8)	–
Semantic fluency (animals)	15.5 (4.9)	−0.5 (1.0)	–
PPTT (/52)	49.9 (1.1)	–	–
Executive functions			
Stroop D-KEFS, inhibition (s)	75.4 (27.2)	0.0 (1.2)	–
Stroop D-KEFS, switching (s)	72.1 (21.8)	0.4 (0.9)	–
Stroop D-KEFS, inhibition (errors)	2.5 (3.7)	0.0 (1.0)	–
Stroop D-KEFS, switching (errors)	4.0 (4.3)	−0.2 (1.2)	–

Note. Z scores and percentiles were obtained from age- and education-adjusted normative data. BNT, Boston Naming Test; BORB, Birmingham Object Recognition Battery; D-KEFS, Delis-Kaplan Executive Function System; DRS, Dementia Rating Scale; GDS, Geriatric Depression Scale; MoCA, Montreal Cognitive Assessment; PPTT, Pyramids and Palm Trees Test; RL/RI, Rappel libre/rappel indicé; ROCFT, Reu-Osterrieth Complex Figure Test; WAIS, Wechsler Adult Intelligence Scale.

was observed was not significant ($\chi_{(15,4)}$ = 5.72, p = 0.22). Similar results were noted for the number of tailgating events (on average, 1.1 events per session; ($\chi_{(15,4)}$ = 6.86, p = 0.143) and for vehicle control at intersections with a traffic light ($\chi_{(15,4)}$ = 4.69, p = 0.319). As for intersections with a stop sign, we looked for major errors and noted two events where drivers stopped at a green light and two events where drivers did not stop at a red light.

Session 6: 6-month Recall

Table 3 shows a summary of the comparisons between the 6-month recall session and the last training session (session 5) and between the 6-month recall session and the first training session. Mean values (and standard errors) are available in **Figure 1**. Overall, the analyses suggest a decrease in the performance between the 6-month recall session and the last training session (as expressed by a significant increased number of errors). This was observed for nearly all variables. The increased number of errors was significant for speeding, verification of the blind spot, omitting to engage in visual search before crossing an intersection with a stop sign, omitting to indicate a lane change, and tailgating. All other comparisons were not significant. Although we noted a decreased performance at the 6-month recall, when comparing the data with the first training session, none of the comparisons were significant.

Although, the number of errors observed for each variable could be considered small, the total number of errors is certainly not negligible. **Figure 2** presents the mean number of errors per driver. For session 1, 21.6 errors were noted. This number decreased to 8.2 at session 5. The main effect of Session was significant ($\chi_{(15,4)}$ = 39.36, p = 0.0001). The number of errors at the 6-month recall session increased to the level observed for Session 1 (21.8). The comparison between session 6 and session 5 was significant (Z = 3.17, p = 0.001) while that between session 6 and session 1 was not (Z = 1.13, p = 0.255). These errors were observed for a relatively short drive (27.48-km long scenario). Although few of these errors were critical (two for stopping at green-light intersections and two red-light crossings), the large numbers (at session 1 and at the recall) suggests that driving is not optimal in MCI individuals.

DISCUSSION

The main goal of this study was to examine if MCI individuals could benefit from a driving training program that provided automated real-time auditory feedback on various aspects of the

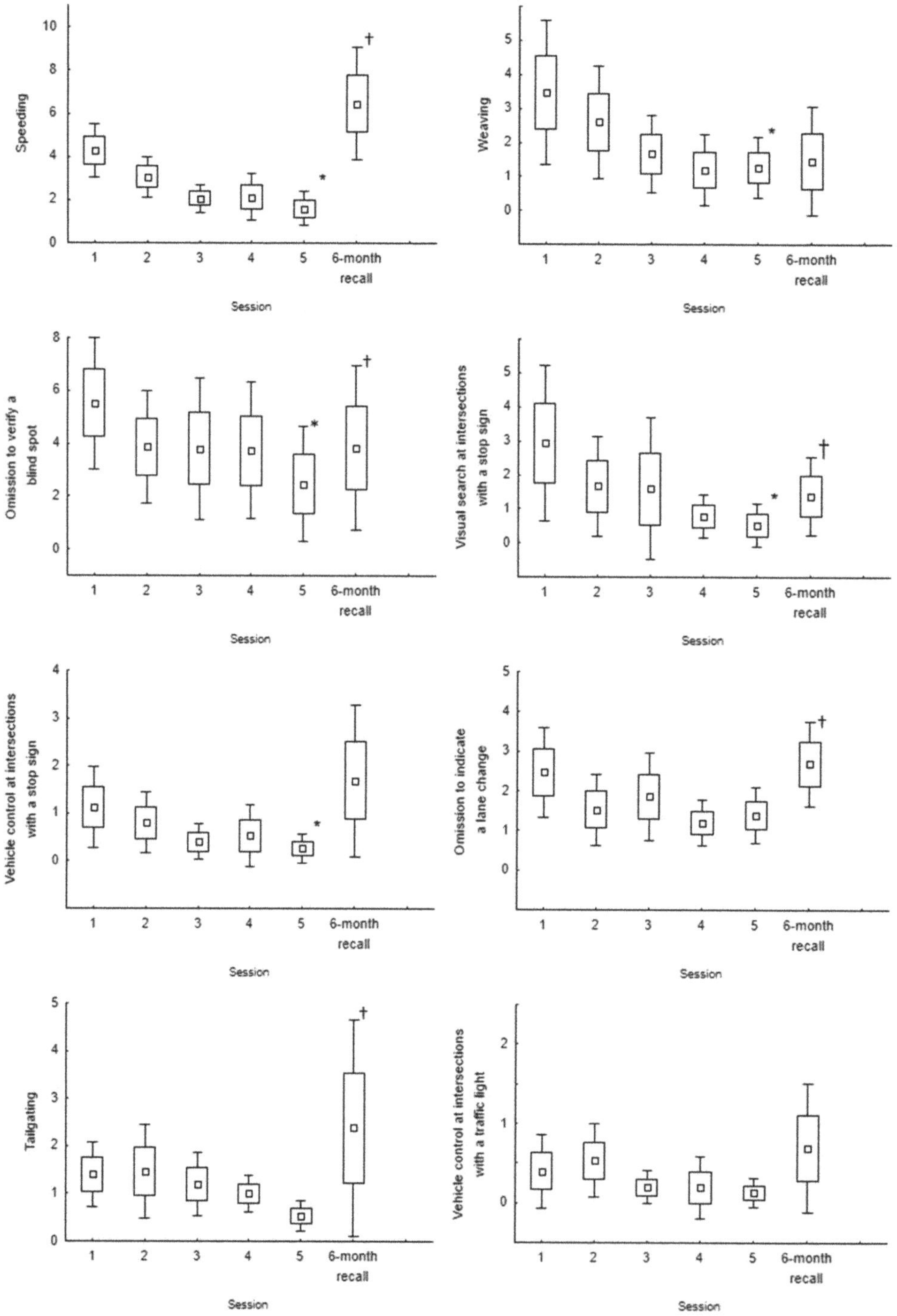

FIGURE 1 | Mean number of errors for the five training sessions and the 6-month recall session for speeding, weaving, omission to verify a blind spot, omission to engage visual search at intersections with a stop sign, vehicle control at intersections with a stop sign, omission to indicate a lane change, tailgating and vehicle control at intersections with a traffic light. Box and Whisker indicate the standard error of the mean (±1.0 and ±1.96, respectively). *Indicates a main effect of Session (Session 1 to Session 5). †Indicates a significant difference between Session 6 and Session 5. None of the comparisons between Session 6 and Session 1 were significant.

driving performance known to be affected in drivers that are cognitively impaired (speeding, weaving, tailgating, omitting to indicate a lane change, omitting to verify a blind spot, vehicle control at intersections with a stop sign, omitting to engage in visual search before crossing maneuvers, crossing an intersection with a stop sign or a traffic light, and weaving). Also, an

TABLE 3 | Summary of the comparisons between the 6-month recall session and the first and last training sessions (Wilcoxon rank-sum tests).

	6-month recall vs. session 5		6-month recall vs. session 1	
Variable	***Z***	***p*-value**	***Z***	***p*-value**
Speeding	2.66	0.007	1.53	0.124
Weaving	0.15	0.878	1.92	0.054
Omission to verify a blind spot	2.03	0.042	0.57	0.563
Visual search at intersections with stop sign	2.2	0.027	0.11	0.905
Vehicle control at intersections with stop sign	1.12	0.262	0.17	0.858
Omission to indicate lane change	2.66	0.007	0.84	0.400
Tailgating	2.366	0.017	0.254	0.798
Vehicle control at intersections with a traffic light	1.21	0.225	0.314	0.753

important objective was to determine if the benefits that could result from the initial training would be maintained at a 6-month recall session.

Overall, MCI individuals showed short-term improvements (five training sessions over a 21-day period). This was observed for speeding, weaving, omitting to verify a blind spot, vehicle control at intersections with a stop sign, and visual search at intersections. There was also a general trend for a decreased number of errors for the other variables that were analyzed (tailgating, omitting to indicate a lane change and vehicle control at red-light intersections). These results corroborate our previous observations also made with another group of MCI participants and a group of healthy older drivers (Teasdale et al., 2016). Contrary to a recent observation made by Pavlou et al. (2016), also in a simulator study, none of our participants drove with an excessively low speed and none maintained a large distance with the preceding vehicle. On the contrary, our participants exceeded the speed limit on several occasions (on average, four errors per driver for the first session with all drivers showing at least one speeding event; all but one driver showed an increased number of speeding events for the recall session) and several drivers also maintained a short time headway (tailgating; 11 out of 15 drivers showed at least one tailgating event on the first session). This was also observed in our previous study (Teasdale et al., 2016). Compared to the study of Pavlou et al. (2016), participants that were tested in our studies were at an earlier stage of MCI. Indeed, their participants included drivers with AD, Parkinson's disease and MCI. Unfortunately, a lack of more specific information about how they diagnosed MCI makes direct comparisons difficult with their study. It may suggest, however, that as MCI progresses, more severe driving errors will come forth (Wheatley et al., 2014; Hird et al., 2016).

The validity of simulator studies is sometimes questioned. Simulator and on-road driving performance have been compared for different populations. These studies have confirmed the relative validity of driving simulators to assess on-road driving performance (Lee et al., 2003; Romoser and Fisher, 2009; Shechtman et al., 2009; Bédard et al., 2010; Mayhew et al., 2011; Lavallière et al., 2012). For example, Bédard et al. (2010) found a correlation of 0.74 between simulator demerit points and on-road demerit points in older drivers. More important, there are studies showing that training in a simulator allowed not only to improve driving in the simulator but also to transfer the learning to a better on-road driving performance. This was shown with healthy older drivers by Romoser and Fisher (2009) and Lavallière et al. (2012) and more recently, by Casutt et al. (2014). The training offered to older drivers in the studies by Romoser and Fisher (2009) and Lavallière et al. (2012) was individualized. Specifically, in Romoser and Fisher (2009), it emphasized visual scanning at intersections while in Lavallière et al. (2012), it emphasized lane change behaviors (indicating a lane change, verification of the mirrors and blind spot prior to changing lanes). In both studies, drivers who received a passive training (no feedback while driving in the simulator and a classroom-like training) showed no improvement in their driving performance. These results (beneficial effect of an active simulator training for improving on-road performance) were replicated by Casutt et al. (2014) in a study where the training consisted of increasing the mental workload by gradually increasing the traffic frequency, the number of virtual drivers ignoring traffic rules and hazardous traffic situations and by providing specific vigilance training. The key result from these three studies is that training improvements observed in a simulator transferred to an improved on-road performance. Furthermore, Lavallière et al. (2011) and Romoser (2013) both reported long lasting effects (2 years post-training) for the on-road performance for most drivers that participated in the active training. These studies are important because they clearly support the suggestion that active training in a simulator can benefit the on-road driving performance. In the current study, we showed clear improvements within the first five sessions and there is a likelihood this training also yielded to safer on-road driving, at least on a short-term basis. Future studies are needed to examine specifically if the improved simulator performance translates into safer on the road driving for MCI individuals.

An important feature of this study was the 6-month recall session. As mentioned in the "Introduction" Section, this last session served the purpose to examine if the participants were able to maintain their improved performance observed within the first five sessions to a new context approximating what is needed in a real-world setting (i.e., driving alone without any additional verbal feedback on the performance; Lee, 1988; Schmidt and Bjork, 1992). Our results show the improvements observed after the first five sessions were not long lasting as

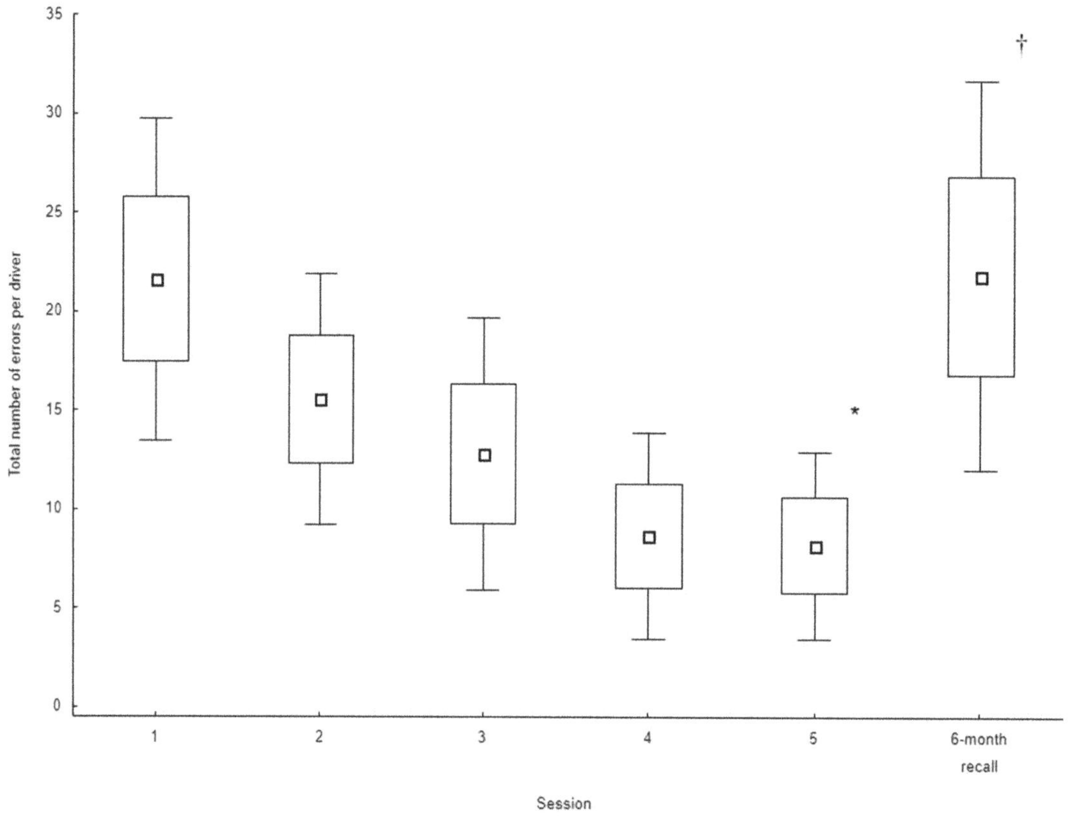

FIGURE 2 | Total number of errors (sum of all maneuvers evaluated) for the five training sessions and the 6-month recall session. Values are the mean of all participants. Box and Whisker indicate the standard error of the mean (±1.0 and ±1.96, respectively). *Indicates a main effect of Session (Session 1 to Session 5). †Indicates a significant difference between Session 6 and Session 5. The comparison between Session 6 and Session 1 was not significant.

we observed a significant increase in the number of errors for four measures (speeding, omission to verify a blind spot, visual search at intersections with a stop sign, and omission to indicate a lane change). The number of tailgating events, which was small and did not vary significantly across the first five sessions, also increased significantly at the recall session. For instance, for speeding events, only one out of 13 participants maintained the level of performance observed at the fifth session (six for weaving, and seven for the omission to indicate a lane change). The performance at the 6-month recall, however, was not different than that observed at the first training session. Considering the large number of errors observed in session 1 and at the recall but the near absence of critical errors, this could indicate that MCI participants showed less than optimal performance. As mentioned in the "Introduction" Section, this fits the general description of the driving of MCI individuals both in simulator (Frittelli et al., 2009; Devlin et al., 2012), and on the road (Wadley et al., 2009). For instance, Devlin et al. (2012) reported an absence of significant differences when comparing the driving performance in a simulator of drivers with MCI to age-matched healthy drivers. In a previous simulator study, we also observed limited differences between MCI and healthy control drivers (Teasdale et al., 2016). The progression of MCI certainly could lead to a decreased performance. The present study opens up the possibility, however, that proper training could contribute to preserve and perhaps enhance driving competencies. This is an important result and future studies should aim at defining the optimal training conditions and regime for inducing safer driving in MCI individuals.

A large randomized, controlled clinical trial examining the long-term effectiveness of cognitive training on enhancing mental abilities (ACTIVE study, Unverzagt et al., 2009) showed that at a 2-year follow-up, MCI individuals did not benefit from interventions that were focused on declarative memory. Our study did not involve any training on issues such as trip planning/scheduling or navigation. These features of naturalistic driving clearly are associated with declarative memory (and with executive functioning) and individuals with MCI may experience more difficulties when driving involves these additional tasks. On the other hand, in the ACTIVE study, MCI individuals, just as healthy older adults, did benefit from training in reasoning and speed of processing, two qualities that are fundamental to driving. This is important as it indicates that future studies should consider establishing a list of driving skills that are pervious and impervious to training. Our study clearly shows, that several important driving skills can be improved in MCI individuals. This opens up possibilities to offer regular training to these individuals to maintain safe driving. At the same time, regular follow-ups may offer a window into the progression of cognitive decline and allow to better identify the limitations MCI drivers face.

The present study involved only 15 individuals with MCI. Although this is a limitation, it replicates previous findings observed for the first five sessions (Teasdale et al., 2016). More importantly, it shows that at a 6-month recall session, the MCI drivers were unable to maintain the level of performance they attained at the end of the training session (**Figure 2**). Our results also show large individual differences. These differences could be related to variability in the progression of cognitive decline and intrinsic differences in the driving style. Only three drivers showed a total number of errors smaller than 10 at the recall session. Two of these drivers exhibited safe driving throughout the training and at the recall (that is, less than 10 errors throughout all sessions). A third one who exhibited 20 errors at session 1 maintained the improved level of performance observed at the end of the training at the recall session. All other drivers showed a large number of errors at the recall session (with two drivers showing more than 50 errors). As a key question associated with the driving performance of MCI drivers relates to the impact of the progression of cognitive decline on the performance, a longitudinal study allowing to understand how the performance degrades with the progression of cognitive decline is much needed. A large randomized controlled trial with a control MCI group exposed to the simulator without any feedback and healthy control groups (with and without feedback) would provide additional and important details about limitations and capabilities of MCI individuals when compared to healthy older drivers. Finally, participants in this study were a convenience sample of individuals with MCI. It would be important to determine if the smaller number of women that volunteered is indicative of a fear of being tested in this population.

In conclusion, this study shows that MCI individuals can be trained in a simulator to improve their driving. This improvement, however, appears to be labile for most MCI individuals that participated. This suggests, that regular rehearsal may be needed to maintain the improved performance. This decreased performance, however, was not beyond the performance observed at the first training session indicating that the MCI individual that were tested had maintained a safe, but not optimal driving performance during this period. Simulator training could be an important means not only for maintaining safe driving in MCI individuals, but also to offer cost-effective and safe means of evaluating how the progression of cognitive decline affects driving until it becomes unsafe.

AUTHOR CONTRIBUTIONS

All authors have fulfilled the criteria for authorship and have approved the final article.

ACKNOWLEDGMENTS

This research has received support from the Alzheimer Society of Canada. CH and SD are both Research Scholars from the Fonds de la Recherche du Québec-Santé.

REFERENCES

Albert, M. S., DeKosky, S. T., Dickson, D., Dubois, B., Feldman, H. H., Fox, N. C., et al. (2011). The diagnosis of mild cognitive impairment due to Alzheimer's disease: recommendations from the national institute on aging-Alzheimer's association workgroups on diagnostic guidelines for Alzheimer's disease. *Alzheimers Dement.* 7, 270–279. doi: 10.1016/j.jalz.2011.03.008

Albouy, G., Sterpenich, V., Balteau, E., Vandewalle, G., Desseilles, M., Dang-Vu, T., et al. (2008). Both the hippocampus and striatum are involved in consolidation of motor sequence memory. *Neuron* 58, 261–272. doi: 10.1016/j.neuron.2008.02.008

Bédard, M., Dickerson, A. E., and National Highway Traffic Safety Administration; American Occupational Therapy Association. (2014). Consensus statements for screening and assessment tools. *Occup. Ther. Health Care* 28, 127–131. doi: 10.3109/07380577.2014.903017

Bédard, M. B., Parkkari, M., Weaver, B., Riendeau, J., and Dahlquist, M. (2010). Assessment of driving performance using a simulator protocol: validity and reproducibility. *Am. J. Occup. Ther.* 64, 336–340. doi: 10.5014/ajot.64.2.336

Bédard, M., Weaver, B., Darzins, P., and Porter, M. M. (2008). Predicting driving performance in older adults: we are not there yet!. *Traffic Inj. Prev.* 9, 336–341. doi: 10.1080/15389580802117184

Betz, M. E., and Lowenstein, S. R. (2010). Driving patterns of older adults: results from the second injury control and risk survey. *J. Am. Geriatr. Soc.* 58, 1931–1935. doi: 10.1111/j.1532-5415.2010.03010.x

Blanchard, R. A., Myers, A. M., and Porter, M. M. (2010). Correspondence between self-reported and objective measures of driving exposure and patterns in older drivers. *Accid. Anal. Prev.* 42, 523–529. doi: 10.1016/j.aap.2009.09.018

Carr, D. B., and Ott, B. R. (2010). The older adult driver with cognitive impairment. *JAMA* 303, 1632–1641. doi: 10.1001/jama.2010.481

Casutt, G., Theill, N., Martin, M., Keller, M., and Jäncke, L. (2014). The drive-wise project: driving simulator training increases real driving performance in healthy older drivers. *Front. Aging Neurosci.* 6:85. doi: 10.3389/fnagi.2014.00085

Dawson, J. D., Anderson, S. W., Uc, E. Y., Dastrup, E., and Rizzo, M. (2009). Predictors of driving safety in early Alzheimer disease. *Neurology* 72, 521–527. doi: 10.1212/01.WNL.0000341931.35870.49

Devlin, A., McGillivray, J., Charlton, J., Lowndes, G., and Etienne, V. (2012). Investigating driving behaviour of older drivers with mild cognitive impairment using a portable driving simulator. *Accid. Anal. Prev.* 49, 300–307. doi: 10.1016/j.aap.2012.02.022

Doyon, J., Orban, P., Barakat, M., Debas, K., Lungu, O., Albouy, G., et al. (2011). Plasticité fonctionnelle du cerveau et apprentissage moteur–Imagerie et cognition (5). *Med. Sci.* 27, 413–420. doi: 10.1051/medsci/2011274018

Dubinsky, R. M., Stein, A. C., and Lyons, K. (2000). Practice parameter: risk of driving and Alzheimer's disease (an evidence-based review): report of the quality standards subcommittee of the american academy of neurology. *Neurology* 54, 2205–2211. doi: 10.1212/wnl.54.12.2205

Elias, M. F., Beiser, A., Wolf, P. A., Au, R., White, R. F., and D'Agostino, R. B. (2000). The preclinical phase of Alzheimer disease: a 22-year prospective study of the Framingham cohort. *Arch. Neurol.* 57, 808–813. doi: 10.1001/archneur.1995.00540290075020

Freund, B., Gravenstein, S., Ferris, R., and Shaheen, E. (2002). Evaluating driving performance of cognitively impaired and healthy older adults: a pilot study comparing on-road testing and driving simulation. *J. Am. Geriatr. Soc.* 50, 1309–1310. doi: 10.1046/j.1532-5415.2002.50325.x

Frittelli, C., Borghetti, D., Iudice, G., Bonanni, E., Maestri, M., Tognoni, G., et al. (2009). Effects of Alzheimer's disease and mild cognitive impairment on driving ability: a controlled clinical study by simulated driving test. *Int. J. Geriatr. Psychiatry* 24, 232–238. doi: 10.1002/gps.2095

Gamache, P.-L., Hudon, C., Teasdale, N., and Simoneau, M. (2010). Alternative avenues in the assessment of driving capacities in older drivers and implications for training. *Curr. Direct. Psychol. Sci.* 19, 370–374. doi: 10.1177/0963721410388641

Gaudreau, G., Monetta, L., Macoir, J., Poulin, S., Laforce, R. J., and Hudon, C. (2015). Mental state inferences abilities contribution to verbal irony comprehension in older adults with mild cognitive impairment. *Behav. Neurol.* 2015:685613. doi: 10.1155/2015/685613

Gheysen, F., Van Opstal, F., Roggeman, C., Van Waelvelde, H., and Fias, W. (2010). Hippocampal contribution to early and later stages of implicit motor sequence learning. *Exp. Brain Res.* 202, 795–807. doi: 10.1007/s00221-010-2186-6

Gobel, E. W., Blomeke, K., Zadikoff, C., Simuni, T., Weintraub, S., and Reber, P. J. (2013). Implicit perceptual-motor skill learning in mild cognitive impairment and Parkinson's disease. *Neuropsychology* 27, 314–321. doi: 10.1037/a0032305

Grace, J., Amick, M. M., D'Abreu, A., Festa, E. K., Heindel, W. C., and Ott, B. R. (2005). Neuropsychological deficits associated with driving performance in Parkinson's and Alzheimer's disease. *J. Int. Neuropsychol. Soc.* 11, 766–775. doi: 10.1017/s1355617705050848

Hird, M. A., Egeto, P., Fischer, C. E., Naglie, G., and Schweizer, T. A. (2016). A systematic review and meta-analysis of on-road simulator and cognitive driving assessment in alzheimer's disease and mild cognitive impairment. *J. Alzheimers Dis.* 53, 713–729. doi: 10.3233/JAD-160276

Hunt, L. A., Murphy, C. F., Carr, D., Duchek, J. M., Buckles, V., and Morris, J. C. (1997). Reliability of the washington university road test. A performance-based assessment for drivers with dementia of the Alzheimer type. *Arch. Neurol.* 54, 707–712. doi: 10.1001/archneur.1997.00550180029008

Hunt, L., Morris, J. C., Edwards, D., and Wilson, B. S. (1993). Driving performance in persons with mild senile dementia of the Alzheimer type. *J. Am. Geriatr. Soc.* 41, 747–752. doi: 10.1111/j.1532-5415.1993.tb07465.x

Jeong, H.-G., Jeong, H., Kim, T. H., Han, J. W., Youn, J. C., Park, J. H., et al. (2012). Association between driving performance and neuropsychological deficits in elderly people with mild cognitive impairment. *Alzheimers Dement.* 8, P359–P359. doi: 10.1016/j.jalz.2012.05.984

Lavallière, M., Simoneau, M., Laurendeau, D., and Teasdale, N. (2011). "Active training to improve older drivers' visual inspections when changing lanes: A 2 year follow-up study," in *40th Annual Scientific and Educational Meeting of the Canadian Association on Gerontology*, (Ottawa).

Lavallière, M., Simoneau, M., Tremblay, M., Laurendeau, D., and Teasdale, N. (2012). Active training and driving-specific feedback improve older drivers' visual search prior to lane changes. *BMC Geriatr.* 12:5. doi: 10.1186/1471-2318-12-5

Lee, T. D. (1988). "Transfer-appropriate processing: a framework for conceptualizing practice effects in motor learning," in *Complex Movement Behaviour: The Motor-Action Controversy*, eds D. C. Meijer and K. Roth (Amsterdam: North-Holland), 201–215.

Lee, H. C., Cameron, D., and Lee, A. H. (2003). Assessing the driving performance of older adult drivers: on-road versus simulated driving. *Accid. Anal. Prev.* 35, 797–803. doi: 10.1016/s0001-4575(02)00083-0

Martin, A. J., Marottoli, R., and O'Neill, D. (2013). Driving assessment for maintaining mobility and safety in drivers with dementia. *Cochrane Database Syst. Rev.* 8:CD006222. doi: 10.1002/14651858.CD006222.pub4

Mayhew, D. R., Simpson, H. M., Wood, K. M., Lonero, L., Clinton, K. M., and Johnson, A. G. (2011). On-road and simulated driving: concurrent and discriminant validation. *J. Safety Res.* 42, 267–275. doi: 10.1016/j.jsr.2011.06.004

McEvoy, C. L., and Patterson, R. L. (1986). Behavioral treatment of deficit skills in dementia patients. *The Gerontologist* 26, 475–478. doi: 10.1093/geront/26.5.475

Metari, S., Prel, F., Moszkowicz, T., Laurendeau, D., Teasdale, N., Beauchemin, S., et al. (2013). A computer vision framework for the analysis and interpretation of the cephalo-ocular behavior of drivers. *Mach. Vis. Appl.* 24, 159–173. doi: 10.1007/s00138-011-0381-5

O'Connor, M. L., Edwards, J. D., and Bannon, Y. (2013). Self-rated driving habits among older adults with clinically-defined mild cognitive impairment, clinically-defined dementia and normal cognition. *Accid. Anal. Prev.* 61, 197–202. doi: 10.1016/j.aap.2013.05.010

O'Connor, M. L., Edwards, J. D., Wadley, V. G., and Crowe, M. (2010). Changes in mobility among older adults with psychometrically defined mild cognitive impairment. *J. Gerontol. B Psychol. Sci. Soc. Sci.* 65B, 306–316. doi: 10.1093/geronb/gbq003

Olsen, K., Taylor, J.-P., and Thomas, A. (2014). Mild cognitive impairment: safe to drive? *Maturitas* 78, 82–85. doi: 10.1016/j.maturitas.2014.03.004

Oosterman, J. M., Vogels, R. L. C., van Harten, B., Gouw, A. A., Scheltens, P., Poggesi, A., et al. (2008). The role of white matter hyperintensities and medial temporal lobe atrophy in age-related executive dysfunctioning. *Brain Cogn.* 68, 128–133. doi: 10.1016/j.bandc.2008.03.006

Owsley, C., Stalvey, B., Wells, J., and Sloane, M. E. (1999). Older drivers and cataract: driving habits and crash risk. *J. Gerontol. A Biol. Sci. Med. Sci.* 54, M203–M211. doi: 10.1093/gerona/54.4.m203

Pavlou, D., Beratis, I., Papadimitriou, E., Antoniou, C., Yannis, G., and Papageorgiou, S. (2016). Which are the critical measures to assess the driving performance of drivers with brain pathologies? *Transp. Res. Procedia* 14, 4393–4402. doi: 10.1016/j.trpro.2016.05.361

Petersen, R. C. (2004). Mild cognitive impairment as a diagnostic entity. *J. Intern. Med.* 256, 183–194. doi: 10.1111/j.1365-2796.2004.01388.x

Porter, M. M., Smith, G. A., Cull, A. W., Myers, A. M., Bédard, M., Gélinas, I., et al. (2015). Older driver estimates of driving exposure compared to in-vehicle data in the Candrive II study. *Traffic InJ. Prev.* 16, 24–27. doi: 10.1080/15389588.2014.894995

Rizzo, M., McGehee, D. V., Dawson, J. D., and Anderson, S. N. (2001). Simulated car crashes at intersections in drivers with Alzheimer disease. *Alzheimer Dis. Assoc. Disord.* 15, 10–20. doi: 10.1097/00002093-200101000-00002

Romoser, M. R. E. (2013). The long-term effects of active training strategies on improving older drivers' scanning in intersections: a two-year follow-up to Romoser and Fisher (2009). *Hum. Factors* 55, 278–284. doi: 10.1177/0018720812457566

Romoser, M. R. E., and Fisher, D. L. (2009). The effect of active versus passive training strategies on improving older drivers' scanning in intersections. *Hum. Factors* 51, 652–668. doi: 10.1177/0018720809352654

Rose, M., Haider, H., Salari, N., and Büchel, C. (2011). Functional dissociation of hippocampal mechanism during implicit learning based on the domain of associations. *J. Neurosci.* 31, 13739–13745. doi: 10.1523/JNEUROSCI.3020-11.2011

Schmidt, R. A., and Bjork, R. (1992). New conceptualizations of practice: common principles in three paradigms suggest new concepts for training. *Psychol. Sci.* 3, 207–217. doi: 10.1111/j.1467-9280.1992.tb00029.x

Shechtman, O., Classen, S., Awadzi, K., and Mann, W. (2009). Comparison of driving errors between on-the-road and simulated driving assessment: a validation study. *Traffic InJ. Prev.* 10, 379–385. doi: 10.1080/15389580902894989

Silverstein, N. M. (2008). Alzheimer's disease and fitness to drive. AAA Foundation for Traffic Safety Conference. (Consulted November 1, 2014). Available online at: http://trid.trb.org/view.aspx?id=864024

Simon, S. S., Yokomizo, J. E., and Bottino, C. M. C. (2012). Cognitive intervention in amnestic mild cognitive impairment: a systematic review. *Neurosci. Biobehav. Rev.* 36, 1163–1178. doi: 10.1016/j.neubiorev.2012.01.007

Staplin, L., Gish, K. W., and Wagner, E. K. (2003). MaryPODS revisited: updated crash analysis and implications for screening program implementation. *J. Safety Res.* 34, 389–397. doi: 10.1016/j.jsr.2003.09.002

Teasdale, N., Simoneau, M., Hudon, L., Moszkowicz, T., Laurendeau, D., Germain Robitaille, M., et al. (2016). Drivers with amnestic mild cognitive impairment can benefit from a multiple-session driving simulator automated training program. *J. Am. Geriatr. Soc.* 64, e16–e18. doi: 10.1111/jgs.14219

Tessier, J., Kaszap, M. E., Lavallière, M., Tremblay, M., and Teadale, N. (2009). Implementing an analog speedometer in STISIM Drive using Parallax BSTAMP microcontroller. *Advances in Transportation Studies: An International Journal, Special Issue* 5, 91–96.

Turcotte, M. (2012). Profil des habitudes liées au transport chez les aînés, Statistique Canada (Tendances sociales canadiennes) No 11-008-X.

Uc, E. Y., Rizzo, M., Anderson, S. W., Shi, Q., and Dawson, J. D. (2005). Driver landmark and traffic sign identification in early Alzheimer's disease. *J. Neurol. Neurosurg. Psychiatry* 76, 764–768. doi: 10.1136/jnnp.2004.049338

Unverzagt, F. W., Smith, D. M., Rebok, G. W., Marsiske, M., Morris, J. N., Jones, R., et al. (2009). The Indiana Alzheimer disease center's symposium on mild cognitive impairment. cognitive training in older adults: lessons from the ACTIVE Study. *Curr. Alzheimer Res.* 6, 375–383. doi: 10.2174/156720509788929345

van Halteren-van Tilborg, I. A. D. A., Scherder, E. J. A., and Hulstijn, W. (2007). Motor-skill learning in Alzheimer's disease: a review with an eye to the clinical practice. *Neuropsychol. Rev.* 17, 203–212. doi: 10.1007/s11065-007-9030-1

Vinter, A., and Perruchet, P. (2002). Implicit motor learning through observational training in adults and children. *Mem. Cognit.* 30, 256–261. doi: 10.3758/bf03195286

Wadley, V. G., Okonkwo, O., Crowe, M., Vance, D. E., Elgin, J. M., Ball, K. K., et al. (2009). Mild cognitive impairment and everyday function: an investigation of driving performance. *J. Geriatr. Psychiatry Neurol.* 22, 87–94. doi: 10.1177/0891988708328215

Ward, A., Arrighi, H. M., Michels, S., and Cedarbaum, J. M. (2012). Mild cognitive impairment: disparity of incidence and prevalence estimates. *Alzheimers Dement.* 8, 14–21. doi: 10.1016/j.jalz.2011.01.002

Wheatley, C. J., Carr, D. B., and Marottoli, R. A. (2014). Consensus statements on driving for persons with dementia. *Occup. Ther. Health Care* 28, 132–139. doi: 10.3109/07380577.2014.903583

Willingham, D. B. (1998). A neuropsychological theory of motor skill learning. *Psychol. Rev.* 105, 558–584. doi: 10.1037/0033-295x.105.3.558

Willingham, D. B., and Goedert-Eschmann, K. (1999). The relation between implicit and explicit learning: evidence for parallel development. *Psychol. Sci.* 10, 531–534. doi: 10.1111/1467-9280.00201

Witt, J. K., and Willingham, D. T. (2006). Evidence for separate representations for action and location in implicit motor sequencing. *Psychonom. Bull. Rev.* 13, 902–907. doi: 10.3758/bf03194017

6

Movement-Related Cortical Potential Amplitude Reduction after Cycling Exercise Relates to the Extent of Neuromuscular Fatigue

Jérôme Nicolas Spring[1], Nicolas Place[2], Fabio Borrani[3], Bengt Kayser[2] and Jérôme Barral[1]*

[1] *Institute of Sport Sciences, Faculty of Social and Political Sciences, University of Lausanne, Lausanne, Switzerland,* [2] *Institute of Sport Sciences and Department of Physiology, Faculty of Biology and Medicine, University of Lausanne, Lausanne, Switzerland,* [3] *Institute of Sport Sciences, Faculty of Biology and Medicine, University of Lausanne, Lausanne, Switzerland*

Edited by:
Claudia Voelcker-Rehage, Technische Universität Chemnitz, Germany

Reviewed by:
Marika Berchicci, University of Rome "Foro Italico" - Rome, Italy
Sahil Bajaj, The Houston Methodist Research Institute, USA

***Correspondence:**
Jérôme Nicolas Spring
jerome.spring@unil.ch

Exercise-induced fatigue affects the motor control and the ability to generate a given force or power. Surface electroencephalography allows researchers to investigate movement-related cortical potentials (MRCP), which reflect preparatory brain activity 1.5 s before movement onset. Although the MRCP amplitude appears to increase after repetitive single-joint contractions, the effects of large-muscle group dynamic exercise on such pre-motor potential remain to be described. Sixteen volunteers exercised 30 min at 60% of the maximal aerobic power on a cycle ergometer, followed by a 10-km all-out time trial. Before and after each of these tasks, knee extensor neuromuscular function was investigated using maximal voluntary contractions (MVC) combined with electrical stimulations of the femoral nerve. MRCP was recorded during 60 knee extensions after each neuromuscular sequence. The exercise resulted in a significant decrease in the knee extensor MVC force after the 30-min exercise ($-10 \pm 8\%$) and the time trial ($-21 \pm 9\%$). The voluntary activation level (VAL; -6 ± 8 and $-12 \pm 10\%$), peak twitch (Pt; -21 ± 16 and $-32 \pm 17\%$), and paired stimuli (P100 Hz; -7 ± 11 and $-12 \pm 13\%$) were also significantly reduced after the 30-min exercise and the time trial. The first exercise was followed by a decrease in the MRCP, mainly above the mean activity measured at electrodes FC1-FC2, whereas the reduction observed after the time trial was related to the FC1-FC2 and C2 electrodes. After both exercises, the reduction in the late MRCP component above FC1-FC2 was significantly correlated with the reduction in P100 Hz ($r = 0.61$), and the reduction in the same component above C2 was significantly correlated with the reduction in VAL ($r = 0.64$). In conclusion, large-muscle group exercise induced a reduction in pre-motor potential, which was related to muscle alterations and resulted in the inability to produce a maximal voluntary contraction.

Keywords: EEG, fatigue, *Bereitschaftspotential*, peripheral nerve stimulation, maximal voluntary contraction

INTRODUCTION

Prolonged exercise increases the difficulty to perform voluntary motor actions by altering motor control or the capacity to sustain an ongoing effort or to generate maximal force or power (Allen et al., 1995; Jaric et al., 1997, 1999; Gandevia, 2001; Bottas et al., 2004) in other words, fatigue develops. Exercise-induced muscle fatigue can be defined as a reduction in the maximal voluntary contraction force (MVC; Gandevia, 2001) and can be related to alterations occurring at different sites along the motor pathway, from the cortex to the muscle fiber. It is typical to distinguish between the central factors located before the neuromuscular junction (central fatigue), which refers to the neural activity that drives the muscle, and the peripheral factors located after the motor plate at the muscle level (peripheral fatigue).

Standardized investigative methods for examining neuromuscular function, such as peripheral nerve stimulation or transcranial magnetic stimulation, have been extensively used to explore the complex relationship between exercise and fatigue (Gandevia, 2001; Taylor et al., 2006; Barry and Enoka, 2007). Peripheral nerve stimulation provides relevant information about muscular properties such as excitation-contraction coupling. This method also allows for the quantification of suboptimal motor drive for force production by the twitch interpolation technique (Merton, 1954). However, peripheral nerve stimulation alone remains ineffective for differentiating between supraspinal and spinal adaptations. Transcranial magnetic stimulation is an alternative stimulation method that consists in applying an electromagnetic field above the motor cortex and/or the cervicomedullary junction, to evoke motor evoked potentials, and as such transcranial magnetic stimulation provides information about changes in corticospinal excitability/inhibition (Goodall et al., 2012). By combining transcranial magnetic stimulation and peripheral nerve stimulation, it is possible to assess the neuromuscular pathway and to gain insight into potential site(s) of impairment during or following exercise (Gruet et al., 2014).

Because any voluntary physical effort begins and ends in the brain (Kayser, 2003), voluntary contraction is not limited by the motor command *per se* but also by processes upstream from the motor cortex that might limit motor drive and thus contribute to central fatigue (Gruet et al., 2013). Indeed, during voluntary movement, cortical and subcortical regions are involved in the final motor output (Ball et al., 1999; Shibasaki, 2012; Tanaka and Watanabe, 2012). For example, peripheral afferents send projections to the cingulate anterior cortex, the premotor area, the lateral prefrontal cortex and the orbitofrontal cortex (Liu et al., 2002; Liu, 2003; Hilty et al., 2011a; Robertson and Marino, 2016) and thereby participate in modulating motivational and executive processes. Hence, the brain integrates the internal state and the perceptual information to finally modulate the motor output.

Electroencephalography (EEG) appears to be a relevant method for investigating exercise-induced changes in brain activity, particularly because it reflects the spontaneous and immediate activity of neural networks from a wide range of brain systems. During voluntary muscle contraction tasks, EEG allows for investigation of the spontaneous cortical activity related to movement production. The movement-related cortical potential (MRCP) is an event-related potential locked to the onset of movement (Shibasaki and Hallett, 2006). It reflects the preparatory brain activity, taking into account the time factor. First described by Kornhuber and Deecke; (1965a, b) as the *Bereitschaftspotential*, this EEG pattern is characterized by a slow negative shift, starting ~2 s before movement, and reflects neural processes involved in preparing the motor command. The MRCP is composed of two main components, distinguished by their change in slopes occurring ~500 ms before movement onset (Deecke, 1996; Shibasaki and Hallett, 2006). The first component (BP: Bereitschaftspotential) has a moderate steepness and is bilaterally distributed at the fronto-central midline above the supplementary motor area (SMA). BP occurs between 1500 and 500 ms before movement onset. The second component (NS′: negative slope) is contralateral dominant, more pronounced above the primary motor cortex (M1) and occurs between 500 ms before movement onset and movement onset. Within NS′, the motor potential (MP) is observed at movement onset and corresponds to the MRCP peak amplitude.

Performing voluntary movement implies dynamic processes that involve multiple areas within the brain, likely with overlapping activities. At present, there is a divergence in opinion regarding whether the MRCP components reflect different processes (Jahanshahi and Hallett, 2012). Nevertheless, the identification of the generators of MRCP and their related intracortical connections suggest different stages in the movement-generating procedure. The main generator of MRCP is not limited to the primary motor cortex; the pre-SMA, SMA, and cingulate cortex have a major contribution (Jahanshahi and Hallett, 2012). The activity of additional subcortical structures, such as the thalamus, the caudate, the putamen, and the pallidum also participate in scalp surface-recorded activity and cannot be excluded. By manipulating motor preparation with specific tasks, neuroimaging studies have shown increased activity in the SMA in self-generated movement, compared with movements directed by external cues (Deiber et al., 1991, 1996; Jenkins et al., 2000). Some evidence supports sequential activation within this neural network, in which the SMA has a driving effect on M1 (Herz et al., 2012). Thus, we can assume that the early MRCP generated above the SMA represents the cognitive process related to the decision to perform a movement and the preparation, whereas the late MRCP recorded above the primary motor cortex is more likely to represent the motor part of movement production (Arai et al., 2012; Hoffstaedter et al., 2013). Although the functional distinction between components is still unclear, their segmentation helps to differentiate the processes related to movement planning from motor execution.

The MRCP is obtained by repeated single-joint contractions protocols. Some studies have reported that repetitions of the same movement are accompanied by an increase in MRCP amplitude (Johnston et al., 2001; Schillings et al., 2006; Morree et al., 2012), which has been interpreted as a way to compensate for peripheral fatigue, whereas others have reported no modifications (Siemionow et al., 2004; Liu et al., 2005). Schillings et al. (2006) observed an increase in MRCP after handgrip contractions, but did not find any correlation between MRCP modulations and the reduction in force or with any peripheral fatigue parameters. The authors postulated that the increase in the motor cortical activity compensated for a reduction in central efficiency. In their study, Freude and Ullsperger (1987) asked participants to perform self-paced contractions for 30 min (i.e., 150–250 contractions) at 20, 50, and 80% of their MVC. MRCP increased when fatigue developed during exercise at 20 and 80% of MVC but decreased when the contractions were performed in the absence of fatigue at 50% of MVC. The increase in MRCP amplitude was interpreted differently according to the intensity of effort. At 80% of MVC, the results suggested an increase in cortical activation to compensate for peripheral fatigue, whereas at 20% of MVC, they indicated the high degree of concentration and attention required to properly perform the task. Conversely, at 50% of MVC, the reduction in MRCP was interpreted as a decrease in intentional involvement because of task monotony. More recently, Berchicci et al. (2013) investigated simultaneously MRCP, perception of effort, muscle twitch force and EMG activity. Eighteen subjects performed four blocks of isometric knee extension at 40% of MVC (240 2 s long contractions). After averaging the early (block 1–2) and late blocks (block 3–4), the authors performed a cluster analysis to create two groups based on the rating of perceived exertion (RPE) and the peripheral fatigue (muscle twitch force loss). MRCP increased in the group with higher RPE and in the group with greater peripheral fatigue. They also observed higher positive activity in the prefrontal cortex in the group with greater RPE. According to the authors, the protocol used required high cognitive effort to properly perform the task, which could explain the frontal positivity. In summary, MRCP modulations appear to be related to global exercise-induced fatigue, not only to peripheral fatigue. Some factors might influence the modulations of the pre-motor potential, such as the cognitive load and the perceived effort (Freude and Ullsperger, 1987; Slobounov et al., 2004).

The present study is the first to investigate the effects of an acute endurance exercise on a motor task (voluntary knee extensions) by combining pre-motor brain activity and neuromuscular measurements. Our strategy was to use a specific fatigue-generating procedure, different from the task used to quantify MRCP changes, to avoid bias from additional and unwanted mental weariness. We asked our subjects to perform a large-muscle-group exercise (cycling) and to participate in a specific MRCP task (repeated knee extension; before and after cycling) to quantify the changes induced by the fatiguing exercise. The aim of the study as two-fold: (1) to assess the effect of cycling exercise intensity (heavy and severe) on MRCP modulations and (2) to relate the exercise-induced MRCP modulations to the extent of central and peripheral fatigue. We hypothesized that large-muscle-group exercise would induce neuromuscular fatigue and an increase in MRCP amplitude above the premotor and motor area.

MATERIALS AND METHODS

Participants

Twenty well-trained male athletes were enrolled in the study after having been informed of the experimental procedure. All the participants completed the Baecke questionnaire to ensure that they were physically active (Baecke et al., 1982). The protocol was approved by the local ethics committee (CERVD: protocol 153/14) and was in agreement with the Declaration of Helsinki. Each subject provided written consent before participation.

Experimental Protocol

The volunteers visited the laboratory on two occasions, for the pre-participation session and for the experimental session. During the pre-participation session, preliminary medical screening confirmed that participants were in good health and had no disorders that could interfere with the experimental procedure. Upon inclusion, they performed a maximal ramp exercise protocol on a cycle ergometer (Lode Excalibur Sport, Groningen, the Netherlands) to measure the first ventilatory threshold (SV_1), peak oxygen consumption ($\dot{V}O_2$ *peak*), and maximal aerobic power (MAP). The participants warmed up for 6 min at 60 W, after which power was incremented by 30 W/min until voluntary exhaustion. Maximality was considered to have been reached when at least three of the following criteria were met: $\dot{V}O_2$ plateau; respiratory quotient (QR) >1.1; maximal heart rate (HR_{max}) >90% of theoretical HR_{max} (i.e., 220-age); or a pedaling rate below 60 rotations per minute despite strong verbal encouragement.

The experimental session occurred within 4 weeks after the pre-participation session. The volunteers were instructed to maintain their usual diet and to avoid severe exercise the day before. They had to avoid alcohol and caffeine consumption over the 12 h preceding the session. The last meal had to be taken at least 2.5 h before the beginning of the test, and water was provided *ad libitum* during the experimental session.

The protocol consisted of heavy exercise, followed 15 min later by severe exercise (**Figure 1**). The heavy exercise consisted in pedaling at a freely chosen cadence on a cycle ergometer (Lode Excalibur Sport, Groningen, the Netherlands) for 30 min at an intensity of ~60% of MAP. The severe exercise was a 10-km all-out time trial (TT) performed on a road bike with the rear wheel mounted on a home trainer (CycleOps, Madison, USA). The objective was to complete the distance as fast as possible, with the distance displayed on a bike computer fixed to the handlebar. The resistance of the roller increased automatically with the force exerted by the cyclist to reproduce field-like sensations. A fan was placed in front of the subject to avoid excessive sweating, and the wind speed was adjusted upon request. A power meter in the rear hub (PowerTap, CycloOps, Madison, USA) allowed the power output to be recorded. Perceived exertion was assessed with the 6–20 Borg scale at the end of the heavy exercise and the TT. Knee extensor neuromuscular function was investigated through the quantification of several parameters. The MVC represents the maximum force that a subject could produce in the isometric knee exercise. The voluntary activation level (VAL) was chosen

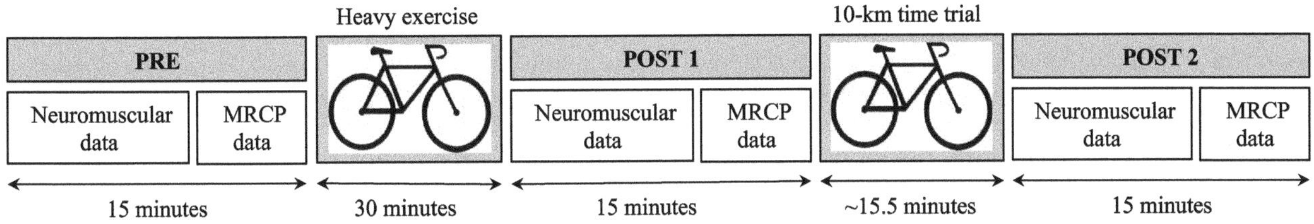

FIGURE 1 | Experimental session design and timeline. PRE, pre-exercise condition; POST1, post-heavy exercise condition; POST2, post-time trial condition; MRCP, movement-related cortical potential.

as an index of central fatigue and is believed to reflect the ability of the motor cortex to drive muscle. The M-wave was recorded to explore neuromuscular transmission/propagation. The paired stimuli force at 100 Hz (P100 Hz) and the muscle twitch force (Pt) reflected the muscle properties and were both chosen as indices of peripheral fatigue. Neuromuscular data were collected before the fatiguing task (PRE), immediately after the 30-min exercise (POST1) and immediately after the 10-km TT (POST2). The MRCP data were recorded after each neuromuscular assessment for these three time points.

Neuromuscular Data Collection

Neuromuscular Assessment

The session began with a warm-up of 10 submaximal voluntary isometric knee extensor contractions (4–5 s) between 20 and 90% of the estimated MVC. After a short recovery period, the participants performed two MVCs (4 s duration) with the right leg, separated by a 1-min rest period. For both trials, P100 Hz were delivered at maximal force, followed by a P100 Hz and a Pt in 2-s intervals.

Evoked Contractions

A constant-current stimulator (DS7AH, Digitimer, Hertfordshire, UK) was used to deliver electrical pulses. The cathode (5 cm diameter) and the anode (5 × 10 cm, Dermatrode, American Imex Irvine, CA) were placed over the femoral nerve at the femoral triangle level below the inguinal ligament and on the lower part of the gluteal fold opposite the cathode, respectively. The optimal intensity for electrical stimulation was determined after the warm-up period by progressively increasing the stimulus intensity in 10-mA increments until there was no further increase in the amplitude of the mechanical or electrical (M-wave) responses. A 20% supplementary increment was added to ensure supramaximal stimulation intensity (Neyroud et al., 2013).

Force Recording

Voluntary and evoked force exerted by the right knee extensors were recorded using an isometric ergometer consisting of a custom-built chair equipped with a strain gauge (Universal Load Cell, model 9363-C3, linear range 0–250 N•m, output sensitivity 2.0 mV•V^{-1}, Vishay, Malvern, US). The calibrated strain gauge was fixed to the chair and strapped to the ankle with a custom-made mold. Subjects were seated with a 90-degree knee angle, the trunk was attached at a 100° angle to the chair back panel with a harness belt, and the arms had to be crossed on the chest to minimize upper body movement. The force signal was recorded at 1 kHz using an AD converter system (MP 150, BIOPAC Systems, Goleta, CA).

EMG Recording

The EMG activity of the right vastus lateralis (VL) was recorded with a pair of silver chloride (Ag/AgCl) circular (1 cm) surface electrodes (MediTrace 100, Kendall, Canada) positioned lengthwise over the middle of the muscle belly according to SENIAM recommendations (Hermens et al., 2000); the inter-electrode distance was 2 cm. The reference electrode was placed over the patella. The VL was chosen as representative of quadriceps muscle activity (Place et al., 2007). Low resistance (<5 kΩ) was obtained by shaving, abrading and cleaning the skin. EMG signals were amplified (gain = 1000) over a frequency bandwidth of 10–500 Hz and digitized at a sampling frequency of 2 kHz using an AD converter system. Force and EMG data were analyzed offline using the software Acknowledge (Biopac System, Santa Barbara CA, USA).

MRCP Data Collection

EEG Recording

Continuous EEG was recorded at a sampling rate of 2048 Hz with a 64-channel Biosemi Active two-amplifier system (Biosemi, Amsterdam, the Netherlands) mounted according to the 10–20 International System. All channels were referenced to the CMS-DRL ground, which functioned as a feedback loop driving the average potential across the montage as close as possible to amplifier zero (Biosemi, Amsterdam, the Netherlands). Impedance was kept below 5 kΩ by using conducting gel. Participants wore the EEG cap during the entire protocol. Post-exercise recordings started 5.5 ± 0.5 min after the end of the heavy exercise and the TT, and lasted 10 min. Offline analyses were performed with BrainVision analyzer software (Brain Products Gmbh, Munich, Germany).

The MRCP data were collected using the same ergometer device used for neuromuscular assessment. To avoid any unknown disturbances induced by the neuromuscular stimulation, the other leg was used for the MRCP task. A string attached to the left ankle ran over a pulley to a free-hanging weighted platform. The subjects were instructed to lift this weight 60 times, equivalent of 20% of their MVC force, by ~10 cm. The contraction duration was not strictly controlled, but participants were instructed to produce a 2-s contraction: a 1-s concentric contraction to lift the weight, and 1-s eccentric contraction to put it down (metronome). The onset of movement was automatically reported on the EEG recording by the release of a trigger placed behind the heel of the subjects. The contractions were self-generated, but to ensure that the duration of the task was identical for each participant in each condition, a beep sounded every 10 s. The participants were instructed to perform the contraction spontaneously between two beeps. The subjects were also instructed to keep their eyes closed during the task to avoid excessive attentional load and artifacts generated by visual feedback.

Data Analysis

Gas Exchange

Breath-by-breath pulmonary gas-exchange data were collected during the maximal ramp test with a metabolic cart (OxyconPro, Jaeger, Germany) and averaged over consecutive 10-s period. The $\dot{V}O_2$ *peak* was taken as the highest value attained during the last 30 s before the subject's volitional exhaustion. SV_1 was determined from the combination of different measurements, including the first disproportionate increase in $\dot{V}CO_2$ from visual inspection of individual plots of $\dot{V}CO_2$ vs $\dot{V}O_2$, an increase in expired ventilation $\dot{V}E/\dot{V}O_2$ with no increase in $\dot{V}E/\dot{V}CO_2$, and an increase in end-tidal O_2 tension with no fall in end-tidal CO_2 tension. The intensity for the 30-min exercise was obtained by adding 20% of the difference between SV_1 and MAP to the power reached at SV_1.

Force Data

MVC force of the knee extensors was reported as the force produced during the maximal voluntary contractions (i.e., peak to peak). Resting P100 Hz and Pt amplitude were analyzed for the trials yielding the highest MVC. The VAL during MVCs was estimated with the superimposed and the potentiated doublets according to the formula proposed by Strojnik and Komi (1998).

$$VAL = \left(1 - \left(superimposed\ 100\ Hz\ doublet\ force \times \left(force\ level\ at\ stimulation\ /MVC\ force\right)\ / \ superimposed\ 100\ Hz\ doublet\ force\right)\right) \times 100$$

EMG Data

The EMG signals recorded during the highest MVC were used for analysis. M-wave peak-to-peak amplitude was measured from the EMG response after the single stimulation.

MRCP Data

The raw EEG data were first down-sampled from 2048 to 512 Hz to reduce computational load and band-pass filtered from 0.1 to 5 Hz. The low-pass filter was set at 5 Hz (Thacker et al., 2014) to avoid bias for alpha rhythm induced by the eyes-closed procedure and to avoid unwanted activity generated by spontaneous physiological and rolandic *mu* rhythms. EEG signals were segmented into 60 epochs of 3000 ms each (from 2500 ms before movement onset to 500 ms after movement onset). All trials were baseline-corrected with −2500 ms to −2000 ms as a reference and averaged using a semi-automatic artifact rejection procedure with a ±80 μV criterion. Artifacted electrodes were interpolated when necessary with a spherical 3D spline, and trials containing periods of muscular artifacts were also rejected. On average, 53 ± 9, 52 ± 11, and 52 ± 9 of 60 trials were available for analysis for the PRE, POST1, and POST2 conditions, respectively. The MRCPs were segmented into four sequential components (Shibasaki and Hallett, 2006; Jahanshahi and Hallett, 2012). The *Bereitschaftspotential* was divided into BP1 and BP2. The BP1 corresponds to the average amplitude between −1500 and −1000 ms. The BP2 corresponds to the average amplitude between −1000 and −500 ms. The third component was the negative slope (NS′), which corresponds to the average amplitude from −500 ms to the onset of movement. The last component was the motor potential (MP), taken as the maximal peak amplitude recorded between −500 ms and movement onset. Those components were calculated for two regions of interest. The first region corresponded to the mean activity of the FC1 and FC2 electrodes and the second region was the mean activity above the C2 electrode. Those electrodes were chosen because they correspond to the area known to generate MRCP, namely the SMA (represented by FC1-FC2 mean activity) for the first part of MRCP and the primary motor cortex (M1; represented by C2 activity) for the late part of MRCP (Shibasaki and Hallett, 2006).

Statistical Analysis

One-way repeated measures ANOVAs with factor Time were used to compare the neuromuscular and MRCP variables between the different times of measurement (PRE, POST1, and POST2, respectively). When ANOVA revealed significant interactions, pairwise contrasts were performed using the Bonferroni correction. Friedman ANOVAs with follow-up Wilcoxon signed rank tests were used in a few cases in which conditions for using parametric tests were not reached. To better understand the mechanisms responsible for the MVC loss, we performed Pearson correlation analyses by using the deltas between PRE-POST1 and PRE-POST2 on the factor MVC explained by VAL and P100 Hz.

Because of the non-normal distributions of EEG variables, Spearman correlations were used to explore the relationship between neuromuscular and MRCP modulations. The three neuromuscular parameters used for the correlation analyses were the reduction in MVC, VAL, and P100 Hz, which were chosen as global, central and peripheral indices of fatigue, respectively. Those parameters were correlated with the four MRCP components modulations (i.e., BP1, BP2, NS′, MP) at the FC1-FC2 and C2 electrodes. All statistical analyses were performed using the software Statistica 12.6 (Statsoft, Tulsa, USA). The level of significance was set to $p < 0.05$. The results are presented as mean ± standard deviation.

RESULTS

Participants

Data from four of the original 20 recruited participants had to be excluded because of heavily artifacted EEG signals. The mean age of the 16 remaining participants was 29 ± 7 (years ± SD), and their body mass index was 22.9 ± 1.6 (kg•m^{-2}). All of them were active road cyclists and/or triathlon athletes, had a total score of 9.2 ± 0.7 on the Baecke questionnaire, and reached a MAP of 385 ± 47 W at a $\dot{V}O_2$ *peak* of 63.8 ± 5.9 ml•min^{-1}•kg^{-1} during the incremental cycling test.

Exercise Data

The mean power output during the 30-min exercise was 231 ± 97 W. The mean duration for the TT was 15.7 ± 1.6 min and the average power was 279 ± 31 W. The RPE was 14.9 ± 1.7 at the end of the heavy exercise, whereas the RPE reached 19.7 ± 0.5 at the end of the TT.

Neuromuscular Data

Force

The sequence of the two cycling exercises caused a significant reduction in the MVC force measured at POST1 and POST2 [$F_{(2, 30)} = 55.34$, $p < 0.001$; **Table 1**]. **Figure 2** shows two representative recordings of a superimposed MVC with a 100 Hz-potentiated doublet in the PRE (A) and POST2 (B) conditions.

Peripheral and Central Fatigue

The peripheral indices of fatigue measured by the Pt force and P100 Hz were significantly reduced [$F_{(2, 30)} = 36.95$, $p < 0.001$ and Chi^2 ($N = 16$, df = 2) = 6.5, $p = 0.039$], respectively after POST1 and POST2 (**Table 1**). For the M-wave amplitude, Friedman ANOVA revealed a significant effect of Time [Chi^2 ($N = 16$, df = 2) = 9.5, $p = 0.008$]. However, although no reduction was observed between PRE and POST1 ($p = 0.3$), the difference in the M-wave amplitude between PRE and POST2 was significant ($p = 0.007$). Concerning central fatigue, a Time effect [$F_{(2, 30)} = 14.21$, $p < 0.001$] was observed for VAL. For all the significant main Time effects, *post-hoc* tests revealed a significant difference between PRE and POST1 (except for M-wave) and between PRE and POST2 (All $p < 0.033$; **Table 1**).

Correlations

At POST1, Pearson correlation analysis showed a trend toward a relationship between the reduction in MVC force and the reduction in P100 Hz ($r = 0.44$, $p = 0.08$), but without reaching the level of significance. No relationship was found between MVC and VAL reduction ($r = 0.32$, $p = 0.22$). At POST2, the results indicated no significant relationship between the decrease in MVC and P100 Hz ($r = 0.27$, $p = 0.3$), whereas a positive relationship was found between the reduction in MVC and VAL ($r = 0.5$, $p = 0.047$).

MRCP Data

The MRCP grand averages between the PRE, POST1, and POST2 conditions at FC1-FC2 and C2 are shown in **Figures 3A,B**. The common MRCP shape can be observed, with a typical increase in slope at ~1000 and 500 ms before movement onset.

Mean Activity at FC1-FC2

ANOVA revealed an effect of Time for FC1-FC2 mean activity for the components BP1 [$F_{(2, 30)} = 3.93$, $p = 0.03$], BP2

TABLE 1 | Neuromuscular indices of central and peripheral fatigue measured before the fatiguing task (PRE), after the heavy exercise (POST1), and after the 10-km time trial (POST2).

	PRE	POST1		POST2	
	Mean ± SD	**Mean ± SD**	**Δ PRE % ± SD**	**Mean ± SD**	**Δ PRE % ± SD**
MVC (N)	306 ± 54	276 ± 55**	−10 ± 8	244 ± 51**	−21 ± 9
VAL (%)	90.9 ± 5.1	85.6 ± 9.5*	−5.9 ± 8.4	80.5 ± 11.5**	−11.6 ± 10.4
Pt (N)	93.3 ± 21.3	72.7 ± 19.4**	−20.9 ± 15.8	61.2 ± 14.2**	−32.4 ± 16.7
P100 Hz (N)	132.7 ± 30.1	122.6 ± 28.8**	−6.9 ± 10.69	116.5 ± 30.9**	−12.1 ± 13.2
M-wave (mV)	4.8 ± 2.3	4.6 ± 2.3	−3.9 ± 15.2	4.3 ± 2.3**	−10 ± 15.5

*MVC, maximal voluntary contraction; VAL, voluntary activation level with reference to the 100 Hz resting peak doublet. Pt, muscle twitch; P100 Hz, resting peak doublet at 100 Hz; M-wave, peak to peak M-wave amplitude. Δ PRE, percentage of difference from PRE. Significant differences from PRE: *p < 0.05; **p < 0.01.*

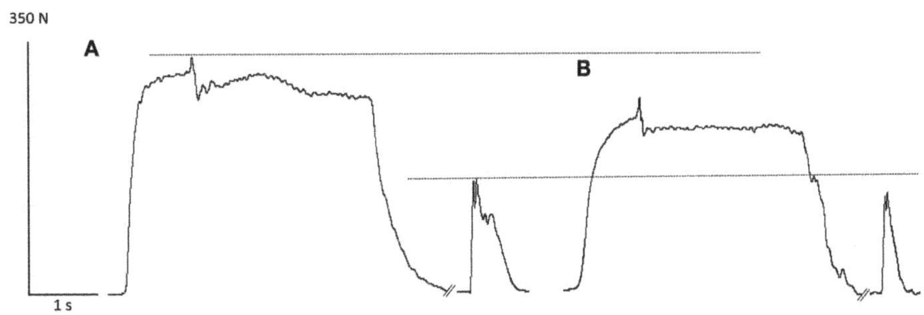

FIGURE 2 | Representative recordings of a superimposed maximal voluntary contraction with a 100 Hz-potentiated doublet in the PRE (A) and POST2 (B) conditions. Note the decrease in MVC force and P100 Hz after the completion of the two fatiguing exercises.

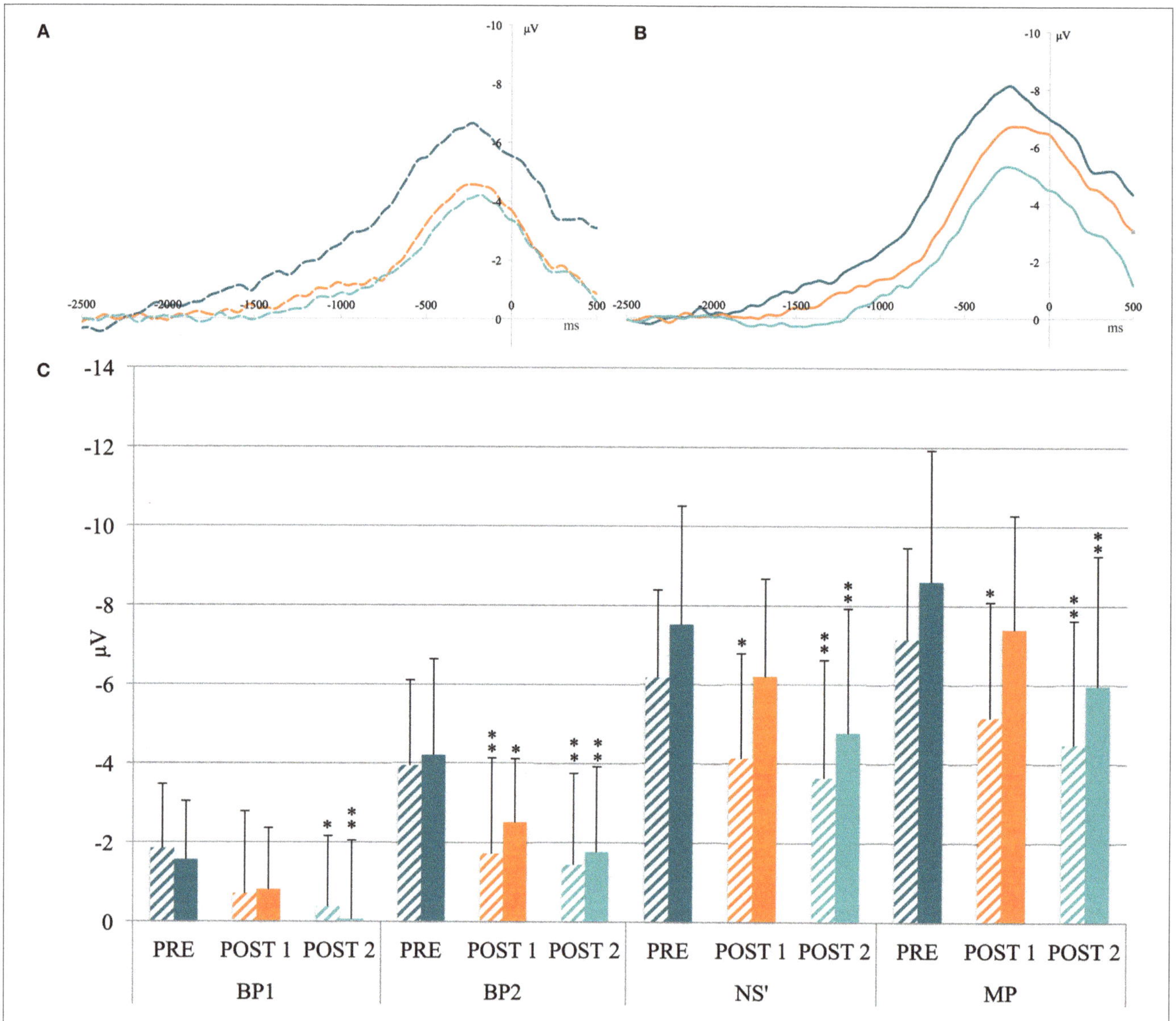

FIGURE 3 | (A) Grand MRCP average recorded above the FC1-FC2 (i.e., above supplementary motor area) and **(B)** C2 electrodes (i.e., above primary motor cortex) in the pre-exercise condition (dark blue curve), after the heavy exercise (orange curve) and after the 10-km time trial (light blue curve). X-axis units: time in milliseconds locked to the movement onset. Y-axis units: amplitude in microvolts. **(C)** Mean activity of movement-related cortical potential components measured before the cycling task (PRE), after the heavy exercise (POST1), and after the 10-km time trial (POST2) on the FC1-FC2 electrodes (shaded column) and the C2 electrode (filled column). BP1, mean activity from −1500 to −1000 ms; BP2, mean activity from −1000 to −500 ms; NS', mean activity from −500 ms to movement onset; MP, peak amplitude. Significant differences from PRE: *$p < 0.05$; **$p < 0.01$.

[$F_{(2, 30)} = 7.73, p = 0.019$], NS′ [$F_{(2, 30)} = 7.17, p = 0.003$], and MP [$F_{(2, 30)} = 7.39, p = 0.002$; **Figure 3C**]. The *post-hoc* tests indicated a significant reduction between PRE and POST1 for BP2 ($p = 0.007$), NS′ ($p = 0.012$), and MP ($p = 0.016$). At POST2, the reduction was significant for the four MRCP components (All $p < 0.04$; **Figure 3C**).

Mean Activity at C2

ANOVA revealed a Time effect on the C2 mean activity for the component BP1 [$F_{(2, 30)} = 4.91, p = 0.014$], BP2 [$F_{(2, 30)} = 8.83, p < 0.001$], NS′ [$F_{(2, 30)} = 9.14, p < 0.001$], and MP [$F_{(2, 30)} = 8.43, p = 0.001$]. The *post-hoc* tests indicated a significant decrease between PRE and POST1 only for B2 ($p = 0.01$), whereas the reduction was significant for the four components between PRE and POST2 (all $p < 0.012$; **Figure 3C**).

Neuromuscular and MRCP Correlations

Bonferroni *post-hoc* tests revealed significant changes for the MRCP components between PRE-POST1 and between PRE-POST2 conditions, whereas no changes were observed between POST1 and POST2 (see **Figure 3**). Therefore, the correlation analyses between MRCP and neuromuscular modulations were based solely on the PRE-POST1 and PRE-POST2 differences.

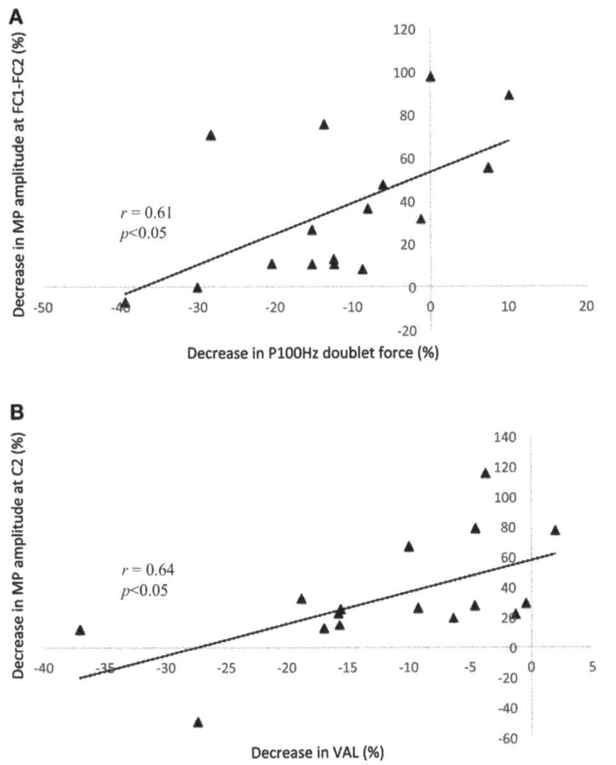

FIGURE 4 | Correlation analyses between the P100 Hz doublet force and the motor potential above the C2 electrode (A) and between the voluntary activation level and the decrease in the motor potential above the FC1-FC2 electrodes (B). Both correlations are based on the differences between the PRE and POST2 conditions. Note that the pre-motor potential is a negative value, and thus, a reduction in the amplitude represents a change toward zero (i.e., the value becomes less negative). MP, motor potential; VAL, voluntary activation level.

No correlation was found between PRE and POST1. In contrast, between PRE and POST2, the reduction in P100 Hz was correlated with the decrease in NS′ ($r = 0.61$) and the MP ($r = 0.61$) amplitude above FC1-FC2 (all $p < 0.05$), whereas the reduction in VAL was correlated with the decrease in BP1 ($r = 0.57$), BP2 ($r = 0.65$), NS′ ($r = 0.72$), and MP ($r = 0.64$) above C2 (all $p < 0.05$). The correlations between the reduction in VAL and MP above FC1-FC2 and between the reduction in P100 Hz and MP amplitude above C2 are illustrated in **Figure 4**. Note that the pre-motor potential is a negative value, and thus, a reduction in the amplitude represents a change toward zero (i.e., the value becomes less negative).

DISCUSSION

The current study was designed to induce neuromuscular fatigue by using two successive cycling exercises, at heavy and severe intensities, and to assess the related effects on MRCP. The second aim was to relate the exercise-induced MRCP modulations with neuromuscular alterations. Although the large-muscle-group exercise induced neuromuscular fatigue, the results indicated a reduction in MRCP amplitude instead of an increase as expected. The cycling exercise induced both peripheral alterations (as indicated by the decreased P100 Hz and Pt) and central impairments (as indicated by the reduction in VAL). The exercise intensity difference between the heavy exercise and the TT was indicated by a higher perception of effort and a greater strength loss after the second exercise. After heavy exercise, MRCP was reduced mainly above the FC1-FC2 electrodes, whereas the MRCP reduction observed at the end of the TT was associated with the FC1-FC2 and C2 electrodes. The relationship found between the reduction in the late MRCP components (i.e., NS′, MP) and P100 Hz above FC1-FC2 and with VAL above C2 indicated a close interaction between neuromuscular fatigue and pre-motor brain activity.

Physical Exercise and Neuromuscular Fatigue

An MVC loss of 10% was observed after the heavy exercise. As expected, this reduction was associated with peripheral alterations characterized by a decrease of 20% in Pt force, without changes in the VL M-wave amplitude and with central fatigue, as reflected by the decrease in VAL. Such neuromuscular changes are very similar to those reported by Lepers et al. (2001). After a cycling exercise lasting 30 min at 80% MAP among trained athletes, the authors reported a decrease of 13% in knee extension force, accompanied by a reduction of 20% in the Pt without changes in the M-wave properties, suggesting alteration of processes located beyond action potential propagation/transmission. Such a reduction in Pt force may be related to intracellular disturbances, such as reduced Ca^{2+} release from the sarcoplasmic reticulum, decreased sensitivity of myofilaments to Ca^{2+}, changes in metabolite (H^+, inorganic phosphate) concentrations within the muscle, and/or reduced force produced by each active cross-bridge (Allen et al., 2008). The absence of significant correlations between MVC force loss and central or peripheral markers of fatigue between PRE and POST1 does not allow for a clear determination of the origin of fatigue. However, relying on other studies demonstrating that peripheral fatigue develops early during such exercise (Decorte et al., 2010), we believe that the trend observed between the MVC force loss and the reduction in P100 Hz in POST1 favors a major role for peripheral alterations.

After the severe intensity exercise, knee extensor MVC force was decreased by 21%. This strength loss is comparable to the results of Lepers et al. (2001), who reported a reduction of 16% after 30 min of cycling at 80% of PMA. As at POST1, peripheral and central alterations participated in knee extensor force impairment at POST2. The additional peripheral fatigue (−32% in Pt at POST2 vs. −21% at POST2) can be attributed to alteration in action potential transmission/propagation, as indirectly indicated by the 10% reduction in VL M-wave amplitude at POST2. The finding that the VL M-wave amplitude decreased at POST2 but not at POST1 confirms the results of Lepers et al. (2002, 2004) suggesting that cycling exercise must be of sufficient intensity and duration to affect muscle excitability.

The purpose of performing the 10-km time trial after having previously performed a heavy exercise lasting 30 min at 60% of MAP (i.e., 67% $\dot{V}O_2$ *peak*), with only a 15-min break (i.e., for data collection), was also to generate greater central fatigue. Indeed, VAL was 91% in PRE condition and decreased to 80% at POST2, in accord with the literature (Lepers et al., 2001; Millet and Lepers, 2004). This finding suggests altered CNS functioning leading to a limitation of descending motor drive. Overall, our results indicate that peripheral mechanisms were mainly involved in the development of fatigue at POST1, whereas central fatigue played a major role in force reduction at POST2.

MRCP Data

Before, between and after exercise, we observed MRCPs with a shape and amplitude similar to those reported in the literature (Shibasaki and Hallett, 2006). The MRCPs were characterized by a slow negative shift starting between 1500 and 2000 ms before movement onset, with a typical change in slope occurring at approximately −500 ms (**Figure 3**). Our data indicate that this inflection occurred slightly earlier (around −750 ms), likely because the trigger was set at the onset of movement instead of the onset of EMG activity. Both fatiguing cycling tasks resulted in a decrease in MRCP amplitude recorded during 60 spontaneous knee extensions at 20% of MVC. A long-term effect on brain activity was already reported by Thacker et al. (2014), who showed MRCP modulations 1 h after the end of an endurance exercise. Our results extend these findings by showing that the large-muscle-group exercise led to distinctive changes in the pre-motor potential during the two 15-min periods post-exercise (POST1 and 2) compared with the fresh condition (PRE).

The present findings do not confirm that pre-motor brain activity increases with muscle fatigue, as expected and as previously reported in repeated single-joint contraction protocols. Our study used a dynamic large-muscle-group-fatiguing task quite different from the task used to quantify changes in MRCP. It is therefore difficult to compare our results with those of previous single-joint contractions protocols. Several authors have asked their experimental subjects to perform repetitive blocks of contractions and have compared pre-motor potential amplitudes between the first and the last blocks. In such designs, fatigue is not experimentally manipulated through a specific fatiguing task. Another difference from our design is the potential for mental load. In most studies, participants have had to achieve a given force level during contraction by using visual feedback. A high degree of concentration must be maintained to correctly perform the task throughout the block of repeated contractions. However, it has been suggested that an increase in attentional load and the mobilization of cognitive resources could be a confounding factor resulting in an increase in MRCP amplitude (Freude and Ullsperger, 1987; Berchicci et al., 2013). Another factor to consider is the contraction force level used during the MRCP task. In the studies of Johnston et al. (2001) and Schillings et al. (2006), the MRCP task consisted of contractions at 70% of the MVC. By comparing the premotor potential amplitude between the first and last blocks of contractions, the authors reported an increase in MRCP. According to the authors, this result suggested that the cortical activity compensated for the reduction in strength capacities (i.e., to provide the same level of force, the brain had to mobilize more resources). In the present study, the load lifted during the MRCP task was kept low (20% of MVC force) and additional cortical activation to compensate for peripheral fatigue did not appear to be required. In a similar vein, Morree et al. (2012) did not observe any increase in pre-motor potential after repeated contractions at 20% of MVC force despite a final maximal force loss of 35%.

The difference in the effects on pre-motor potential observed in this study and others (i.e., a reduction in pre-motor vs. an increase, respectively) may arise from the differing fatiguing task features. The effect of single-joint contraction tasks on motor cortex excitability measured by transcranial magnetic stimulation has been reported to be different from the effect observed for locomotor exercises. The excitability of the motor cortex increases after a fatiguing single-joint contraction task, but after a 30-min steady-state sustained cycling exercise, Sidhu et al. (2012) reported no increase in the responsiveness of the motor cortex. Modulation of cortical excitability is likely task-specific and may be related to the systemic physiological consequences of large-muscle-group exercise. The reduction in MRCP could be related to input from group III and IV muscle afferents to the brain. Indeed, fatiguing voluntary contraction lengthens the cortical silent period, as measured by transcranial magnetic stimulation, which is believed to reflect intracortical inhibitory activity (Gruet et al., 2013). However, when the activation of group III and IV muscle afferents are artificially blocked with an anesthetic solution (fentanyl) injection, the cortical silent period is not prolonged, indicating a modulation of intracortical inhibitions (Hilty et al., 2011b). Similarly, maintaining muscle afferent activity at the end of a fatiguing task with ischemia reduces motor cortex output that maximally activates the muscle (Gandevia et al., 1996). More generally, endurance exercise modulates several additional parameters that might play a role in the reduction of the pre-motor potential, such as cerebral oxygenation (Ide and Secher, 2000), brain catecholamines (Nybo and Secher, 2004), or hyperthermia (Périard et al., 2011).

To the best of our knowledge, only one study has investigated MRCP modulations after a large-muscle-group endurance exercise (Thacker et al., 2014). The exercise consisted in pedaling for 20 min at 70% of the age-predicted maximum heart rate on a cycle ergometer. To remove confounding and fatigue factors, the authors used an MRCP task involving the upper limbs (i.e., wrist extension). The results indicated no changes in MRCP amplitude or onset immediately after the end of exercise. We assume that the absence of modification was caused by insufficient exercise intensity or durations and/or because the muscle group used for the MRCP task was different from that mobilized for the fatiguing task.

In our protocol, a reduction in MRCP was observed during movement preparation, initiation, and movement onset, as reflected by the reduction in the BP, NS′, and MP components, respectively. The heavy exercise induced a decrease in MRCP amplitude for the components BP2, NS′, and MP above FC1-FC2, whereas only BP2 decreased significantly above C2. After the TT, all MRCP components decreased significantly from the PRE condition above the FC1-FC2 and C2 electrodes. Our results indicate that heavy exercise affects the MRCP differently if it is recorded above SMA or M1. The SMA is connected to the subcortical region, relays sensory feedback received from the muscle and sends direct signals to the M1 (Dum and Strick, 1991; Cadoret and Smith, 1997; Colebatch, 2007), such that the neurons in the SMA are activated several milliseconds before activity within the pyramidal tract (Eccles, 1982). Thus, it appears that the modulations observed above the SMA are more closely related to the integration of peripheral mechanisms, whereas the modulations above the primary motor cortex are more likely to reflect the cortico-motor command. The positive correlation between the increase in peripheral fatigue measured by P100 Hz and the reduction in MRCP (i.e., NS′ and MP) above the SMA strengthens the assumption that this area may be under the modulatory influence of muscle activity, likely via type III and IV afferents. This assumption is also supported by the studies of Gandevia (2001) and Amann et al. (2011) which showed that type III/IV muscle afferents are likely to exert an inhibitory effect on central motor drive during whole-body exercise.

At POST1, the components related to movement preparation are first altered without affecting the execution period of movement production, as reflected by no differences in NS′ and MP amplitude above M1. When neuromuscular fatigue is more pronounced, as observed at POST2, the components related to movement preparation and execution are both modulated, showing a growing impact of fatigue on all the components involved in movement production. The activation of the corticospinal tract via the primary motor cortex is the final step of movement production. Thus, when exercise-induced fatigue decreases the MP above the SMA and M1, it is possible that the motor cortex does not reach the level of activity required to produce the same level of voluntary activation, resulting in a greater decrease in MVC force, as observed at POST2. The positive correlation between the decrease in VAL and the reduction in MRCP above M1 support this assumption, as well as the positive correlation between the drop in MP amplitude above M1 and the reduction in MVC force. Interestingly, some authors have reported neural plasticity between the SMA and M1. By using transcranial magnetic stimulation, Arai et al. (2012) showed that the motor-evoked potential generated by stimulating M1 can be modulated by an SMA-conditioning stimulation procedure. Recently, Bajaj et al. (2015) also showed that the neural connectivity between the SMA and M1 could be modulated by therapy in stroke survivors. It is not unlikely that the acute fatiguing task performed in our study reorganized the connectivity between the SMA and M1 and that the neural impulses sent from SMA to M1 were reduced under the influence of afferent projections.

The limits of our study concern the factors related to movement characteristics, such as strength, accuracy, or rate of force development, all of which are known to modulate the MRCP (Shibasaki and Hallett, 2006). In our protocol, the range of motion was the same between trials. However, the movement duration was not controlled, and we cannot exclude that the duration between the onset of muscle activity and the onset of movement did not change with fatigue. In addition, the MRCP modulations reported in this study are specific to well-trained athletes and cannot be extended to the general population. Because neuroelectric activity could be related to physical fitness (Kamijo et al., 2010), further studies have to be repeated in different populations to determine the impact of fitness on MRCP, especially after endurance exercises.

In conclusion, the MRCP reflects the intention to move and the preparatory period for the intended movement. The results of our study indicate that a cycling exercise induces peripheral and central fatigue and reduces MRCP amplitude. The MRCP components related to movement planning and initiation above the SMA area first altered by heavy exercise-related fatigue, likely by peripheral muscle activity. When neuromuscular fatigue is substantial, as observed after the TT, the overall reduction in MRCP, especially the reduction in the brain component related to movement execution above the primary motor cortex (i.e., MP), is associated with the reduction in the maximal voluntary level, resulting in a decrease in maximal voluntary force.

Finally, large-muscle-group exercise induces neuromuscular fatigue, resulting in an alteration of the corticospinal command. Because this study indicates that this command is modulated by pre-motor cortical activity, we now suggest taking a step backwards to investigate post-exercise resting state electro-cortical dynamics, from which the intention to move emerges.

AUTHOR CONTRIBUTIONS

JNS, FB, JB: Contributions to the conception of the work. JNS, FB, NP, BK, JB: Contributions the acquisition and interpretation of data. JNS, FB, NP, BK, JB: Revising the content. JNS, FB, NP, BK, JB: Final approval of the version.

REFERENCES

Allen, D. G., Lamb, G. D., and Westerblad, H. (2008). Skeletal muscle fatigue: cellular mechanisms. *Physiol. Rev.* 88, 287–332. doi: 10.1152/physrev.00015.2007

Allen, G. M., Gandevia, S. C., and McKenzie, D. K. (1995). Reliability of measurements of muscle strength and voluntary activation using twitch interpolation. *Muscle Nerve* 18, 593–600. doi: 10.1002/mus.880180605

Amann, M., Blain, G. M., Proctor, L. T., Sebranek, J. J., Pegelow, D. F., and Dempsey, J. A. (2011). Implications of group III and IV muscle afferents for high-intensity endurance exercise performance in humans. *J. Physiol.* 589, 5299–5309. doi: 10.1113/jphysiol.2011.213769

Arai, N., Lu, M.-K., Ugawa, Y., and Ziemann, U. (2012). Effective connectivity between human supplementary motor area and primary motor cortex: a paired-coil TMS study. *Exp. Brain Res.* 220, 79–87. doi: 10.1007/s00221-012-3117-5

Baecke, J. A., Burema, J., and Frijters, J. E. (1982). A short questionnaire for the measurement of habitual physical activity in epidemiological studies. *Am. J. Clin. Nutr.* 36, 936–942.

Bajaj, S., Butler, A. J., Drake, D., and Dhamala, M. (2015). Brain effective connectivity during motor-imagery and execution following stroke and rehabilitation. *Neuroimage Clin.* 8, 572–582. doi: 10.1016/j.nicl.2015.06.006

Ball, T., Schreiber, A., Feige, B., Wagner, M., Lucking, C. H., and Kristeva-Feige, R. (1999). The role of higher-order motor areas in voluntary movement as revealed by high-resolution EEG and fMRI. *Neuroimage* 10, 682–694. doi: 10.1006/nimg.1999.0507

Barry, B. K., and Enoka, R. M. (2007). The neurobiology of muscle fatigue: 15 years later. *Integr. Comp. Biol.* 47, 465–473. doi: 10.1093/icb/icm047

Berchicci, M., Menotti, F., MacAluso, A., and Di Russo, F. (2013). The neurophysiology of central and peripheral fatigue during sub-maximal lower limb isometric contractions. *Front. Hum. Neurosci.* 7:135. doi: 10.3389/fnhum.2013.00135

Bottas, R., Linnamo, V., Nicol, C., and Komi, P. V. (2004). Repeated maximal eccentric actions causes long-lasting disturbances in movement control. *Eur. J. Appl. Physiol.* 94, 62–69. doi: 10.1007/s00421-004-1253-8

Cadoret, G., and Smith, A. M. (1997). Comparison of the neuronal activity in the SMA and the ventral cingulate cortex during prehension in the monkey. *J. Neurophysiol.* 77, 153–166.

Colebatch, J. G. (2007). Bereitschaftspotential and movement-related potentials: origin, significance, and application in disorders of human movement. *Mov. Dis.* 22, 601–610. doi: 10.1002/mds.21323

Decorte, N., Lafaix, P. A., Millet, G. Y., Wuyam, B., and Verges, S. (2010). Central and peripheral fatigue kinetics during exhaustive constant-load cycling. *Scand. J. Med. Sci. Sports* 22, 381–391. doi: 10.1111/j.1600-0838.2010.01167.x

Deecke, L. (1996). Planning, preparation, execution, and imagery of volitional action. *Cogn. Brain Res.* 3, 59–64. doi: 10.1016/0926-6410(95)00046-1

Deiber, M. P., Ibañez, V., and Sadato, N. (1996). Cerebral structures participating in motor preparation in humans: a positron emission tomography study. *J. Neurophysiol.* 75, 233–247.

Deiber, M. P., Passingham, R. E., and Colebatch, J. G. (1991). Cortical areas and the selection of movement: a study with positron emission tomography. *Exp. Brain Res.* 84, 393–402. doi: 10.1007/BF00231461

Dum, R. P., and Strick, P. L. (1991). The origin of corticospinal projections from the premotor areas in the frontal lobe. *J. Neurosci.* 11, 667–689.

Eccles, J. C. (1982). The initiation of voluntary movements by the supplementary motor area. *Arch. Psychiatr. Nervenkr.* 231, 423–441. doi: 10.1007/BF00342722

Freude, G., and Ullsperger, P. (1987). Changes in Bereitschaftspotential during fatiguing and non-fatiguing hand movements. *Eur. J. Appl. Physiol. Occup. Physiol.* 56, 105–108. doi: 10.1007/BF00696384

Gandevia, S. C. (2001). Spinal and supraspinal factors in human muscle fatigue. *Physiol. Rev.* 81, 1725–1789. Available online at: http://physrev.physiology.org/content/81/4/1725.short

Gandevia, S. C., Allen, G. M., Butler, J. E., and Taylor, J. L. (1996). Supraspinal factors in human muscle fatigue: evidence for suboptimal output from the motor cortex. *J. Physiol.* 490, 529–536. doi: 10.1113/jphysiol.1996.sp021164

Goodall, S., González-Alonso, J., Ali, L., Ross, E. Z., and Romer, L. M. (2012). Supraspinal fatigue after normoxic and hypoxic exercise in humans. *J. Physiol.* 590, 2767–2782. doi: 10.1113/jphysiol.2012.228890

Gruet, M., Temesi, J., Brisswalter, J., Millet, G. Y., and Verges, S. (2014). Stimulation magnétique transcrânienne:application à la physiologie de l'exercice. *Sci. Sports* 29, 173–187. doi: 10.1016/j.scispo.2014.04.002

Gruet, M., Temesi, J., Rupp, T., Levy, P., Millet, G. Y., and Verges, S. (2013). Stimulation of the motor cortex and corticaospinal tract to assess human muscle fatigue. *Neuroscience* 231, 384–399. doi: 10.1016/j.neuroscience.2012.10.058

Hermens, H. J., Freriks, B., and Disselhorst-Klug, C. (2000). Development of recommendations for SEMG sensors and sensor placement procedures. *J. Electromyogr. Kinesiol.* 10, 361–374. doi: 10.1016/S1050-6411(00)00027-4

Herz, D. M., Christensen, M. S., Reck, C., Florin, E., Barbe, M. T., Stahlhut, C., et al. (2012). Task-specific modulation of effective connectivity during two simple unimanual motor tasks: a 122-channel EEG study. *Neuroimage* 59, 3187–3193. doi: 10.1016/j.neuroimage.2011.11.042

Hilty, L., Langer, N., Pascual-Marqui, R., Boutellier, U., and Lutz, K. (2011a). Fatigue-induced increase in intracortical communication between mid/anterior insular and motor cortex during cycling exercise. *Eur. J. Neurosci.* 34, 2035–2042. doi: 10.1111/j.1460-9568.2011.07909.x

Hilty, L., Lutz, K., Maurer, K., Rodenkirch, T., Spengler, C. M., Boutellier, U., et al. (2011b). Spinal opioid receptor-sensitive muscle afferents contribute to the fatigue-induced increase in intracortical inhibition in healthy humans. *Exp. Physiol.* 96, 505–517. doi: 10.1113/expphysiol.2010.056226

Hoffstaedter, F., Grefkes, C., Zilles, K., and Eickhoff, S. B. (2013). The "What" and "When" of self-initiated movements. *Cereb. Cortex* 23, 520–530. doi: 10.1093/cercor/bhr391

Ide, K., and Secher, N. H. (2000). Cerebral blood flow and metabolism during exercise. *Prog. Neurobiol.* 61, 397–414. doi: 10.1016/S0301-0082(99)00057-X

Jahanshahi, M., and Hallett, M. (2012). *The Bereitschaftspotential.* New York, NY: Springer Science & Business Media.

Jaric, S., Blesic, S., Milanovic, S., and Radovanovic, S. (1999). Changes in movement final position associated with agonist and antagonist muscle fatigue. *Eur. J. Appl. Physiol.* 80, 467–471. doi: 10.1007/s004210050619

Jaric, S., Radovanovic, S., and Milanovic, S. (1997). A comparison of the effects of agonist and antagonist muscle fatigue on performance of rapid movements. *Eur. J. Appl. Physiol.* 76, 41–47. doi: 10.1007/s004210050210

Jenkins, I. H., Jahanshahi, M., Jueptner, M., Passingham, E. R., and Brook, J. D. (2000). Self-initiated versus externally triggered movements. *Brain* 123, 1216–1228. doi: 10.1093/brain/123.6.1216

Johnston, J., Rearick, M., and Slobounov, S. (2001). Movement-related cortical potentials associated with progressive muscle fatigue in a grasping task. *Clin. Neurophysiol.* 112, 68–77. doi: 10.1016/S1388-2457(00)00452-1

Kamijo, K., O'leary, K. C., Pontifex, M. B., Themanson, J. R., and Hillman, C. H. (2010). The relation of aerobic fitness to neuroelectric indices of cognitive and motor task preparation. *Psychophysiology* 47, 814–821. doi: 10.1111/j.1469-8986.2010.00992.x

Kayser, B. (2003). Exercise starts and ends in the brain. *Eur. J. Appl. Physiol.* 90, 411–419. doi: 10.1007/s00421-003-0902-7

Kornhuber, H. H., and Deecke, L. (1965a). Changes in the brain potential in voluntary movementa and passive movements in man: readiness potential and reafferent potentials. *Pflügers Arch.* 284, 1–17.

Kornhuber, H. H., and Deecke, L. (1965b). Hirnpotentialänderungen bei Willkürbewegungen und passiven Bewegungen des Menschen: Bereitschaftspotential und reafferente Potentiale. *Pflügers Arch.* 284, 1–17. doi: 10.1007/BF00412364

Lepers, R., Maffiuletti, N. A., and Millet, G. (2004). Étiologie et cinétique d'apparition de la fatigue neuromusculaire lors d'exercices prolongés de cyclisme. *Mov. Sport Sci.* 52, 83–107. doi: 10.3917/sm.052.0083

Lepers, R., Maffiuletti, N. A., Rochette, L., Brugniaux, J., and Millet, G. Y. (2002). Neuromuscular fatigue during a long-duration cycling exercise. *J. Appl. Physiol. (1985).* 92, 1487–1493. doi: 10.1152/japplphysiol.00880.2001

Lepers, R., Millet, G. Y., and Maffiuletti, N. A. (2001). Effect of cycling cadence on contractile and neural properties of knee extensors. *Med. Sci. Sports Exer.* 33, 1882–1888. doi: 10.1097/00005768-200111000-00013

Liu, J. Z. (2003). Human brain activation during sustained and intermittent submaximal fatigue muscle contractions: an fMRI study. *J. Neurophysiol.* 90, 300–312. doi: 10.1152/jn.00821.2002

Liu, J. Z., Dai, T. H., Sahgal, V., Brown, R. W., and Yue, G. H. (2002). Nonlinear cortical modulation of muscle fatigue: a functional MRI study. *Brain Res.* 957, 320–329. doi: 10.1016/S0006-8993(02)03665-X

Liu, J. Z., Yao, B., Siemionow, V., Sahgal, V., Wang, X., Sun, J., et al. (2005). Fatigue induces greater brain signal reduction during sustained than preparation phase of maximal voluntary contraction. *Brain Res.* 1057, 113–126. doi: 10.1016/j.brainres.2005.07.064

Merton, P. A. (1954). Voluntary strength and fatigue. *J. Physiol. (Lond).* 123, 553–564. doi: 10.1113/jphysiol.1954.sp005070

Millet, G. Y., and Lepers, R. (2004). Alterations of neuromuscular function after prolonged running, cycling and skiing exercises. *Sports Med.* 34, 105–116. doi: 10.2165/00007256-200434020-00004

Morree, H. M., Klein, C., and Marcora, S. M. (2012). Perception of effort reflects central motor command during movement execution. *Psychophysiology* 49, 1242–1253. doi: 10.1111/j.1469-8986.2012.01399.x

Neyroud, D., Vallotton, A., Millet, G. Y., Kayser, B., and Place, N. (2013). The effect of muscle fatigue on stimulus intensity requirements for central and peripheral fatigue quantification. *Eur. J. Appl. Physiol.* 114, 205–215. doi: 10.1007/s00421-013-2760-2

Nybo, L., and Secher, N. H. (2004). Cerebral perturbations provoked by prolonged exercise. *Prog. Neurobiol.* 72, 223–261. doi: 10.1016/j.pneurobio.2004.03.005

Périard, J. D., Caillaud, C., and Thompson, M. W. (2011). Central and peripheral fatigue during passive and exercise-induced hyperthermia. *Med. Sci. Sports Exer.* 43, 1657–1665. doi: 10.1249/MSS.0b013e3182148a9a

Place, N., Maffiuletti, N. A., Martin, A., and Lepers, R. (2007). Assessment of the reliability of central and peripheral fatigue after sustained maximal voluntary contraction of the quadriceps muscle. *Muscle Nerve* 35, 486–495. doi: 10.1002/mus.20714

Robertson, C. V., and Marino, F. E. (2016). A role for the prefrontal cortex in exercise tolerance and termination. *J. Appl. Physiol. (1985),* 120, 464–466. doi: 10.1152/japplphysiol.00363.2015

Schillings, M. L., Kalkman, J. S., van der Werf, S. P., Bleijenberg, G., van Engelen, B. G. M., and Zwarts, M. J. (2006). Central adaptations during repetitive contractions assessed by the readiness potential. *Eur. J. Appl. Physiol.* 97, 521–526. doi: 10.1007/s00421-006-0211-z

Shibasaki, H. (2012). Cortical activities associated with voluntary movements and involuntary movements. *Clin. Neurophysiol.* 123, 229–243. doi: 10.1016/j.clinph.2011.07.042

Shibasaki, H., and Hallett, M. (2006). What is the Bereitschaftspotential? *Clin. Neurophysiol.* 117, 2341–2356. doi: 10.1016/j.clinph.2006.04.025

Sidhu, S. K., Cresswell, A. G., and Carroll, T. J. (2012). Motor cortex excitability does not increase during sustained cycling exercise to volitional exhaustion. *J. Appl. Physiol. (1985),* 113, 401–409. doi: 10.1152/japplphysiol.00486.2012

Siemionow, V., Fang, Y., Calabrese, L., Sahgal, V., and Yue, G. H. (2004). Altered central nervous system signal during motor performance in chronic fatigue syndrome. *Clin. Neurophysiol.* 115, 2372–2381. doi: 10.1016/j.clinph.2004.05.012

Slobounov, S., Hallett, M., and Newell, K. M. (2004). Perceived effort in force production as reflected in motor-related cortical potentials. *Clin. Neurophysiol.* 115, 2391–2402. doi: 10.1016/j.clinph.2004.05.021

Strojnik, V., and Komi, P. V. (1998). Neuromuscular fatigue after maximal stretch-shortening cycle exercise. *J. Appl. Physiol.* 84, 344–350.

Tanaka, M., and Watanabe, Y. (2012). Supraspinal regulation of physical fatigue. *Neurosci. Biobehav. Rev.* 36, 727–734. doi: 10.1016/j.neubiorev.2011.10.004

Taylor, J. L., Todd, G., and Gandevia, S. C. (2006). Evidence for a supraspinal contribution to human muscle fatigue. *Clin. Exp. Pharmacol. Physiol.* 33, 400–405. doi: 10.1111/j.1440-1681.2006.04363.x

Thacker, J. S., Middleton, L. E., McIlroy, W. E., and Staines, W. R. (2014). The influence of an acute bout of aerobic exercise on cortical contributions to motor preparation and execution. *Physiol. Rep.* 2:e12178. doi: 10.14814/phy2.12178

7

Mediators of Physical Activity on Neurocognitive Function: A Review at Multiple Levels of Analysis

Chelsea M. Stillman[1,2]*, *Jamie Cohen*[2,3], *Morgan E. Lehman*[3] *and Kirk I. Erickson*[1,2,3]*

[1] *Department of Psychiatry, School of Medicine, University of Pittsburgh Medical Center, Pittsburgh, PA, USA,* [2] *Center for the Neural Basis of Cognition, University of Pittsburgh, Pittsburgh, PA, USA,* [3] *Department of Psychology, University of Pittsburgh, Pittsburgh, PA, USA*

Edited by:
Louis Bherer,
Université de Montréal, Canada

Reviewed by:
Arun Bokde,
Trinity College, Dublin, Ireland
Cédric T. Albinet,
Jean-François Champollion University Center for Teaching and Research, France

****Correspondence:***
Chelsea M. Stillman
cms289@pitt.edu
Kirk I. Erickson
kiericks@pitt.edu

Physical activity (PA) is known to maintain and improve neurocognitive health. However, there is still a poor understanding of the mechanisms by which PA exerts its effects on the brain and cognition in humans. Many of the most widely discussed mechanisms of PA are molecular and cellular and arise from animal models. While information about basic cellular and molecular mechanisms is an important foundation from which to build our understanding of how PA promotes cognitive health in humans, there are other pathways that could play a role in this relationship. For example, PA-induced changes to cellular and molecular pathways likely initiate changes to macroscopic properties of the brain and/or to behavior that in turn influence cognition. The present review uses a more macroscopic lens to identify potential brain and behavioral/socioemotional mediators of the association between PA and cognitive function. We first summarize what is known regarding cellular and molecular mechanisms, and then devote the remainder of the review to discussing evidence for brain systems and behavioral/socioemotional pathways by which PA influences cognition. It is our hope that discussing mechanisms at multiple levels of analysis will stimulate the field to examine both brain and behavioral mediators. Doing so is important, as it could lead to a more complete characterization of the processes by which PA influences neurocognitive function, as well as a greater variety of targets for modifying neurocognitive function in clinical contexts.

Keywords: brain, cognition, exercise, physical activity, mechanisms, mediation

INTRODUCTION

Physical activity (PA) is important for maintaining *physical* health. PA has also been shown to maintain and improve *neurocognitive* health, but we know much less about the mechanisms by which it exerts its salutary effects on brain and cognition in humans (e.g., see Tomporowski and Ellis, 1986; Hillman et al., 2008; Gomez-Pinilla and Hillman, 2013 for reviews). However, research has found that physical *inactivity* is a risk factor for cognitive impairment, which has stimulated interest in examining whether PA can act to improve neurocognitive function, as well as the mechanisms by which it might work.

What are the cellular and molecular, brain systems, and behavioral mechanisms by which PA influences cognitive function, and how can they be identified? There are two frameworks that are typically used for causal inference—one is related to the design of the study, and the other is related to the statistical approach used for analysis (Imai et al., 2011).

The gold standard for assessing causality is through an **experimental manipulation**. A study is "experimental" when an independent variable (i.e., PA) is manipulated to examine its influence on a dependent variable (i.e., cognition). In the context of exercise studies, human or animal subjects are randomly assigned to an experimental condition (i.e., exercise treatment) or control group (i.e., standard care), and the outcome of interest is assessed in each group while all other factors are held constant. In the context of PA, this type of causal evidence comes almost exclusively from *exercise training* studies when studying humans, or from animal models of exercise in which one group of animals is permitted to exercise while another group is treated as a control. Causality is established if the outcome variable (e.g., cognition) changes to a greater extent in the treatment (e.g., exercise training) group relative to the control group.

Of course, it is not always feasible or practical to randomly assign participants to groups and experimentally manipulate treatment variables such as exercise, especially when studying humans. In this case, an alternative framework for causal inference can be used. **Statistical mediation** is used to test the plausibility of causal models not only in experimental studies, but also in observational, longitudinal, or quasi-experimental designs in which random assignment did not occur and/or the treatment variable of interest was not directly manipulated. Further, statistical mediation can be used in at least two different contexts. It is important to distinguish between these contexts as they influence the type of conclusions that can be drawn from the model's results.

In the first context (i.e., observational, longitudinal, and quasi-experimental studies), mediation models allow us to evaluate alternative causal mechanisms between the treatment and outcome variables by examining the roles of several intermediate variables that lie in the causal path. The benefit of using statistical mediation models in this context is that we are able to obtain evidence of a potential causal pathway using data or designs that are inherently non-experimental. Importantly, however, it is still not possible to rule out whether some third, confounding factor is driving the pattern of statistical mediation observed in a non-experimental design.

In the second context, a "gold standard" experimental design is used alongside a statistical mediation model. Using statistical models in experimental designs allows us to further examine intermediate factors that might covary with the treatment and outcome variables, and to test their plausibility as causal paths. Significant statistical mediation in this latter context provides more definitive evidence of a causal path because random assignment minimizes the influence of confounders and the direction of the relationships in the model can be established (i.e., it is possible to demonstrate that a manipulation caused changes in the mediator and outcome, rather than the reverse).

In both contexts described above where statistical mediation models can be used, the intermediate variable is considered a *mediator* if the coefficient describing the strength of the treatment-outcome relationship through the mediating variable (i.e., the indirect effect) is statistically significant (Preacher and Hayes, 2008). In other words, the significance of the indirect effects examines whether the mediator is a viable mechanism by which the independent (i.e., treatment) variable influences the outcome. Although statistical mediation can, and perhaps should, routinely be used in experimental studies, this approach is most frequently used to infer possible causal relationships from non-experimental data.

For the purposes of the present review, both types of causal evidence—design-related and statistical mediation—are relevant and will be discussed in the context of understanding mechanisms by which PA influences cognitive function. However, a critical caveat of the statistical mediation approach in quasi-experimental and observational studies is that causal relationships between a predictor and outcome through the mediator cannot be definitively determined, even in the case of significant statistical mediation. This is because random assignment did not occur, thus there could be pre-existing differences between the groups. However, statistical mediation approaches *can* provide evidence that one mediation pattern is more plausible than another, and they provide valuable theoretical insight for the design of future experimental studies.

Based on the description of causality outlined above, mechanisms can be conceived at multiple levels. However, most studies have taken a reductionist approach to mechanisms. To date, for example, most systematic reviews focusing on the causal mechanisms by which PA affects cognition have focused on cellular and molecular mechanisms, hereafter referred to as those at *Level 1 of analysis*. Consequently, there is a wealth of evidence (the majority from animal models) indicating that PA likely improves cognition by promoting various cellular and molecular pathways, including those responsible for neurogenesis and angiogenesis (van Praag et al., 2005), while decreasing others, such as inflammation (e.g., Parachikova et al., 2008). While information about basic cellular and molecular mechanisms is an important foundation from which to build our understanding of how PA promotes cognitive health in humans, there are other possible ways of thinking about mechanisms.

Just as mechanisms can be assessed in multiple ways (e.g., statistically or experimentally), they can also be assessed at multiple levels, ranging from the cellular and molecular level (i.e., Level 1) up to other, more macroscopic levels of analysis (see **Figure 1** for conceptual model). We will refer to brain systems and behavioral mechanisms as those at *Level 2* and *Level 3 of analysis*, respectively, and describe them further below. Separating mediators into different levels of analysis may be informative because PA-induced changes to cellular and molecular pathways (Level 1) likely initiate changes to macroscopic properties of the brain (Level 2) and behavior (Level 3) that in turn influence cognition. For example, changes in brain structure and function (Level 2) and behaviors, such as in socioemotional functions (e.g., mood, motivation, or sleep) (Level 3) could mediate improvements in cognitive performance following PA. Crucially, our choice to organize potential mediators into different levels is not meant to imply that the mechanisms at each level are mutually exclusive. In fact, pathways identified using Levels 2 and 3 analyses are necessarily invoked by changes at lower levels of analysis, and bidirectional effects likely exist between levels (e.g., feedback loops from higher levels influencing lower levels of analysis).

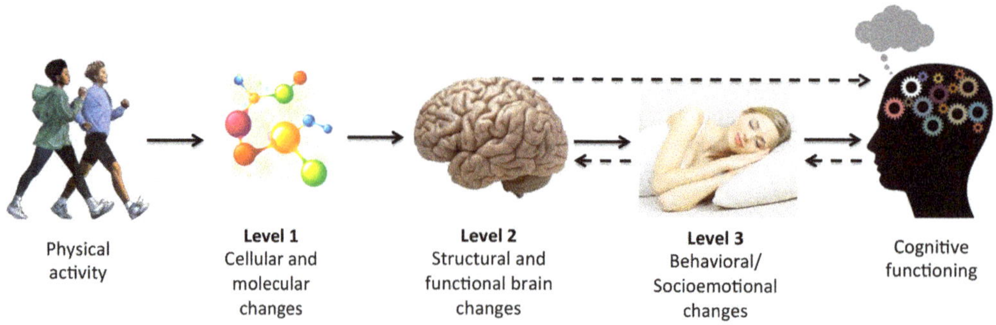

FIGURE 1 | Conceptual model of mechanisms of physical activity (PA) at multiple levels of analysis. There are various possible mediating pathways and bidirectional effects. Several possibilities are denoted with dotted arrows.

For conceptual purposes, however, we have chosen to discuss evidence for mediators at each level of analysis separately.

Prior reviews have focused almost entirely on Level 1 mechanisms at the expense of the other levels. The goal of this review is to use a more macroscopic lens that attempts to identify Levels 2 and 3 mediators of the association between PA and cognitive function. To accomplish this, we will briefly summarize what is known regarding cellular and molecular mechanisms and will devote the remainder of the review to discussing the brain systems and behavioral/socioemotional mechanisms at Levels 2 and 3 of analysis. It is our hope that discussing mechanisms at multiple levels of analysis will stimulate the field to examine systems and socioemotional mediators, leading to a more complete characterization of the processes by which PA influences neurocognitive function, and a greater variety of targets for modifying neurocognitive function.

In summary, the main aim of the present review is to summarize the evidence that macroscopic brain and behavioral/psychological changes can be mediators of the effects of exercise. We define high quality evidence of mediation as either coming from randomized controlled trials (RCT) or from correlational/cross-sectional work in which a statistical mediation model is tested after finding a pattern of correlations consistent with mediation. We are not aware of any other reviews to date considering such macroscopic (i.e., non-molecular) brain and behavior changes as mediators of exercise.

Key Definitions

Before we discuss the evidence for mechanisms at each level of analysis, we will first define several terms related to cognition and PA, as they will be used throughout the following sections. *Neurocognition* is a broad term referring broadly to the brain and its cognitive functions. We will use this term when referring to general observations about the effects of PA on both brain and cognitive outcomes. *Cognition* is a slightly more specific term. We will use this when referring to particular behavioral performance measures, such as those frequently used to assess the effects of PA in experimental studies.

Physical activity (PA) is a broad term referring to an activity that raises heart rate above resting levels (Caspersen et al., 1985). This could include anything from housework or gardening, to walking or lifting weights. Importantly, the term PA has also been used to refer to coordinative activities, such as those requiring balance and higher-order cognitive processes (Voelcker-Rehage and Niemann, 2013). However, it is the former definition of PA—that referring to aerobic, heart-rate-raising activity–that will be the focus of the present review as the PA field in the context of neurocognitive function is dominated by research using this definition. Further, different types of PA may have overlapping and distinct mechanisms (Voelcker-Rehage et al., 2010; Voelcker-Rehage and Niemann, 2013; Niemann et al., 2014). Aerobic PA, hereafter referred to as "PA," is often assessed subjectively in research studies, but it can also be measured objectively using devices such as accelerometers. Regular participation in PA influences aerobic fitness. Aerobic *fitness* (hereafter just "fitness") is a measure of cardiovascular efficiency and is often measured with a graded maximal exercise test. The main outcome measure from graded exercise tests is VO_{2max}, a metric describing a person's maximal oxygen uptake. VO_{2max} is widely accepted as the gold standard of the functional limit of the cardiovascular system. As such, it is often used as the primary objective outcome of fitness in non-experimental studies, or to assess whether a PA intervention was effective. Both PA and fitness are often used to describe the results of non-experimental designs. *Exercise* refers to any structured activity that is intended to improve physical fitness. This term is often used to describe the type of PA occurring in training studies. For the purposes of this review, we will use *PA* or *fitness* when referring to study outcomes and will use PA when discussing overall concepts or discussing mechanisms more generally. We will use *exercise* exclusively when referring to studies employing a randomized, controlled experimental design.

LEVEL 1: MOLECULAR AND CELLULAR MECHANISMS

PA and Cognitive Functioning

Much of what is known about the cellular and molecular mechanisms linking PA to cognitive functioning comes from animal models. This is because animals (most often mice or rats) can be randomly assigned to an exercise or control group while the external environments are controlled for the duration of the study. This experimental manipulation examines whether outcomes between groups can be attributed to the exercise and not to other unmeasured factors. In a typical study, animals in the exercise group are given free access to a running wheel (i.e., voluntary exercise), while those in the control group are not given access to a running wheel to ensure they are comparatively inactive; all other environmental conditions (e.g., diet) are held constant. Cognitive function is assessed at the conclusion of the study (typically lasting 2–8 weeks), and physiological and brain changes are evaluated shortly after during autopsy.

Experimental studies employing animal models have established that PA (in particular, aerobic exercise) improves cognitive function, especially in cognitive domains dependent on the hippocampus, such as spatial or relational learning and memory, object recognition (e.g., Hopkins and Bucci, 2010; Bechara and Kelly, 2013), and avoidance learning (e.g., Baruch et al., 2004; Chen et al., 2008) (see van Praag, 2008 for review). In addition, exercise increases long-term potentiation, a cellular analog of learning and memory, in a hippocampal sub-region known as the dentate gyrus (e.g., van Praag et al., 1999). Animal models have been critical in establishing that the changes initiated by exercise extend beyond behavior into cognition, prompting further research into the mechanisms underlying exercise-induced synaptic, and downstream cognitive, changes.

Molecular Mechanisms

Exercise exerts its salutary effects on learning and memory by modulating key growth factor cascades responsible for energy maintenance and synaptic plasticity (**Figure 2**). Currently, the two pathways most studied in relation to the PA-neurocognition link are brain-derived neurotropic factor (BDNF) and insulin-like growth factor-1 (IGF-1) (for reviews of mechanisms see Cotman et al., 2007; Gomez-Pinilla and Hillman, 2013). Exercise increases BDNF and IGF-1 gene expression and protein levels, both in the periphery, as well as in several brain regions, with the most robust and long-lasting changes in the hippocampus (Voss et al., 2013b; Duzel et al., 2016). BDNF and IGF-1 signaling are considered to be causal pathways underlying exercise-related neurocognitive improvements because they are *necessary* to observe exercise-induced cellular effects. That is, experimentally blocking signaling in these pathways (e.g., with receptor-blocking ligands) eliminates or attenuates the beneficial effects of exercise on cellular and molecular pathways related to cognition (e.g., long-term potentiation) (Cotman et al., 2007). Most of the initial studies manipulating the action of BDNF or IGF-1 pathways have focused on the cellular consequences of this manipulation, and not on cognition itself. However, there is evidence suggesting that blocking BDNF attenuates behavioral learning and memory improvements following exercise (Vaynman et al., 2004). Therefore, exercise-related increases in at least one of these growth factors has been directly linked to both cellular and cognitive changes.

Blocking IGF-1 signaling also prevents exercise-induced increases in BDNF, suggesting that the two pathways converge at certain points in their cascades (Carro et al., 2000; Ding et al., 2006). Thus, the results of experimental animal studies have established that both BDNF and IGF-1 are mediators of exercise-induced cognitive improvements and that their relationship may be interdependent, and also involve other molecules and cascades. Therefore, while BDNF and IGF-1 are two molecular pathways affected by exercise, there are likely many others involved. Nonetheless, the heavy theoretical focus on these two molecular pathways has spurred research into other possible cellular mechanisms underlying effects of exercise on neurocognition, such as vascular endothelial growth factor (VEGF) and various neurotransmitters (e.g., serotonin) (Fabel et al., 2003; Cotman et al., 2007; Hamilton and Rhodes, 2015).

Cellular Mechanisms

Angiogenesis, the development of new blood vessels, and neurogenesis, the development of new neurons, are complex cellular changes that result from increased growth factor production and up-regulated molecular cascades. Both processes have emerged as viable candidates mediating the relationship between exercise and cognition (Cotman et al., 2007) (**Figure 2**). Changes in neurovasculature precede neurogenesis in rodents, particularly in the hippocampus (van Praag, 2008). Therefore, improvements in cognition following exercise may be due, in part, to increased growth of blood vessels, which in turn stimulates cell proliferation and survival.

Neurogenesis, particularly that which occurs in the dentate gyrus, is one of the most replicated cellular changes linked to

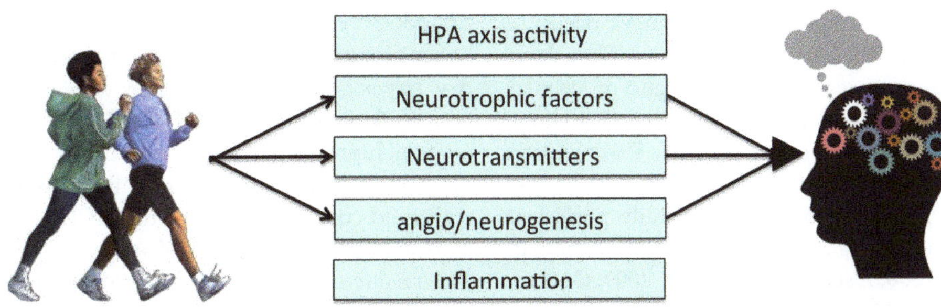

FIGURE 2 | Level 1 of analysis: Possible molecular and cellular mechanisms of PA. HPA, Hypothalamic-pituitary-adrenal axis activity.

exercise (van Praag, 2008). The mediating role of neurogenesis to exercise-related cognitive changes was once controversial (Leuner et al., 2006; Meshi et al., 2006), but it is now more accepted as a viable mechanism underlying learning and memory improvements (Clark et al., 2008; van Praag, 2008). Following 2–3 weeks of voluntary exercise in rodents, there is an increase in dendritic length and complexity of existing neurons, as well as neural progenitor proliferation, in the dentate gyrus compared to control animals (Eadie et al., 2005; Cotman and Berchtold, 2007). Importantly, exercise-induced increases in the number of newborn, dividing neurons occurs in regions that overlap with those showing enhanced synaptic plasticity and growth factor expression following exercise (e.g., dentate gyrus). Exercise-induced changes in vasculature are less regionally specific (Cotman et al., 2007; Voss et al., 2011; Vivar et al., 2013). Moreover, abolishing the division of new neurons during environmental enrichment manipulations that include exercise, or inhibiting the integration of these neurons into the existing hippocampal cell structure, eliminates the learning and memory improvements typically observed following such manipulations (Bruel-Jungerman et al., 2005; Vivar et al., 2012). Thus, animal studies have suggested that neurogenesis and the survival and integration of new neurons into existing cellular networks are *necessary* to observe some cognitive improvements, particularly in the domain of learning and memory, following exercise. Yet, several studies have suggested that neurogenesis alone is not enough to induce cognitive changes, and that cognitive changes only arise when the new neurons successfully integrate themselves within an existing body of cells. This pattern of results establishes neurogenesis – potentially by way of angiogenesis – as another, slightly more macroscopic mechanism at Level 1 of analysis and further highlights the importance of examining mechanisms from multiple perspectives, even within our conceptualized three levels of analysis.

The bulk of evidence for the molecular and cellular mechanisms of exercise comes from animal models. One limitation of animal models is that the results cannot always be directly extrapolated to humans. Indeed, the cellular and molecular mechanisms of exercise-induced improvements to cognitive functioning in humans (not only in regards to learning and memory, but also other cognitive domains) remain largely unknown. This is, in part, because there are limited techniques available to measure *cellular and molecular pathways* in the human brain.

Despite these limitations, animal models have been critical in establishing that molecular and cellular changes occur in response to PA, particularly in the hippocampus. They have provided evidence that changes in molecular and/or cellular pathways mediate cognitive changes, supporting that these pathways are underlying mechanisms of the PA-cognition link. We have spoken about Level 1 mechanisms in brevity above because of the multitude of reviews already published summarizing this literature (e.g., Cotman et al., 2007; Hillman et al., 2008; van Praag, 2008; Lista and Sorrentino, 2009; Gomez-Pinilla and Hillman, 2013). However, these molecular and cellular mechanisms likely invoke more macroscopic changes in the brain, which leads us to Level 2 of analysis.

LEVEL 2: MACROSCOPIC BRAIN SYSTEMS

Statistical Mediation – Cross-Sectional Studies

The molecular and cellular mechanisms of exercise in humans have been difficult to establish because it is not possible to experimentally manipulate or measure cellular and molecular processes in humans in the same way we do in animals – through the use of brain tissue samples. Fortunately, advances in neuroimaging have allowed us to examine, *in vivo* and non-invasively, more macroscopic effects of PA on the structure and function of brain regions and circuits. But this leads to a critical question: Do the effects of exercise and fitness on neuroimaging markers (e.g., volume) have a mediating effect on cognitive outcomes, or are they just a meaningless by-product of increased exercise?

Most studies assessing mechanisms at Level 2 of analysis have examined how gray and white matter morphology are associated with PA and, in turn, whether these associations mediate differences in cognitive performance. We use the term *morphology* as a broad way to refer to changes in brain structure, most often assessed by measuring the volume of gray and/or white matter, or white matter integrity. Separate bodies of literature have demonstrated that brain morphology relates to cognitive function (e.g., Madden et al., 2012; Zhang et al., 2015) *or* to PA (e.g., Burzynska et al., 2014; Smith et al., 2014). However, it is a comparatively new concept to test brain morphology as a mechanism through which PA or fitness influences cognition. For example, in a cross-sectional study, Erickson et al. (2009) examined the possibility that links between fitness and memory function could be accounted for by hippocampal volume. Using statistical mediation modeling, they demonstrated that hippocampal volume significantly mediated the relationship between fitness and spatial memory. The authors used a statistical framework to test their mechanistic hypothesis because the study was not an experimental manipulation of PA (i.e., a randomized controlled trial). However, the results provide insight into a possible casual role of the hippocampus that would be further tested in later experimental manipulations, as described below.

Similar statistical mediation has been reported across the lifespan, suggesting that these associations may be independent of age. For example, in a group of 49 preadolescent children, Chaddock et al. (2010) found that higher-fit children had larger hippocampal volumes compared to lower-fit children, and that larger hippocampal volumes were associated with superior relational memory performance. Importantly, they found that bilateral hippocampal volume mediated the relationship between fitness and memory task performance. A study of older adults with mild cognitive impairment (MCI) reported similar pattern of results using hippocampal volume (Makizako et al., 2015). The results of these studies are consistent with animal studies demonstrating that the cognitive-enhancing effects of exercise can be traced to changes in the molecular and cellular architecture of the hippocampus. However, one limitation from human studies is that we cannot determine which molecular and cellular pathways are mediating the associations with hippocampal volume (Braun and Jessberger, 2014).

Importantly, PA research in humans has also revealed that the hippocampus is not the only region mediating the link between exercise and cognition. Recent work suggests that changes to regions other than the hippocampus (e.g., prefrontal cortex) mediate some cognitive improvements in humans. For example, in a cross-sectional study, Weinstein et al. (2012) demonstrated that higher cardiorespiratory fitness levels were associated with better performance on both executive control and working memory tasks. Fitness levels were also associated with greater gray matter volume in several prefrontal brain regions. Further, the volume of these prefrontal regions statistically mediated the relationship between fitness and executive function and working memory performance. Similarly, Verstynen et al. (2012) found that caudate nucleus volume statistically mediated the relationship between fitness and cognitive flexibility, a function known to be supported by this region. Thus, in addition to the hippocampus, volumetric differences in the prefrontal cortex and caudate nucleus may mediate fitness- or exercise-related improvements in executive control and cognitive flexibility. These results demonstrate, as would be expected, that brain regions that support certain cognitive processes are the same regions that also statistically mediate associations between fitness or PA and cognitive performance in particular domains.

In addition to the cross-sectional studies showing that gray matter volume may statistically mediate the fitness-cognition relationship, the integrity of white matter tracts may also mediate the link between PA and cognitive functioning. The first line of evidence for this idea comes from studies showing that white matter integrity has a clear association with cognitive performance across a number of domains (Fjell et al., 2011; Bennett and Madden, 2014). The second line of evidence comes from studies showing that higher levels of PA are associated with greater white matter integrity (Smith et al., 2016). Given these patterns of findings, white matter integrity is another potential mediator of the link between PA and cognitive performance. This mechanism has only recently been tested. In two independent samples with a total of 267 healthy older adults, Oberlin et al. (2016) reported that white matter integrity in diffuse tracts statistically mediated the relationship between cardiorespiratory fitness (as measured by a VO_{2max} test) and spatial working memory performance. These tracts included those connecting the medial temporal to prefrontal cortices – the same brain regions discussed above that have been found to be associated with fitness and PA in studies examining gray matter volume. Overall, these results extend the research on brain volume by demonstrating that aerobic fitness may also be associated with cognition through its associations with white matter microstructure.

The studies described above provide evidence that changes in the structure of both gray and white matter statistically mediate the relationship between PA (or fitness, in the case of cross-sectional work) and cognition. However, PA could also induce changes to the functioning, most often operationalized as functional activation or connectivity, of certain brain regions as a result, *or independent of*, changes in brain structure. Functional MRI (fMRI) markers have been found to differ between groups or change in response to an intervention; the question is if these changes mediate improvements in cognition. Several recent, cross-sectional studies examined functional activation as a statistical mediator of the effects of PA on cognition. Building on evidence of a relationship between fitness, executive control, and prefrontal functioning (Colcombe et al., 2004), Wong et al. (2015) examined the relationship between cardiorespiratory fitness (via VO_{2max}), executive functioning (via dual-task processing), and prefrontal cortex activation. A statistical mediation model revealed that activation of a region in the anterior cingulate/prefrontal cortex significantly mediated the relationship between cardiorespiratory fitness and dual task performance, such that those who were more fit had more activation in this region. Similarly, Hyodo et al. (2016) found that the level of activation in the left dorsolateral prefrontal cortex statistically mediated the association between higher fitness and less cognitive interference (via a Stroop task). A recent study reported a pattern of relationships consistent with a mediating role of prefrontal cortex activation to the fitness-executive control relationship using (functional Near Infrared Spectroscopy; fNIRS) (Albinet et al., 2014). The pattern of results reported in these cross-sectional studies supports the argument that PA influences cognition through its effects on the functional allocation of neural resources (i.e., functional activation) during cognitive tasks. The results of several other cross-sectional studies assessing links between fitness, neural functioning, and cognition provide support for this general idea (Dupuy et al., 2015; Gauthier et al., 2015). However, these studies did not fully test for mediation because they either did not observe or did not test for the prerequisite correlations amongst the variables.

Cross-sectional studies utilizing statistical mediation provide a theoretical and mechanistic foundation about the relationships between cardiorespiratory fitness, brain, and cognition. However, their correlational nature leaves open the possibility that the observed behavioral and structural fitness-related differences between high and low-fit groups are caused by some unmeasured factor. RCTs are necessary to account for potential selection bias, as well as to establish a direct, causal relationship in humans between aerobic fitness, brain structure, and cognitive functioning.

Experimental Mediation – Randomized Controlled Trials

There have been numerous RCT examining the effects of exercise on cognition *or* on brain outcomes (Kramer et al., 2006; Hillman et al., 2008; Smith et al., 2010). However, only a small subset has examined both brain *and* cognitive outcomes in the same study, allowing for causal inference (**Table 1**). Even fewer of the existing RCTs on this topic have included both cognitive and brain changes within a statistical model in order to definitively demonstrate a mechanism of exercise at Level 2 of analysis. In fact, while many of the RCTs that will be discussed below have shown promising patterns, only one tested for statistical mediation.

TABLE 1 | Evidence for mechanisms of PA at Level 2 of analysis.

Lead author	Year	Sample	Mechanistic finding	Type mediation
Albinet	2014	34 older adults (all female)	Increases in cerebral oxygen responses in the right DLPFC partially mediate relationship between aerobic fitness and executive control performance	Statistical
Chaddock	2010	49 preadolescent children	Hippocampal volume mediates relationship between aerobic fitness and relational memory	Statistical
Chaddock-Heyman	2013	23 preadolescent children	Increases in prefrontal activation and executive functioning following a 9-month aerobic exercise intervention	Experimental
Colcombe	2004	41 older adults (study 1); 29 older adults (study 2)	Greater activation in prefrontal, parietal, and anterior cingulate cortex, and well as increased cognitive control performance in higher aerobically fit (Study 1) or aerobically trained (Study 2) individuals	Statistical (Study 1); Experimental (Study 2)
Erickson	2009	165 older adults	Hippocampal volume mediates relationship between cardiorespiratory fitness and spatial memory	Statistical
Erickson	2011	120 older adults	Volume of the hippocampus and memory performance increase following a 12-month aerobic exercise intervention	Experimental
Hillman	2014	221 preadolescent children	Frontal activation, cognitive inhibition, and flexibility increases following 9-month aerobic exercise intervention	Experimental
Hyodo	2015	60 male older adults	Activation of left dorsolateral prefrontal cortex mediates relationship between fitness and cognitive control	Statistical
Kamijo	2011	43 preadolescent children	Increases in cognitively relevant frontal ERP component (CNV) and in working memory following a 9-month aerobic exercise intervention	Experimental
Kraft	2014	43 overweight children	Activity increases in the anterior cingulate cortex and decreases in precentral gyrus and parietal cortex following 8-month aerobic exercise intervention; Improved cognitive control performance	Experimental *No group × Time interactions for any neurocognitive outcome
Krogh	2014	79 clinically depressed older adults	Positive association between change in hippocampal volume and changes in memory following a 3-month aerobic exercise intervention	Experimental *Issues with adherence; no group × Time interactions
Maass	2015	40 older adults	Hippocampal volume, perfusion, and memory increases following a 3-month aerobic exercise intervention; Changes in perfusion statistically mediate relationship between volume and memory	Experimental and Statistical
Makizako	2015	310 older adults with MCI	Hippocampal volume mediates the association between PA and memory in older adults with MCI	Statistical
Oberlin	2016	241 older adults across two studies	White matter integrity mediates relationship between fitness and spatial working memory	Statistical
Pajonk	2010	24 schizophrenic patients	Hippocampal volume and short-term memory improve following 3-month aerobic exercise intervention; Changes in volume correlate with changes in memory	Experimental
Ruscheweyh	2012	62 older adults	Positive association between changes in PA and episodic memory following a 6 months mixed-intensity intervention no longer significant after accounting for the variance associated with change in anterior cingulate gray matter volume	Experimental *No group × Time interactions
Ten Brinke	2015	86 female older adults	Hippocampal volume increases following 6-month aerobic exercise intervention. Changes in volume negatively associated with changes in short-term memory	Experimental
Verstynen	2012	179 older adults	Volume of the caudate nucleus mediates relationship between fitness and cognitive flexibility	Statistical
Voss	2010	62 older adults	Connectivity of large-scale brain networks and executive functioning improve following 6-month aerobic exercise intervention; changes in connectivity correlate with changes in executive functioning.	Experimental

(Continued)

TABLE 1 | Continued

Lead author	Year	Sample	Mechanistic finding	Type mediation
Voss	2013a	70 older adults	Improved fitness is associated with changes in prefrontal and temporal white matter integrity following a 12-month aerobic exercise intervention; no changes in short-term memory performance reported between groups; no mediation model could be tested	Experimental *No group × Time interaction for neurocognitive outcome
Weinstein	2012	142 older adults	Volume of prefrontal cortex mediates the relationship between cardiorespiratory fitness and working memory, as well as that between fitness and inhibitory control	Statistical
Wong	2015	128 older adults	Greater anterior cingulate cortex activation mediates relationship between fitness and dual task performance	Statistical

Changes in Brain Structure

As in the human cross-sectional work, most RCTs examining mechanisms of PA at Level 2 of analysis have focused on its effects on brain structure, particularly on gray matter volume. In general, this literature has shown that exercise training increases brain volume particularly in the hippocampus, and these volumetric changes partially account for cognitive improvements following the intervention. In a seminal study on this topic, 120 inactive older adults were randomly assigned to a 12-month aerobic walking (experimental) group, or to a stretching and toning (control) group (Erickson et al., 2011). Following the intervention, the aerobic exercise group showed greater gray matter volume in the anterior hippocampus compared to the control group. These findings represent the first experimental evidence linking changes in exercise to changes in both gray matter volume and cognitive performance in aging humans in the context of a RCT. Further, the findings are consistent with animal models of regional specificity for the effects of exercise on the brain, such that volume changes are particularly robust in the anterior portion of the hippocampus.

One limitation of the Erickson et al. (2011) study was that they did not test whether the relation between changes in fitness levels and spatial memory could be statistically accounted for by changes in hippocampal volume. It is therefore possible that another factor associated with both changes in fitness and gray matter volume accounted for the cognitive changes. In fact, the control group in this study also showed improvements in memory performance, despite showing *decreases* in hippocampal volume, making the causal links between changes in fitness and changes in hippocampal volume and spatial memory in the experimental group tenuous. Further, only the volumes of subcortical regions were assessed; potential changes in cortical regions, such as the prefrontal cortex, were not examined (but see Colcombe et al., 2006; Ruscheweyh et al., 2011 for evidence of cortical volume changes). Nonetheless, these results are important, as they were the first experimental evidence to suggest that exercise training can increase the volume of the hippocampus and improve memory in older adults.

In addition to examining mechanisms of exercise in healthy older adults, RCTs have also examined whether exercise can increase gray matter volume and cognition in clinical samples. The patient groups studied are those in which there are well-known hippocampal deficits, including schizophrenia (Pajonk et al., 2010), major depressive disorder (Krogh et al., 2014), and MCI (Ten Brinke et al., 2015). Each of these studies reported increases in gray matter volume in the hippocampus, but results were mixed regarding whether the exercise intervention improved cognition. For example, Pajonk et al. (2010) conducted a study with 24 participants, 16 of whom had schizophrenia. Eight of the patients and all of the healthy participants ($n = 8$) were enrolled in an aerobic (cycling) exercise intervention ($n = 16$), while the other eight patients played table tennis as a low-aerobic control activity. The authors found that hippocampal volume increased and short-term memory improved in the exercise group following the intervention, but not in the non-exercising control group. Short-term memory and schizophrenic symptom severity improved with changes in hippocampal volume in schizophrenics, suggesting a possible mediating role of hippocampal changes on behavioral outcomes. Unfortunately, these associations were not tested using a statistical mediation framework (see Firth et al., 2015 for mixed findings).

Increased cerebral perfusion has also been suggested as a possible mechanism for the cognitive-enhancing effects of exercise. For example, Maass et al. (2015) combined brain volume, perfusion, and memory change outcomes from their 3-month intervention and found that changes in gray matter volume could be accounted for by changes in cerebral perfusion. These results suggest that perfusion changes may mediate the effects of exercise on both gray matter volume *and* memory performance. Thus, while gray matter volume is the most widely studied Level 2 mechanism of exercise on cognitive outcomes, there are other neuroimaging modalities tapping into different components of brain health that could shed light on the mechanisms of volumetric and cognitive changes (e.g., see Zimmerman et al., 2014).

Changes in white matter microstructure may be another mechanism for the effects of PA on cognition because white matter supports communication between brain regions. Greater PA is linked to white matter preservation (Sexton et al., 2016) and decreased white matter integrity is linked to cognitive deficits (Roberts et al., 2013). This pattern raises the possibility that white matter health is a mechanism underlying the effects of PA on cognition. In the first RCT to examine this possibility, Voss et al. (2013a) evaluated the effects of a 12-month exercise intervention on white matter integrity and cognitive performance in healthy older adults. Seventy older adults were randomly assigned to either an aerobic walking or toning/stretching group; the groups participated in their respective activities for 40 min per day, 3 days per week. Increases in temporal and prefrontal white matter integrity, assessed via fractional anisotropy (FA), and memory were positively associated with improvements in fitness. However, the exercise-induced changes in FA were not associated with changes in memory performance. One possible explanation for this null finding is that the sample size was too small, limiting the statistical power to detect a relationship between FA and memory. This is a limitation that applies to many of the RCTs conducted to date.

Exercise-Induced Changes in Brain Function

Changes in brain function in response to exercise, as measured by fMRI, could potentially precede changes in brain structure. It is also possible that exercise induces changes in brain function that are independent of changes in structure (i.e., not simply a byproduct of structural changes). Functional imaging studies of exercise therefore offer information about another potential brain mechanism underlying cognitive changes in response to exercise. Although less studied compared to structural change, exercise-related changes in brain function have been examined in the context of several RCTs (e.g., Voss et al., 2010; Kamijo et al., 2011; Chaddock-Heyman et al., 2013; Hillman et al., 2014; Krafft et al., 2014). Unlike RCTs examining structural outcomes, however, most of the RCTs focusing on functional outcomes have focused on changes in prefrontal cortex functioning, rather than the hippocampus. For example, using fMRI, Chaddock-Heyman et al. (2013) observed that children participating in a 9-month exercise intervention, 5 days per week, showed improved executive control performance and increased prefrontal activation patterns following the intervention, similar to the pattern seen in a healthy adult comparison group. Krafft et al. (2014) reported a similar pattern of findings in obese children: Following an 8-month intervention, obese children showed improved cognitive control and increased activation in a comparable set of prefrontal brain regions to those reported by Chaddock-Heyman et al. (2013). Further, using similarly aged (i.e., childhood) samples, two additional studies by Kamijo et al. (2011) and Hillman et al. (2014) observed that exercise improved cognitive performance (i.e., working memory and cognitive flexibility, respectively) and increased frontal electrophysiological indices of cognitive preparation and flexibility (i.e., contingent negative variation and P3 amplitude, respectively) following 9-month exercise interventions. Thus, in the pre-pubescent, developing brain, exercise has been shown to improve executive functioning, and these improvements have been associated with increased activation or neural responsiveness in prefrontal brain regions.

At least two RCTs suggest that the functional changes induced by exercise extend to older adults, although perhaps in a less regionally specific manner. Using fMRI, Voss et al. (2010) showed that a 12-month walking intervention increased functional connectivity among regions within two large-scale brain networks: The default mode and the frontal executive networks (FEN). The increased functional connectivity in the FEN, a network that includes several prefrontal brain regions, was associated with improvements in executive control performance. A seminal study by Colcombe et al. (2004) reported similar findings in the functioning and recruitment of the FEN following a shorter, 6-month exercise intervention in older adults, supporting the claim that changes to large scale brain networks may occur relatively soon after the commencement of exercise training. Since large-scale brain networks are known to become less efficient and less flexible with age, these results suggest that exercise may exert more global effects on the efficiency and flexibility in which networks of brain regions interact in older adults, leading to preserved cognitive performance.

There have been a number of RCTs examining the effects of exercise on both brain outcomes and cognition. While many have demonstrated brain *or* cognitive changes following an exercise intervention, few have gone on to test for statistical mediation after finding a pattern of results consistent with a causal mechanism. Doing so, however, is important to establish the behavioral relevance of changes in neuroimaging metrics in PA-induced improvements in cognitive functioning (**Figure 3**). Further, the various differences in study design, measurement techniques, analytic approach, and study samples employed across the existing RCTs limit the mechanistic conclusions that can be drawn and highlight the need for more RCTs in this area. In particular, there is a need for RCTs to include larger samples and multiple imaging modalities in order to tease apart mechanistic questions related to temporal precedence. There is also a need to look at the activation of networks of brain regions, as well as the connectivity between them, as potential mediators. Given the recent shift in the field to focus on functional brain networks, it seems unlikely that any single brain region works in isolation to mediate cognitive improvements. More complex mediation models may prove useful for more fully capturing the mechanisms underlying the effects of PA on cognition. Nonetheless, the results of the existing body of literature are promising in that they indicate that exercise has multi-modal effects on the brain that likely underlie improvements in cognition. Further, the convergence of results, despite various differences across the studies, speaks to the robustness of the effects of exercise on both brain and cognition, and pinpoints PA as an effective tool to preserve and promote neurocognitive functioning across the lifespan.

LEVEL 3: BEHAVIORAL AND SOCIOEMOTIONAL MECHANISMS

The evidence described above implicates a number of molecular, cellular, and brain processes involved in PA, but it is likely that PA also exerts changes in other behaviors that contribute to cognitive improvements (**Figure 4**). Unfortunately, few studies have examined how mechanisms at Level 3 of analysis might underlie the effects of exercise on cognitive performance. From a clinical standpoint, however, changes in human behavior are much easier to observe and may reflect a cost-effective approach to understanding behavioral mechanisms by which exercise improves cognitive function. Thus, there is added practical value

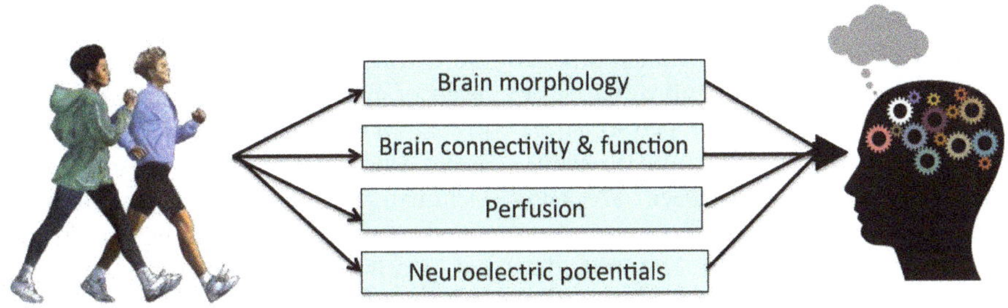

FIGURE 3 | Level 2 of Analysis: Possible brain systems-level mechanisms of PA.

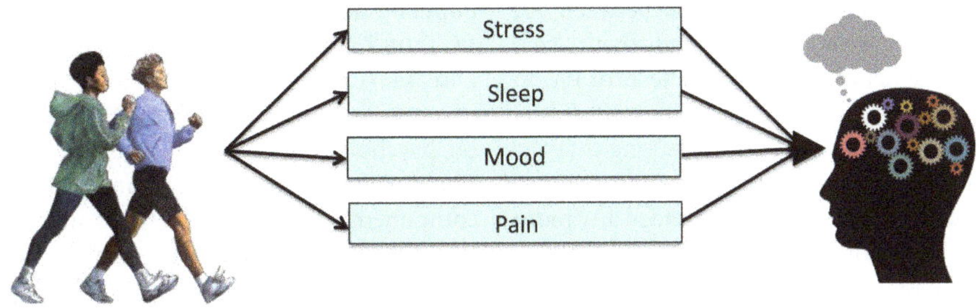

FIGURE 4 | Level 3 of analysis: Possible behavioral mechanisms of PA.

in understanding potential mechanisms at the behavioral and socioemotional level.

Sleep as a Mediator

Sleep quantity and quality are important for healthy cognitive function (Yaffe et al., 2014). For example, both the amount and quality of sleep are considered to be important in memory consolidation and learning processes (Walker, 2009). There is also a wealth of cross-sectional and experimental evidence that supports the idea that high quality sleep leads to better performance on a variety of cognitive tasks (see Ellenbogen, 2005 for review). Sleep is therefore a critical contributor to cognitive performance.

There is also evidence that increased PA improves sleep quality. The first RCTs to examine this demonstrated that relatively brief (e.g., 10-week) exercise interventions boosted self-reported sleep quality in older adults compared to non-exercise control groups (King et al., 1997; Singh et al., 1997). These studies did not include measures of cognitive performance, so the effects of exercise-induced sleep improvements on cognition could not be determined. However, given the connections between sleep and cognition, and between sleep and PA, it is possible that PA improves cognitive outcomes by influencing sleep quality and efficiency.

The only study to date that included PA, sleep, and cognition in one model tested the hypothesis that sleep mediates the relationship between PA and executive functioning in 109 young ($n = 59$) and older adults (Wilckens et al., in press). Both PA and sleep were objectively measured with accelerometry. Wilckens et al. (in press) found that PA energy expenditure was positively associated with sleep efficiency, as well as executive functioning and processing speed. Further, sleep efficiency statistically mediated the relationship between PA and several measures of cognitive performance. Although limited by the cross-sectional nature of the design, these findings provide evidence that sleep may be a behavioral mechanism by which PA influences cognitive performance. Future RCTs in which participants are randomly assigned to multiple sleep and exercise conditions are needed to test this hypothesis directly.

Mood as a Mediator

Low mood, often assessed using measures of depressive symptomology, is associated with poorer performance on a variety of cognitive tests (see Lichtenberg et al., 1995; Austin et al., 2001 for reviews). These cognitive deficits typically manifest in the domains of executive functioning, attention, and memory—the same domains that are most affected by PA (McClintock et al., 2010).

Increased PA is associated with improved mood, and is an efficacious approach to reduce symptoms of depression and anxiety (Byrne and Byrne, 1993; Fox, 1999; Penedo and Dahn, 2005; Ströhle, 2009; see for review Bridle et al., 2012). In fact, PA is increasingly being used as an adjunct treatment for clinically significant depression (Mead et al., 2008). Interestingly, there is also evidence that the relationship between PA and mood is bidirectional, such that poorer mood may lead to decreased PA (Roshanaei-Moghaddam et al., 2009).

Despite the fact that mood has been linked both to PA and cognitive function, only a handful of studies have considered mood as a mediating pathway through which PA influences cognition. For example, Vance et al. (2005) and Robitaille et al. (2014) both used statistical mediation in cross-sectional studies to examine the effects of several socioemotional factors (i.e., social support, depressive symptoms, cognitive activity) on the relationship between PA and cognitive performance. Consistent with their predictions and results from previous work, there were positive relationships between PA and tests of cognition, specifically in the domains of memory, processing speed, and visuospatial functioning. However, the two studies found disparate results when examining the behavioral predictors. In particular, Vance et al. (2005) found that physical inactivity had significant indirect associations with cognitive functioning through depressive symptomology and social support, while Robitaille et al. (2014) did not find that depression scores mediated the associations between PA and cognitive performance. Instead, they found that social support and cognitive engagement mediated the effects of PA on cognition (Robitaille et al., 2014). However, the indirect effects of these factors varied by cognitive outcome, suggesting that the mechanisms may vary across cognitive domains.

Unfortunately, the results of RCTs have not provided any more clarity regarding the role of factors, such as mood, on the PA-cognition relationship. One RCT examined mood as a mediating pathway with 64 younger adults randomly assigned to an exercise or control group (Lichtman and Poser, 1983). Following the intervention, the exercise group performed significantly better on an executive control test (i.e., a Stroop task) compared to the control group. The exercise group also showed a significant decrease in their depression and anxiety symptoms compared to baseline. However, the control group also exhibited decreases in depression and anxiety. Albinet et al. (2016) found similar results in a sample of 36 older adults who either participated in aerobic exercise or stretching control intervention for 21 weeks (Albinet et al., 2016). While both groups showed improvement in self-reported depressive symptomology, only the exercise group showed neurocognitive improvements. This pattern of results indicates that exercise was not the primary mechanism for the mood or cognitive improvements.

There are also studies in which mood changes following an exercise RCT, but no cognitive effects are observed. Another early RCT examined changes in psychological (including mood) and neuropsychological functioning following a 4-month aerobic exercise intervention in older adults (Blumenthal et al., 1989). Participants across three randomized groups (i.e., aerobic exercise, yoga and flexibility control, or waitlist control) did not show any clear pattern of differences on neuropsychological tests following the intervention. However, males in the aerobic exercise group showed a significant decline in depression and anxiety scores compared the control groups. There was still no clear pattern of cognitive improvements following exercise, even after training was extended for up to 10 months (Madden et al., 1989; Blumenthal et al., 1991).

Conversely, there are RCTs in which neurocognition changes, but mood does not. For example, Williams and Lord (1997) conducted an RCT examining the effects of a 42-week exercise intervention on mood and cognitive functioning in a group of older, community-dwelling women. Following the intervention, the exercise group performed better than the control group on measures of memory and processing speed. In addition, within the exercise group, individuals who reported higher baseline levels of anxiety and depression showed greater improvements in cognitive performance compared to individuals in the exercise group who reported lower baseline levels. However, as with Lichtman and Poser (1983), there were no group differences in mood symptoms following the intervention, and so exercise may not be driving the cognitive changes they observed. While none of these correlational studies were conclusive regarding whether mood mediates exercise-induced cognitive improvements, the results provide evidence that the relationship between exercise, cognition, and mood merits further exploration.

Testing the influence of exercise on cognition in clinical populations has not been as common in the literature. In a RCT of 73 older adults with Chronic Obstructive Pulmonary Disease (COPD), Emery et al. (1998) examined the effects of exercise, education about COPD, and stress management on psychological and cognitive functioning. Participants were randomized to three groups, only one of which had an exercise component (in addition to stress management and education). Post-intervention analyses revealed that the group receiving exercise (hereafter referred to as the "exercise group") showed lower depressive symptomatology compared to their baseline scores and to the post-intervention scores of the education-only group. Participants in the exercise group also showed improved verbal fluency scores, while the other two groups' scores did not change from their pre-intervention levels. While Emery et al. (1998) did not directly test a mediation model in this RCT, the fact that only the exercise group showed improvements in both mood and cognitive performance suggests a possible mediating link between exercise, changes in mood, and changes in cognition. However, it is difficult to interpret the exact nature of these effects because there was no group that *only* engaged in exercise. Thus, it is unclear whether the mood and cognitive improvements were due to exercise alone or to some synergistic effect of exercise, education, and stress management. Further, given that these results—the only experimental evidence to date to show both mood and cognitive changes in an exercising group—were reported in a clinical sample with known disturbances in mood (Maurer et al., 2008) and cognitive functioning (Liesker et al., 2004), it remains an open question whether the same mechanisms would underlie exercise-related changes to cognition in healthy populations. These results of the studies of PA and mood reviewed indicate that we do not yet understand whether, to what extent, and how changes to mood mediate the effects of PA on cognition.

DISCUSSION

The main motivation for writing the present review was to highlight the basic idea that mechanisms of PA on cognitive outcomes can be conceptualized on multiple levels, and it is possible to examine them using a variety of study designs. Historically, the discussion of mechanisms of PA or exercise on cognitive outcomes has been limited to Level 1 of analysis.

There have been numerous reviews in the past decade that have described in detail the molecular and cellular mechanisms of PA. Since excellent evidence for these mechanisms already exists, we did not explain them in detail. Instead, we focused on evidence for mechanisms of PA on cognition at Level 2 and took stock of the (limited) evidence for mechanisms of PA on cognition at Level 3 of analysis.

Mechanisms at Level 2 (i.e., structural and functional brain changes) are only just beginning to be discussed in the scientific literature. Our review suggests that regional gray matter volume statistically mediates the relationship between cardiorespiratory fitness or PA and cognitive functioning, but most of these studies have been limited to cross-sectional designs. In addition, white matter microstructure and functional brain activity may also be mediating associations between fitness or PA and cognition (e.g., Wong et al., 2015; Oberlin et al., 2016). Across the studies, brain changes do not occur equally or uniformly throughout the brain; rather, they seem specific to several brain regions in particular, namely, the hippocampus and prefrontal cortex. The regional specificity of PA-related structural and functional brain changes is important because it mirrors some of the regional specificity observed in animal models (i.e., hippocampus).

Consistent with the cross-sectional work, RCTs also support the argument that changes in brain structure and function may be mechanisms underlying the relationship between PA and cognitive performance. Specifically, the majority of RCTs have reported changes in brain structure or function, as well as in cognition following the exercise intervention. However, of the 13 RCTs including both cognitive and neuroimaging measures conducted to date, only 1 has used a statistical mediation model. Thus, it has not been possible in the majority of RCTs to rule out the possibility that another, unmeasured factor that covaries with both the treatment and outcome is underlying the intervention effects observed in the brain and/or cognitive performance.

The search for mechanisms at Level 2 is further complicated for several reasons. First, while the volume or function of specific brain regions (again, mostly the hippocampus and prefrontal cortex) consistently change following exercise interventions, the evidence has been less consistent with regard to cognitive performance. For example, although the majority of RCTs discussed above report cognitive changes that are exclusive to the exercise group following training, several reported cognitive improvements in both the exercise *and* control groups—i.e., a lack of group-by-time interaction (Erickson et al., 2011; Ruscheweyh et al., 2011; Voss et al., 2013a; Krafft et al., 2014). This makes it difficult to link exercise and brain changes exclusively to the cognitive changes observed. It also highlights a key limitation of RCTs in humans: It is extremely difficult to control the behavior of participants outside of the context of the RCT. Thus, even using this gold standard design, extra-training behaviors (e.g., those in the "control" condition might inadvertently increase their PA) could lead to unexpected effects. Second, there is variability in the design of the existing RCTs in terms of, for example, activity level/engagement of the control group, intervention length, type and frequency of PA, adherence, exclusionary criteria, neurocognitive outcomes assessed, and analytic techniques. It is therefore difficult to know whether null findings are the result of this inter-study variability or a true lack of effect. Finally, there are many factors that may moderate the effects of PA on neurocognition. Despite the favorable effects of PA and cardiorespiratory fitness on brain health and cognitive function reviewed above, there is significant inter-individual variability within studies regarding the extent to which any one individual will reap the physical and cognitive benefits of PA. Thus, it is likely that mediators are being moderated by other factors, such as the presence of pathology, age, genotype, gender, and diet (see Leckie et al., 2012 for review). However, the convergence of the effects of PA on brain health, despite this wide range of variability, speaks to the robustness of PA on both brain health outcomes and cognitive function.

Along these lines, if PA is thought to enhance cognition by improving brain structure and function, then eliminating PA should have the opposite effect. Examination of the effects of PA cessation has been comparatively unexplored to date. However, there have been two recent studies on this topic that support this idea (Alfini et al., 2016; Thomas et al., 2016). Alfini et al. (2016), showed that cortical and hippocampal resting brain perfusion decreases following PA cessation after just 10 days in older adult athletes. In addition, Thomas et al. (2016) found that hippocampal volume gains following an exercise intervention in young-middle aged adults, were abolished following 2-weeks of exercise cessation. These results are interesting and important for the field because they support PA as the causal variable in mechanistic models (i.e., removing PA reverses the brain effects attributed to this behavior). However, Alfini et al. (2016) did not administer a full cognitive battery, thereby limiting an interpretation of their results with regard to cognition. Thomas et al. (2016) administered a brief cognitive battery, but found no change in cognition following their 6-week intervention. It was therefore not possible to thoroughly evaluate whether cognition (our outcome variable of interest) also decreased following PA cessation. Such evidence is needed, as it would further strengthen the causal role Level 2 mediators play in PA-related cognitive effects.

Mechanisms of PA on cognition at Level 3 of analysis have not been frequently considered or assessed. However, there are a handful of studies suggesting that this level may be important to consider for future studies (**Table 2**). Changes in sleep quality, for example, are linked to both cognition and to PA. However, only one study to date (Wilckens et al., in press) has combined all three variables in a statistical model to test whether sleep can account for the relationship between PA and cognitive performance—the results of this initial study suggest that it can. Similarly, mood is linked both to cognitive performance and PA. While several studies have considered mood along with other behavioral or socioemotional factors in statistical models assessing mechanisms of PA, virtually none have considered the unique or independent contribution of mood to the PA-cognition relationship.

We highlighted sleep and mood as two examples of potential mechanisms at Level 3 because there are literatures linking

TABLE 2 | Evidence for mechanisms of PA at Level 3 of analysis.

Lead author	Year	Sample	Mechanistic finding	Type of mediation
Albinet	2016	36 older adults	Improvements in cognition following a 21-week exercise intervention are independent of improvements in mood	Experimental
Blumenthal	1989	101 older adults	A 4-month exercise intervention improves mood symptoms in males, but does not show any clear pattern of improvements in cognition	Experimental
Blumenthal	1991	101 older adults	4, 8, or 14 months of exercise training does not improve cognitive task performance	Experimental
Emery	1998	73 Chronic Obstructive Pulmonary Disorder patients	Exercise improves verbal fluency and reduces depressive symptoms compared to baseline scores and non-exercising groups	Experimental
King	1997	43 older adults	Improvements in self-rated sleep quality in exercising group following 16-week exercise intervention	Statistical
Lichtman	1983	64 young and mid-life adults	A 4-month exercise intervention improves performance on the Stroop Task	Statistical
Madden	1989	85 older adults and 24 younger adults	4 or 8 months of exercise does not improve cognitive task performance	Experimental
Robitaille	2014	470 older adults	Social support and cognitive engagement mediate the effects of PA on cognition	Statistical
Singh	1997	32 older adults	Exercise improves self-rated sleep quality following a 10-week intervention	Statistical
Vance	2005	158 older adults	Sedentary behavior has significant indirect associations with neurocognitive functioning through depression and social support	Statistical
Wilckens	in press	109 adults (59 younger, 50 older)	Sleep mediates the relationship between PA and executive functioning	Statistical
Williams	1997	187 older women	Exercise improves performance on tests of memory and processing speed following a 12-month intervention. Depression and anxiety symptoms decrease following the intervention for participants reporting the highest symptoms at baseline, though not differently from the non-exercising group.	Experimental *No group × Time interaction for mood outcomes

these factors to both cognition and PA, thus making them candidate mediators. However, it is important to note that there are likely many other possible behavioral mechanisms (e.g., self-efficacy, motivation, and fatigue, pain) that should be examined in future work (e.g., see relevant reviews McAuley and Blissmer, 2000; Mullen et al., 2012; Teixeira et al., 2012). Identifying such mechanisms is important, as they would provide additional outcome targets to assess the effectiveness of PA interventions. These additional possible behavioral mechanisms were not addressed in the current review because, to our knowledge, there are no studies to date examining them as potential mediators of the PA-cognition relationship. Additional studies including both psychological and neurocognitive functioning as outcome variables are needed to enhance our understanding of this level of analysis.

The studies reviewed above suggest that the individual pieces of a model from PA to cognitive functioning through behavioral changes, such as sleep or mood, exist, but they have not been succinctly combined in one cohesive model. Future work should address the gaps in our understanding of how behavioral mechanisms modulate the effects of PA on cognition by conducting RCTs with participants aged across the lifespan and measuring both behavioral and cognitive outcomes at multiple time points. Designs with these components would allow us to test not only for experimental mediation, but also for statistical mediation following exercise interventions.

CONCLUSION AND LIMITATIONS

One important point of consideration/limitation for studies examining the mechanisms of PA relates to the sample size needed to test for mediation. There are a number of publications addressing this topic (Cerin et al., 2006; Fritz and Mackinnon, 2007; MacKinnon et al., 2007). These articles suggest that the sample size needed to detect mediation effects depends on the size of the effect expected and the statistical method used to test for mediation. Effect sizes generally decrease with increasing variability of the outcome and so, although not always practical, larger samples are likely needed to detect mediation effects when outcome measures are highly variable (i.e., as is often the case in neuroimaging data) (Preacher and Kelley, 2011). RCTs in which groups are made to more extremely differ on a manipulated independent variable is one possible way to decrease variability (by the making groups differ extremely) and therefore increase power to detect mediation. Thus, RCTs might be the best context in which to test for Level 2 mediators. In terms of analytical method, bootstrapping methods of testing mediation generally require smaller samples, while causal-steps approaches require the most (Cerin et al., 2006). The recommended sample size to test for a small-moderate mediation effect range from as few as $N =$ 50–100 people using bootstrapping methods (e.g., Cerin et al., 2006) to anywhere from 400 to >20,000 people using more conservative causal-steps approaches (e.g., Fritz and Mackinnon, 2007). Many of the studies of PA cited above do not meet these recommended power requirements, increasing the likelihood of Types I and II error. Future studies should keep these guidelines in mind when budgeting and planning for recruitment.

Despite these considerations, there are many studies that implicate mechanisms of PA on cognition at Levels 2 and 3 of analysis that have given us the groundwork to construct our proposed mechanistic models (**Figures 2** and **3**), but very few have actually tested for statistical mediation. Doing so is critically important in order to rule out the possibility that the more macroscopic brain and socioemotional changes linked to PA are meaningless byproducts of PA. While we currently have the foundation to think about more macroscopic mechanisms that may mediate the relationship between PA and cognition, and potentially provide new, clinically relevant targets, these components need to be combined in testable models in future studies.

AUTHOR CONTRIBUTIONS

CS, JC, ML, and KE have seen and approved this manuscript for submission and are accountable for all aspects of the work. CS, JC, ML, and KE made substantial contributions to conceptualizing, drafting, and revising the manuscript.

ACKNOWLEDGMENT

The authors would like to thank BACH Lab undergraduate, Melanie Cieciuch, for assistance with the literature search for this review.

REFERENCES

Albinet, C. T., Abou-Dest, A., André, N., and Audiffren, M. (2016). Executive functions improvement following a 5-month aquaerobics program in older adults: role of cardiac vagal control in inhibition performance. *Biol. Psychol.* 115, 69–77. doi: 10.1016/j.biopsycho.2016.01.010

Albinet, C. T., Mandrick, K., Bernard, P. L., Perrey, S., and Blain, H. (2014). Improved cerebral oxygenation response and executive performance as a function of cardiorespiratory fitness in older women: a fNIRS study. *Front. Aging Neurosci.* 6:272. doi: 10.3389/fnagi.2014.00272

Alfini, A. J., Weiss, L. R., Leitner, B. P., Smith, T. J., Hagberg, J. M., and Smith, J. C. (2016). Hippocampal and cerebral blood flow after exercise cessation in master athletes. *Front. Aging Neurosci.* 8:184. doi: 10.3389/fnagi.2016.00184

Austin, M.-P., Mitchell, P., and Goodwin, G. M. (2001). Cognitive deficits in depression. *Br. J. Psychiatry* 178, 200–206. doi: 10.1192/bjp.178.3.200

Baruch, D. E., Swain, R. A., and Helmstetter, F. J. (2004). Effects of exercise on Pavlovian fear conditioning. *Behav. Neurosci.* 118, 1123–1127. doi: 10.1037/0735-7044.118.5.1123

Bechara, R. G., and Kelly, ÁM. (2013). Exercise improves object recognition memory and induces BDNF expression and cell proliferation in cognitively enriched rats. *Behav. Brain Res.* 245, 96–100. doi: 10.1016/j.bbr.2013.02.018

Bennett, I. J., and Madden, D. J. (2014). Disconnected aging: cerebral white matter integrity and age-related differences in cognition. *Neuroscience* 276, 187–205. doi: 10.1016/j.neuroscience.2013.11.026

Blumenthal, J. A., Emery, C. F., Madden, D. J., George, L. K., Coleman, R. E., Riddle, M. W., et al. (1989). Cardiovascular and behavioral effects of aerobic exercise training in healthy older men and women. *J. Gerontol.* 44, M147-157. doi: 10.1093/geronj/44.5.M147

Blumenthal, J. A., Emery, C. F., Madden, D. J., Schniebolk, S., Walsh-Riddle, M., George, L. K., et al. (1991). Long-term effects of exercise on psychological functioning in older men and women. *J. Gerontol.* 46, 352–361. doi: 10.1093/geronj/46.6.P352

Braun, S. M. G., and Jessberger, S. (2014). Adult neurogenesis: mechanisms and functional significance. *Development* 141, 1983–1986. doi: 10.1242/dev.104596

Bridle, C., Spanjers, K., Patel, S., Atherton, N. M., and Lamb, S. E. (2012). Effect of exercise on depression severity in older people: systematic review and meta-analysis of randomised controlled trials. *Br. J. Psychiatry* 201, 180–185. doi: 10.1192/bjp.bp.111.095174

Bruel-Jungerman, E., Laroche, S., and Rampon, C. (2005). New neurons in the dentate gyrus are involved in the expression of enhanced long-term memory following environmental enrichment. *Eur. J. Neurosci.* 21, 513–521. doi: 10.1111/j.1460-9568.2005.03875.x

Burzynska, A. Z., Chaddock-Heyman, L., Voss, M. W., Wong, C. N., Gothe, N. P., Olson, E. A., et al. (2014). Physical activity and cardiorespiratory fitness are beneficial for white matter in low-fit older adults. *PLoS ONE* 9:e107413. doi: 10.1371/journal.pone.0107413

Byrne, A., and Byrne, D. G. (1993). The effect of exercise on depression, anxiety and other mood states: a review. *J. Psychosom. Res.* 37, 565–574. doi: 10.1016/0022-3999(93)90050-P

Carro, E., Nuñez, A., Busiguina, S., and Torres-Aleman, I. (2000). Circulating insulin-like growth factor I mediates effects of exercise on the brain. *J. Neurosci.* 20, 2926–2933.

Caspersen, C. J., Powell, K. E., and Christenson, G. M. (1985). Physical activity, exercise, and physical fitness: definitions and distinctions for health-related research. *Public Health Rep.* 100, 126–131.

Cerin, E., Taylor, L. M., Leslie, E., and Owen, N. (2006). Small-scale randomized controlled trials need more powerful methods of mediational analysis than the Baron–Kenny method. *J. Clin. Epidemiol.* 59, 457–464. doi: 10.1016/j.jclinepi.2005.11.008

Chaddock, L., Erickson, K. I., Prakash, R. S., Kim, J. S., Voss, M. W., VanPatter, M., et al. (2010). A neuroimaging investigation of the association between aerobic fitness, hippocampal volume, and memory performance in preadolescent children. *Brain Res.* 1358, 172–183. doi: 10.1016/j.brainres.2010.08.049

Chaddock-Heyman, L., Erickson, K. I., Voss, M. W., Knecht, A. M., Pontifex, M. B., Castelli, D. M., et al. (2013). The effects of physical activity on functional MRI activation associated with cognitive control in children: a randomized controlled intervention. *Front. Hum. Neurosci.* 7:72. doi: 10.3389/fnhum.2013.00072

Chen, H.-I., Lin, L.-C., Yu, L., Liu, Y.-F., Kuo, Y.-M., Huang, A.-M., et al. (2008). Treadmill exercise enhances passive avoidance learning in rats: the role of down-regulated serotonin system in the limbic system. *Neurobiol. Learn. Mem.* 89, 489–496. doi: 10.1016/j.nlm.2007.08.004

Clark, P. J., Brzezinska, W. J., Thomas, M. W., Ryzhenko, N. A., Toshkov, S. A., and Rhodes, J. S. (2008). Intact neurogenesis is required for benefits of exercise on spatial memory but not motor performance or contextual fear conditioning in C57BL/6J mice. *Neuroscience* 155, 1048–1058. doi: 10.1016/j.neuroscience.2008.06.051

Colcombe, S. J., Erickson, K. I., Scalf, P. E., Kim, J. S., Prakash, R., McAuley, E., et al. (2006). Aerobic exercise training increases brain volume in aging humans. *J. Gerontol. A Biol. Sci. Med. Sci.* 61, 1166–1170. doi: 10.1093/gerona/61.11.1166

Colcombe, S. J., Kramer, A. F., Erickson, K. I., Scalf, P., McAuley, E., Cohen, N. J., et al. (2004). Cardiovascular fitness, cortical plasticity, and aging. *Proc. Natl. Acad. Sci. U.S.A.* 101, 3316–3321. doi: 10.1073/pnas.0400266101

Cotman, C. W., and Berchtold, N. C. (2007). Physical activity and the maintenance of cognition: learning from animal models. *Alzheimers Dement.* 3(2 Suppl.), S30-7. doi: 10.1016/j.jalz.2007.01.013

Cotman, C. W., Berchtold, N. C., and Christie, L.-A. (2007). Exercise builds brain health: key roles of growth factor cascades and inflammation. *Trends Neurosci.* 30, 464–472. doi: 10.1016/j.tins.2007.06.011

Ding, Q., Vaynman, S., Akhavan, M., Ying, Z., and Gomez-Pinilla, F. (2006). Insulin-like growth factor I interfaces with brain-derived neurotrophic factor-mediated synaptic plasticity to modulate aspects of exercise-induced cognitive function. *Neuroscience* 140, 823–833. doi: 10.1016/j.neuroscience.2006.02.084

Dupuy, O., Gauthier, C. J., Fraser, S. A., Desjardins-Crèpeau, L., Desjardins, M., Mekary, S., et al. (2015). Higher levels of cardiovascular fitness are associated with better executive function and prefrontal oxygenation in younger and older women. *Front. Hum. Neurosci.* 9:66. doi: 10.3389/fnhum.2015.00066

Duzel, E., van Praag, H., and Sendtner, M. (2016). Can physical exercise in old age improve memory and hippocampal function? *Brain* 139, 662–673. doi: 10.1093/brain/awv407

Eadie, B. D., Redila, V. A., and Christie, B. R. (2005). Voluntary exercise alters the cytoarchitecture of the adult dentate gyrus by increasing cellular proliferation, dendritic complexity, and spine density. *J. Comp. Neurol.* 486, 39–47. doi: 10.1002/cne.20493

Ellenbogen, J. M. (2005). Cognitive benefits of sleep and their loss due to sleep deprivation. *Neurology* 64, E25-7. doi: 10.1212/01.WNL.0000159942.64562.AD

Emery, C. F., Schein, R. L., Hauck, E. R., and MacIntyre, N. R. (1998). Psychological and cognitive outcomes of a randomized trial of exercise among patients with chronic obstructive pulmonary disease. *Health Psychol.* 17, 232–240. doi: 10.1037/0278-6133.17.3.232

Erickson, K. I., Prakash, R. S., Voss, M. W., Chaddock, L., Hu, L., Morris, K. S., et al. (2009). Aerobic fitness is associated with hippocampal volume in elderly humans. *Hippocampus* 19, 1030–1039. doi: 10.1002/hipo.20547

Erickson, K. I., Voss, M. W., Prakash, R. S., Basak, C., Szabo, A., Chaddock, L., et al. (2011). Exercise training increases size of hippocampus and improves memory. *Proc. Natl. Acad. Sci. U.S.A.* 108, 3017–3022. doi: 10.1073/pnas.1015950108

Fabel, K., Fabel, K., Tam, B., Kaufer, D., Baiker, A., Simmons, N., et al. (2003). VEGF is necessary for exercise-induced adult hippocampal neurogenesis. *Eur. J. Neurosci.* 18, 2803–2812. doi: 10.1111/j.1460-9568.2003.03041.x

Firth, J., Cotter, J., Elliott, R., French, P., and Yung, A. R. (2015). A systematic review and meta-analysis of exercise interventions in schizophrenia patients. *Psychol. Med.* 45, 1343–1361. doi: 10.1017/S0033291714003110

Fjell, A. M., Westlye, L. T., Amlien, I. K., and Walhovd, K. B. (2011). Reduced white matter integrity is related to cognitive instability. *J. Neurosci.* 31, 18060–18072. doi: 10.1523/JNEUROSCI.4735-11.2011

Fox, K. R. (1999). The influence of physical activity on mental well-being. *Public Health Nutr.* 2, 411–418. doi: 10.1017/S1368980099000567

Fritz, M. S., and Mackinnon, D. P. (2007). Required sample size to detect the mediated effect. *Psychol. Sci.* 18, 233–239. doi: 10.1111/j.1467-9280.2007.01882.x

Gauthier, C. J., Lefort, M., Mekary, S., Desjardins-Crépeau, L., Skimminge, A., Iversen, P., et al. (2015). Hearts and minds: linking vascular rigidity and aerobic fitness with cognitive aging. *Neurobiol. Aging* 36, 304–314. doi: 10.1016/j.neurobiolaging.2014.08.018

Gomez-Pinilla, F., and Hillman, C. (2013). The influence of exercise on cognitive abilities. *Compr. Physiol.* 3, 403–428. doi: 10.1002/cphy.c110063

Hamilton, G. F., and Rhodes, J. S. (2015). Exercise regulation of cognitive function and neuroplasticity in the healthy and diseased brain. *Prog. Mol. Biol. Transl. Sci.* 135, 381–406. doi: 10.1016/bs.pmbts.2015.07.004

Hillman, C. H., Erickson, K. I., and Kramer, A. F. (2008). Be smart, exercise your heart: exercise effects on brain and cognition. *Nat. Rev. Neurosci.* 9, 58–65. doi: 10.1038/nrn2298

Hillman, C. H., Pontifex, M. B., Castelli, D. M., Khan, N. A., Raine, L. B., Scudder, M. R., et al. (2014). Effects of the FITKids randomized controlled trial on executive control and brain function. *Pediatrics* 134, e1063-71. doi: 10.1542/peds.2013-3219

Hopkins, M. E., and Bucci, D. J. (2010). BDNF expression in perirhinal cortex is associated with exercise-induced improvement in object recognition memory. *Neurobiol. Learn. Mem.* 94, 278–284. doi: 10.1016/j.nlm.2010.06.006

Hyodo, K., Dan, I., Kyutoku, Y., Suwabe, K., Byun, K., Ochi, G., et al. (2016). The association between aerobic fitness and cognitive function in older men mediated by frontal lateralization. *Neuroimage* 125, 291–300. doi: 10.1016/j.neuroimage.2015.09.062

Imai, K., Keele, L., Tingley, D., and Yamamoto, T. (2011). Unpacking the black box of causality: learning about causal mechanisms from experimental and observational studies. *Am. Polit. Sci. Rev.* 105, 765–789. doi: 10.1017/S0003055411000414

Kamijo, K., Pontifex, M. B., O'Leary, K. C., Scudder, M. R., Wu, C.-T., Castelli, D. M., et al. (2011). The effects of an afterschool physical activity program on working memory in preadolescent children. *Dev. Sci.* 14, 1046–1058. doi: 10.1111/j.1467-7687.2011.01054.x

King, A. C., Oman, R. F., Brassington, G. S., Bliwise, D. L., and Haskell, W. L. (1997). Moderate-intensity exercise and self-rated quality of sleep in older adults. A randomized controlled trial. *JAMA* 277, 32–37.

Krafft, C. E., Schwarz, N. F., Chi, L., Weinberger, A. L., Schaeffer, D. J., Pierce, J. E., et al. (2014). An 8-month randomized controlled exercise trial alters brain activation during cognitive tasks in overweight children. *Obesity* 22, 232–242. doi: 10.1002/oby.20518

Kramer, A. F., Erickson, K. I., and Colcombe, S. J. (2006). Exercise, cognition, and the aging brain. *J. Appl. Physiol.* 101, 1237–1242. doi: 10.1152/japplphysiol.00500.2006

Krogh, J., Rostrup, E., Thomsen, C., Elfving, B., Videbech, P., and Nordentoft, M. (2014). The effect of exercise on hippocampal volume and neurotrophines in patients with major depression–a randomized clinical trial. *J. Affect. Disord.* 165, 24–30. doi: 10.1016/j.jad.2014.04.041

Leckie, R. L., Weinstein, A. M., Hodzic, J. C., and Erickson, K. I. (2012). Potential moderators of physical activity on brain health. *J. Aging Res.* 2012: e948981. doi: 10.1155/2012/948981

Leuner, B., Gould, E., and Shors, T. J. (2006). Is there a link between adult neurogenesis and learning? *Hippocampus* 16, 216–224. doi: 10.1002/hipo.20153

Lichtenberg, P. A., Ross, T., Millis, S. R., and Manning, C. A. (1995). The relationship between depression and cognition in older adults: a cross-validation study. *J. Gerontol. B Psychol. Sci. Soc. Sci.* 50, 25–32. doi: 10.1093/geronb/50B.1.P25

Lichtman, S., and Poser, E. G. (1983). The effects of exercise on mood and cognitive functioning. *J. Psychosom. Res.* 27, 43–52. doi: 10.1016/0022-3999(83)90108-3

Liesker, J. J. W., Postma, D. S., Beukema, R. J., Ten Hacken, N. H. T., Van der Molen, T., Riemersma, R. A., et al. (2004). Cognitive performance in patients with COPD. *Respir. Med.* 98, 351–356. doi: 10.1016/j.rmed.2003.11.004

Lista, I., and Sorrentino, G. (2009). Biological mechanisms of physical activity in preventing cognitive decline. *Cell Mol. Neurobiol.* 30, 493–503. doi: 10.1007/s10571-009-9488-x

Maass, A., Düzel, S., Goerke, M., Becke, A., Sobieray, U., Neumann, K., et al. (2015). Vascular hippocampal plasticity after aerobic exercise in older adults. *Mol. Psychiatry* 20, 585–593. doi: 10.1038/mp.2014.114

MacKinnon, D. P., Fairchild, A. J., and Fritz, M. S. (2007). Mediation analysis. *Annu. Rev. Psychol.* 58, 593–614. doi: 10.1146/annurev.psych.58.110405.085542

Madden, D. J., Bennett, I. J., Burzynska, A., Potter, G. G., Chen, N., and Song, A. W. (2012). Diffusion tensor imaging of cerebral white matter integrity in cognitive aging. *Biochim. Biophys. Acta* 1822, 386–400. doi: 10.1016/j.bbadis.2011.08.003

Madden, D. J., Blumenthal, J. A., Allen, P. A., and Emery, C. F. (1989). Improving aerobic capacity in healthy older adults does not necessarily lead to improved cognitive performance. *Psychol. Aging* 4, 307–320. doi: 10.1037/0882-7974.4.3.307

Makizako, H., Liu-Ambrose, T., Shimada, H., Doi, T., Park, H., Tsutsumimoto, K., et al. (2015). Moderate-intensity physical activity, hippocampal volume, and memory in older adults with mild cognitive impairment. *J. Gerontol. A Biol. Sci. Med. Sci.* 70, 480–486. doi: 10.1093/gerona/glu136

Maurer, J., Rebbapragada, V., Borson, S., Goldstein, R., Kunik, M. E., Yohannes, A. M., et al. (2008). Anxiety and depression in COPD. *Chest* 134(4 Suppl.), 43S–56S. doi: 10.1378/chest.08-0342

McAuley, E., and Blissmer, B. (2000). Self-efficacy determinants and consequences of physical activity. *Exerc. Sport Sci. Rev.* 28, 85–88.

McClintock, S. M., Husain, M. M., Greer, T. L., and Cullum, C. M. (2010). Association between depression severity and neurocognitive function in major depressive disorder: a review and synthesis. *Neuropsychology* 24, 9–34. doi: 10.1037/a0017336

Mead, G. E., Morley, W., Campbell, P., Greig, C. A., McMurdo, M., and Lawlor, D. A. (2008). Exercise for depression. *Cochrane Database Syst. Rev.* 4: CD004366. doi: 10.1002/14651858.CD004366.pub3

Meshi, D., Drew, M. R., Saxe, M., Ansorge, M. S., David, D., Santarelli, L., et al. (2006). Hippocampal neurogenesis is not required for behavioral effects of environmental enrichment. *Nat. Neurosci.* 9, 729–731. doi: 10.1038/nn1696

Mullen, S. P., McAuley, E., Satariano, W. A., Kealey, M., and Prohaska, T. R. (2012). Physical activity and functional limitations in older adults: the influence of self-efficacy and functional performance. *J. Gerontol. B Psychol. Sci. Soc. Sci.* 67B, 354–361. doi: 10.1093/geronb/gbs036

Niemann, C., Godde, B., and Voelcker-Rehage, C. (2014). Not only cardiovascular, but also coordinative exercise increases hippocampal volume in older adults. *Front. Aging Neurosci.* 6:170. doi: 10.3389/fnagi.2014.00170

Oberlin, L. E., Verstynen, T. D., Burzynska, A. Z., Voss, M. W., Prakash, R. S., Chaddock-Heyman, L., et al. (2016). White matter microstructure mediates the relationship between cardiorespiratory fitness and spatial working memory in older adults. *Neuroimage* 131, 91–101. doi: 10.1016/j.neuroimage.2015.09.053

Pajonk, F.-G., Wobrock, T., Gruber, O., Scherk, H., Berner, D., Kaizl, I., et al. (2010). Hippocampal plasticity in response to exercise in schizophrenia. *Arch. Gen. Psychiatry* 67, 133–143. doi: 10.1001/archgenpsychiatry.2009.193

Parachikova, A., Nichol, K. E., and Cotman, C. W. (2008). Short-term exercise in aged Tg2576 mice alters neuroinflammation and improves cognition. *Neurobiol. Dis.* 30, 121–129. doi: 10.1016/j.nbd.2007.12.008

Penedo, F. J., and Dahn, J. R. (2005). Exercise and well-being: a review of mental and physical health benefits associated with physical activity. *Curr. Opin. Psychiatry* 18, 189–193. doi: 10.1097/00001504-200503000-00013

Preacher, K. J., and Hayes, A. F. (2008). Asymptotic and resampling strategies for assessing and comparing indirect effects in multiple mediator models. *Behav. Res. Methods* 40, 879–891. doi: 10.3758/BRM.40.3.879

Preacher, K. J., and Kelley, K. (2011). Effect size measures for mediation models: quantitative strategies for communicating indirect effects. *Psychol. Methods* 16, 93–115. doi: 10.1037/a0022658

Roberts, R. E., Anderson, E. J., and Husain, M. (2013). White matter microstructure and cognitive function. *Neuroscientist* 19, 8–15. doi: 10.1177/1073858411421218

Robitaille, A., Muniz, G., Lindwall, M., Piccinin, A. M., Hoffman, L., Johansson, B., et al. (2014). Physical activity and cognitive functioning in the oldest old: within- and between-person cognitive activity and psychosocial mediators. *Eur. J. Ageing* 11, 333–347. doi: 10.1007/s10433-014-0314-z

Roshanaei-Moghaddam, B., Katon, W. J., and Russo, J. (2009). The longitudinal effects of depression on physical activity. *Gen. Hosp. Psychiatry* 31, 306–315. doi: 10.1016/j.genhosppsych.2009.04.002

Ruscheweyh, R., Willemer, C., Krüger, K., Duning, T., Warnecke, T., Sommer, J., et al. (2011). Physical activity and memory functions: an interventional study. *Neurobiol. Aging* 32, 1304–1319. doi: 10.1016/j.neurobiolaging.2009.08.001

Sexton, C. E., Betts, J. F., Demnitz, N., Dawes, H., Ebmeier, K. P., and Johansen-Berg, H. (2016). A systematic review of MRI studies examining the relationship between physical fitness and activity and the white matter of the ageing brain. *Neuroimage* 131, 81–90. doi: 10.1016/j.neuroimage.2015.09.071

Singh, N. A., Clements, K. M., and Fiatarone, M. A. (1997). Sleep, sleep deprivation, and daytime activities. A randomized controlled trial of the effect of exercise on sleep. *Sleep* 20, 95–101.

Smith, J. C., Lancaster, M. A., Nielson, K. A., Woodard, J. L., Seidenberg, M., Durgerian, S., et al. (2016). Interactive effects of physical activity and APOE-ε4 on white matter tract diffusivity in healthy elders. *Neuroimage* 131, 102–112. doi: 10.1016/j.neuroimage.2015.08.007

Smith, J. C., Nielson, K. A., Woodard, J. L., Seidenberg, M., Durgerian, S., Hazlett, K. E., et al. (2014). Physical activity reduces hippocampal atrophy in elders at genetic risk for Alzheimer's disease. *Front. Aging Neurosci.* 6:61. doi: 10.3389/fnagi.2014.00061

Smith, P. J., Blumenthal, J. A., Hoffman, B. M., Cooper, H., Strauman, T. A., Welsh-Bohmer, K., et al. (2010). Aerobic exercise and neurocognitive performance: a meta-analytic review of randomized controlled trials. *Psychosom. Med.* 72, 239–252. doi: 10.1097/PSY.0b013e3181d14633

Ströhle, A. (2009). Physical activity, exercise, depression and anxiety disorders. *J. Neural Transm. (Vienna)* 116, 777–784. doi: 10.1007/s00702-008-0092-x

Teixeira, P. J., Carraça, E. V., Markland, D., Silva, M. N., and Ryan, R. M. (2012). Exercise, physical activity, and self-determination theory: a systematic review. *Int. J. Behav. Nutr. Phys. Act.* 9:78. doi: 10.1186/1479-5868-9-78

Ten Brinke, L. F., Bolandzadeh, N., Nagamatsu, L. S., Hsu, C. L., Davis, J. C., Miran-Khan, K., et al. (2015). Aerobic exercise increases hippocampal volume in older women with probable mild cognitive impairment: a 6-month randomised controlled trial. *Br. J. Sports Med.* 49, 248–254. doi: 10.1136/bjsports-2013-093184

Thomas, A. G., Dennis, A., Rawlings, N. B., Stagg, C. J., Matthews, L., Morris, M., et al. (2016). Multi-modal characterization of rapid anterior hippocampal volume increase associated with aerobic exercise. *Neuroimage* 131, 162–170. doi: 10.1016/j.neuroimage.2015.10.090

Tomporowski, P. D., and Ellis, N. R. (1986). Effects of exercise on cognitive processes: A review. *Psychol. Bull.* 99, 338–346. doi: 10.1037/0033-2909.99.3.338

van Praag, H. (2008). Neurogenesis and exercise: past and future directions. *Neuromolecular Med.* 10, 128–140. doi: 10.1007/s12017-008-8028-z

van Praag, H., Christie, B. R., Sejnowski, T. J., and Gage, F. H. (1999). Running enhances neurogenesis, learning, and long-term potentiation in mice. *Proc. Natl. Acad. Sci. U.S.A.* 96, 13427–13431. doi: 10.1073/pnas.96.23.13427

van Praag, H., Shubert, T., Zhao, C., and Gage, F. H. (2005). Exercise enhances learning and hippocampal neurogenesis in aged mice. *J. Neurosci.* 25, 8680–8685. doi: 10.1523/JNEUROSCI.1731-05.2005

Vance, D. E., Wadley, V. G., Ball, K. K., Roenker, D. L., and Rizzo, M. (2005). The effects of physical activity and sedentary behavior on cognitive health in older adults. *J. Aging Phys. Act.* 13, 294–313. doi: 10.1123/japa.13.3.294

Vaynman, S., Ying, Z., and Gomez-Pinilla, F. (2004). Hippocampal BDNF mediates the efficacy of exercise on synaptic plasticity and cognition. *Eur. J. Neurosci.* 20, 2580–2590. doi: 10.1111/j.1460-9568.2004.03720.x

Verstynen, T. D., Lynch, B., Miller, D. L., Voss, M. W., Prakash, R. S., Chaddock, L., et al. (2012). Caudate nucleus volume mediates the link between cardiorespiratory fitness and cognitive flexibility in older adults, caudate nucleus volume mediates the link between cardiorespiratory fitness and cognitive flexibility in older adults. *J. Aging Res.* 2012, e939285. doi: 10.1155/2012/939285

Vivar, C., Potter, M. C., Choi, J., Lee, J.-Y., Stringer, T. P., Callaway, E. M., et al. (2012). Monosynaptic inputs to new neurons in the dentate gyrus. *Nat. Commun*, 3: 1107. doi: 10.1038/ncomms2101

Vivar, C., Potter, M. C., and van Praag, H. (2013). All about running: synaptic plasticity, growth factors and adult hippocampal neurogenesis. *Curr. Top. Behav. Neurosci.* 15, 189–210. doi: 10.1007/7854_2012_220

Voelcker-Rehage, C., Godde, B., and Staudinger, U. M. (2010). Physical and motor fitness are both related to cognition in old age. *Eur. J. Neurosci.* 31, 167–176. doi: 10.1111/j.1460-9568.2009.07014.x

Voelcker-Rehage, C., and Niemann, C. (2013). Structural and functional brain changes related to different types of physical activity across the life span. *Neurosci. Biobehav. Rev.* 37(9 Pt B), 2268–2295. doi: 10.1016/j.neubiorev.2013.01.028

Voss, M. W., Heo, S., Prakash, R. S., Erickson, K. I., Alves, H., Chaddock, L., et al. (2013a). The influence of aerobic fitness on cerebral white matter integrity and cognitive function in older adults: results of a one-year exercise intervention. *Hum. Brain Mapp.* 34, 2972–2985. doi: 10.1002/hbm.22119

Voss, M. W., Nagamatsu, L. S., Liu-Ambrose, T., and Kramer, A. F. (2011). Exercise, brain, and cognition across the life span. *J. Appl. Physiol.* 111, 1505–1513. doi: 10.1152/japplphysiol.00210.2011

Voss, M. W., Prakash, R. S., Erickson, K. I., Basak, C., Chaddock, L., Kim, J. S., et al. (2010). Plasticity of brain networks in a randomized intervention trial of exercise training in older adults. *Front. Aging Neurosci.* 2:32. doi: 10.3389/fnagi.2010.00032

Voss, M. W., Vivar, C., Kramer, A. F., and van Praag, H. (2013b). Bridging animal and human models of exercise-induced brain plasticity. *Trends Cogn. Sci.* 17, 525–544. doi: 10.1016/j.tics.2013.08.001

Walker, M. P. (2009). The role of sleep in cognition and emotion. *Ann. N. Y. Acad. Sci.* 1156, 168–197. doi: 10.1111/j.1749-6632.2009.04416.x

Weinstein, A. M., Voss, M. W., Prakash, R. S., Chaddock, L., Szabo, A., White, S. M., et al. (2012). The association between aerobic fitness and executive function is mediated by prefrontal cortex volume. *Brain Behav. Immun.* 26, 811–819. doi: 10.1016/j.bbi.2011.11.008

Wilckens, K., Erickson, K. I., and Wheeler, M. E. (in press). Physical activity and cognition: a mediating role of efficient sleep. *Behav. Sleep Med.*

Williams, P., and Lord, S. R. (1997). Effects of group exercise on cognitive functioning and mood in older women. *Aust. N. Z. J. Public Health* 21, 45–52. doi: 10.1111/j.1467-842X.1997.tb01653.x

Wong, C. N., Chaddock-Heyman, L., Voss, M. W., Burzynska, A. Z., Basak, C., Erickson, K. I., et al. (2015). Brain activation during dual-task processing is associated with cardiorespiratory fitness and performance in older adults. *Front. Aging Neurosci.* 7:154. doi: 10.3389/fnagi.2015.00154

Yaffe, K., Falvey, C. M., and Hoang, T. (2014). Connections between sleep and cognition in older adults. *Lancet Neurol.* 13, 1017–1028. doi: 10.1016/S1474-4422(14)70172-3

Zhang, S., Chen, Y., Liu, Z., Zhang, J., Li, X., Cui, R., et al. (2015). Association of white matter integrity and cognitive functions in chinese non-demented elderly with the APOE 4 allele. *J. Alzheimers Dis.* 48, 781–791. doi: 10.3233/JAD-150357

Zimmerman, B., Sutton, B. P., Low, K. A., Fletcher, M. A., Tan, C. H., Schneider-Garces, N., et al. (2014). Cardiorespiratory fitness mediates the effects of aging on cerebral blood flow. *Front. Aging Neurosci.* 6:59. doi: 10.3389/fnagi.2014.00059

8

No Overt Effects of a 6-Week Exergame Training on Sensorimotor and Cognitive Function in Older Adults: A Preliminary Investigation

Madeleine Ordnung [1], ***Maike Hoff*** [1], ***Elisabeth Kaminski*** [1], ***Arno Villringer*** [1, 2] **and** ***Patrick Ragert*** [1, 3*]

[1] Department of Neurology, Max Planck Institute for Human Cognitive and Brain Sciences, Leipzig, Germany, [2] Mind and Brain Institute, Charité and Humboldt University, Berlin, Germany, [3] Institute for General Kinesiology and Exercise Science, University of Leipzig, Leipzig, Germany

Edited by:
Claudia Voelcker-Rehage, Technische Universität Chemnitz, Germany

Reviewed by:
Tongjian You, University of Massachusetts, USA
Eling D. De Bruin, ETH Zurich, Switzerland

***Correspondence:**
Patrick Ragert
patrick.ragert@uni-leipzig.de

Several studies investigating the relationship between physical activity and cognition showed that exercise interventions might have beneficial effects on working memory, executive functions as well as motor fitness in old adults. Recently, movement based video games (exergames) have been introduced to have the capability to improve cognitive function in older adults. Healthy aging is associated with a loss of cognitive, as well as sensorimotor functions. During exergaming, participants are required to perform physical activities while being simultaneously surrounded by a cognitively challenging environment. However, only little is known about the impact of exergame training interventions on a broad range of motor, sensory, and cognitive skills. Therefore, the present study aims at investigating the effects of an exergame training over 6 weeks on cognitive, motor, and sensory functions in healthy old participants. For this purpose, 30 neurologically healthy older adults were randomly assigned to either an experimental (ETG, $n = 15$, 1 h training, twice a week) or a control group (NTG, $n = 15$, no training). Several cognitive tests were performed before and after exergaming in order to capture potential training-induced effects on processing speed as well as on executive functions. To measure the impact of exergaming on sensorimotor performance, a test battery consisting of pinch and grip force of the hand, tactile acuity, eye-hand coordination, flexibility, reaction time, coordination, and static balance were additionally performed. While we observed significant improvements in the trained exergame (mainly in tasks that required a high load of coordinative abilities), these gains did not result in differential performance improvements when comparing ETG and NTG. The only exergaming-induced difference was a superior behavioral gain in fine motor skills of the left hand in ETG compared to NTG. In an exploratory analysis, within-group comparison revealed improvements in sensorimotor and cognitive tasks (ETG) while NTG only showed an improvement in a static balance test. Taken together, the present study indicates that even though exergames might improve gaming performance, our behavioral assessment was probably not sensitive enough to capture exergaming-induced improvements. Hence, we suggest to use more tailored outcome measures in future studies to assess potential exergaming-induced changes.

Keywords: exergames, healthy aging, sensorimotor, cognition, video games, aerobic fitness, motor skills

INTRODUCTION

In the last decades, great effort has been put into understanding how to improve healthy and successful aging, since a prolonged lifespan has major implications for our health care and social system.

Typically, aging is accompanied with a decline in cognitive (Park et al., 2002; Verhaeghen and Cerella, 2002; Salthouse, 2004) and sensorimotor functions (Stevens and Choo, 1996; Konrad et al., 1999; Smith et al., 1999; Krampe, 2002; Li and Lindenberger, 2002). However, there are substantial individual differences in how much people are affected by age-related decline. And it seems that some people are relatively spared of age-related alterations and disabilities (Nelson and Dannefer, 1992; Morse, 1993; Christensen et al., 1994; Fozard et al., 1994; Stewart et al., 2014). In this regard, successful aging has become a familiar term and is defined by three components: being actively engaged in life, the absence of disease as well as physical and mental fitness (Rowe and Kahn, 1997). More importantly, these components are not acting independently; they rather contribute in an interrelated fashion. Accordingly, many studies emphasized the key role of physical activities in preventing as inevitable seeming age-related chronic diseases, neurodegenerative, and psychiatric disorders (Sacco et al., 1998; Franklin et al., 2001; Strawbridge et al., 2002; Ravaglia et al., 2008; Ciolac, 2013). Being engaged in physical activity can further contribute significantly to life satisfaction and happiness in later life (Menec, 2003; Liffiton et al., 2012). Moreover, there is compelling evidence that exercising is an effective approach to prevent cognitive decline associated with increasing age (Hertzog et al., 2008; Bherer et al., 2013). For instance, it is well established that aerobic training not only improves motor fitness, it also positively influences cognitive performance, such as working memory and executive functions. Furthermore, these behavioral benefits are accompanied by structural and functional brain adaptations (Kramer et al., 1999; Colcombe et al., 2006; Angevaren et al., 2008; Erickson et al., 2011; Voelcker-Rehage et al., 2011; Voss et al., 2013; Bamidis et al., 2014), like volume changes in cortical motor and frontal areas as well as in subcortical structures. Interestingly, these changes are not exclusively induced by cardiovascular training. Coordination training combining balance, limb coordination, spatial orientation and reaction time tasks are also effective in modulating brain structure and function that are associated with improvements in cognition and motor performance (Voelcker-Rehage et al., 2010, 2011). Comparative studies revealed that combining motor and cognitive demands during exercising can even lead to greater enhancements in cognition than training the domains separately (Fabre et al., 2002; Oswald et al., 2006; Lauenroth et al., 2016). It has been argued that enhanced neuronal metabolic processes induced by physical activity can only be exploited efficiently when the brain is simultaneously challenged by cognitive demands (Oswald et al., 2006; Bamidis et al., 2014). Moreover, it is thought that multi-modal training interventions resemble real-life demands and therefore yield higher chances of successful transfer to other tasks and every-day life situations (Lustig et al., 2009). In line with this, recent studies have highlighted the capacity of lifestyle interventions, like dancing (Kattenstroth et al., 2013; Coubard et al., 2014) or playing video games (Maillot et al., 2012; Pichierri et al., 2012), to enhance sensorimotor and cognitive functions in older adults. Investigating the potential of video games in preventing age-related cognitive decline has gained great research interest within the last years (Green and Seitz, 2015). It has been frequently shown that cognitive video game training can have beneficial effects on several cognitive functions in older adults, including memory, attention, and reaction time (Lampit et al., 2014; Toril et al., 2014). While classical video games being played sedentarily, movement based video games (exergames) require the performance of physical activities while being simultaneously surrounded by a cognitively challenging environment. Studies were able to show that exergaming for instance can promote executive functions and cognitive processing speed in older adults (Maillot et al., 2012; Schoene et al., 2013). Furthermore, a recent review article could show that various studies using exergame trainings, show beneficial effects on cognitive, as well as on dual-task performance, which potentially reduces the risk of falls in older adults (Ogawa et al., 2016). Nevertheless, exergame intervention studies attempting to examine effects on motor performance, investigated mainly the effect on balance, which showed rather mixed results (Bisson et al., 2007; Nicholson et al., 2015). The same holds true for improvements in muscle strength of lower and upper limbs (Nitz et al., 2010; Jorgensen et al., 2013). Moreover, benefits are mostly shown for trained tasks but only limited transfer effects to other tests (Bisson et al., 2007; Pichierri et al., 2012; Baniqued et al., 2014; Sato et al., 2014). Video game characteristics might contribute to this since most of the video games used are tailor-made, representing predominantly highly controlled laboratory conditions and therefore missing a multi-modal environment promoting transfer (Lustig et al., 2009; Baniqued et al., 2014). In contrast, commercial video games which, for instance, include different sport disciplines, require fast reactions and the ability to shift the attentional focus for performing appropriate and well timed movements. Up do date, studies examining commercial video games were mostly conducted using different applications of Nintendo®, for instance Nintendo Wii™ (Nintendo Co. Ltd., Kyoto, Japan). This system is equipped with a hand remote controller which requires to play the game in performing physical gestures by moving upper limbs. A more recent development are consoles using a camera system, for instance Xbox™ 360 Kinect™ (Microsoft corp., Redmond, WA), which recognizes gestures and therefore requires whole body movements for playing (van Diest et al., 2013). Up to now, only a few studies examined the effects of a whole-body exergame training and they have indicated improvements in balance (van Diest et al., 2016) and lower extremity muscle strength (Sato et al., 2014). In fact, to date little is known about the impact of a whole-body and multi-modal exergame training intervention on a broad range of sensorimotor and cognitive skills, such as aerobic fitness, fine motor skills, tactile acuity, and working memory. Furthermore, sample characteristics between studies differ to a great extent and ranging from hospitalized, community dwelling (Jorgensen et al., 2013; Schoene et al., 2013; Sato et al., 2014; Nicholson et al., 2015; van Diest et al., 2016) to independent living sedentary participants (Maillot et al., 2012). Until now, it is not known whether healthy active older adults would also benefit from exergame training. Likewise, there is a huge difference in study design of previously performed studies. They differ in duration and frequency of the training program and the standardization of the setting (home-based or under supervision in the lab; Maillot et al., 2012; Schoene et al., 2013; van Diest et al., 2016). Typically, studies so far were taken place within training periods up to 12 weeks, with a training frequency of 2–3 sessions per week (Hall et al., 2012; Marston and Smith, 2012). Interestingly, Colcombe and Kramer (2003) stated that effects of physical training on cognition can already be found after 1 month of training, while longer training periods show substantially larger effects. Therefore, the current study aimed to investigate the effect of a whole-body exergame training intervention using the console Xbox™ 360 Kinect™ over a rather short training period of 6 weeks. Based on previous findings from the aforementioned studies, we expected that a multi-domain video exergame training combining endurance, coordination, strength as well as demands on cognitive processing will translate into overall, and therefore generalized enhancements of a broad range of sensorimotor as well as cognitive functions. Following on this, we further wanted to examine the potential benefits of exergame training for provoking benefits in a healthy, active sample of older adults. We therefore hypothesized that exergaming will induce significant improvements in the performance of sensorimotor and cognitive functions compared with a group receiving no training. We further expected that the exergame training group will show significant practice effects during exergaming and that these online improvements will be associated with the baseline performance in the sensorimotor and cognitive tests.

MATERIALS AND METHODS

Participants

A total number of 30 healthy participants were enrolled in the present study after giving written informed consent. To exclude any evidence for neurological disease and contraindications with respect to the study procedures, all participants were neurologically examined by a physician. All participants were free of taking any central-acting drugs and completed the Mini-Mental State Examination (MMSE; Folstein et al., 1983). We further did not include highly skilled musicians, typists, or sportsmen. Nevertheless, some of the participants were experienced in playing a musical instrument or did sports on a regular basis as assessed by a questionnaire (for group characteristics also see **Table 1**). Handedness was assessed using the Edinburgh Handedness Inventory (Oldfield, 1971). According to this questionnaire, three participants were considered ambidextrous (mean score: 2; range −10–26) and therefore excluded for the analysis on hand function, grip strength and pinch force, as well as touch sensitivity. The remaining participants were all right handed (91.81; range 70–100). None of the participants reported to have experiences in playing exergames. The participants were randomly assigned to a passive no training group ($n = 15$, 8 female, mean age: 68.6 ± 4.67) or the exergame training group ($n = 14$, 7 female, mean age: 69.79 ± 6.34). All subjects gave written informed consent in accordance with the declaration of Helsinki. The protocol was approved by the local ethics committee of the University of Leipzig (ref no. 376-15-24082015).

Experimental Procedure

We used a between groups, pretest-training-posttest design for which participants were randomly assigned to either the exergame training group (ETG) or a passive no training group (NTG). All participants completed cognitive tests as well as sensorimotor tests before and after the respective intervention (see also **Figure 1**). The tests were administered each time in a random order over 2 days. Prior to the pre and post-tests for both groups as well as before each session for the ETG, level of attention, fatigue and discomfort was examined using a visual analog scale (VAS) ranging from 1 to 10 (1 = very inattentive to 10 = very attentive; 1 = high fatigue to 10 low fatigue; 1 = no discomfort to 10 = high discomfort). For the ETG, motivation to train was administered at the beginning of each training session (1 = very unmotivated to 10 = very motivated). Between pre and post assessments, participants from the ETG performed

TABLE 1 | Group demographics.

Variable	ETG		NTG		p-value
	M	SD	M	SD	
Age	69.79	6.34	68.6	4.67	0.569
Education	1.93	0.83	1.47	0.74	0.125
MMSE	29.36	1.22	28.73	1.1	0.158
BMI	25.54	3.84	26.36	4.85	0.665
Physical activity	1.64	1.22	1.73	2.22	0.894
Musical training	0.21	0.43	0.33	0.49	0.491

Education: years of school; total score range 1–3 (1 = at least 12 years; 2 = 10 years, 3 = 8 years). MMSE, Mini Mental State Examination; total score range of 1–30; cut-off score for exclusion: <26. BMI, Body Mass Index; Physical Activity: average hours of sport activity per week. Music training: average hours of playing a musical instrument. All values are depicted as mean ± standard deviation of the mean. ETG, Exergame Training Group; NTG, No Training Group.

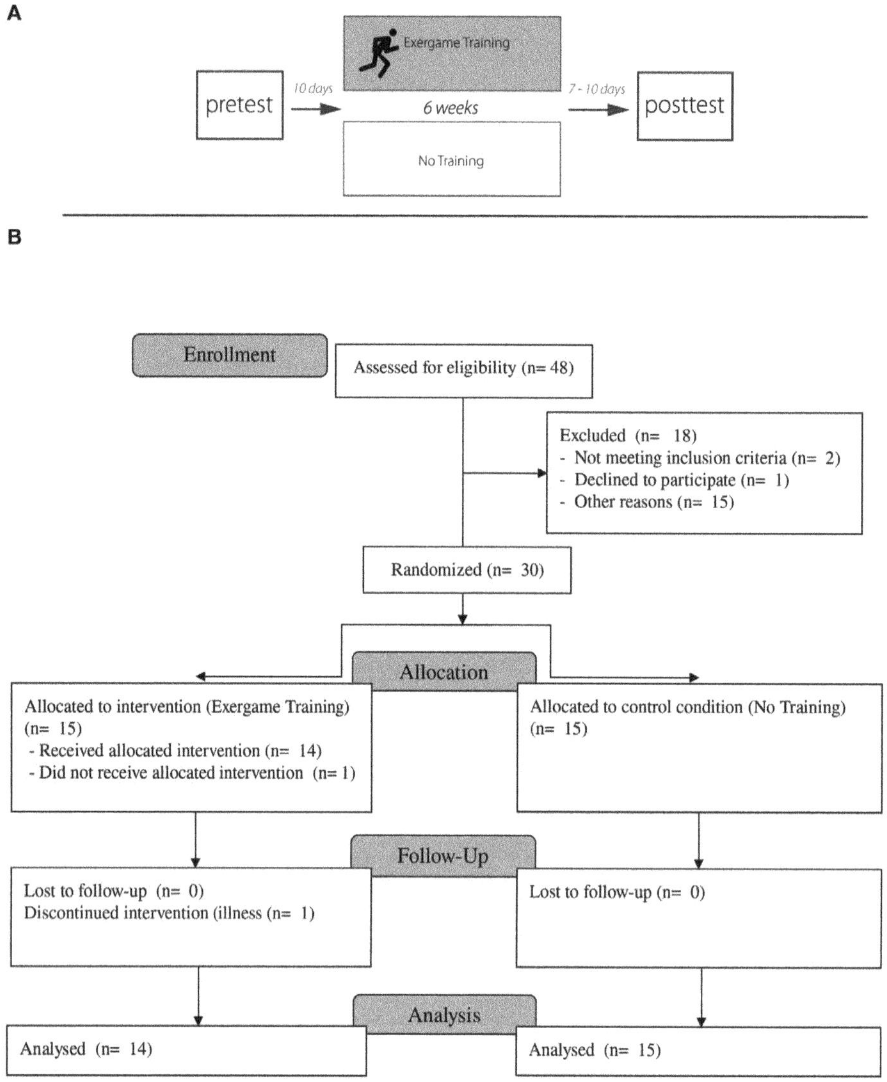

FIGURE 1 | Experimental setup and design. (A) Subjects were randomly assigned to a intervention group (exergame training), participating in a exergame training over 6 weeks, or a passive control group (no training group). All participants completed cognitive as well as sensorimotor tests 10 days before (pretest) the intervention. The same tests were administered with cognitive testings 10 days and sensorimotor testings 7 days after the intervention. **(B)** Flow diagram presenting the enrollment, intervention allocation, follow-up, and data analysis with the respective number of participants.

in total 12 exergame training sessions over 6 weeks, with 2 sessions per week. Each session lasted 60 min resulting in a total training time of 12 h. For avoiding potential influences by social interactions, each participant received personal training sessions. At the beginning of each session pulse at rest was measured using a pulse oximeter, placed at the index finger. In order to reduce the risk of injuries a standardized warm-up of 5 min was performed prior to the exergame training.

Outcome Variables

Aerobic Fitness and Sensorimotor Performance

Aerobic fitness

To characterize aerobic fitness, we used the 3 Min Step Test (ACSM, 2010) measuring pulse recovery to a functional activity (step climbing). The test was performed on an aerobic platform (heights: 24 cm) and step cadence was controlled using a metronome which was set to 84 beats per minute (bpm). Prior to the test, resting pulse (RP) on the index finger was measured with a finger-tip pulse oximeter (PULOX® PO-200, Novidion GmbH, Germany). Following the demonstration by an instructor, the participants performed the test for 3 min. Immediately after finishing the test, strained pulse (ST) and 1 min later recovery pulse (ReP) were measured. For the analysis we computed the Ruffier performance index (Rodríguez Cabrero, 2015) using the following formula: [(RP + ST + ReP) − 200]/10. Participants were excluded from the analysis if they could not keep the given cadence or if they had to stop the test due to exhaustion. For those reasons, data of three participants had to be excluded from the analysis.

Upper body muscular endurance

For measuring muscular endurance of the upper body, participants were asked to lie prone on an exercise mattress with the forehead resting on a wedge pillow. The participants were given a dumbbell in each hand and were instructed to perform a rowing motion simultaneously with both arms (stretching and bending of the arms) between two markers. The movement frequency was determined by a metronome which was set to 60 bpm. Upper arms and elbows had to form an angle of 90°, slightly touching a marker on the back. For performing the stretching movement, the hands with the dumbbells were supposed to touch the front marker. The number of movement repetitions served as outcome measurement. The test was stopped if the participants were touching the mattress with the dumbbells, if they could not keep the movement frequency or if they were not able to touch the two markers (front or back) anymore. Female participants had to move dumbbells with a weight of 1 kg each; males were tested using 2 kg dumbbells. Data of two participants could not be collected due to non-attendance.

Grip strength

The maximum strength of the hand and forearm muscle was analyzed using a hydraulic dynamometer (SEAHAN®, SEAHAN Corporation, S. Korea). Participants sat in an upright position and were instructed to hold the dynamometer in the hand while keeping the elbow by the side of the body and the arm at right angles. For the testing, participants had to squeeze the dynamometer for 5 s applying maximum isometric effort. Left and right hand were measured three times in a randomized order. Grip strength was measured in kg and for the final analysis mean performance of each side was used. Due to non-attendance, data from one participant could not be collected.

Pinch force

Maximum pinch force of the thumb was evaluated using a hydraulic pinch gauge (SEAHAN®, SEAHAN Corporation, S. Korea). Participants were asked to take an upright position with the arm forming an angle of 90° while keeping the elbow on the side. Participants were holding the pinch gauge between the proximal interphalangeal joint of the index finger and the thumb. The pinch gauge had to be squeezed with maximum force three times each side. Each trial lasted 5 s with a break of 10 s in between. The dependent variable was mean performance of each side in kg.

Motor reaction time

For measuring motor reaction time we used the Ruler Drop Test (Del Rossi et al., 2014). Participants were seated sideways on a chair with the forearm placed over the edge of the chair. The bottom of the measuring stick was placed perpendicular between the thumb and the index finger of the participant. After an acoustic warning signal, the stick was dropped and the participant had to catch it as fast as possible. We recorded the number on the measuring stick displayed just over the thumb representing the reaction time. The test was performed with the dominant hand. Due to non-attendance, data from one participant could not be collected.

Hand motor skills

Fine motor skills of the upper extremities were evaluated using the Jebson-Taylor Hand Function Test (JTT) (Jebsen et al., 1969). Originally the JTT consists of seven different subtests from which six were included in this study: turning over cards, picking up small objects and placing them in a can, picking up small objects with a teaspoon and placing them in a can, stacking chequers, moving large light-weighted cans, and moving heavy-weighted cans. Participants were instructed to perform the tasks as fast and accurate as possible. All subtests were performed separately with left and right hand with left-hand performance always evaluated first. For the analysis, we recorded times for completion of each task and each hand.

Flexibility

Flexibility was characterized using the Back Scratch Test (Konopack et al., 2008) which was performed in a sitting position. Participants had to place one hand behind the head and back over the shoulder and reaching down the back as far as possible. The palm was supposed to touch the body and the fingers were directed downwards. The other arm was also moved behind the back under the shoulder with the palm turned outward and fingers upward reaching the fingers from the other hand. The movements of the arms had to be performed without any momentum. As the dependent variable, distance or overlap in centimeter from the two middle fingers was assessed. If there was a distance between the fingers, participants received a negative score while, for overlapping fingers, a positive score was attributed. If the fingertips were exactly touching, the given score was zero. Due to non-attendance data from one participant could not be collected.

Static balance

For investigating static balance we used the Wii Balanceboard© (Nintendo Co. Ltd., Kyoto, Japan) which has been shown to reliable measure balance in the elderly (Chang et al., 2013). Static stance was assessed under four different conditions: standing still on both legs eyes open and closed, on the right leg and left leg eyes open. Each condition lasted for 15 s. Subjects were instructed to stand as quietly as possible on the platform. Prior the testing, individual center of pressure was calibrated. For all conditions, the average body sway in anterior-posterior (AP) and medio-lateral (ML) direction was analyzed using the STABLE software from pro-WISS© (Bochum, Germany).

Tactile performance

Tactile performance was measured using Touch-Test™ Sensory Evaluators (Semmes-Weinstein Monofilaments, North Coast Medical, Inc., CA). The test kit contained 20 filaments differing in length and diameter, therefore resulting in a specific buckling force. Hence, the applied forces were ranging between 0.008 and 300 mN. The filaments were pressed in a 90° angle against the tip of the index finger until they bowed and were hold in place for approximately 2 s. The participants were asked to close their eyes and respond as soon as the stimulus was felt. The test was performed using a staircase procedure starting with the filament representing the highest force by decreasing until the participant could not perceive the stimulus anymore (lower boundary). The forces then were increased until the participant reported an indentation again (upper boundary). In order to receive the absolute touch threshold, this procedure was repeated for three times and the resulting six values were averaged.

Cognition

Cognitive performance was measured using subtests from the TAP 2.3 (Test of Attentional Performance, PsyTest, Herzogenrath), a computer-based neuropsychological test-battery for analyzing different aspects of attention (Zimmermann and Fimm, 1995). Therefore, the participants were seated in front of a computer screen with hands placed in front of two response keys (left and right). For familiarizing the participants with each subtest, a short exercise session followed the instructions. Subtests were presented in randomized order.

Alertness and simple reaction time

Reaction time was measured under two conditions. The first condition concerned simple reaction time to a visual stimuli (greek cross) appearing in random intervals on the screen. Participants had to respond as quickly as possible by pressing a key. In the second condition, the visual stimuli was preceded by a cue in form of a warning tone. The cross followed the warning tone in random intervals. Mean reaction times in ms for both conditions were assessed.

Working memory

Working memory capacity and information flow was evaluated by using a N-back task ($N = 2$). Therefore, a sequence of numbers was presented on the screen. Participants were instructed to press the key if the given number was the same as the last but one number. We assessed the number of correct trials out of 15 in 5 min. Due to technical problems, data of one participant was discarded for the final analysis.

Response inhibition

This paradigm was used to measure the participant's capability to inhibit a response triggered by an external stimulus. For this either an upright cross (Go-stimulus) or a diagonal cross (NoGo-stimulus) was presented on the screen. Participants were instructed to press a key as fast as possible only when the Go-stimulus appeared. The average of correct answers out of 20 in 2 min was used as dependent variable.

Exergame Training

For the training we used the Microsoft X box 360^{TM}, a commercial video game console, in combination with the Microsoft Kinect Sensor^{TM}. The Kinect sensor is a horizontal bar which is connected to a motorized base. Equipped with a RGB camera, a depth sensor and a multi-array microphone the Kinect sensor provides full-body 3D motion capture. Hence, without any need for a game controller the sensor enables exergaming via whole body movements. Connected to a screen the Kinect sensor was placed in 2 ms distance frontal to the participants. While training, the Kinect sensor was tracking the participants' movements and therefore allowed them to control their avatars, a graphical representation of the user, in the game. Every training session included different sport games from the commercial video game *Summer Stars 2012* (DEEP SILVER GmbH, Munich Germany). Based on their primarily required motor proficiency, the games were categorized as endurance (freestyle and butterfly swimming, hammer throwing), strength (hurdles, javelin throwing, 100 meter running), and coordination (trampoline, high diving, archery, mountain biking) disciplines. Each participant was playing two times eight disciplines which were presented in a fixed order. Gaming scores for each discipline and every session were noted to examine practice effects. For motivating adherence and enjoyment, 100 meter running and butterfly swimming were replaced by hurdles and freestyle swimming after 6 training sessions, due to similarly required skills. To prevent overexertion pulse was monitored throughout each training session, assessed before and right after every discipline. Each training session was supervised by an instructor ensuring the participants safety and the correct performance of the required movements. For this purpose participants practiced only half of the training program during the first week of training. The participants in the NTG were instructed to keep their usual lifestyle over the entire time of the study.

Data Analysis

Statistical analyses of the data were performed using the statistical software package for social sciences (IBM SPSS v22), figures were made using RStudio 3.3.1 (RStudio Team, 2015). As an initial step, data-sets were checked for normal distribution using the Kolmogorov-Smirnov Test. Since behavioral data were not normally distributed for some outcome measures, we subsequently performed non-parametric statistical tests to evaluate performance improvements within- and between-groups. Effect-sizes were analyzed accordingly, using effect-size measurement r. Comparing VAS, we performed parametric statistical tests using an rmANOVA with factor TIME × GROUP. Sample demographics were compared using two-sample t-Tests. Effect size for ANOVA was reported as η_p^2. Effect size for T-tests as Cohen's d.

One participant was excluded from the final analysis due to non-attendance of at least 80 percent of all training sessions. Therefore, the data of 29 participants (mean age: 69.17 ± 5.47 years; range 60–78 years; 15 females) were included in the final analysis.

Group Comparisons of Sensorimotor and Cognitive Performance Measures

To unravel potential pre-training differences, we compared the baseline scores from both groups in the sensorimotor and cognitive performance measures using the Mann-Whitney U-Test for two independent samples. Based on significant pre-training differences between both groups, we then computed a gain score of each subtest representing the percentage performance improvement using the following formula:

$$[(\text{post} - \text{pre})/\text{pre}]^{*}100$$

pre (raw test score before the training period), post (raw test score after the training period).

Thereby, we assured that performance gain was evaluated independent from potential baseline differences between groups. In order to examine offline effects induced by the exergame training, gain scores were subsequently compared between-groups using Mann-Whitney *U*-test for two independent samples.

Practice Effects and Baseline Dependency of Exergaming Performance

For excluding influences on gaming performance, we analyzed the average VAS scores and motivation to train before and after each training session using paired *t*-tests. To characterize online training effects, gain scores (see formula above) out of the noted raw game scores from the first (pre) and last session (post) for each sport discipline were calculated. Statistical evaluation was carried out using one sample Wilcoxon signed rank test. Bonferroni correction was applied if necessary to account for multiple comparisons. Within- and between-group comparisons were assessed at the 5% level of significance.

RESULTS

Demographics

According to independent samples *t*-tests, there were no significant between-group differences regarding age [$t_{(27)} = -0.57$, $p = 0.569$, $d = -0.21$], years of education [$t_{(27)} = -1.58$, $p = 0.125$, $d = -0.59$], MMSE scores [$t_{(27)} = -1.45$, $p = 0.158$, $d = -0.54$], body mass index [$t_{(20)} = 0.44$, $p = 0.665$, $d = 0.19$], hours of physical activity [$t_{(27)} = 0.14$, $p = 0.894$, $d = 0.05$] and hours of playing a musical instrument per week [$t_{(27)} = 0.70$, $p = 0.491$, $d = 0.27$] (see also **Table 1** for mean values). RM-ANOVA revealed no group differences in fatigue [$F_{(1,25)} = 1.23$, $p = 0.279$, $\eta_p^2 = 0.047$] and discomfort [$F_{(1,25)} = 0$, $p = 0.946$, $\eta_p^2 = 0.001$] but a significant TIME × GROUP interaction for attention [$F_{(1,25)} = 7.17$, $p = 0.013$, $\eta_p^2 = 0.223$]. Nevertheless, considering the mean values (see also **Table 2**), we believe that there was no impact from attention on the post-performance of the NTG.

Group Comparisons of Sensorimotor and Cognitive Performance Measures

We found significant between-group baseline differences in JTT performance of the left hand (Mann-Whitney *U*-Test for two independent samples, ETG Mdn: 5.91 s, NTG Mdn: 5.34 s, $U = -3.275$, $p = 0.001$, $r = 0.61$), as well as in the touch test of the right hand (ETG Mdn: 3.32 mN, NTG Mdn: 3.03 mN, $U = -2.389$, $p = 0.016$, $r = 0.44$). Please see **Table 3** for details on all variables tested. When comparing the gain scores of both groups, we found significantly greater improvements for the ETG in the JTT performance of the left hand (ETG Mdn: 14.747%, NTG Mdn: 2.538%, $U = -3.230$, $p = 0.001$, see also **Figure 2**). However, all other variables showed no significant differences between groups. The descriptives and inferentials for all variables are given in **Table 4**.

TABLE 2 | Visual Analogue Scale (VAS).

Variable	ETG		NTG		
	M	SD	M	SD	*p*-value
Attention	8.46	0.77	8.89	1	0.075
Fatigue	8.61	0.84	9.18	1.15	0.065
Discomfort	1.1	0.79	1.03	0.73	0.521

A visual analog scale was used to assess attention, fatigue and discomfort before the pre-training and post-training measurements. Attention scale ranging from 1 to 10 (1 = very inattentive to 10 = very attentive). Fatigue scale, from 1 to 10 (1 = high fatigue to 10 low fatigue) and discomfort scale ranging from 1 to 10 (1 = no discomfort to 10 = high discomfort). All values are expressed as mean ± standard deviation. ETG, Exergame Training Group; NTG, No Training Group.

Within-Group Comparisons of Sensorimotor and Cognitive Performance Measures

Within-group comparison were done in an exploratory fashion, to investigate potential training effects and their effect sizes, in the ETG and NTG separately. The ETG showed significant performance improvements from baseline to post-measurement in pinch force of both hands (Wilcoxon-Test for two related samples, Pinch Force Test right, Mdn pre: 6.16 kg, Mdn post: 7.40 kg, $W = -2.542$, $p = 0.011$, $r = 0.68$, Pinch Force Test left, Mdn pre: 6.61, Mdn post:6.95, $W = -2.982$, $p = 0.003$, $r = 0.80$), in fine motor function of both hands as assessed with the JTT (JTT right hand Mdn pre: 4.91 s, Mdn post:4.62 s, $W = -3.296$, $p = 0.00$, $r = 0.88$, JTT left hand Mdn pre: 5.91 s. Mdn post: 5.27 s, $W = -3.107$, $p = 0.002$, $r = 0.83$), in the assessment of static balance with eyes closed (COP AP Mdn pre: 7.05 mps, Mdn post: 6.00 mps, $W = -2.010$, $p = 0.044$, $r = 0.54$, COP ML Mdn pre: 2.90 mps, Mdn post: 2.10, $W = -1.992$, $p = 0.046$, $r = 0.53$) and in two cognitive assessments (Alertness Mdn pre: 273.75 ms, Mdn post: 241.10 ms, $W = -2.291$, $p = 0.022$, $r = 0.61$, simple reaction time Mdn pre: 274.55 ms, Mdn post: 251.60 ms, $W = -2.040$, $p = 0.041$, $r = 0.55$). However, the NTG only showed significant performance improvements in one assessment of static balance (COP AP Mdn pre: 6.60 mps, Mdn post: 6.00 mps, $W = -2.786$, $p = 0.005$, $r = 0.72$). Please see **Table 5** for details.

Practice Effects and Baseline Dependency of Exergaming Performance

The overall adherence to the training was 97% with 163 out of 168 sessions (14 participants for 6 weeks/2 sessions per week). The ETG did not show significant differences in their level of attention [$t_{(13)} = -1.94$, $p = 0.075$, $d = 0.47$], fatigue [$t_{(13)} = -2.01$, $p = 0.065$, $d = 0.56$] and discomfort [$t_{(13)} = 0.66$, $p = 0.520$, $d = 0.09$] before and after each training session as assessed by paired *t*-tests. On average, participants showed a high motivation to train at the beginning of each session (mean: 8.77 ± 0.84). Participants of the ETG showed significant online practice improvements in six of the performed disciplines. Two of the strength and all coordination dominated disciplines showed significant performance improvements already after the

TABLE 3 | Baseline characteristics of both groups.

Variables	ETG		NTG		U	*p*-value	Effect-size r
	Median	Min–Max	Median	Min–Max			
AEROBIC FITNESS AND SENSORIMOTOR PERFORMANCE							
Step test (Index)	10.60	0.0–14.40	7.50	0–18.2	−0.917	0.377	0.17
Upper body muscular endurance test (rep.)	26.00	0.0–40.00	22.00	0–77.0	−0.529	0.621	0.10
Grip strength test R (kg)	21.32	16.53–49.59	27.83	0–48.08	−0.568	0.591	0.11
Grip strength test L (kg)	21.09	16.18–42.03	27.67	0–45.51	−0.371	0.715	0.07
Pinch force test R (kg)	6.16	4.54–12.70	7.12	0–12.4	−0.044	0.983	0.01
Pinch force test L (kg)	6.61	4.55–11.17	6.65	0–12.25	−0.284	0.780	0.05
Motor reaction time test (cm)	17.00	0.00–28.00	17.0	9.50–32.50	−0.459	0.652	0.09
JTT R (s)	4.91	4.38–6.69	4.80	0–5.27	−1.179	0.252	0.22
JTT L (s)	5.91	4.48–8.08	5.34	0–5.91	−3.275	0.001*	0.61
Back scratch test R (cm)	−12.50	−30.00–12.00	−2.0	−38.0–12.0	−0.415	0.683	0.08
Back scratch test L (cm)	−16.00	−39.00–6.00	−8.0	−35.0–12.0	−1.026	0.310	0.19
COP AP EO (mps)	3.90	2.10–6.30	4.8	2.90–11.0	−1.719	0.077	0.32
COP AP EC (mps)	7.05	3.20–13.50	6.60	3.0–11.80	−0.175	0.880	0.03
COP ML EO (mps)	2.15	1.00–4.10	1.80	1.10–3.40	−1.116	0.270	0.21
COP ML EC (mps)	2.90	1.30–9.00	2.80	1.10–5.90	−0.459	0.652	0.09
Touch-test R (mN)	3.32	3.09–3.60	3.03	0.0–3.90	−2.389	0.016	0.44
Touch-test L (mN)	3.22	2.43–4.06	3.16	0.0–3.74	−0.918	0.377	0.17
COGNITION							
Alertness (ms)	273.75	237.40–390.70	254.0	229.50–330.70	−1.746	0.085	0.32
Simple reaction time (ms)	274.55	230.60–391.30	254.90	227.10–329.60	−1.200	0.234	0.22
Working memory (correct)	9.00	−26.00–15.00	13.0	−1.0–15.0	−1.744	0.085	0.32
Response inhibition (correct)	19.00	10.00–20.00	19.0	16.0–20.0	−1.021	0.331	0.19

*ETG, Exergame Training Group; NTG, No Training Group; Min, Minimum; Max, Maximum; COP, Center of pressure deviation; AP, Anterior-Posterior; ML, medio-lateral; EO, eyes open; EC, eyes closed; U-Test-statistic for Mann-Whitney-U nonparametric test for the comparison of two independent samples, Effect-size r: $r = |z/\sqrt{n}|$; r = 0.01: small effect, r = 0.30: medium effect; r = 0.50: large effect. *indicate significant finding.*

first half of the training period (Wilcoxon signed rank test for one sample, hurdles Mdn middle session: 6.00% improvement, $Z = 2.551$, $p = 0.011$, $r = 0.68$), (javelin throwing Mdn middle session: 14.69% improvement, $Z = 2.794$, $p = 0.005$, $r = 0.75$), (archery Mdn middle session: 23.29% improvement, $Z = 3.110$, $p = 0.002$, $r = 0.83$), (high diving Mdn middle session: 24.68% improvement, $Z = 2.605$, $p = 0.009$, $r = 0.69$), (trampoline Mdn middle session: 7.30% improvement, $Z = 3.269$, $p = 0.001$, $r = 0.87$), (mountain biking Mdn middle session: 19.08% improvement, $Z = 3.233$, $p = 0.001$, $r = 0.86$) while there were no significant in-game improvements in the endurance-based disciplines. For detailed description see **Table 6**.

DISCUSSION

The main objective of the current study was to investigate whether an exergame training is able to induce changes in cognitive, as well as sensorimotor performance in healthy older adults. Recent exergame studies addressed this question by using rather long training periods and specific tailor-made training regimes. Hence, our main aim was to elaborate effects based on a multi-modal video game combining endurance, coordination, strength and cognitive demands after a short training period of 6 weeks. We observed significant exergaming induced improvements in fine motor skills of the left hand when comparing performance gains between ETG and NTG. Participants in the intervention group showed significant improvements in online gaming performance across the training sessions for most of the strength and all of the coordination based disciplines. However, these online training effects did not seem to translate into overall performance improvements on the assessed cognitive and sensorimotor functions. While we observed significant improvements in the trained exergame (mainly in tasks that required a high load of coordinative abilities), these gains did not result in differential performance improvements when comparing ETG and NTG.

In an exploratory analysis, within-group comparison revealed improvements in sensorimotor and cognitive tasks (ETG) while NTG only showed an improvement in a static balance test. Taken together, the present study indicates that even though exergames might improve gaming performance, our behavioral assessment was probably not sensitive enough to capture exergaming-induced improvements. To which amount different training parameters such as duration, frequency, or study population contribute to the absence of effect regarding cognition and parameters of motor activity, can not be tested with the given

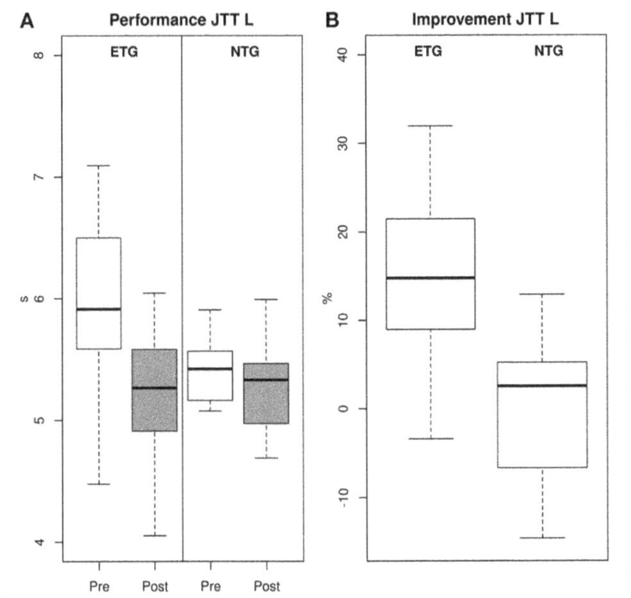

FIGURE 2 | Exergame training-induced improvements in motor performance. (A) Mean performance in JTT (left hand). There were significant differences at baseline for the JTT (left hand) indicating that both groups started at different performance levels. After the exergame training the ETG were able to complete the JTT faster than the NTG. **(B)** Relative improvement in JTT (left hand). In order to account for baseline differences performance was analyzed independently from baseline measures by calculating a relative gain score. When comparing the relative gains score between both groups, we observed significant improvements for the ETG compare to the NTG.

study design. However, different aspects will be discussed in the next sections.

To date, the beneficial effects of exergames on fine motor skills have primarily been shown in clinical studies (Sin and Lee, 2013; Pietrzak et al., 2014; da Silva Ribeiro et al., 2015; Wittmann et al., 2016). For example, Paquin et al. (2015) could show that a 15 min Wii-based training over 8 weeks enhanced upper limb fine motor performance in stroke patients, as assessed by the JTT which was also used in the present study. In a study by McNulty et al. (2011), stroke patients performed a Wii-based training over 10 consecutive days and improved significantly in the Wolf Motor Function Test (WMFT). They concluded that improvements in Wii gaming skills might have generalized to more functional tasks as assessed by the WMFT. The WMFT includes several functional and timed tasks to quantify upper extremity motor ability and is therefore similar to the JTT (Jebsen et al., 1969; Wolf et al., 2001). In the present study, the ETG was able to complete the JTT significantly faster after participating in an exergame training over 6 weeks compared to the NTG, at least in left hand performance. Except from video game training interventions, other lifestyle interventions have already been shown to be effective in enhancing motor performance in healthy older adults (Van Roie et al., 2010; Wu et al., 2010; Kattenstroth et al., 2013; van het Reve and de Bruin, 2014; Eggenberger et al., 2015, 2016). For example, Kattenstroth et al. (2013) performed a 6-month dance intervention in healthy older adults and found beneficial effects in hand-arm steadiness, control precision, and wrist movements compared to a passive control group. Comparable to dancing, playing exergames is based on complex upper body movements and it is therefore assumable that exergaming would also translate into enhanced fine motor skills. The exergame training used in the present study required an intensive use of upper limbs for performing strength and endurance dominated disciplines as well as fine adjusted movements of upper extremity inter-limb coordination. Hence, our findings of improved fine motor performance after 6 weeks of exergame training could be interpreted as transfer of newly acquired motor skills to functional tasks which were not directly practiced during exergaming. Interestingly, exergame induced effects were only visible in significant performance improvements of the non-dominant left hand. This transfer of bilateral training to unilateral improvements has already been well documented in previous studies (Schulze et al., 2002; Burgess et al., 2007; McCombe Waller and Whitall, 2008; Hinder et al., 2013). A study by Schulze et al. (2002) revealed that a bimanual training of the pegboard task leads to improvements in unimanual performance with, however, no difference for the left or right hand. Middleton et al. (2013) demonstrated that after a Wii-based training over 2 weeks young participants performed significantly better in a bimanual and eye-hand coordination task simulating surgical procedures using their non-dominant left hand. One could speculate that task characteristics might explain this effect since performing surgery-like movements require complex functional skills and are therefore visuo-motor and cognitively more demanding compared to a simple motor task. In older adults it has been shown that the performance of unimanual and bimanual tasks requires more neural resources compared to young participants which is known as neural "overactivation" (Mattay et al., 2002; Ward, 2006; Heuninckx et al., 2008; Goble et al., 2010). In a study by Goble et al. (2010), it was shown that older adults exhibited elaborated brain activity in several motor and frontal brain regions during a wrist coordination task compared to younger adults. Moreover, the elaborated brain activation in the supplementary motor area and the somatosensory cortex was positively correlated with higher coordination task demands during antiphasic movements and can therefore be considered a marker for increased task complexity. Hinder et al. (2013) demonstrated a strong transfer of bimanual and unimanual contexts for young and old adults with, however, a release of intracortical inhibition only by older participants. During the exergame training, participants had to perform various bimanual movements. Thus, one could argue that a more elaborated bihemispheric activation while performing the required movements during exergaming might explain the significant improvements in the JTT for the left hand. Nevertheless, the absence of effects in the dominant hand might also be due to an already relatively high skill level compared to the less used hand.

Moreover, Kattenstroth et al. (2013) attributed the enhanced effects in fine motor skills not only to increased sensorimotor coordination but also to muscle strength. Our results corroborate this assumption by showing, that when comparing the within-group effects of the ETG, there is not only a significant

TABLE 4 | Group comparisons of sensormimotor and cognitive performance gains.

Variables	ETG		NTG		U	p-value	Effect-size r
	Median	Min–max	Median	Min–max			
AEROBIC FITNESS AND SENSORIMOTOR PERFORMANCE							
Step test (Index)	10.047	−52.73–70.00	−2.236	−104.41–45.05	−1.878	0.063	0.35
Upper body muscular endurance test (rep.)	−2.00	−47.06–87.50	−3.226	−81.48–100.00	−0.568	0.591	0.11
Grip strength test R (kg)	2.475	−16.56–19.17	−6.232	−14.03–25.44	−1.615	0.112	0.30
Grip strength test L (kg)	1.159	−32.14–19.50	−8.807	−26.80–9.35	−1.746	0.081	0.32
Pinch force test R (kg)	12.512	−20.74–78.69	18.494	−16.12–58.28	−0.611	0.561	0.11
Pinch force test L (kg)	28.077	−5.13–48.61	17.411	−18.35–42.23	−1.571	0.123	0.29
Motor reaction time test (cm)	0.00	−41.94–23.21	−21.053	−115.79–37.84	0.590	0.561	0.11
JTT R (s)	6.652	0.04–28.87	5.566	−18.00–18.37	−0.567	0.561	0.11
JTT L (s)	14.747	−3.40–31.94	2.538	−14.64–12.90	−3.230	0.001*	0.60
Back scratch test R (cm)	−5.556	−110.00–75.00	−5.263	−275.00–500.00	−0.611	0.561	0.11
Back scratch test L (cm)	−3.571	−1900.00–80.00	0.00	−230.00–200.00	−0.655	0.533	0.12
COP AP EO (mps)	−4.021	−121.05–50.00	5.00	−56.25–71.11	−1.135	0.270	0.21
COP AP EC (mps)	0.00	−135.48–60.98	−20.69	−81.82–64.00	−0.131	0.914	0.02
COP ML EO (mps)	23.132	−94.34–50.79	11.11	−6.98–42.37	−0.873	0.400	0.16
COP ML EC (mps)	25.238	−119.35–65.56	7.692	−36.36–65.52	−0.458	0.652	0.09
Touch-test R (mN)	2.104	−13.91–20.60	1.979	−16.67–27.34	−0.306	0.780	0.06
Touch-test L (mN)	3.074	−13.94–11.43	3.881	−14.10–35.44	−0.284	0.780	0.05
COGNITION							
Alertness (ms)	4.500	−27.08–25.70	2.026	−32.62–24.97	−1.047	0.310	0.19
Simple reaction time (ms)	10.185	−14.90–32.35	5.398	−15.35–18.97	−1.571	0.123	0.29
Working memory (correct)	0.00	−66-67–200.00	0.00	−400.00–16.67	−1.263	0.217	0.23
Response inhibition (correct)	0.00	−5.26–50.00	0.00	−10.53–18.75	−1.230	0.234	0.23

*ET, Exergame Training Group; NTG, No Training Group; Min, Minimum; Max, Maximum; COP, Center of pressure deviation; AP, Anterior-Posterior; ML, medio-lateral; EO, eyes open; EC, eyes closed; Effect-size r: $r = |z/\sqrt{n}|$; r = 0.01; small effect; r = 0.30: medium effect; r = 0.50: large effect. *indicate significant finding.*

performance improvement of fine motor skills of the hand, but also in pinch force of both hands, after 6 weeks of exergame training.

However, since a direct comparison between ETG and NTG did not reach significance, our within-group findings need to be interpreted with caution since sample size might be to small to reach significant between-group effects. The impact on strength by exergame training has been reported mainly in clinical studies with mixed results (Yavuzer et al., 2008; McNulty et al., 2011; Lee, 2013; Sin and Lee, 2013; Laver et al., 2015). In fact, Lee (2013) reported that after 6 weeks of exergame training stroke patients improved in upper body muscle strength which were, however, not significantly different to a control group who received occupational therapy. Up to date, only a few studies were examining exergame trainings using healthy populations with preliminary results indicating that video game training can promote lower limb muscle strength in middle aged woman (Nitz et al., 2010) and older adults (Jorgensen et al., 2013). However, since we only assessed muscle strength of the upper limbs, this assessment might have been not specific enough to capture differential training effects between the ETG and NTG.

The investigated exergame training had no differential effects on aerobic fitness when comparing ETG with NTG. This is in contrast to Maillot et al. (2012) where older adults exhibited improvements in aerobic fitness assessed by a reduction in maximum and mean heart rate in a 6-min walking test after 12 weeks of Wii-based training. While Maillot et al. (2012) were using more stationary games without the necessity of leaving the ground with one foot, in the present study, sport disciplines which required pronounced efforts in running (100 meter running) or walking on the spot while performing additional arm movements (javelin throwing, freestyle swimming, hammer throwing) were given.

Effects of rather classical aerobic training regimes have been intensively investigated within the last years, with results indicating strong associations between cardio-respiratory fitness and performance in cognition (Kramer et al., 1999; Colcombe et al., 2006; Erickson et al., 2011; Leckie et al., 2014). Only a small number of studies have focused on this relationship using exergame training interventions. These studies showed that exergames have beneficial effects on executive functions, processing speed and dual-task-performance which is consistent with findings on aerobic training (Maillot et al., 2012; Schoene et al., 2013). Interestingly, in our study we found no significant between-group evidence for a transfer of exergaming on response inhibition (in a Go/NoGo task) or on reaction time.

However, when looking at the within-group comparison in only the ETG, we found significant performance improvements

TABLE 5 | Within-group comparison from pre to post.

	ETG					NTG				
	Pre median	Post median	W	*p*-value	Effect-size r	Pre	Post	W	*p*-value	Effect-size r
AEROBIC FITNESS AND SENSORIMOTOR PERFORMANCE										
Step test (Index)	10.60	8.05	−1.363	0.173	0.36	7.50	10.00	−0.943	0.345	0.24
Upper body muscular endurance test (rep.)	26.00	24.00	−0.236	0.813	0.06	22.00	20.00	−1.473	0.141	0.38
Grip strength test R (kg)	21.32	21.17	0.847	0.397	0.23	27.82	35.00	−0.568	0.570	0.15
Grip strength test L (kg)	21.09	22.33	−0.094	0.925	0.03	27.67	32.67	−0.682	0.496	0.18
Pinch force test R (kg)	6.16	7.40	−2.542	0.011*	0.68	7.11	7.60	−1.817	0.069	0.47
Pinch force test L (kg)	6.61	6.95	−2.982	0.003*	0.80	6.65	7.33	−1.761	0.078	0.45
Motor reaction time test (cm)	17.00	17.75	−0.045	0.964	0.01	17.00	17.00	−0.483	0.629	0.12
JTT R (s)	4.91	4.62	−3.296	0.001*	0.88	4.79	4.68	0.00	1.00	0.00
JTT L (s)	5.91	5.27	−3.107	0.002*	0.83	5.34	5.33	−1.477	0.140	0.38
Back scratch test R (cm)	−12.50	−11.00	−1.429	0.153	0.38	−2.00	−4.00	−0.399	0.690	0.10
Back scratch test L (cm)	−16.00	−13.50	−1.102	0.271	0.29	−8.00	−11.00	−0.537	0.591	0.14
COP AP EO (mps)	3.90	3.85	−0.440	0.660	0.12	4.80	5.00	−1.221	0.222	0.32
COP AP EC (mps)	7.05	6.00	−2.010	0.044*	0.54	6.60	6.00	−2.786	0.005*	0.72
COP ML EO (mps)	2.15	1.80	−0.707	0.480	0.19	1.80	1.80	−0.566	0.572	0.15
COP ML EC (mps)	2.90	2.10	−1.992	0.046*	0.53	2.80	2.00	−2.328	0.020*	0.60
Touch-test R (mN)	3.32	3.25	−1.014	0.311	0.27	3.025	3.22	−0.824	0.410	0.21
Touch-test L (mN)	3.22	3.12	−1.400	0.162	0.37	3.16	3.16	−0.398	0.691	0.10
COGNITION										
Alertness (ms)	273.75	241.10	−2.291	0.022*	0.61	254.00	238.90	−1.647	0.10	0.43
Simple reaction time (ms)	274.55	251.60	−2.040	0.041*	0.55	254.90	241.10	−1.022	0.307	0.26
Working memory (correct)	9.00	10.00	−1.101	0.271	0.29	13.00	11.00	−1.630	0.103	0.42
Response inhibition (correct)	19.00	19.00	−1.706	0.088	0.46	19.00	19.00	−0.203	0.839	0.05

*Wilcoxon-Test for two dependent samples, W, Test-statistic for Wilcoxon-test; ETG, Exergame Training Group; NTG, No Training Group; COP, Center of pressure deviation; AP, Anterior-Posterior; ML, medio-lateral; EO, eyes open; EC, eyes closed; Effect-size r: $r = |z/\sqrt{n}|$; r = 0.01: small effect; r = 0.30: medium effect; r = 0.50: large effect. *indicate significant finding.*

from before to after the exergame training in alertness and simple reaction time. Interestingly, this effect was absent in the NTG. Accordingly, one could speculate that a training period of 6 weeks might have been too short for inducing distinct changes in cognition, or that the selected cognitive tests were not sensitive enough for capturing these. On the other hand, sample characteristics might have also crucially contributed. Indeed, while participants of the aforementioned studies were living a sedentary lifestyle, our study sample was characterized by an according to their age, healthy and physical active sample of older adults.

It is well established that poor balance and the risk of falling seems to be associated with executive functions and attention since keeping balance requires the integration of somatosensory informations and is further associated with the control and shift of attentional resources (Woollacott and Shumway-Cook, 2002; Granacher et al., 2008; Yogev-Seligmann et al., 2008; Mirelman et al., 2012; Kearney et al., 2013). Consequently, recent research suggest that an effective balance training should include more complex exercises as well as cognitive demands (Halvarsson et al., 2015). The used exergame sport disciplines required the performance of highly demanding movements covering multiple domains within a cognitively challenging environment. Interestingly, we found significant performance improvements in static balance tasks, after 6 weeks of exergame training, in the ETG as well as in the NTG. This effect was however, only visible in within-group pre to post comparisons and did not reach significance for the differential between-group comparisons.

Studies suggested that static (e.g., in quiet stance) and dynamic postural control (e.g., in perturbation or locomotion) are governed by different neuromuscular mechanisms. In a study by Kang and Dingwell (2006) significant differences and no correlation between dynamic stability properties of walking and standing have been found. Interestingly, while participants in the study of Bisson et al. (2007) improved in functional balance, as assessed by the Community Balance and Mobility Scale, no significant changes in postural sway during quite stance were found. A meta analysis on exergaming for balance training pointed out that instrumental assessments of balance often fails to detect small changes whereas more functional clinical tests are too global. van Diest et al. (2013) therefore concluded that only the usage of both functional and objective-instrumental measures of balance is reliable for capturing effects on balance induced by exergame interventions. In the present study, static balance was administered in an objective-instrumental fashion by using a force plate. As a consequence, the absence of specific

TABLE 6 | Online learning effects in gaming performance.

Variables	% Improvement from FS to										% Improvement from MS to LS				
	MS					LS					LS vs. MS				
	Median	Min–max	Z	*p*-value	Effect-size r	Median	Min–max	Z	*p*-value	Effect-size r	Median	Min–max	Z	*p*-value	Effect-size r
STRENGTH															
100 Meter running	6.46	−1.07–16.84	2.132	0.033	0.57	3.00	−18–21	1.572	0.116	0.42	2.00	−21–12	−0.549	0.583	0.15
Hurdles	6.00	−9–39	2.551	0.011	0.68	7.00	−8–33	2.552	0.011	0.68	0.00	−16–6	−0.78	0.937	0.21
Javelin throwing	14.69	−17.56–101.18	2.794	0.005	0.75	19.2	−20.74–109.66	2.62	0.009	0.70	−3.00	−14–25	−0.454	0.650	0.12
ENDURANCE															
Freestyle swimming	4.00	−8–35	1.572	0.116	0.42	1.00	−7–26	0.863	0.388	0.23	−2.00	−13–8	−1.782	0.075	0.48
Butterfly swimming	0.55	−5.48–4.65	1.036	0.300	0.28	2.36	−11.18–6.37	1.852	0.064	0.49	0.79	−12.71–6.48	1.161	0.245	0.31
Hammer throwing	2.78	−6.29–23.60	1.664	0.096	0.44	6.00	−4–19.00	2.132	0.033	0.57	−2.00	−5–4	−1.363	0.73	0.36
COORDINATION															
Archery	23.29	−8.52–40.10	3.110	0.002	0.83	32	−7–48	3.040	0.002	0.81	−2.00	−11–6	−2.213	0.021	0.59
High diving	24.68	−32.93–68.45	2.605	0.009	0.69	35	−38–149	2.621	0.009	0.70	−7.00	−48– 25	−0.943	−0.345	0.25
Trampoline	7.30	2.15–43.95	3.269	0.001	0.87	8	3–46	3.180	0.001	0.85	−1.00	−4–1	−2.621	0.009	0.70
Mountain biking	19.08	−2.10–48.82	3.233	0.001	0.86	22.00	12–51	3.180	0.001	0.85	5.00	−9–16	1.992	0.046	0.53

FS, First Session; MS, Middle Session; LS, Last Session. All disciplines were trained over 12 sessions, except butterfly and freestyle swimming, as well as hurdles and 100 meter running which were trained only over 6 weeks. For those disciplines the scores for the MS therefore represent the performance from the 4th session. Scores from the LS represent the performance from the 6th session. For the remaining disciplines MS refers to the score from 6th session and LS to the 12th session. All values are given in percentage. After Bonferroni correction, a p-value of $p < 0.017$ was considered as significant.

training-induced effects on balance performance could be due to the applied test which might have not been able to detect slight improvements of our training participants.

The sense of touch is essential for daily life since sensorimotor performance such as keeping balance or motor hand function depends on afferent tactile informations (Lord et al., 1991; Tremblay et al., 2003). To date, the potential training of tactile performance has been mostly investigated using passive stimulation paradigms such as tactile coactivation where small skin portions of the finger are directly stimulated for a few hours. While studies using this procedure demonstrated that tactile acuity can be restored in older adults (Dinse et al., 2006; Kalisch et al., 2008), the potential of exercise interventions is yet largely unexplored. One study reported that an enriched training environment in the form of dancing activities over 6 month can induce changes in tactile performance in healthy elderly (Kattenstroth et al., 2013). Likewise, exergames provide simultaneous sensorimotor and cognitive demands and can therefore be considered as environmental enrichment. Nevertheless, after 6 weeks of exergame training, the ETG in the present study did not exhibit improvements in tactile performance. Our result is in line with the study of Nitz et al. (2010) which could not find significant changes after 10 weeks of Wii-based training in middle aged woman. Interestingly, it has been proposed that long term practice in Tai Chi, a whole-body sensory-attentional exercise, is associated with superior tactile skills (Kerr et al., 2008, 2016). Hence, it seems that exercise interventions could provoke benefits in tactile performance but a training duration of 6 weeks might have been to short for inducing effects, or the assessment procedure used, was not specific enough to capture training-induced improvements in tacile performance in older adults

Context Interference and Timing of Post Assessments Crucial for Capturing Training-Induced Effects

In the present study, we especially were interested in whether a multi-domain exergame training is able to foster transfer effects to untrained tasks resulting in significant improvements in a variety of sensorimotor and cognitive assessments. Lustig et al. (2009) reviewed different training types with respect to their effectiveness in improving cognitive functioning in older adults. They pointed out that multi-modal approaches often exhibit broad benefits with, however, relatively small effect sizes. Most of the reviewed multi-modal studies did not include longitudinal follow-up assessments and therefore cannot exclude the possibility that results might have been influenced by interference. The context interference effect suggests that learning of multiple tasks will lead to a poorer initial practice performance but induce superior gains in subsequent retention tests as well as transfer to untrained tasks (Magill and Hall, 1990). Numerous studies investigating simple motor paradigms (Lee and Magill, 1983; Albaret and Thon, 1998; Giuffrida et al., 2002; Sidaway et al., 2016) or more complex real-life motor skills (Bortoli et al., 1992; Hall et al., 1994; Sherwood, 1996; Tsutsui et al., 1998; Babo et al., 2008) concluded that a random compared to a blocked order training of multiple tasks seems to promote learning and transfer more efficiently. For the exergame training used in the present study, participants played different sport disciplines from which each combined different quantities of sensorimotor and cognitive demands. Hence, the training procedure was similar to a random design and we therefore assumed that the exergame training will translate into pronounced gains in the post-tests. After 6 weeks of exergame training, we found improvements in fine motor skill of the left hand in the ETG with, however, no overall enhancements. In general, during exercising various peripheral and central acting physiological processes occur and proceed on different time scales (Adkins et al., 2006). Thus, for capturing training induced changes, timing of post-test assessments seems to be crucial. There are conflicting results regarding the amount of time separating acquisition and retention tests. John dos Santos et al. (2014) confirmed superior performance of a practice group, randomly training a dart throwing task, compared to a block training group, 24 h after the training. However, no significant differences in radial distance from the dart to the inner bull were found 7 and 30 days after training. Contradictory to that, in a study by Pauwels et al. (2014), the interleaved practice group outperformed the block group even 1 week after training in a bimanual tracking task. Moreover, superior performance in retention tests has been found even 2 weeks after training of a throwing task (Granda Vera and Montilla, 2003). According to Lee and Magill (1983) better results in retention following interleaved practice can be explained by higher cognitive demands during the acquisition phase since action plans have to be reconstructed constantly. In the present study, post-tests in motor performance measures were administered 7 days after finishing the exergame training intervention. Despite the fact that we did not have a control group for comparing contextual practice effects, one could speculate that interference between the single tasks took place mediated by a information processing overload. Accordingly, post-test measurements were probably administered too late or too early for capturing overall changes in the sensorimotor and cognitive variables.

Limitations

As a consequence, one limitation of the present study is that we did not examine performance changes in retention tests 2 weeks after training completion. Therefore, it is not possible to draw conclusions about the persistence as well as about the dynamics of behavioral benefits induced by the exergame training. Hence, to draw a comprehensive picture, future studies should include long term retention tests. Furthermore, we did not enroll additional comparison groups to distinguish the domains which were potentially driving the improvements. With the used passive control group, we have accounted for test-retest effects. When investigating effects on motor and cognitive outcome variables manipulated by exergaming, future studies should include a physical activity and cognitive training group for controlling the contribution of each of those domains. Hall et al. (2012) reviewed studies about exergaming in the elderly and consequently emphasized the high potential on physical and mental health outcomes such as enhanced physical mobility, balance, attention, and information processing. Nevertheless, concerns have been addressed regarding methodological issues especially about differences in frequency and duration of interventions as well as the low number of participants. Regarding the duration of physical training interventions, Colcombe and Kramer (2003) stated that a short training period between 1 up to 3 month already showed moderate effects on cognitive function, while longer training periods show substantially larger effects. Accordingly, studies applying the exergame training within this period were able to show significant effects on cognition as well as motor performance (Nitz et al., 2010; Maillot et al., 2012). However, these studies were using participants having a predominantly sedentary lifestyle. In the present study, a sample of active older adults has been used and it is therefore conceivable that the training period of 6 weeks might have been too short for inducing overall effects in active elderly.

However, since we were rather interested in the exploratory investigation on the effects of an commercially available exergame, which is not specificially designed to enhance sensorimotor and cognitive functions, it is possible, that the behavioral improvements only resulted in significant in-game improvements and did not translate into improvements of the specific assessments of sensorimotor and cognitive functions. Finally, for some of our outcome measures (e.g., endurance tests, back scratch test, COP measures), there is no information about the reliability of the respective test available. Hence, our results should be interpreted with caution especially because our study might in fact be underpowered.

CONCLUSIONS

In summary, the present study was the first which addressed the question whether a whole-body exergame training can promote a broad range of sensorimotor and cognitive functions in healthy and active older adults. Interestingly, we observed significant in-game improvements of the exergame training, which was mainly present in disciplines requiring high coordination skills. However, the only exergaming-induced difference was a superior behavioral gain in fine motor skills of the left hand. However, when assessing behavioral improvements of the ETG alone, we saw significant improvements in pinch force, fine motor skills, static balance, and cognitive function, while the assessment of the NTG alone only showed significant improvements in static balance. In conclusion, we found evidence, that 6 weeks of exergame training result in improved gaming performance, but our behavioral assessment was probably not sensitive enough to capture rather global improvements on sensorimotor and cognitive function in older adults.

Therefore, future studies should control for potential driving variables with simultaneous and careful consideration of sample characteristics. Additionally, more knowledge is needed about the underlying neuronal adaptations induced by exergaming which could be of high relevance in preventing pathological age-related brain alterations. Future studies should therefore include neuroimaging assessments in order to identify key regions and significant mental processes acting in multi-domain exergames.

AUTHOR CONTRIBUTIONS

MO, AV, and PR designed the study. MH and EK helped during data acquisition. MO analyzed the data. MO, MH, EK, and PR wrote the manuscript. All authors were involved in discussing data.

ACKNOWLEDGMENTS

We wish to thank Sophia Rose, Pauline Bassler, Claudia Predel, Rouven Kenville as well as Tom Maudrich for helpful support in conducting the study.

REFERENCES

Adkins, D. L., Boychuk, J., Remple, M. S., and Kleim, J. A. (2006). Motor training induces experience-specific patterns of plasticity across motor cortex and spinal cord. *J. Appl. Physiol.* 101, 1776–1782. doi: 10.1152/japplphysiol.00515.2006

Albaret, J. M., and Thon, B. (1998). Differential effects of task complexity on contextual interference in a drawing task. *Acta Psychol.* 100, 9–24.

American College of Sports Medicine (2010). *ACSM's Resource Manual for Guidelines for Exercise Testing and Prescription*, 6th Edn. New York, NY: Lippincott, Williams and Wilkins.

Angevaren, M., Aufdemkampe, G., Verhaar, H. J. J., Aleman, A., and Vanhees, L. (2008). Physical activity and enhanced fitness to improve cognitive function in older people without known cognitive impairment. *Cochrane Database Syst. Rev.* 16:CD005381. doi: 10.1002/14651858.CD005381.pub3

Babo, A. G. F., Azevedo Neto, R. M., and Teixeira, L. A. (2008). Adaptability from contextual interference in the learning of an open skill is context dependent. *Open Sports Med. J.* 2, 56–59. doi: 10.2174/1874387000802010056

Bamidis, P. D., Vivas, A. B., Styliadis, C., Frantzidis, C., Klados, M., Schlee, W., et al. (2014). A review of physical and cognitive interventions in aging. *Neurosci. Biobehav. Rev.* 44, 206–220. doi: 10.1016/j.neubiorev.2014.03.019

Baniqued, P. L., Kranz, M. B., Voss, M. W., Lee, H., Cosman, J. D., Severson, J., et al. (2014). Cognitive training with casual video games: points to consider. *Front. Psychol.* 4:1010. doi: 10.3389/fpsyg.2013.01010

Bherer, L., Erickson, K. I., and Liu-Ambrose, T. (2013). A review of the effects of physical activity and exercise on cognitive and brain functions in older adults. *J. Aging Res.* 2013:657508. doi: 10.1155/2013/657508

Bisson, E., Contant, B., Sveistrup, H., and Lajoie, Y. (2007). Functional balance and dual-task reaction times in older adults are improved by virtual reality and biofeedback training. *Cyberpsychol. Behav.* 10, 16–23. doi: 10.1089/cpb.2006.9997

Bortoli, L., Robazza, C., Durigon, V., and Carra, C. (1992). Effects of contextual interference on learning technical sports skills. *Percept. Mot. Skills* 75, 555–562. doi: 10.2466/pms.1992.75.2.555

Burgess, J. K., Bareither, R., and Patton, J. L. (2007). Single limb performance following contralateral bimanual limb training. *IEEE Trans. Neural Syst. Rehabil. Eng.* 15, 347–355. doi: 10.1109/TNSRE.2007.903908

Chang, W.-D., Chang, W.-Y., Lee, C.-L., and Feng, C.-Y. (2013). Validity and reliability of wii fit balance board for the assessment of balance of healthy young adults and the elderly. *J. Phys. Ther. Sci.* 25, 1251–1253. doi: 10.1589/jpts.25.1251

Christensen, H., Mackinnon, A., Jorm, A. F., Henderson, A. S., Scott, L. R., and Korten, A. E. (1994). Age differences and interindividual variation in cognition in community-dwelling elderly. *Psychol. Aging* 9, 381–390.

Ciolac, E. G. (2013). Exercise training as a preventive tool for age-related disorders: a brief review. *Clinics (Saao Paulo)* 68, 710–717. doi: 10.6061/clinics/2013(05)20

Colcombe, S. J., Erickson, K. I., Scalf, P. E., Kim, J. S., Prakash, R., McAuley, E., et al. (2006). Aerobic exercise training increases brain volume in aging humans. *J. Gerontol. A Biol. Sci. Med. Sci.* 61, 1166–1170. doi: 10.1093/gerona/61.11.1166

Colcombe, S., and Kramer, A. F. (2003). Fitness effects on the cognitive function of older adults: a meta-analytic study. *Psychol. Sci.* 14, 125–130. doi: 10.1111/1467-9280.t01-1-01430

Coubard, O. A., Ferrufino, L., Nonaka, T., Zelada, O., Bril, B., and Dietrich, G. (2014). One month of contemporary dance modulates fractal posture in aging. *Front. Aging Neurosci.* 6:17. doi: 10.3389/fnagi.2014.00017

da Silva Ribeiro, N. M., Ferraz, D. D., Pedreira, É., Pinheiro, Í., da Silva Pinto, A. C., Neto, M. G., et al. (2015). Virtual rehabilitation via Nintendo Wii® and conventional physical therapy effectively treat post-stroke hemiparetic patients. *Top. Stroke Rehabil.* 22, 299–305. doi: 10.1179/1074935714Z.0000000017

Del Rossi, G., Malaguti, A., and Del Rossi, S. (2014). Practice effects associated with repeated assessment of a clinical test of reaction time. *J. Athl. Train.* 49, 356–359. doi: 10.4085/1062-6059-49.2.04

Dinse, H. R., Kleibel, N., Kalisch, T., Ragert, P., Wilimzig, C., and Tegenthoff, M. (2006). Tactile coactivation resets age-related decline of human tactile discrimination. *Ann. Neurol.* 60, 88–94. doi: 10.1002/ana.20862

Eggenberger, P., Theill, N., Holenstein, S., Schumacher, V., and de Bruin, E. D. (2015). Multicomponent physical exercise with simultaneous cognitive training to enhance dual-task walking of older adults: a secondary analysis of a 6-month randomized controlled trial with 1-year follow-up. *Clin. Interv. Aging* 10, 1711–1732. doi: 10.2147/CIA.S91997

Eggenberger, P., Wolf, M., Schumann, M., and de Bruin, E. D. (2016). Exergame and balance training modulate prefrontal brain activity during walking and enhance executive function in older adults. *Front. Aging Neurosci.* 8:66. doi: 10.3389/fnagi.2016.00066

Erickson, K. I., Voss, M. W., Prakash, R. S., Basak, C., Szabo, A., Chaddock, L., et al. (2011). Exercise training increases size of hippocampus and improves memory. *Proc. Natl. Acad. Sci. U.S.A.* 108, 3017–3022. doi: 10.1073/pnas.1015950108

Fabre, C., Chamari, K., Mucci, P., Massé-Biron, J., and Préfaut, C. (2002). Improvement of cognitive function by mental and/or individualized aerobic training in healthy elderly subjects. *Int. J. Sports Med.* 23, 415–421. doi: 10.1055/s-2002-33735

Folstein, M. F., Robins, L. N., and Helzer, J. E. (1983). The mini-mental state examination. *Arch. Gen. Psychiatry* 40:812. doi: 10.1016/0022-3956(75)90026-6

Fozard, J. L., Vercryssen, M., Reynolds, S. L., Hancock, P. A., and Quilter, R. E. (1994). Age differences and changes in reaction time: the Baltimore Longitudinal Study of Aging. *J. Gerontol.* 49, P179–P189.

Franklin, S. S., Larson, M. G., Khan, S. A., Wong, N. D., Leip, E. P., Kannel, W. B., et al. (2001). Does the relation of blood pressure to coronary heart disease risk change with aging? The Framingham Heart Study. *Circulation* 103, 1245–1249. doi: 10.1161/01.CIR.103.9.1245

Giuffrida, C., Lare, G., Shea, J. B., and Fairbrother, J. T. (2002). Differential transfer benefits of increased practice for constant, blocked, and serial practice schedules. *J. Mot. Behav.* 34, 353–365. doi: 10.1080/00222890209601953

Goble, D. J., Coxon, J. P., Van Impe, A., De Vos, J., Wenderoth, N., and Swinnen, S. P. (2010). The neural control of bimanual movements in the elderly: brain regions exhibiting age-related increases in activity, frequency-induced neural modulation, and task-specific compensatory recruitment. *Hum. Brain Mapp.* 31, 1281–1295. doi: 10.1002/hbm.20943

Granacher, U., Zahner, L., and Gollhofer, A. (2008). Strength, power, and postural control in seniors: considerations for functional adaptations and for fall prevention. *Eur. J. Sport Sci.* 8, 325–340. doi: 10.1080/17461390802478066

Granda Vera, J., and Montilla, M. M. (2003). Practice schedule and acquisition, retention, and transfer of a throwing task in 6-yr.-old children. *Percept. Motor Skills* 96(3 Pt 1), 1015–1024. doi: 10.2466/pms.2003.96.3.1015

Green, C. S., and Seitz, A. R. (2015). The impacts of video games on cognition (and how the government can guide the industry). *Policy Insights Behav. Brain Sci.* 2, 101–110. doi: 10.1177/2372732215601121

Hall, A. K., Chavarria, E., Maneeratana, V., Chaney, B. H., and Bernhardt, J. M. (2012). Health benefits of digital videogames for older adults: a systematic review of the literature. *Games Health J.* 1, 402–410. doi: 10.1089/g4h.2012.0046

Hall, K. G., Domingues, D. A., and Cavazos, R. (1994). Contextual interference effects with skilled baseball players. *Percept. Motor Skills* 78(3 Pt 1), 835–841. doi: 10.2466/pms.1994.78.3.835

Halvarsson, A., Oddsson, L., Franzén, E., and Ståhle, A. (2015). Long-term effects of a progressive and specific balance-training programme with multi-task exercises for older adults with osteoporosis: a randomized controlled study. *Clin. Rehabil.* 30, 1049–1059. doi: 10.1177/0269215515605553

Hertzog, C., Kramer, A. F., Wilson, R. S., and Lindenberger, U. (2008). Enrichment effects on adult cognitive development: can the functional capacity of older adults be preserved and enhanced? *Psychol. Sci. Public Interest* 9, 1–65. doi: 10.1111/j.1539-6053.2009.01034.x

Heuninckx, S., Wenderoth, N., and Swinnen, S. P. (2008). Systems neuroplasticity in the aging brain: recruiting additional neural resources for successful motor performance in elderly persons. *J. Neurosci.* 28, 91–99. doi: 10.1523/JNEUROSCI.3300-07.2008

Hinder, M. R., Carroll, T. J., and Summers, J. J. (2013). Transfer of ballistic motor skill between bilateral and unilateral contexts in young and older adults: neural adaptations and behavioral implications. *J. Neurophysiol.* 109, 2963–2971. doi: 10.1152/jn.00535.2012

Jebsen, R. H., Taylor, N., Trieschmann, R. B., Trotter, M. J., and Howard, L. A. (1969). An objective and standardized test of hand function. *Arch. Phys. Med. Rehabil.* 50, 311–319.

John dos Santos, J., Henrique Bastos, F., de Oliveira Souza, T., and Cesar Corrêa, U. (2014). Contextual interference effect depends on the amount of time separating acquisition and testing. *Adv. Phys. Educ.* 4, 102–109. doi: 10.4236/ape.2014.42014

Jorgensen, M. G., Laessoe, U., Hendriksen, C., Nielsen, O. B. F., and Aagaard, P. (2013). Efficacy of Nintendo Wii training on mechanical leg muscle function and postural balance in community-dwelling older adults: a randomized controlled trial. *J. Gerontol. A Biol. Sci. Med. Sci.* 68, 845–852. doi: 10.1093/gerona/gls222

Kalisch, T., Tegenthoff, M., and Dinse, H. R. (2008). Improvement of sensorimotor functions in old age by passive sensory stimulation. *Clin. Interv. Aging* 3, 673–690. doi: 10.2147/CIA.S3174

Kang, H. G., and Dingwell, J. B. (2006). A direct comparison of local dynamic stability during unperturbed standing and walking. *Exp. Brain Res.* 172, 35–48. doi: 10.1007/s00221-005-0224-6

Kattenstroth, J.-C., Kalisch, T., Holt, S., Tegenthoff, M., and Dinse, H. R. (2013). Six months of dance intervention enhances postural, sensorimotor, and cognitive performance in elderly without affecting cardio-respiratory functions. *Front. Aging Neurosci.* 5:5. doi: 10.3389/fnagi.2013.00005

Kearney, F. C., Harwood, R. H., Gladman, J. R. F., Lincoln, N., and Masud, T. (2013). The relationship between executive function and falls and gait abnormalities in older adults: a systematic review. *Dement. Geriatr. Cogn. Disord.* 36, 20–35. doi: 10.1159/000350031

Kerr, C. E., Agrawal, U., and Nayak, S. (2016). The effects of tai chi practice on intermuscular beta coherence and the rubber hand illusion. *Front. Hum. Neurosci.* 10:37. doi: 10.3389/fnhum.2016.00037

Kerr, C. E., Shaw, J. R., Wasserman, R. H., Chen, V. W., Kanojia, A., Bayer, T., et al. (2008). Tactile acuity in experienced Tai Chi practitioners: evidence for use dependent plasticity as an effect of sensory-attentional training. *Exp. Brain Res.* 188, 317–322. doi: 10.1007/s00221-008-1409-6

Konopack, J. F., Marquez, D. X., Hu, L., Elavsky, S., McAuley, E., and Kramer, A. F. (2008). Correlates of functional fitness in older adults. *Int. J. Behav. Med.* 15, 311–318. doi: 10.1080/10705500802365557

Konrad, H. R., Girardi, M., and Helfert, R. (1999). Balance and aging. *Laryngoscope* 109, 1454–1460. doi: 10.1097/00005537-199909000-00019

Kramer, A. F., Hahn, S., Cohen, N. J., Banich, M. T., McAuley, E., Harrison, C. R., et al. (1999). Ageing, fitness and neurocognitive function. *Nature* 400, 418–419. doi: 10.1038/22682

Krampe, R. T. (2002). Aging, expertise and fine motor movement. *Neurosci. Biobehav. Rev.* 26, 769–776. doi: 10.1016/S0149-7634(02)00064-7

Lampit, A., Hallock, H., and Valenzuela, M. (2014). Computerized cognitive training in cognitively healthy older adults: a systematic review and meta-analysis of effect modifiers. *PLoS Med.* 11:e1001756. doi: 10.1371/journal.pmed.1001756

Lauenroth, A., Ioannidis, A. E., and Teichmann, B. (2016). Influence of combined physical and cognitive training on cognition: a systematic review. *BMC Geriatr.* 16:141. doi: 10.1186/s12877-016-0315-1

Laver, K. E., George, S., Thomas, S., Deutsch, J. E., and Crotty, M. (2015). Virtual reality for stroke rehabilitation. *Cochrane Database Syst. Rev.* CD008349. doi: 10.1002/14651858.CD008349.pub3

Leckie, R. L., Oberlin, L. E., Voss, M. W., Prakash, R. S., Szabo-Reed, A., Chaddock-Heyman, L., et al. (2014). BDNF mediates improvements in executive function following a 1-year exercise intervention. *Front. Hum. Neurosci.* 8:985. doi: 10.3389/fnhum.2014.00985

Lee, G. (2013). Effects of training using video games on the muscle strength, muscle tone, and activities of daily living of chronic stroke patients. *J. Phys. Ther. Sci.* 25, 595–597. doi: 10.1589/jpts.25.595

Lee, T. D., and Magill, R. A. (1983). The locus of contextual interference in motor-skill acquisition. *J. Exp. Psychol.* 9, 730–746. doi: 10.1037/0278-7393.9.4.730

Li, K. Z. H., and Lindenberger, U. (2002). Relations between aging sensory/sensorimotor and cognitive functions. *Neurosci. Biobehav. Rev.* 26, 777–783. doi: 10.1016/S0149-7634(02)00073-8

Liffiton, J. A., Horton, S., Baker, J., and Weir, P. L. (2012). Successful aging: how does physical activity influence engagement with life? *Eur. Rev. Aging Phys. Act.* 9, 103–108. doi: 10.1007/s11556-012-0098-0

Lord, S. R., Clark, R. D., and Webster, I. W. (1991). Postural stability and associated physiological factors in a population of aged persons. *J. Gerontol.* 46, M69–M76.

Lustig, C., Shah, P., Seidler, R., and Reuter-Lorenz, P. A. (2009). Aging, training, and the brain: a review and future directions. *Neuropsychol. Rev.* 19, 504–522. doi: 10.1007/s11065-009-9119-9

Magill, R. A., and Hall, K. G. (1990). A review of the contextual interference effect in motor skill acquisition. *Hum. Mov. Sci.* 9, 241–289. doi: 10.1016/0167-9457(90)90005-X

Maillot, P., Perrot, A., and Hartley, A. (2012). Effects of interactive physical-activity video-game training on physical and cognitive function in older adults. *Psychol. Aging* 27, 589–600. doi: 10.1037/a0026268

Marston, H. R., and Smith, S. T. (2012). Interactive videogame technologies to support independence in the elderly: a narrative review. *Games Health J.* 1, 139–152. doi: 10.1089/g4h.2011.0008

Mattay, V. S., Fera, F., Tessitore, A., Hariri, A. R., Das, S., Callicott, J. H., et al. (2002). Neurophysiological correlates of age-related changes in human motor function. *Neurology* 58, 630–635. doi: 10.1212/WNL.58.4.630

McCombe Waller, S., and Whitall, J. (2008). Bilateral arm training: why and who benefits? *NeuroRehabil.* 23, 29–41.

McNulty, P., Mouawad, M., Doust, C., and Max, M. (2011). Wii-based movement therapy to promote improved upper extremity function post-stroke: a pilot study. *J. Rehabil. Med.* 43, 527–533. doi: 10.2340/16501977-0816

Menec, V. H. (2003). The relation between everyday activities and successful aging: a 6-year longitudinal study. *J. Gerontol. B Psychol. Sci. Soc. Sci.* 58, S74–S82. doi: 10.1093/GERONB/58.2.S74

Middleton, K. K., Hamilton, T., Tsai, P.-C., Middleton, D. B., Falcone, J. L., and Hamad, G. (2013). Improved nondominant hand performance on a laparoscopic virtual reality simulator after playing the Nintendo Wii. *Surg. Endosc.* 27, 4224–4231. doi: 10.1007/s00464-013-3027-z

Mirelman, A., Herman, T., Brozgol, M., Dorfman, M., Sprecher, E., Schweiger, A., et al. (2012). Executive function and falls in older adults: new findings from a five-year prospective study link fall risk to cognition. *PLoS ONE* 7:e40297. doi: 10.1371/journal.pone.0040297

Morse, C. K. (1993). Does variability increase with age? An archival study of cognitive measures. *Psychol. Aging* 8, 156–164.

Nelson, E. A., and Dannefer, D. (1992). Aged heterogeneity: fact or fiction? The fate of diversity in gerontological research. *Gerontologist* 32, 17–23.

Nicholson, V. P., McKean, M., Lowe, J., Fawcett, C., and Burkett, B. (2015). Six weeks of unsupervised Nintendo Wii Fit gaming is effective at improving balance in independent older adults. *J. Aging Phys. Act.* 23, 153–158. doi: 10.1123/japa.2013-0148

Nitz, J. C., Kuys, S., Isles, R., and Fu, S. (2010). Is the Wii Fit a new-generation tool for improving balance, health and well-being? A pilot study. *Climacteric* 13, 487–491. doi: 10.3109/13697130903395193

Ogawa, E. F., You, T., and Leveille, S. G. (2016). Potential benefits of exergaming for cognition and dual-task function in older adults: a systematic review. *J. Aging Phys. Act.* 24, 332–336. doi: 10.1123/japa.2014-0267

Oldfield, R. C. (1971). The assessment and analysis of handedness: the Edinburgh inventory. *Neuropsychologia* 9, 97–113. doi: 10.1016/0028-3932(71)90067-4

Oswald, W. D., Gunzelmann, T., Rupprecht, R., and Hagen, B. (2006). Differential effects of single versus combined cognitive and physical training with older adults: the SimA study in a 5-year perspective. *Eur. J. Ageing* 3, 179–192. doi: 10.1007/s10433-006-0035-z

Paquin, K., Ali, S., Carr, K., Crawley, J., McGowan, C., and Horton, S. (2015). Effectiveness of commercial video gaming on fine motor control in chronic stroke within community-level rehabilitation. *Disabil. Rehabil.* 37, 2184–2191. doi: 10.3109/09638288.2014.1002574

Park, D. C., Lautenschlager, G., Hedden, T., Davidson, N. S., Smith, A. D., and Smith, P. K. (2002). Models of visuospatial and verbal memory across the adult life span. *Psychol. Aging* 17, 299–320. doi: 10.1037/0882-7974.17.2.299

Pauwels, L., Swinnen, S. P., and Beets, I. A. M. (2014). Contextual interference in complex bimanual skill learning leads to better skill persistence. *PLoS ONE* 9:e100906. doi: 10.1371/journal.pone.0100906

Pichierri, G., Murer, K., and de Bruin, E. D. (2012). A cognitive-motor intervention using a dance video game to enhance foot placement accuracy and gait under dual task conditions in older adults: a randomized controlled trial. *BMC Geriatr.* 12:74. doi: 10.1186/1471-2318-12-74

Pietrzak, E., Cotea, C., and Pullman, S. (2014). Using commercial video games for upper limb stroke rehabilitation: is this the way of the future? *Top. Stroke Rehabil.* 21, 152–162. doi: 10.1310/tsr2102-152

Ravaglia, G., Forti, P., Lucicesare, A., Pisacane, N., Rietti, E., Bianchin, M., et al. (2008). Physical activity and dementia risk in the elderly: findings from a prospective Italian study. *Neurology* 70(19 Pt 2), 1786–1794. doi: 10.1212/01.wnl.0000296276.50595.86

Rodríguez Cabrero, M. (2015). Physical activity and leisure habits and heir relation with the ruffier index in adolescents. *Rev. Int. Med. Cienc Act. Física Deporte* 15:165. doi: 10.15366/rimcafd2015.57

Rowe, J. W., and Kahn, R. L. (1997). Successful aging. *Gerontologist* 37, 433–440. doi: 10.1093/geront/37.4.433

RStudio Team (2015). *RStudio: Integrated Developement for R.* Boston, MA; RStudio, Inc. Availble online at: http://www.rstudio.com

Sacco, R. L., Gan, R., Boden-Albala, B., Lin, I. F., Kargman, D. E., Hauser, W., et al. (1998). Leisure-time physical activity and ischemic stroke risk: the Northern Manhattan Stroke Study. *Stroke* 29, 380–387. doi: 10.1161/01.STR.29.2.380

Salthouse, T. A. (2004). What and when of cognitive aging. *Curr. Dir. Psychol. Sci.* doi: 10.1111/j.0963-7214.2004.00293.x

Sato, K., Kuroki, K., Saiki, S., and Nagatomi, R. (2014). The effects of exercise intervention using KinectTM on healthy elderly individuals: a quasi-experimental study. *Open J. Ther. Rehabil.* 2, 38–44. doi: 10.4236/ojtr.2014.21008

Schoene, D., Lord, S. R., Delbaere, K., Severino, C., Davies, T. A., and Smith, S. T. (2013). A randomized controlled pilot study of home-based step training in older people using videogame technology. *PLoS ONE* 8:e57734. doi: 10.1371/journal.pone.0057734

Schulze, K., Lüders, E., and Jäncke, L. (2002). Intermanual transfer in a simple motor task. *Cortex* 38, 805–815. doi: 10.1016/S0010-9452(08)70047-9

Sherwood, D. E. (1996). The benefits of random variable practice for spatial accuracy and error detection in a rapid aiming task. *Res. Q. Exerc. Sport* 67, 35–43. doi: 10.1080/02701367.1996.10607923

Sidaway, B., Ala, B., Baughman, K., Glidden, J., Cowie, S., Peabody, A., et al. (2016). Contextual interference can facilitate motor learning in older adults and in individuals with Parkinson's Disease. *J. Mot. Behav.* 48, 509–518. doi: 10.1080/00222895.2016.1152221

Sin, H., and Lee, G. (2013). Additional virtual reality training using xbox kinect in stroke survivors with hemiplegia. *Am. J. Phys. Med. Rehabil.* 92, 871–880. doi: 10.1097/PHM.0b013e3182a38e40

Smith, C. D., Umberger, G. H., Manning, E. L., Slevin, J. T., Wekstein, D. R., Schmitt, F. A., et al. (1999). Critical decline in fine motor hand movements in human aging. *Neurology* 53, 1458–1461. doi: 10.1212/WNL.53.7.1458

Stevens, J. C., and Choo, K. K. (1996). Spatial acuity of the body surface over the life span. *Somatosens. Mot. Res.* 13, 153–166. doi: 10.3109/089902296090 51403

Stewart, J. C., Tran, X., and Cramer, S. C. (2014). Age-related variability in performance of a motor action selection task is related to differences in brain function and structure among older adults. *Neuroimage* 86, 326–34. doi: 10.1016/j.neuroimage.2013.10.016

Strawbridge, W. J., Deleger, S., Roberts, R. E., and Kaplan, G. A. (2002). Physical activity reduces the risk of subsequent depression for older adults. *Am. J. Epidemiol.* 156, 328–334. doi: 10.1093/AJE/KWF047

Toril, P., Reales, J. M., and Ballesteros, S. (2014). Video game training enhances cognition of older adults: a meta-analytic study. *Psychol. Aging* 29, 706–716. doi: 10.1037/a0037507

Tremblay, F., Wong, K., Sanderson, R., and Coté, L. (2003). Tactile spatial acuity in elderly persons: assessment with grating domes and relationship with manual dexterity. *Somatosens. Mot. Res.* 20, 127–132. doi: 10.1080/0899022031000105154

Tsutsui, S., Lee, T. D., and Hodges, N. J. (1998). Contextual interference in learning new patterns of bimanual coordination. *J. Mot. Behav.* 30, 151–157. doi: 10.1080/00222899809601332

van Diest, M., Lamoth, C. J. C., Stegenga, J., Verkerke, G. J., and Postema, K. (2013). Exergaming for balance training of elderly: state of the art and future developments. *J. Neuroeng. Rehabil.* 10:101. doi: 10.1186/1743-0003-10-101

van Diest, M., Stegenga, J., Wörtche, H. J., Verkerke, G. J., Postema, K., and Lamoth, C. J. C. (2016). Exergames for unsupervised balance training at home: a pilot study in healthy older adults. *Gait Posture* 44, 161–167. doi: 10.1016/j.gaitpost.2015.11.019

van het Reve, E., and de Bruin, E. D. (2014). Strength-balance supplemented with computerized cognitive training to improve dual task gait and divided attention in older adults: a multicenter randomized-controlled trial. *BMC Geriatr.* 14:134. doi: 10.1186/1471-2318-14-134

Van Roie, E., Delecluse, C., Opdenacker, J., De Bock, K., Kennis, E., and Boen, F. (2010). Effectiveness of a lifestyle physical activity versus a structured exercise intervention in older adults. *J. Aging Phys. Act.* 18, 335–352. doi: 10.1123/japa.18.3.335

Verhaeghen, P., and Cerella, J. (2002). Aging, executive control, and attention: a review of meta-analyses. *Neurosci. Biobehav. Rev.* 26, 849–857. doi: 10.1016/S0149-7634(02)00071-4

Voelcker-Rehage, C., Godde, B., and Staudinger, U. M. (2010). Physical and motor fitness are both related to cognition in old age. *Eur. J. Neurosci.* 31, 167–176. doi: 10.1111/j.1460-9568.2009.07014.x

Voelcker-Rehage, C., Godde, B., and Staudinger, U. M. (2011). Cardiovascular and coordination training differentially improve cognitive performance and neural processing in older adults. *Front. Hum. Neurosci.* 5:26. doi: 10.3389/fnhum.2011.00026

Voss, M. W., Heo, S., Prakash, R. S., Erickson, K. I., Alves, H., Chaddock, L., et al. (2013). The influence of aerobic fitness on cerebral white matter integrity and cognitive function in older adults: results of a one-year exercise intervention. *Hum. Brain Mapp.* 34, 2972–2985. doi: 10.1002/hbm. 22119

Ward, N. S. (2006). Compensatory mechanisms in the aging motor system. *Ageing Res. Rev.* 5, 239–254. doi: 10.1016/j.arr.2006.04.003

Wittmann, F., Held, J. P., Lambercy, O., Starkey, M. L., Curt, A., Höver, R., et al. (2016). Self-directed arm therapy at home after stroke with a sensor-based virtual reality training system. *J. Neuroeng. Rehabil.* 13:75. doi: 10.1186/s12984-016-0182-1

Wolf, S. L., Catlin, P. A., Ellis, M., Archera, L., Morgan, B., and Piacentino, A. (2001). Assessing Wolf motor function test as outcome measure for research in patients after stroke. *Stroke* 32, 1635–1639. doi: 10.1161/01.STR.32.7.1635

Woollacott, M., and Shumway-Cook, A. (2002). Attention and the control of posture and gait: a review of an emerging area of research. *Gait Posture* 16, 1–14. doi: 10.1016/S0966-6362(01)00156-4

Wu, W., Wei, T.-S., Chen, S.-K., Chang, J.-J., Guo, L.-Y., and Lin, H.-T. (2010). The effect of chinese yuanji-dance on dynamic balance and the associated attentional demands in elderly adults. *J. Sports Sci. Med.* 9, 119–126.

Yavuzer, G., Senel, A., Atay, M. B., and Stam, H. J. (2008). Playstation eyetoy games improve upper extremity-related motor functioning in subacute stroke: a randomized controlled clinical trial. *Eur. J. Phys. Rehabil. Med.* 44, 237–244.

Yogev-Seligmann, G., Hausdorff, J. M., and Giladi, N. (2008). The role of executive function and attention in gait. *Mov. Disord.* 23, 329–342; quiz 472. doi: 10.1002/mds.21720

Zimmermann, P., and Fimm, B. (1995). *Test for Attentional performance (TAP).* Herzogenrath: PsyTest. 76–77.

9

Cognitive Resources Necessary for Motor Control in Older Adults are Reduced by Walking and Coordination Training

Ben Godde[1,2,3]* *and Claudia Voelcker-Rehage*[2,3,4]

[1]*Department of Psychology and Methods, Jacobs University Bremen, Bremen, Germany,* [2]*Jacobs Center on Lifelong Learning and Institutional Development, Jacobs University Bremen, Bremen, Germany,* [3]*Center for Cognitive Science, Bremen University, Bremen, Germany,* [4]*Institute of Human Movement Science and Health, Technische Universität Chemnitz, Chemnitz, Germany*

Edited by:
Klaus Gramann,
Technische Universität Berlin, Germany

Reviewed by:
Brenda Malcolm,
The Graduate Center (CUNY), USA
Karen Zown-Hua Li,
Concordia University, Canada
Eling D. De Bruin,
ETH Zurich, Switzerland

Correspondence:
Ben Godde
b.godde@jacobs-university.de

We examined if physical exercise interventions were effective to reduce cognitive brain resources recruited while performing motor control tasks in older adults. Forty-three older adults (63–79 years of age) participated in either a walking (n = 17) or a motor coordination (n = 15) intervention (1 year, 3 times per week) or were assigned to a control group (n = 11) doing relaxation and stretching exercises. Pre and post the intervention period, we applied functional MRI to assess brain activation during imagery of forward and backward walking and during counting backwards from 100 as control task. In both experimental groups, activation in the right dorsolateral prefrontal cortex (DLPFC) during imagery of forward walking decreased from pre- to post-test (Effect size: −1.55 and −1.16 for coordination and walking training, respectively; Cohen's d). Regression analysis revealed a significant positive association between initial motor status and activation change in the right DLPFC ($R^2 = 0.243$, $F_{(3,39)} = 4.18$, $p = 0.012$). Participants with lowest motor status at pretest profited most from the interventions. Data suggest that physical training in older adults is effective to free up cognitive resources otherwise needed for the control of locomotion. Training benefits may become particularly apparent in so-called dual-task situations where subjects must perform motor and cognitive tasks concurrently.

Keywords: motor imagery, functional MRI, motor status, cognitive aging, physical fitness, locomotion

INTRODUCTION

It has been demonstrated that gait and balance are increasingly in need of cognitive control and supervision with advancing age (Hausdorff et al., 2005; Yogev-Seligmann et al., 2008; Berchicci et al., 2014; Van Swearingen and Studenski, 2014). Such need for a certain amount of cognitive resources for movement coordination or control in older adults (Loewenstein and Acevedo, 2010) has been indicated by expanded brain networks and increased brain activation while performing a single motor task as compared with young adults (for reviews see Seidler et al., 2010; Papegaaij et al., 2014; Hamacher et al., 2015).

Due to the impossibility of performing larger movements in the MR or PET scanner, in recent years, motor imagery has been established as a method to investigate cortical activations during locomotion (Miyai et al., 2001; Malouin et al., 2003; Jahn et al., 2004; la Fougère et al., 2010; Peterson et al., 2014). Numerous studies confirmed that when imagining a movement similar and identical brain areas are activated as if the movement was actually being performed (Stephan et al., 1995; Jeannerod and Frak, 1999; Lotze et al., 1999; Sahyoun et al., 2004; Solodkin et al., 2004; la Fougère et al., 2010; for review see Lafleur et al., 2002; Allali et al., 2014). The locomotor network, as revealed by motor imagery, includes the supplementary and primary motor areas, right prefrontal cortex the basal ganglia, brainstem, tegmentum and cerebellum (Miyai et al., 2001; Jahn et al., 2004; la Fougère et al., 2010; Allali et al., 2014).

With respect to age differences, Allali et al. (2014) observed an age-related increase in brain activity in the right supplementary motor area (BA6), the right orbitofrontal cortex (BA11), and the left dorsolateral frontal cortex (BA10; Allali et al., 2014). Higher activations in older as compared to young adults were also observed in the middle temporal visual area MT/V5 (Wai et al., 2012; Zwergal et al., 2012) and subcortical regions including putamen and substantia nigra (Allali et al., 2014). The resulting use of frontal cortical resources also leads to lower cognitive and motor performance during dual-task situations in older adults (Kahnemann, 1973; Lindenberger et al., 2000; Huxhold et al., 2008; Malcolm et al., 2015).

The amount of cognitive control required for performing a motor task is not only affected by a person's age but also by her or his motor fitness status (Godde and Voelcker-Rehage, 2010; Berchicci et al., 2014). Using electroencephalography, Berchicci et al. (2014) revealed that older adults who regularly exercise reveal less reliance on extra cognitive control resources during basic visuo-motor functions. In a previous cross-sectional study, using motor imagery, we investigated with functional MRI brain activation in simple and complex walking tasks (walking forward and backward on a treadmill) and analyzed if the motor status of older adults influenced these activation patterns. Motor high-fit individuals showed more activations and larger BOLD signals in motor-related areas compared to low-fit participants but demonstrated lower activity in the dorsolateral prefrontal cortex (DLPFC). Moreover, parietal activation in high-fit participants remained stable throughout the movement period whereas low-fit participants revealed an early drop in activity in this area accompanied by increasing activity in frontal brain regions (Godde and Voelcker-Rehage, 2010).

Based on these findings, one could assume that interventions targeted to improve motor fitness could be a reasonable approach to free up prefrontal (cognitive) brain resources otherwise used for cognitive control of locomotion in older adults. To confirm this assumption, we examined the effects of 1 year of physical exercise interventions on brain activation in the same simple and complex walking tasks (walking forward and backward on a treadmill) as in our previous cross-sectional study. As we could also show previously that different dimensions of physical fitness (cardiovascular and motor fitness) and different types of physical exercise interventions (cardiovascular and motor coordination training) had different positive effects on brain functioning during performance of cognitive tasks (Voelcker-Rehage et al., 2010, 2011), we were also interested whether such interventions would differ in their effect on cognitive control of imagined walking movements. As in the previous study, we used motor imagery of walking forward and backward to assess brain activation patterns during locomotion with functional MRI.

MATERIALS AND METHODS

This study was part of the *Old Age on the Move* intervention study at Jacobs University Bremen (see Voelcker-Rehage et al., 2011) that examined effects of different kinds of physical exercise on cognitive, motor, and emotional functioning. Motor status and brain processing during motor imagery were assessed before the start of the intervention (t1) and after 12 months (t2).

Participants

In total, for the *Old Age on the Move* study, 91 older adults between 63 and 79 years from the Bremen (Germany) area were recruited through the member registry of a German health insurance company (DAK) or through newspaper articles. All participants took part voluntarily and provided written informed consent to the procedures of the study. They received compensation for their travel expenses at the end of the 1-year study amounting to Euro 100. The study conformed to the Code of Ethics of the World Medical Association (Declaration of Helsinki) and was approved by the ethics committee of the German Psychological Society (DGPs; Voelcker-Rehage_072006).

Participants had medical clearance and were screened for health restrictions before inclusion in the study by means of a telephone interview. They were excluded from study participation if they had a history of cardiovascular diseases, any neurological disorder (e.g., self-report of neurological diseases such as a brain tumor, Parkinson's disease, stroke), any other motor or cognitive restrictions (e.g., a score of less than 27 in the Mini Mental Status Examination, MMSE, Folstein and Van Petten, 2008), or metal devices in the body. Further, participants were screened for number of falls in the year before study participation (no falls: n = 38; one fall: n = 4, two falls: n = 1). Participants who were absent for more than one test day or more than 25% of the training sessions (calculated independently for each half year of the study) were excluded from data analysis (n = 47). One participant had to be excluded due to incomplete brain imaging data. None of the included participants experienced change in health status during the 1 year study interval. To assess the subjective ability to perform the requested imagery tasks, the Movement imagery questionnaire MIQ-R (Hall and Martin, 1997) was applied during debriefing directly after the scanning session. The MIQ-R is a rating scale to assess the capacity to elicit mental images. It asks for the clarity of image (scale from 1 very hard to see/feel to 7 very easy to see/feel) and the intensity in which participants could feel themselves making movements (Hall and Martin, 1997). No further participant had to be excluded because of not answering to or scoring less than 4 on the 7-point vividness scale of the questionnaire.

TABLE 1 | Demographic information for participants of the two experimental groups (cardiovascular and coordination training) and the control group.

Characteristic	Cardiovascular training		Coordination training		Control group	
	M	*SD*	*M*	*SD*	*M*	*SD*
Age	68.47	3.06	71.33	4.67	69.27	3.29
Education	13.00	2.96	12.06	3.77	12.09	2.34
IQ	51.42	5.77	47.83	5.36	49.93	5.91
Health	1.35	0.93	1.33	1.18	1.36	1.75
Subj. health	3.94	0.90	3.67	0.49	3.27	0.65
Activity index	1223.38	685.29	1028.29	609.55	1610.55	1044.56
BMI	27.44	4.31	25.88	2.60	26.25	3.43
Hypertension	0.12	0.33	0.50	0.52	0.18	0.41
ERT	0.24	0.44	0.33	0.49	0.09	0.31
Positive affect	3.74	0.67	3.68	0.53	3.76	0.54
VO2 peak	1.62	0.35	1.60	0.31	1.76	0.42

Age (average age in years), Education (years of education), IQ, Health (number of diseases), Activity Index (kcal expended per week by leisure time and physical activities, see Huy et al., 2008), Body Mass Index (BMI), hypertension (proportion of participants who had been diagnosed with hypertensive disorder), estrogene replacement therapy (ERT, proportion of participants who participated in an estrogene replacement therapy), and positive affect (affect questionnaire encompassing high and low arousal (Kessler and Staudinger, 2009). There was no significant group effect for any of the measures.

The final sample consisted of 43 participants between 63 and 79 years of age (28 women and 16 men, mean age = 69.6, SD = 3.8). Detailed demographic information as well as information about cognitive and fitness status of the participants is summarized in **Table 1**. Participants of the experimental and the control groups did not differ statistically on measures of age, years of formal education, intelligence index, health, physical activity index, BMI, hypertension, estrogen replacement therapy (for women only) and positive affect (always $p > 0.10$).

As describe in Voelcker-Rehage et al. (2011), only small sample selectivity was found for age (remaining participants were older), health (remaining participants were healthier), and positive affect (remaining participants were more positive). Given the size of the effects, it seems viable to conclude that findings obtained with the post-test sample may be generalized to the pre-test parent sample.

Interventions

Participants were assigned to two experimental groups and one control group. Not all interventions could be offered at all training facilities and thus randomization of group assignment was restricted by residency of the participants. Training groups were led by an experienced exercise leader, three times a week and 1 h each for 12 months (Voelcker-Rehage et al., 2011). Participants of the cardiovascular training group (N = 17, 12 women, 5 men, mean age = 69.3, SD = 3.3) participated in a walking intervention designed to improve cardiorespiratory fitness (aerobic endurance). Training intensity prescriptions were based on HR responses to spiroergometry exercise testing and was aimed to meet a moderate level. Participants of the second intervention group (N = 15, 10 women, 5 men, mean age = 71.3, SD = 4.7) received coordination training designed to improve fine and gross-motor body coordination. This program focused on the improvement of complex movements for the whole body such as balance, eye-hand coordination, leg-arm coordination as well as spatial orientation and reaction to moving objects/persons. The active control group (N = 11, 6 women, 5 men, mean age = 68.5, SD = 3.1) performed a program of relaxation techniques, stretching and limbering for the whole body especially designed for older adults. This group served as a control group to evaluate the potential effects of being involved in a guided group activity for 12 months as well as controlling for retest effects. For details of the intervention programs, see Voelcker-Rehage et al. (2011).

Assessment of Motor Status

The motor status of the participants was assessed at t1 and t2 by a heterogeneous motor test battery comprising tests of the five dimensions movement speed, balance, fine coordination, flexibility and strength (Godde and Voelcker-Rehage, 2010): movement speed was assessed by use of the following four tests: hand tapping (Oja and Tuxworth, 1995; cronbachs α = 0.88), feet tapping (Voelcker-Rehage and Wiertz, 2003; cronbachs α = 0.97), 30-s chair stand test (Rikli and Jones, 1999; single trial), and agility test (Adrian, 1981; cronbachs α = 0.95). Balance was assessed by backwards beam walk (Kiphard and Schilling, 1974; cronbachs α = 0.90) and one-leg-stand with eyes open and closed (Ekdahl et al., 1989, cronbachs α = 0.88). Further we assessed fine coordination by use of the Purdue Pegboard test (Tiffin and Asher, 1948; cronbachs α = 0.93), flexibility by the shoulder flexibility test (Rikli and Jones, 1999; cronbachs α = 0.95) and strength by measuring grip force (Igbokwe, 1992; cronbachs α = 0.97). An overall index for the motor status (mean of the z-transformed individual performances within the five domains) was calculated using a z-transformed sum score of the five fitness dimensions. This index was normally distributed at T1 (Shapiro-Wilk test: $W_{(43)}$ = 0.978, p = 0.564).

Movement Imagery

At t1 and t2, participants performed three imagery tasks with eyes closed and in first-person perspective: (i) walking forward with an individual moderate speed (2.5–3.5 km/h); (ii) walking backward in tandem walk (1 km/h); (iii) standing still and relaxed (baseline condition); and (iv) counting backward from 100 was chosen as a non-movement control condition. Outside the MR scanner, before the test sessions, a standardized description of the imagery tasks was provided and participants completed a task familiarization exercise. Participants were trained in the two experimental motor tasks (walking forward and backward) and the two control tasks (standing and counting backward). First, participants performed the real tasks and the imagination on a treadmill (Model Lode Valiant, Groningen Netherland). Walking forward was trained with an individual moderate speed (2.5–3.5 km/h) and easy swinging of the arms and walking backward was trained in tandem walk (1 km/h). All participants were trained as long as they needed to feel comfortable on the treadmill. The range was between 10 min and 20 min in total. We used a treadmill instead of real-world walking to provide constant visual input and ground. After executing the real and imagined movements on the treadmill participants trained imagination of these movements (including gait initiation) in a horizontal position in periods of 20 s each until they felt well experienced with the tasks. Participants were instructed to close their eyes and to use a first-person perspective to perform the imagery tasks. Then, at another day, participants first repeated the movement imagination outside the MRI scanner until they felt confident again and then performed the tasks within the scanner (first person perspective, eyes closed).

Functional MRI

Functional MRI scans were performed at pre- and post-test in a randomized block design with six blocks of 20 s for each of the four conditions in a randomized order without any break between the blocks resulting in a total of 24 blocks lasting for 480 s.

We used a 3T head scanner (Siemens Magnetom Allegra, Erlangen, Germany). A T2*-weighted gradient echo multislice sequence (EPI, TR 2500 ms, TE 60 ms, voxel size 3 × 3 × 3 mm, matrix 64 × 64) was used to acquire 48 slices covering the whole brain and the cerebellum. Additionally, a high-resolution T1-weighted anatomical 3D-dataset containing 172 sagittal slices (1 × 1 × 1 mm^3) was acquired for each subject.

Analysis of fMRI data was performed using Brain Voyager (Brain Innovation B.V., Maastricht, Netherlands). FMRI data were first corrected for motion artifacts and linear trends, smoothed in the temporal (2.8 s) and spatial (6 mm) domain, and normalized to Talairach space. The BOLD responses were modeled with a delayed box-car function convolved with a canonical hemodynamic response and a general linear model (GLM) was applied to the time course of each voxel. A random effects analysis was performed, considering the inter-subject variability; the results can therefore be generalized to other samples. On the first level, weighted beta-images were computed for every condition (forward walking, backward walking, and counting backward from 100) relative to baseline (standing still). On the second level, these individual beta values were then entered into a 3 (INTERVENTION groups) × 2 (SESSION: t1 vs. t2) × 3 (CONDITION) random effects analysis of variance *P*-values were corrected for multiple comparisons by false discovery rate (FDR, $P < 0.05$) and cluster threshold estimation using Monte Carlo simulations (alpha level < 0.05; Forman et al., 1995; Goebel et al., 2006). Effect sizes of group differences (intervention groups vs. control group) in cortical activation changes (t2–t1) were calculated as Cohen's *d* (based on sample size; Hedge's Adjustment and weighted average).

Further Statistical Analysis

Statistical analyses were performed using SPSS for Windows version 20 (IBM Corp., Armonk, NY, USA). From those regions revealing a significant INTERVENTION × SESSION × CONDITION interaction effect we selected those which in our previous cross-sectional study also revealed to be related to fitness (Godde and Voelcker-Rehage, 2010). BOLD values and beta estimates of the individual peak voxels in these regions were extracted and subjected to linear regression analysis with following regressors: group (experimental or control, dummy coded as 1 or −1, respectively; because both intervention groups did not differ in their effect on brain activation change in these regions we combined them in this analysis), the interaction term of group and initial motor status at t1, and the interaction term of group and change in motor status from t1 to t2 (**Table 2**). For that purpose, motor status indices at t1 and t2 were *z*-transformed. T2 values were transformed relative to t1 and change in motor status was defined as the difference t2−t1 of these *z*-transformed indices. For calculating the interaction terms with factor group both indices were centered. The level of significance was set to $p < 0.05$.

RESULTS

To answer our research questions, fMRI data obtained during motor imagery were analyzed in a two-step procedure. First, we identified regions that revealed significant INTERVENTION × SESSION × CONDITION interaction effects. This interaction effect was revealed for a variety of frontal, parietal, and subcortical brain regions. These regions included frontally the right DLPFC and middle frontal cortex, bilaterally the superior and medial frontal gyrus (MeFG), the precentral gyrus (PrCG) and the left anterior cingulate. Further the postcentral gyrus (PoCG) and the left caudate revealed such interaction effects (**Table 3**).

In the second step, from those regions, we selected only regions that had also been activated stronger in less- than in higher motor fit participants in our previous cross-sectional study (Godde and Voelcker-Rehage, 2010), thus indicating

TABLE 2 | Effects of interventions on motor fitness (*z*-scores related to t1).

	Cardiovascular training		Coordination training		Control group	
	M	***SD***	***M***	***SD***	***M***	***SD***
Motor fit t1	0.11	2.63	−0.19	2.49	0.09	1.49
Motor fit t2	1.13	3.06	1.31	2.73	1.33	2.06

TABLE 3 | Regions of interests (ROI) with significant SESSION × INTERVENTION × CONDITION interaction Effects ($P < 0.05$, cluster threshold: 37 voxels).

Brain area	*n* Vox	Tal *X*	Tal *Y*	Tal *Z*	*F*	*p*
Right DLPFC BA9	1025	54	13	36	4.708	0.002
Right SFG BA9	19	17	52	25	2.860	0.029
Right SFG BA8	34	2	31	45	3.013	0.023
Right MFG BA6	236	29	19	48	5.021	0.001
Right MeFG BA6	24	3	37	36	3.172	0.018
Right PrCG BA4	7	15	−26	69	2.711	0.036
Left MeFG BA8	36	−1	28	38	3.379	0.013
Left SFG BA6	21	−13	−8	69	3.993	0.005
Left MeFG BA6	1	−1	−26	54	2.500	0.049
Left PrCG BA6	52	−22	−16	66	3.377	0.013
Left ACC BA24	37	−1	34	9	3.304	0.015
Left PoCG BA3	5	−9	−35	69	2.955	0.025
Left caudate	90	−10	−2	15	4.006	0.005

Listed are the anatomical descriptions (DLPFC, dorsolateral prefrontal cortex; SFG, superior frontal gyrus; MFG, middle frontal gyrus; MeFG, medial frontal gyrus; PrCG, precentral gyrus; ACC, anterior cingulate cortex; PoCG, postcentral gyrus) and Brodmann areas (BA), numbers of voxels (n Vox), Talairach coordinates (Tal X, Tal Y, Tal Z), and F and p-values for the peaks of the respective ROI. The first ROI is marked in gray as it is the only ROI that also revealed significant effects of motor fitness status on brain activation during walking imagery at baseline (Godde and Voelcker-Rehage, 2010).

increased need for cognitive control of motor imagery in low-fit older adults. Only the right DLPFC (Brodmann area 9) met this second criterion.

Follow-up analyses revealed significant reductions in right DLPFC activation from t1 to t2 for both intervention groups as compared to the control group for imagery of walking forward. Even activation for backward walking was reduced in both intervention groups, but not significantly. Interestingly, DLPFC activation was increased for the walking group but not for the coordination group as compared to the control group for counting backward from 100 (**Figure 1**). There were no differences in effect size between the two interventions as revealed by direct comparison of both intervention groups (pairwise two-tailed paired samples *t*-test, $p > 0.13$).

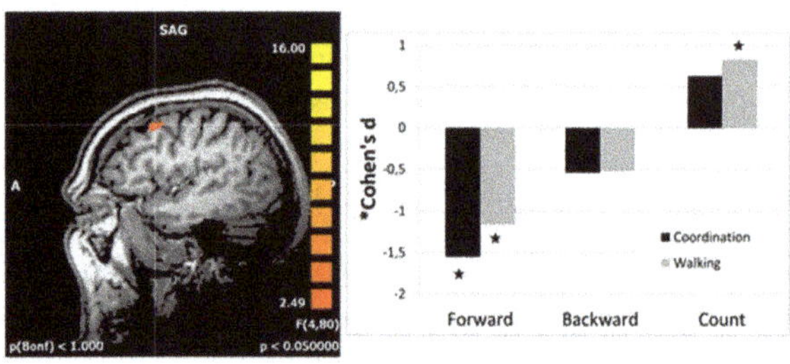

FIGURE 1 | Effect sizes for group differences in activation change (change in beta estimates) in the right dorsolateral prefrontal cortex (DLPFC; left panel). Effect sizes of intervention groups (coordination and walking group) relative to the control group were calculated as Cohen's d (based on sample size; Hedge's Adjustment and weighted average). Stars indicate significant effects of the intervention groups.

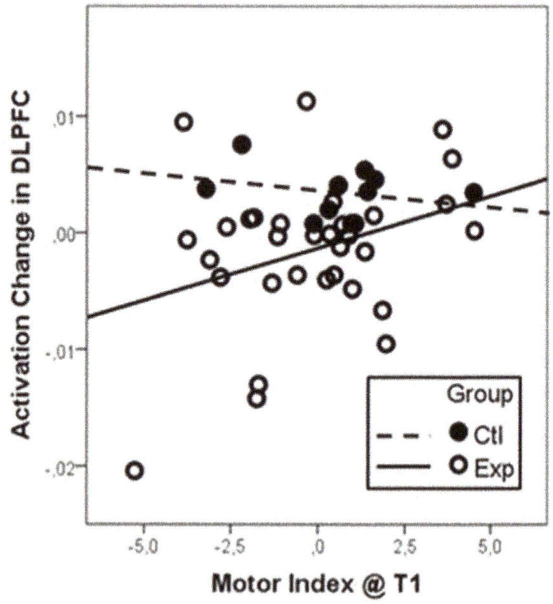

FIGURE 2 | Activation change in the right DLPFC dependent on baseline motor fitness as indicated as the motor index at t1. Data were centered and *z*-transformed. Since we did not find differential effects of the two intervention types (walking and coordination), data from both groups were pooled and compared to the control group. Particularly participants with low motor index at t1 (low motor index) revealed the strongest reduction in DLPFC activation after the intervention (negative change values).

Regression analysis with initial motor status at T1 and change in motor status from T1 to T2 as regressors revealed a significant positive association of the initial motor status and activation change in right DLPFC for pooled intervention groups. The overall linear regression model was significant ($R^2 = 0.243$, $F_{(3,39)} = 4.18$, $p = 0.012$). Besides the factor group (standardized beta coefficient = −0.39, $T = -2.76$, $p = 0.009$), the interaction of group and baseline motor index (standardized beta coefficient = 0.33, $T = 2.30$, $p = 0.027$) were revealed as significant predictors for change in right DLPFC activation. As illustrated in **Figure 2**, participants with low motor status at t1 profited most from the intervention. Because of the small sample size, however, these results must be taken with care.

DISCUSSION

Our study addressed the question whether physical training interventions are effective to reduce the need for cognitive control of locomotion in older adults. Results confirm that both walking and coordination training reduced frontal brain activation during imagery of walking forward and backward. Moreover, participants with lower baseline motor status profited most from the intervention. Our data suggest that physical interventions not only have direct effects on cognitive and brain function in older adults as reported earlier (Colcombe and Kramer, 2003; Colcombe et al., 2004; Hillman et al., 2008; Lustig et al., 2009; Voelcker-Rehage et al., 2011; Hayes et al.,

2013; Voelcker-Rehage and Niemann, 2013; Schättin et al., 2016), but also indirect effects by freeing up frontal brain resources otherwise needed for the control of motor actions. Herewith our findings are also in line with a recent study using near-infrared spectroscopy revealing that video game dancing training and balance training reduce left and right PFC oxygenation during fast walking (Eggenberger et al., 2016). With decreasing reserve capacity in older adults, these effects may become increasingly important and become especially apparent in so-called dual-task situations where subjects have to perform motor and cognitive tasks concurrently, for example, during crossing a street while observing the traffic flow or walking by talking (Lindenberger et al., 2000; Yogev-Seligmann et al., 2010; Al-Yahya et al., 2011; Neider et al., 2011).

We found INTERVENTION × SESSION × CONDITION interaction effects for a variety of frontal cortical areas belonging to the motor imagery network as described earlier (Allali et al., 2014; Hamacher et al., 2015), indicating altered use of cognitive resources for motor control after the training interventions. Interestingly, these effects were also found for the right but not the left DLPFC which has also been shown to be involved in motor imagery in previous studies (e.g., Malouin et al., 2003; Jahn et al., 2004), particularly in older adults (Allali et al., 2014). These studies, however, did not consider the motor fitness status of the participants. When the motor fitness status was considered, as in our previous cross-sectional study (Godde and Voelcker-Rehage, 2010), more activity in the right DLPFC was revealed in low-fit as compared to high-fit older adults. We explained this finding in the sense that the control condition (standing still) also requires some attentional control and thus the right DLPFC activity particularly seen in low-fit participants only mirrors additional activation that can be interpreted as compensatory. Such additional activity in homologs contralateral frontal areas in older adults has repeatedly been put into the context of compensatory mechanisms of age-related changes (e.g., "Hemispheric asymmetry reduction in older adults (HAROLD)" hypothesis; Cabeza, 2002). However, it is not possible to measure motor performance using a motor imagery paradigm, and therefore it must remain open if this additional frontal activation reflects compensation, dedifferentiation or just the higher task complexity for low as compared to high-fit participants. Increased involvement of prefrontal cortex in older adults during complex gait tasks or in imagined walking conditions with high cognitive load was also confirmed by recent reviews (Holtzer et al., 2014; Hamacher et al., 2015).

Interestingly, the interventions did not differ (but they differed from the control group) in respect to their effects on cognitive resources allocated in the DLPFC for the control of walking movements. One explanation might be that the effect in the walking group similar to the coordination group was due to better motor control abilities rather than enhanced cardiovascular fitness, i.e., due to the extensive walking experience walking became more automated (Ross et al., 2003; Wei and Luo, 2010). This is supported by the finding that effects are stronger for imagery of walking forward, what has specifically been trained in the walking group, than walking backwards, what is the more complex task. Indeed, recent MR studies revealed motor training-induced gray and white matter changes in motor-related areas such as the supplementary and presupplementary motor cortex (SMA/pre-SMA) and increased functional connectivity to prefrontal and parietal brain regions, even in older adults (for review see Taubert et al., 2012). Further, coordinative exercise as applied here leads to increased basal ganglia volume in older adults (Niemann et al., 2014).

It might be that (additionally) increase in cardiovascular fitness also could have led to some positive effects on cognitive processing based on more efficient use of frontal brain resources (Voelcker-Rehage et al., 2011). With the paradigms tested here, however, that does not seem to play a role. This might be different under dual-task conditions but must remain speculative here.

We aimed to assure clarity and intensity of motor imagery during scanning. For that purpose, we applied the MIQ-R only. A chronometric test in which the time needed to complete real walking and walking imagery is compared for the two conditions could have given supportive evidence on better forward walking abilities in the walking group.

The motor fitness status of the control group greatly improved from time 1 to time 2, even more so than the cardiovascular training group (**Table 2**) and one might wonder why this improvement in actual motor fitness was not reflected by a change in brain activity (specifically in right DLPFC) for imagined movements in the control group as well. It could well be that stretching and relaxation as exercised in the control group might improve proprioceptive function and self-perception. However, the control group did not explicitly train walking or actively controlled movements. This might explain why they generally performed better in the motor test battery but did not reveal activation changes related to specific motor control in frontal brain regions.

The reader might also wonder about positive effect sizes for counting (**Figure 1**) which seems to indicate increased activation after the intervention and thus more need for cognitive resources. However, all effects were calculated in contrast to the standing condition as baseline condition. Thus, this positive effect for counting might be due to a negative effect for standing (though much less than for walking backwards or even more so walking forward).

Further experiments using electroencephalography or near-infrared spectroscopy during real movements might add additional evidence that frontal brain resources used for cognitive control can be reduced by specific motor training in older adults (Eggenberger et al., 2016; Schättin et al., 2016). Overall physical activity that stress the motor system (here either by regular walking or coordination training) might be beneficial to preserve or enhance cognitive resources (see Voelcker-Rehage et al., 2011), but also to preserve motor functioning—at least in the practiced tasks (here walking forward) leading to less cognitive resources needed to perform a motor task and having resources available in complex situations of daily life.

Based on our results, it is difficult to favor one intervention (walking vs. coordination training) over the other and it might be advised to combine both exercise dimensions in training programs for older adults.

AUTHOR CONTRIBUTIONS

BG and CVR designed and performed the study and acquired, analyzed and interpreted the data. They together drafted the manuscript and agreed to be accountable for all aspects of the work in terms of accuracy and integrity.

ACKNOWLEDGMENTS

Our work was supported by the Robert Bosch Foundation (12.5.1366.0005.0) and the German health insurance company DAK. We thank Peter Erhard, Ekkehard Küstermann and Melanie Löbe (Center for Advanced Imaging, University of Bremen) for support with functional MR imaging.

REFERENCES

Adrian, M. J. (1981). "Flexibility in the aging adult," in *Exercises and Aging: The Scientific Basic*, eds E. L. Smith and R. C. Serfass (Hillside, NJ: Enslow Publishers), 45–58.

Allali, G., van der Meulen, M., Beauchet, O., Rieger, S. W., Vuilleumier, P., and Assal, F. (2014). The neural basis of age-related changes in motor imagery of gait: an fMRI study. *J. Gerontol. A Biol. Sci. Med. Sci.* 69, 1389–1398. doi: 10.1093/gerona/glt207

Al-Yahya, E., Dawes, H., Smith, L., Dennis, A., Howells, K., and Cockburn, J. (2011). Cognitive motor interference while walking: a systematic review and meta-analysis. *Neurosci. Biobehav. Rev.* 35, 715–728. doi: 10.1016/j.neubiorev.2010.08.008

Berchicci, M., Lucci, G., Perri, R. L., Spinelli, D., and Di Russo, F. (2014). Benefits of physical exercise on basic visuo-motor functions across age. *Front. Aging Neurosci.* 6:48. doi: 10.3389/fnagi.2014.00048

Cabeza, R. (2002). Hemispheric asymmetry reduction in older adults: the HAROLD model. *Psychol. Aging* 17, 85–100. doi: 10.1037/0882-7974.17.1.85

Colcombe, S., and Kramer, A. F. (2003). Fitness effects on the cognitive function of older adults: a meta-analytic study. *Psychol. Sci.* 14, 125–130. doi: 10.1111/1467-9280.t01-1-01430

Colcombe, S. J., Kramer, A. F., Erickson, K. I., Scalf, P., McAuley, E., Cohen, N. J., et al. (2004). Cardiovascular fitness, cortical plasticity, and aging. *Proc. Natl. Acad. Sci. U S A* 101, 3316–3321. doi: 10.1073/pnas.0400266101

Eggenberger, P., Wolf, M., Schumann, M., and de Bruin, E.D. (2016). Exergame and balance training modulate prefrontal brain activity during walking and enhance executive function in older adults. *Front. Aging Neurosci.* 8:66. doi: 10.3389/fnagi.2016.00066

Ekdahl, C., Jarnlo, G. B., and Andersson, S. I. (1989). Standing balance in healthy subjects. Evaluation of a quantitative test battery on a force platform. *Scand. J. Rehabil. Med.* 21, 187–195.

Folstein, J. R., and Van Petten, C. (2008). Influence of cognitive control and mismatch on the N2 component of the ERP: a review. *Psychophysiology* 45, 152–170. doi: 10.1111/j.1469-8986.2007.00602.x

Forman, S. D., Cohen, J. D., Fitzgerald, M., Eddy, W. F., Mintun, M. A., and Noll, D. C. (1995). Improved assessment of significant activation in functional magnetic resonance imaging (fMRI): use of a cluster-size threshold. *Magn. Reson. Med.* 33, 636–647. doi: 10.1002/mrm.1910330508

Godde, B., and Voelcker-Rehage, C. (2010). More automation and less cognitive control of imagined walking movements in high-versus low-fit older adults. *Front. Aging Neurosci.* 2:139. doi: 10.3389/fnagi.2010.00139

Goebel, R., Esposito, F., and Formisano, E. (2006). Analysis of functional image analysis contest (FIAC) data with Brainvoyager QX: from single-subject to cortically aligned group general linear model analysis and self-organizing group independent component analysis. *Hum. Brain Mapp.* 27, 392–401. doi: 10.1002/hbm.20249

Hall, C. R., and Martin, K. A. (1997). Measuring movement imagery abilities: a revision of the movement imagery questionnaire. *J. Ment. Imagery* 21, 143–154.

Hamacher, D., Herold, F., Wiegel, P., Hamacher, D., and Schega, L. (2015). Brain activity during walking: a systematic review. *Neurosci. Biobehav. Rev.* 57, 310–327. doi: 10.1016/j.neubiorev.2015.08.002

Hausdorff, J. M., Yogev, G., Springer, S., Simon, E. S., and Giladi, N. (2005). Walking is more like catching than tapping: gait in the elderly as a complex cognitive task. *Exp. Brain Res.* 164, 541–548. doi: 10.1007/s00221-005-2280-3

Hayes, S. M., Hayes, J. P., Cadden, M., and Verfaellie, M. (2013). A review of cardiorespiratory fitness-related neuroplasticity in the aging brain. *Front. Aging Neurosci.* 5:31. doi: 10.3389/fnagi.2013.00031

Hillman, C. H., Erickson, K. I., and Kramer, A. F. (2008). Be smart, exercise your heart: exercise effects on brain and cognition. *Nat. Rev. Neurosci.* 9, 58–65. doi: 10.1038/nrn2298

Holtzer, R., Epstein, N., Mahoney, J. R., Izzetoglu, M., and Blumen, H. M. (2014). Neuroimaging of mobility in aging: a targeted review. *J. Gerontol. A Biol. Sci. Med. Sci.* 69, 1375–1388. doi: 10.1093/gerona/glu052

Huxhold, O., Schäfer, S., and Lindenberger, U. (2008). Wechselwirkungen zwischen sensomotorik und kognition im alter. *Z. Gerontol. Geriat.* 42, 93–98. doi: 10.1007/s00391-008-0566-3

Huy, C., Becker, S., Gomolinsky, U., Klein, T., and Thiel, A. (2008). Health, medical risk factors, and bicycle use in everyday life in the over-50 population. *J. Aging Phys. Act.* 16, 454–464. doi: 10.1123/japa.16.4.454

Igbokwe, N. U. (1992). Hand grip dynamometer and arm muscle size in teenage boys and girls. *J. Phys. Educ. Sport Sci.* 4, 15–19.

Jahn, K., Deutschländer, A., Stephan, T., Strupp, M., Wiesmann, M., and Brandt, T. (2004). Brain activation patterns during imagined stance and locomotion in functional magnetic resonance imaging. *Neuroimage* 22, 1722–1731. doi: 10.1016/j.neuroimage.2004.05.017

Jeannerod, M., and Frak, V. (1999). Mental imaging of motor activity in humans. *Curr. Opin. Neurobiol.* 9, 735–739. doi: 10.1016/s0959-4388(99)00038-0

Kahnemann, D. (1973). *Attention and Effort.* Englewood Cliffs, NJ: Prentice Hall.

Kessler, E. M., and Staudinger, U. M. (2009). Affective experience in adulthood and old age: the role of affective arousal and perceived affect regulation. *Psychol. Aging* 24, 349–362. doi: 10.1037/a0015352

Kiphard, E. J., and Schilling, F. (1974). *Körperkoordinationstest Für Kinder [Body Coordination Test for Children].* Weinheim: Beltz.

Lafleur, M. F., Jackson, P. L., Malouin, F., Richards, C. L., Evans, A. C., and Doyon, J. (2002). Motor learning produces parallel dynamic functional changes during the execution and imagination of sequential foot movements. *Neuroimage* 16, 142–157. doi: 10.1006/nimg.2001.1048

la Fougère, C., Zwergal, A., Rominger, A., Förster, S., Fesl, G., Dieterich, M., et al. (2010). Real versus imagined locomotion: a [^{18}F]-FDG PET-fMRI comparison. *Neuroimage* 50, 1589–1598. doi: 10.1016/j.neuroimage.2009.12.060

Lindenberger, U., Marsiske, M., and Baltes, P. B. (2000). Memorizing while walking: increase in dual-task costs from young adulthood to old age. *Psychol. Aging* 15, 417–436. doi: 10.1037/0882-7974.15.3.417

Loewenstein, D., and Acevedo, A. (2010). "The relationship between instrumental activities of daily living and neuropsychological performance," in *Neuropsychology of Everyday Functioning*, eds T. D. Marcotte and I. Grant (New York, NY: The Guilford Press), 93–112.

Lotze, M., Montoya, P., Erb, M., Hülsmann, E., Flor, H., Klose, U., et al. (1999). Activation of cortical and cerebellar motor areas during executed and imagined hand movements: an fMRI study. *J. Cogn. Neurosci.* 11, 491–501. doi: 10.1162/089892999563553

Lustig, C., Shah, P., Seidler, R., and Reuter-Lorenz, P. A. (2009). Aging, training, and the brain: a review and future directions. *Neuropsychol. Rev.* 19, 504–522. doi: 10.1007/s11065-009-9119-9

Malcolm, B. R., Foxe, J. J., Butler, J. S., and De Sanctis, P. (2015). The aging brain shows less flexible reallocation of cognitive resources during dual-task walking: a mobile brain/body imaging (MoBI) study. *Neuroimage* 117, 230–242. doi: 10.1016/j.neuroimage.2015.05.028

Malouin, F., Richards, C. L., Jackson, P. L., Dumas, F., and Doyon, J. (2003). Brain activations during motor imagery of locomotor-related tasks: a PET study. *Hum. Brain Mapp.* 19, 47–62. doi: 10.1002/hbm.10103

Miyai, I., Tanabe, H. C., Sase, I., Eda, H., Oda, I., Konishi, I., et al. (2001). Cortical mapping of gait in humans: a near-infrared spectroscopic topography study. *Neuroimage* 14, 1186–1192. doi: 10.1006/nimg.2001.0905

Neider, M. B., Gaspar, J. G., McCarley, J. S., Crowell, J. A., Kaczmarski, H., and Kramer, A. F. (2011). Walking and talking: dual-task effects on street crossing behavior in older adults. *Psychol. Aging* 26, 260–268. doi: 10.1037/a0021566

Niemann, C., Godde, B., Staudinger, U., and Voelcker-Rehage, C. (2014). Exercise-induced changes in basal ganglia volume and cognition in older adults. *Neuroscience* 281, 147–163. doi: 10.1016/j.neuroscience.2014.09.033

Oja, P., and Tuxworth, B. (1995). *Eurofit for Adults—Assessment of Health-Related Fitness.* Tampere: Council of Europe Publishing.

Papegaaij, S., Taube, W., Baudry, S., Otten, E., and Hortobágyi, T. (2014). Aging causes a reorganization of cortical and spinal control of posture. *Front. Aging Neurosci.* 6:28. doi: 10.3389/fnagi.2014.00028

Peterson, D. S., Pickett, K. A., Duncan, R. P., Perlmutter, J. S., and Earhart, G. M. (2014). Brain activity during complex imagined gait tasks in Parkinson disease. *Clin. Neurophysiol.* 125, 995–1005. doi: 10.1016/j.clinph.2013.10.008

Rikli, R. E., and Jones, C. J. (1999). Development and validation of a functional fitness test for community-residing older adults. *J. Aging Phys. Act.* 7, 129–161. doi: 10.1123/japa.7.2.129

Ross, J. S., Tkach, J., Ruggieri, P. M., Lieber, M., and Lapresto, E. (2003). The mind's eye: functional MR imaging evaluation of golf motor imagery. *AJNR Am. J. Neuroradiol.* 24, 1036–1044.

Sahyoun, C., Floyer-Lea, A., Johansen-Berg, H., and Matthews, P. M. (2004). Towards an understanding of gait control: brain activation during the anticipation, preparation and execution of foot movements. *Neuroimage* 21, 568–575. doi: 10.1016/j.neuroimage.2003.09.065

Schättin, A., Arner, R., Gennaro, F., and de Bruin, E. D. (2016). Adaptations of prefrontal brain activity, executive functions, and gait in healthy elderly following exergame and balance training: a randomized controlled study. *Front. Aging Neurosci.* 8:278. doi: 10.3389/fnagi.2016.00278

Seidler, R. D., Bernard, J. A., Burutolu, T. B., Fling, B. W., Gordon, M. T., Gwin, J. T., et al. (2010). Motor control and aging: links to age-related brain structural, functional, and biochemical effects. *Neurosci. Biobehav. Rev.* 34, 721–733. doi: 10.1016/j.neubiorev.2009.10.005

Solodkin, A., Hlustik, P., Chen, E. E., and Small, S. L. (2004). Fine modulation in network activation during motor execution and motor imagery. *Cereb. Cortex* 14, 1246–1255. doi: 10.1093/cercor/bhh086

Stephan, K. M., Fink, G. R., Passingham, R. E., Silbersweig, D., Ceballos-Baumann, A. O., Frith, C. D., et al. (1995). Functional anatomy of the mental representation of upper extremity movements in healthy subjects. *J. Neurophysiol.* 73, 373–386.

Taubert, M., Villringer, A., and Ragert, P. (2012). Learning-related gray and white matter changes in humans an update. *Neuroscientist* 18, 320–325. doi: 10.1177/1073858411419048

Tiffin, J., and Asher, E. J. (1948). The Purdue pegboard; norms and studies of reliability and validity. *J. Appl. Psychol.* 32, 234–247. doi: 10.1037/h0061266

Van Swearingen, J. M., and Studenski, S. A. (2014). Aging, motor skill, and the energy cost of walking: implications for the prevention and treatment of mobility decline in older persons. *J. Gerontol. A Biol. Sci. Med. Sci.* 69, 1429–1436. doi: 10.1093/gerona/glu153

Voelcker-Rehage, C., Godde, B., and Staudinger, U. M. (2011). Cardiovascular and coordination training differentially improve cognitive performance and neural processing in older adults. *Front. Hum. Neurosci.* 5:26. doi: 10.3389/fnhum.2011.00026

Voelcker-Rehage, C., Godde, B., and Staudinger, U. M. (2010). Physical and motor fitness are both related to cognition in old age. *Eur. J. Neurosci.* 31, 167–176. doi: 10.1111/j.1460-9568.2009.07014.x

Voelcker-Rehage, C., and Niemann, C. (2013). Structural and functional brain changes related to different types of physical activity across the life span. *Neurosci. Biobehav. Rev.* 37, 2268–2295. doi: 10.1016/j.neubiorev.2013.01.028

Voelcker-Rehage, C., and Wiertz, O. (2003). *Die Lernfaehigkeit Sportmotorischer Fertigkeiten im Lichte der Entwicklungspsychologie der Lebensspanne [Motor Skill Learning in Focus of Lifespan Developmental Psychology].* Bielefeld: Bielefelder Reihe, Universität Bielefeld.

Wai, Y.-Y., Wang, J.-J., Weng, Y.-H., Lin, W.-Y., Ma, H.-K., Ng, S.-H., et al. (2012). Cortical involvement in a gait-related imagery task: comparison between Parkinson's disease and normal aging. *Parkinsonism Relat. Disord.* 18, 537–542. doi: 10.1016/j.parkreldis.2012.02.004

Wei, G., and Luo, J. (2010). Sport expert's motor imagery: functional imaging of professional motor skills and simple motor skills. *Brain Res.* 1341, 52–62. doi: 10.1016/j.brainres.2009.08.014

Yogev-Seligmann, G., Hausdorff, J. M., and Giladi, N. (2008). The role of executive function and attention in gait. *Mov. Disord.* 23, 329–342; quiz 472. doi: 10.1002/mds.21720

Yogev-Seligmann, G., Rotem-Galli, Y., Mirelman, A., Dickstein, R., Giladi, N., and Hausdorff, J. (2010). How does explicit prioritization alter walking during dual-task performance? Effects of age and sex on gait speed and variability. *Phys. Ther.* 90, 177–186. doi: 10.2522/ptj.20090043

Zwergal, A., Linn, J., Xiong, G., Brandt, T., Strupp, M., and Jahn, K. (2012). Aging of human supraspinal locomotor and postural control in fMRI. *Neurobiol. Aging* 33, 1073–1084. doi: 10.1016/j.neurobiolaging.2010.09.022

10

White Matter Plasticity Keeps the Brain in Tune: Axons Conduct While Glia Wrap

*Zahraa Chorghay[1], Ragnhildur Thóra Káradóttir[2] and Edward S. Ruthazer[1]**

[1] *Department of Neurology and Neurosurgery, Montreal Neurological Institute, McGill University, Montreal, QC, Canada,*
[2] *Department of Veterinary Medicine, Wellcome Trust - Medical Research Council Stem Cell Institute, University of Cambridge, Cambridge, United Kingdom*

Edited by:
Egidio D'Angelo, University of Pavia, Italy

Reviewed by:
Lester Melie-Garcia, Lausanne University Hospital (CHUV), Switzerland
Davide Lecca, Università degli Studi di Milano, Italy

***Correspondence:**
Edward S. Ruthazer
edward.ruthazer@mcgill.ca

Precise timing of neuronal inputs is crucial for brain circuit function and development, where it contributes critically to experience-dependent plasticity. Myelination therefore provides an important adaptation mechanism for vertebrate circuits. Despite its importance to circuit activity, the interplay between neuronal activity and myelination has yet to be fully elucidated. In recent years, significant attention has been devoted to uncovering and explaining the phenomenon of white matter (WM) plasticity. Here, we summarize some of the critical evidence for modulation of the WM by neuronal activity, ranging from human diffusion tensor imaging (DTI) studies to experiments in animal models. These experiments reveal activity-dependent changes in the differentiation and proliferation of the oligodendrocyte lineage, and in the critical properties of the myelin sheaths. We discuss the implications of such changes for synaptic function and plasticity, and present the underlying mechanisms of neuron–glia communication, with a focus on glutamatergic signaling and the axomyelinic synapse. Finally, we examine evidence that myelin plasticity may be subject to critical periods. Taken together, the present review aims to provide insights into myelination in the context of brain circuit formation and function, emphasizing the bidirectional interplay between neurons and myelinating glial cells to better inform future investigations of nervous system plasticity.

Keywords: activity-dependent, myelin, plasticity, oligodendrocyte, axon, conduction velocity, glutamate

Myelin is the lipid-rich insulatory material that ensheathes axons in the central nervous system, increasing the speed of signal conduction and providing precise temporal control over the propagation of action potentials within brain networks. Despite the importance of myelination in circuit activity, relatively little is known about how myelination may itself be influenced by neuronal activity. Initial observations that myelination may be altered by changes in neural activity have spawned a growing interest in the phenomenon of myelin plasticity in recent years. This article will expand upon a number of excellent, recent reviews (e.g., Wang and Young, 2014; Fields, 2015; Purger et al., 2016; De Faria et al., 2017; Mount and Monje, 2017) to highlight how myelination may contribute to circuit function, to discuss some of the key evidence for activity-dependent changes in myelination, and to explore the underlying glia–neuron communication that makes this possible.

MYELINATION FINE-TUNES TIMING TO PROMOTE CIRCUIT FUNCTIONALITY AND PLASTICITY

Precise timing of the transmission of neuronal activity is critical for proper circuit function and also plays an important role in the experience-dependent plasticity that modulates brain wiring during development and throughout an organism's lifetime. By preventing current leakage and reducing membrane capacitance, myelination of axons enables action potentials to depolarize more distant sites along the axonal membrane. Consequently, an action potential can rapidly propagate in a saltatory manner from one exposed gap in the myelin sheath, called a node of Ranvier, to the next, with ion flux restricted to the ion channels within the node (**Figure 1C**). Even if some nodes are inactivated, myelination can increase the length constant sufficiently to depolarize adjacent nodes (Tasaki, 1939). Greater internodal distances, along with more rapid membrane depolarization, allow for faster axonal conduction velocity. Thus, myelination of rapidly conducting axons enhances the speed and fidelity of information transmission. In any given axon, the speed at which an action potential travels is dependent upon a number of factors: (1) axon diameter, (2) myelin thickness, measured by g-ratio, which is ratio of the inner to the outer diameter of the sheath (Rushton, 1951; Waxman, 1975; Campbell et al., 2017), (3) length of continuous axonal segment that is wrapped (i.e., the internode distance) (Rushton, 1951; Brill et al., 1977), as well as (4) the nodal geometry itself (Arancibia-Cárcamo et al., 2017; **Figure 1E**). Interestingly, theoretical calculations based on measurements of these biophysical parameters have estimated that myelinated peripheral nerve is indeed optimized for maximum conduction velocity (Waxman, 1975). In contrast, the presence of diverse unmyelinated axons and myelinated axons that differ in these properties confers large heterogeneity in the conduction velocities in central nervous system circuits, implying a more elaborate role for central myelination in the temporal precision of functional circuits. Recent experimental evidence clearly indicates that rather than merely optimizing for high speed and fidelity of transmission along axonal tracts, myelination exerts a fundamental influence over the precise relative timing of signals, contributing to their integration into the network and even to their potential to drive changes in synaptic strength.

Within the early visual system, there are striking differences in conduction velocity along the optic nerve versus the optic tract demonstrating that axons are capable of locally regulating properties such as axon diameter (Baker and Stryker, 1990). In the thalamocortical projections of the somatosensory system, axons appear to regulate myelination to produce remarkably uniform latencies from thalamus to cortex despite a wide range of axonal distances to their different cortical target sites (Salami et al., 2003). Furthermore, these axons exhibit 10-fold differences in conduction velocity for their myelinated segments in the white matter (WM) compared to gray matter terminals where the same axons are not myelinated. This fine-tuning of signal propagation along axonal fibers allows information transmitted from wide-ranging locations across the brain to impinge onto higher order areas nearly simultaneously, permitting downstream neurons to integrate and process diverse inputs within millisecond timescales, unhindered by the different lengths of the individual axons themselves.

Precise timing in the transduction and transmission of sensory inputs is essential for accurate sound localization performed by circuits in the auditory hindbrain (Seidl, 2014). Because the ears are on opposite sides of the head, sound waves will arrive at each ear with interaural time differences (ITD) on the order of microseconds, depending on the relative proximity of each ear to the site from which the sound originated. Cochlear stimulation in response to the arrival of sound waves results in high fidelity activation of neurons in the cochlear nuclei associated with each ear. Bilaterally the relevant cochlear nucleus, called the nucleus magnocellularis in the avian auditory system, extends a bifurcating axon which innervates nucleus laminaris on both sides of the hindbrain. Nucleus laminaris is the first brain area that receives binaural inputs and it is organized such that relevant ITDs are represented along its width. This is accomplished by the implementation of a coincidence detector called a Jeffress model, in which inputs from the two cochlear nuclei enter opposite sides of nucleus laminaris and the coincident arrival of action potentials representing the two ears is detected by the postsynaptic neurons (Jeffress, 1948; Sullivan and Konishi, 1986; Overholt et al., 1992). What is truly remarkable here is that the much greater lengths that must be traversed by axons from the contralateral side of the brain would effectively cause all those inputs to arrive too late to coincide with ipsilateral signals, yet because of dramatic differences in myelin internodal lengths and relative axon diameters of the ipsilateral and contralateral branches of the bifurcating magnocellularis axons, coincident arrival with microsecond accuracy is achieved (Seidl et al., 2010). Fine-tuning of the relative speeds of signal propagation can also be found in the mammalian auditory system (Ford et al., 2015), where it has been shown that sensory deprivation through ear-plugging results in significant reductions in myelin sheath thickness (Sinclair et al., 2017). Thus, auditory brainstem fibers exploit differences in myelination, including gradations in nodal diameter, internodal length, and myelin thickness, to optimize their relative speed and synchronization.

These studies support the notion that the control of myelination along and between axons might be a strategy for modulating conduction velocity to regulate the functional integration of inputs into neuronal circuits (**Figure 2**). Both in development and in adulthood, plasticity mechanisms also rely critically on precise timing (Sjöström and Gerstner, 2010). Hebb (1949) postulated that synapses could be strengthened when a presynaptic neuron "repeatedly or persistently" participates in exciting its postsynaptic partner to fire action potentials, implying temporal correlation of inputs. Conversely, synapses might be expected to weaken when a presynaptic neuron consistently fails to help drive its postsynaptic partner (Stent, 1973). These Hebbian rules of plasticity constitute cellular level manifestations of the cooperativity and competition that guide the development, refinement, and maintenance of circuits at the system level. They underlie the activity-dependent self-organization of developing

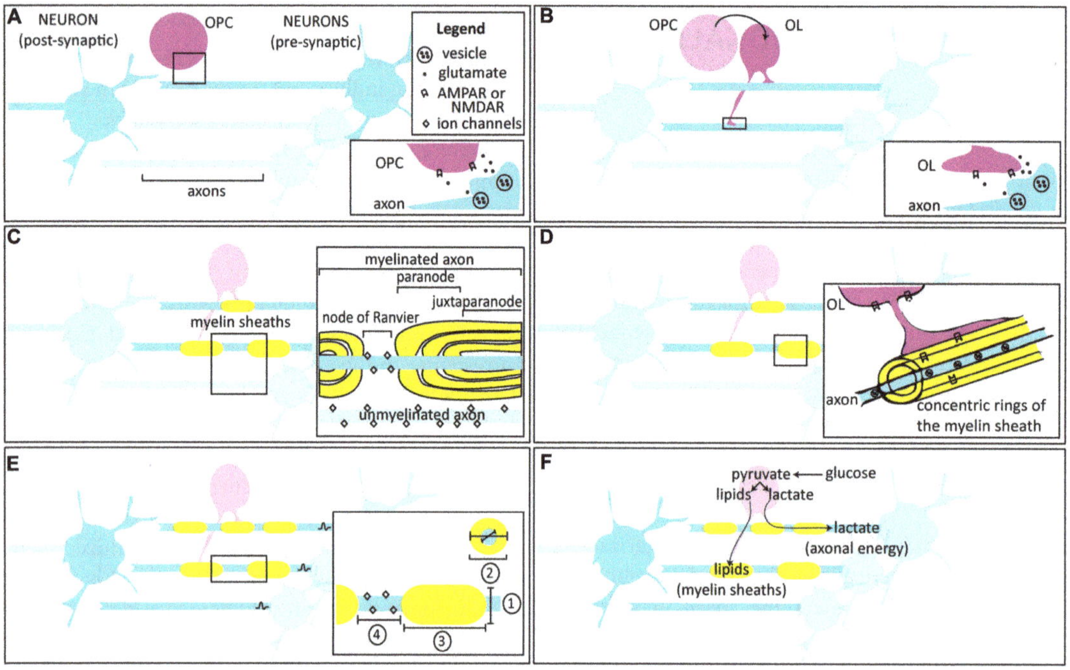

FIGURE 1 | Activity-dependent myelination. **(A)** Oligodendrocyte progenitor / precursor cells (OPCs) are found in the developing circuit alongside neurons, and are thought to interact through glutamatergic signaling. Inset: Following an action potential, glutamate released from the axon is thought to bind to AMPARs and NMDARs on OPCs, either at a synapse or extrasynaptically. **(B)** OPCs differentiate into oligodendrocytes (OLs), which also interact with neurons in the developing circuit. Inset: Following an action potential, glutamate released from the axon is thought to bind to AMPARs and NMDARs on OLs, either at the axomyelinic synapse or extrasynaptically. **(C)** OLs enwrap concentric myelin sheaths around axons. One OL can enwrap multiple axons, while individual myelin sheaths along the same axon are wrapped by different OLs. The most important factor for myelin initiation is axon diameter, but neuronal activity may bias axon selection. Inset: In unmyelinated fibers, ion channels are distributed throughout the axon. Myelin ensheathment prevents current leakage by restricting ion flow primarily to particular, unmyelinated regions called the nodes of Ranvier. Immediately adjacent to the nodes are regions called paranodes, where the myelin loops contact the axons, and the regions further interior are called the juxtaparanodes. Nodes, paranodes, and juxtaparanodes are enriched with specific proteins to support their structural composition and function. **(D)** Over time, the concentric sheaths become compact myelin. In the adaptive myelination phase, changes to the extant myelin may occur in an activity-dependent manner. Inset: Glutamatergic receptors may be found within the sheathes themselves, where they are thought to respond to vesicular release and allow for myelinic calcium influx. **(E)** By varying the conduction velocity of the action potential, myelination can influence the arrival of axonal spikes, acting as a mechanism for regulating precise timing and synchrony in circuits. Mature, more myelinated circuits show inter- and intra-axonal variation in conduction velocity, depending on four factors (inset): ① the axon diameter, ② the myelin thickness, measured by g-ratio: a ratio of the inner to the outer diameter of the sheath, ③ the length of continuous axonal segment that is wrapped, or the internode distance, and ④ the node itself, including its geometry, and the composition and number of ion channels. **(F)** Other than plasticity, activity-dependent myelination is also thought to be important in maintaining circuits. Neuronal activity is detected by receptors in axons and cells of the OL lineage, which use their metabolites for maintenance of the myelin sheaths (e.g., through lipid synthesis) or for providing metabolic support (e.g., by shuttling lactate). This likely corresponds with a development switch in OLs from an earlier mode of myelin formation that utilizes mitochondrial-dependent aerobic respiration to a later, glycolysis-dependent mode that meets the energy demands for survival of the OL and of the associated axon especially during periods of increased activity.

circuits, which calls for the selection of an increasingly restrictive subset of inputs as functional maps refine over time.

The precise timing of the asymmetry between the arrival of presynaptic spikes and the firing of postsynaptic cells is the basis of a type of Hebbian learning called spike-timing-dependent plasticity (STDP; for a comprehensive overview, see the e-book by Markram et al., 2012). STDP is defined by timing windows within which a presynaptic cell that fires *before* its postsynaptic partner undergoes synaptic strengthening, whereas activation of the presynaptic cell *after* its postsynaptic partner weakens the synapse. The specific direction of the synaptic modification may differ between brain areas, but in most cases the timing window to induce the change lasts only a few tens of milliseconds (Dan and Poo, 2004). The first *in vivo* demonstration of STDP was performed in the developing retinotectal system of the *Xenopus laevis* tadpole (Zhang et al., 1998). In the *Xenopus* visual system, STDP has since been implicated in activity-dependent motion selectivity (Engert et al., 2002; Mu and Poo, 2006), receptive field refinement (Tao and Poo, 2005; Vislay-Meltzer et al., 2006; Dong et al., 2009), and recurrent excitation (Pratt et al., 2008). Across different systems, including mammalian somatosensory (Feldman, 2000) and visual (Yao and Dan, 2001; Sjöström et al., 2003) cortices, STDP is an important contributor to the activity-dependent development and refinement of sensory computations (Richards et al., 2010), particularly in circuits that process fast timescales and correlations (Butts and Kanold, 2010). Importantly, it has been observed that the activity requirements for STDP vary considerably across brain regions, among synapse types, and even within the same cell at different dendrites, and this variability is thought to be important for coordinating

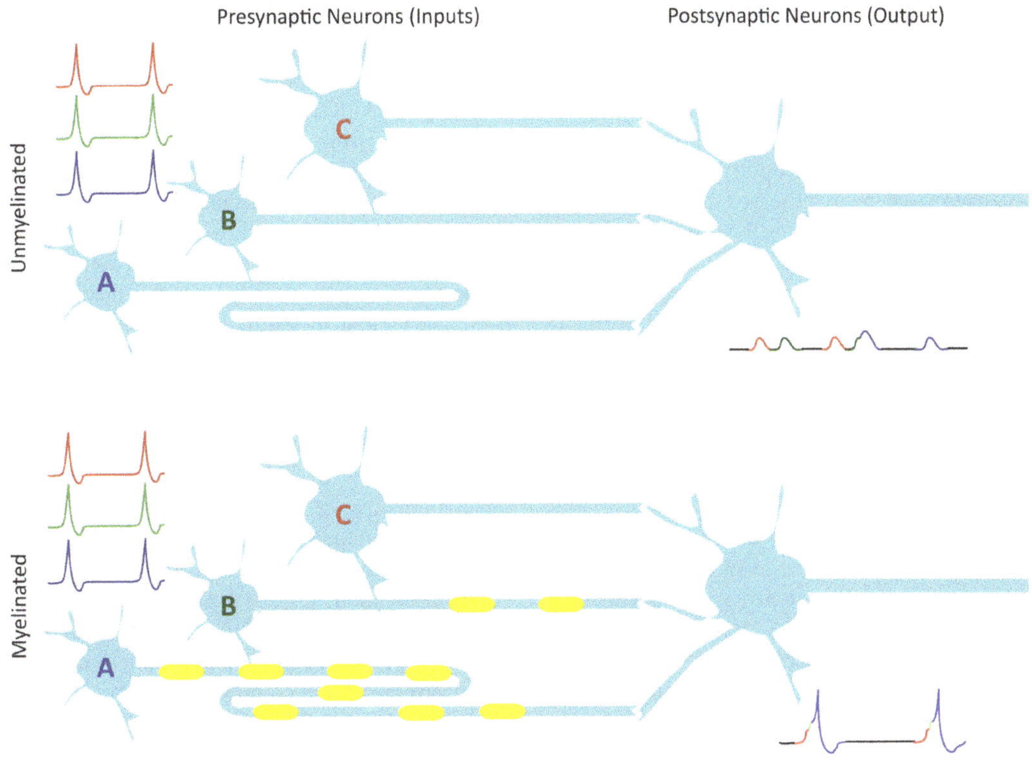

FIGURE 2 | Myelination improves synchrony. Presynaptic neurons A, B, and C provide input to their postsynaptic partner. Although they fire simultaneously, A has a longer axon length than B, which is longer than C. All three presynaptic axons have the same diameter so if they are unmyelinated, they have a constant conduction velocity, which results in non-synchronous activation of excitatory postsynaptic potentials due to conduction delays along the axons. Myelination could modulate conduction velocities in such a way as to allow for synchronous spike arrival at synapses. With spikes from the myelinated inputs arriving coincidentally, summation in the postsynaptic neuron reaches threshold on multiple occasions, leading to a number of action potentials. Small shifts in arrival time could also modulate STDP of inputs.

circuit development (reviewed by Caporale and Dan, 2008; Sjöström and Gerstner, 2010). For example, at the same spatial locations, over the course of development, the spatiotemporal window for neighboring inputs to cooperatively elicit plastic changes at synapses becomes increasingly narrow, conducive to progressively exacting fine-tuning of the circuit (Tao et al., 2001; Takahashi et al., 2012). Timing is integral to plasticity, and therefore mechanisms that control the timing of impulses will influence plasticity.

A study by Yamazaki et al. (2007) recorded from myelinating cells, the oligodendrocytes, in the alveus of rat hippocampal CA1, and showed that they exhibited membrane depolarization in response to high frequency and theta burst stimulation of neuronal fibers, mediated by glutamate receptor activation. Remarkably, they found that depolarization of oligodendrocytes could shorten conduction velocities of CA1 pyramidal cell axons by nearly 10% within a matter of seconds. Such changes in axonal conduction velocity, in conjunction with STDP mechanisms, could result in dramatic changes in synaptic strengths, potentially even converting a synapse that had been undergoing synaptic depression to one that strengthened instead. Moreover, even small changes in conduction velocity can have profound effects on oscillatory network activity, converting synchronous inputs into sources of destructive interference that can disrupt the entrainment of network oscillations (Pajevic et al., 2014), such as the theta-gamma coupling in the hippocampus that has been shown to be essential for effective learning and memory recall (Tort et al., 2009). Examples of how changes in myelin form or function may regulate conduction velocity to affect synaptic plasticity are still largely absent from the literature, but this rather unconventional hypothesis that dynamic control of conduction velocity may function as a potent form of metaplasticity is gaining traction.

EXPERIENCE AND TRAINING INDUCE WM CHANGES

Myelin changes may be reflected at the gross level as WM changes, which have been extensively observed in the human brain using diffusion tensor imaging (DTI) to measure fractional anisotropy (FA) (reviewed by Zatorre et al., 2012; Fields, 2015; Sampaio-Baptista and Johansen-Berg, 2017). FA is a measure of the directional dependence of water diffusion, ranging from isotropic (free) diffusion to diffusion confined to one direction. It is based on the assumption that axonal and myelin membranes within fiber tracts constrain the normally random diffusion of water molecules to instead diffuse anisotropically along the lengths of the fibers. It has therefore been widely used to reveal differences in anatomical characteristics, such as axon dimensions, fiber density, and myelination (Beaulieu, 2002). To date, WM changes have been observed to occur during development, adulthood, and aging. Aging in particular has been linked to changes in WM volume (reduction), WM lesions as seen by hyperintensities, and WM microstructure as measured by FA decreases, with social and cognitive activities acting in a neuroprotective fashion to decrease the magnitude of these changes (meta-analysis by Anatürk et al., 2018), hinting that WM neuroanatomy may be altered by experience over the lifetime of an organism.

Cross-sectional studies comparing experts to novices have revealed FA increases in WM tracts connecting brain regions previously identified as the neuronal correlate of the cognitive domains being studied. Cognitive studies of WM have shown FA increases related to memory, reading ability, grammar learning, and mental rotation (Sampaio-Baptista and Johansen-Berg, 2017). FA increases have been particularly well-characterized in musicians, making the case for musical training as a model of studying plasticity, and especially WM plasticity, with neuroimaging (Herholz and Zatorre, 2012). As a specific example, consider how piano practice in different stages of life has been associated with FA increases in WM. In childhood, FA increases are seen in the following WM regions: (1) the internal capsule carrying corticospinal tracts from the primary sensorimotor and premotor cortices; (2) the superior and inferior frontal regions, including areas of the premotor cortices needed for bimanual coordination and movement sequences; and (3) the corpus callosum connecting auditory regions of the cortex and superior frontal regions (Bengtsson et al., 2005), especially its isthmus in musicians who begin training prior to 7 years of age (Steele et al., 2013). In addition to the FA increases in parts of the internal capsule, piano practicing in adulthood but not in childhood leads to FA increases in fiber bundles of the arcuate fasciculus connecting the temporal and frontal lobes (Bengtsson et al., 2005). However, cross-sectional studies have a caveat: even though they may attempt to reduce confounds by matching participants, such as, for culture when examining reading skills (Carreiras et al., 2009) or for years of training and experience in musicians (Steele et al., 2013), by design, they cannot parse out pre-existing from experience-dependent structural changes.

This disadvantage can be reduced using a longitudinal approach to examine activity-dependent WM changes, since structural images acquired before and after task-specific training can be compared. In one of the first longitudinal studies of myelin plasticity, Scholz et al. (2009) showed that 6 weeks of juggling training led to a FA increase in WM underlying the right posterior intraparietal sulcus. This sulcus has been well characterized in its role in integrating sensorimotor information for the guidance of motor behavior, such as to mediate reaching and grasping behavior in macaques (Borra and Luppino, 2016). The positive correlation between training and FA was, similarly, observed for working memory training, including FA increases in WM regions adjacent to the intraparietal sulcus, around the body of the corpus callosum and adjacent frontal lobe, and near the border between the frontal and parietal lobes that have been previously implicated in working memory (Takeuchi et al., 2010). Using FA as a readout of myelination in human neuroimaging has been validated with animal studies that also observed changes in a molecular marker of myelin called myelin basic protein (MBP): rats showed increases in both FA and MBP expression, as compared to controls, in the corpus callosum after 5 days of training on the Morris water maze (Blumenfeld-Katzir et al., 2011), and in the motor cortex WM tracts contralateral to the limb trained to grasp a food pellet reward (Sampaio-Baptista et al., 2013). The link between task demands and FA increases in corresponding brain regions tends to be correlated with the amount of training rather than outcome (final skill level), perhaps pointing to different anatomical correlates of learning versus performance (Scholz et al., 2009; Takeuchi et al., 2010). Additionally, in these studies, gray versus WM structural changes seem to be relatively independent, both spatially and temporally. These observations suggest that learning (training) but not doing (performing a learned task) involves strengthening of functional connectivity, actively recruiting myelination mechanisms.

However, experience does not always induce FA increases. While most research in musicians reported FA increases, studies in dance and other whole-body motor activities showed decreased FA in WM tracts like the corticospinal tract, superior longitudinal fasciculus, and corpus callosum (Giacosa et al., 2016). Improvement on a car-racing game in humans (and on the Morris water maze in 4 months old rats) led to FA decreases in the fornix (Hofstetter et al., 2013), a WM structure that carries efferents from the hippocampus, a structure implicated in spatial learning and other tasks. FA decreases in WM connectivity of motor and association cortical areas were also observed in a whole-body balancing task: FA was negatively correlated with learning the task and performance improvement in the left lateral prefrontal cortex (PFC) and right motor cortex, and with muscular imbalances in the left superior parietal and right occipital WM and in the left cingulum (Taubert et al., 2010). The authors suggested that these inverse FA changes may be due to the proportion of crossing versus non-crossing fibers that are recruited in a task. FA is a direction-dependent measure, so its readouts regarding WM changes can be confounded by whether local versus distributed networks were recruited. Imaging whole mouse brains for FA changes as well as MBP immunolabeling showed a correlation between the two measures in WM regions of coherent fiber orientations and low fiber dispersion, but not in areas of crossing or complex fiber architecture (Chang et al., 2017). Therefore, some studies show FA decreases rather than increases because FA values are modulated but not necessarily dictated by myelination (Beaulieu, 2002), also reflecting myelin-independent factors like fiber organization (especially crossing fibers), astrocyte number and activity, and angiogenesis (Zatorre et al., 2012; Sampaio-Baptista and Johansen-Berg, 2017). Taken together, research over the last decade-or-so successfully challenges our traditional notions of experience-dependent changes in brain circuits, by showing that not just synapses but also myelin and WM can be altered by experience, and therefore, deserve attention in studies of plasticity. Examining WM with FA and other neuroimaging measures has its caveats requiring careful consideration and interpretation, but nonetheless provide us with insight into human functional neuroanatomy and plasticity. Continued investigations with neuroimaging should be complemented where possible with reductionist cellular and molecular approaches to further enhance our understanding of experience-dependent modulation of WM connectivity.

NEURONAL ACTIVITY IS ASSOCIATED WITH MYELINATION CHANGES AT THE CELLULAR AND MOLECULAR LEVELS

Cellular Markers of Oligodendrocyte Differentiation and Myelination

Myelin is produced and ensheathed around axons by glial cells called oligodendrocytes (OL). The OL lineage arises from embryonic neural progenitors, which give rise to OL precursor or progenitor cells (OPC), finally differentiating into OLs (**Figures 1A,B**). Single-cell transcriptomics show that although early progenitors of the OL lineage converge in terms of their transcriptional identities, OL heterogeneity can nonetheless be observed at later stages (Marques et al., 2016; Zeisel et al., 2018). This suggests that OL diversity arises from secondary diversification rather than developmental patterning, hinting at the role of the local environment in maturation of the OL lineage.

The unique expression profiles of the OL lineage provide useful molecular markers for studying myelination (see reviews by Mitew et al., 2014; Ackerman and Monk, 2016). For example, expression of the transcription factors Sox10, Olig1, and Olig2 turns on as OPCs first appear and stays on as they further develop and differentiate. OPCs are often identified distinctly from OLs by the proteoglycan neuron-glial antigen 2 (NG2) or platelet-derived growth factor α receptor (PDGFαR), and earlier studies also use the expression of O-2A for OPCs though it is slightly less restricted to the OL lineage. These markers can be used to determine the number and proliferation of OPCs, and to study oligondendrogenesis. An antibody commonly used to label OL cell bodies is CC1, which detects anti-adenomatous polyposis coli (APC) (Bin et al., 2016). Pre-myelinating and myelinating OLs express proteolipid protein (PLP), and the enzyme 2′,3′-cyclic-nucleotide 3′-phosphodiesterase (CNP). Only myelinating OLs express myelin associated glycoprotein (MAG) and MBP, enriched in their ensheathing myelin processes. There is a wide array of antigens beyond those noted here, and we will mention these as necessary throughout this review.

Myelin Levels and Morphology Are Influenced by Neuronal Activity

The process of myelination is thought to be subject to both activity-independent and activity-dependent influences. The most prominent cue for myelin initiation is considered to be axon diameter, since even engineered nanofibers can become ensheathed with a physiologically appropriate sheath length reflecting the regional identity of the OL – cortical OLs produce shorter ensheathed segments than spinal cord OLs (Bechler et al., 2015). Other cues intrinsic to heterogeneous populations of OPCs and OLs are more difficult to parse out, but may nonetheless underlie the variation in myelin initiation, with neuronal activity and experience fine-tuning this myelination later on (see review by Bechler et al., 2018), akin to guidance cues establishing the initial coarse neuronal circuit which then undergoes activity-dependent refinement.

The idea that changes in neural activity may alter myelin itself is not new. One of the first reports of the effect on myelination of visual experience came from experiments involving dark-rearing of mice, which delayed differentiation of their optic nerve fibers. Mice reared in complete darkness until postnatal day (P) 20 had a reduced number of myelinated fibers compared to controls, especially in the number of coarser, heavily-myelinated fibers, which were reduced by almost 60% (Gyllensten and Malmfors, 1963). In transgenic mice engineered to express green fluorescent protein in myelin, monocular deprivation from P15 to P32 resulted in a higher proportion of short myelin internodes and slower conduction velocity in the deprived ON, compared to the non-deprived control optic nerve (Etxeberria et al., 2016). Conversely, artificial early eye opening in rabbits at P5 accelerated optic nerve myelination between P7 and P10, compared to controls with normal eye opening, although the myelination reached equal levels in both groups by 3 weeks (Tauber et al., 1980). The change in myelination was observed as increased levels of MBP and PLP, and as increased activity of CNP. Numerous other deprivation experiments have produced a wide range of outcomes depending critically on the exact conditions and brain areas studied (reviewed in De Faria et al., 2017).

In addition to consequences on visual processing, myelin-related changes may also underlie more complex behaviors. MBP expression levels change in the corpus callosum following Morris water maze (Blumenfeld-Katzir et al., 2011) and motor (Sampaio-Baptista et al., 2013) training. Mice that were socially isolated from P21 showed changes in myelination analyzed in the medial PFC at P65, which correlated with deficits in PFC-dependent behavior at P50, including in social interaction and working memory tasks (Makinodan et al., 2012). Specifically, in the medial PFC of isolated mice, OLs had shorter, less-branched processes, fewer internodes per cell, reduced mRNA levels of MBP and MAG, and reduced myelin thickness as assessed by electron microscopy.

Experimentally manipulating electrical activity and vesicular release in neurons also modulates myelination. In dissociated embryonic mouse cultures, administration of the voltage-gated Na^+ channel blocker, tetrodotoxin (TTX), during a period immediately prior to the onset of myelination, reduced the number of myelinated segments (Demerens et al., 1996). Conversely, alpha-scorpion toxin, a drug that slows Na^+ channel inactivation, increased the number of myelinated segments. In dorsal root ganglion neurons co-cultured with OPCs, blocking synaptic vesicle exocytosis by pre-treating the neurons with botulinum toxin or tetanus toxin led to fewer myelin segments, lower MBP expression, and restricted MBP mobility that was visualized by tagging MBP with photoactivatable green fluorescent protein (Wake et al., 2011). A number of studies have investigated activity-dependent myelination in the spinal cord of the zebrafish *(Danio rerio),* an ideal model system for *in vivo* studies, amenable to genetic and pharmacological manipulation together with live imaging. Neurons expressing tetanus toxin light chain to impair vesicular release were less likely to be selected for myelination, and those that were myelinated had reduced sheath lengths compared to controls (Hines et al., 2015; Mensch et al., 2015). Competition between neurons may bias axon selection for myelination: Tetanus toxin-expressing neurons exhibited sheath lengths comparable to untransfected axons when treated with TTX to prevent competition (Hines et al., 2015). Treatment with γ-amino-butyric acid (GABA)-A receptor antagonist, pentylenetetrazole, increased myelin sheath number, presumably by elevating neural activity, as the increase was prevented by tetanus toxin expression (Mensch et al., 2015). In subsequent work, although the impairment in myelination of tetanus toxin-expressing axons was robust for reticulospinal neurons, there was no effect on commissural primary ascending neurons, highlighting that myelin plasticity differs from tract to tract (Koudelka et al., 2016). Elucidating activity-dependent mechanisms underlying axon selection for myelination will be an important direction for future investigations.

Myelinating Glia Number Is Regulated by Neuronal Activity

Other than direct changes to the extant myelin sheaths, an important way that myelin plasticity may be regulated is through the genesis, differentiation, and proliferation of myelinating glia. In the rat visual system, in optic nerve transected at P8, blocking action potentials of retinal ganglion cells (RGCs) with TTX led to a reduced number of mitotic OPCs (Barres and Raff, 1993). Unlike in the optic nerve, TTX administration to cerebellar slice cultures had the opposite effect of increasing OPC proliferation and differentiation into OLs (Fannon et al., 2015). In a toxin-induced focal demyelination lesion of the caudal cerebellar peduncle, TTX treatment increased OPC proliferation but impaired remyelination, indicating differentiation of OPC that failed to properly myelinate axons (Gautier et al., 2015). The decreases in OPC and OL numbers following axonal activity blockade are transient with OL numbers recovering by a later time point (Barres and Raff, 1993; Demerens et al., 1996). In the corticospinal tract, 10 days of daily unilateral stimulation with an implanted electrode increased OPC differentiation and proliferation (Li et al., 2010). Optogenetic stimulation of layer V projection neurons in the mouse premotor cortex promoted OPC proliferation, oligodendrogenesis, and increased myelin sheath thickness (Gibson et al., 2014). This increase in oligodendrogenesis and myelin sheath thickness was also observed in cortical pyramidal neurons, which were stimulated by administering clozapine-*N*-oxide to activate hM3Dq DREADDs (designer receptor exclusively activated by designer drug) electroporated *in utero* in mice (Mitew et al., 2018). Of note, in this study, immunogold labeling of the green fluorescent protein that was co-expressed with the hM3Dq DREADDs showed that the increase in myelin thickness was preferential to stimulated rather than unstimulated axons.

Physiological sensory experience can also modulate myelinating glia number. Whisker clipping decreased the density of CC1+ OLs in the deprived somatosensory cortex, likely through reduced survival or increased apoptosis of NG2+ OPCs that were differentiating into CC1+ OLs (Hill et al., 2014). The barrel cortex is organized such that CNP+ NG2+ cell density is higher in the barrel septa than in the barrel cores where thalamocortical afferents terminate. However, following removal and cauterization of whiskers in mice, which induces reorganization of inputs to the corresponding barrel cortex, NG2+ cell proliferation becomes more uniform across the septa and cores (Mangin et al., 2012). In the same study, dark-rearing was shown not to alter NG2+ cell distribution and density in the primary visual cortex. In contrast, monocular deprivation decreased OPCs and increased mature OLs in the corresponding optic nerve and optic tract (Etxeberria et al., 2016). These studies reveal that the effects of sensory deprivation on OPCs and OLs vary depending on the type of sensory deprivation, modality, and specific brain region.

Physical exercise has also been shown to increase differentiation of NG2+ OPCs into mature OLs and decrease cell proliferation (Simon et al., 2011). When mice were trained to run on a complex wheel, which has irregularly-spaced rungs, learning this task coincided with increased OPC proliferation and OL production in the corpus callosum (McKenzie et al., 2014). This study was particularly convincing regarding the involvement of glia in motor learning: preventing oligodendrogenesis after complex wheel training, using a tamoxifen-inducible Cre deletion of the myelin regulating factor (Myrf), did not lead to the learning impairments seen when oligodendrogenesis was prevented prior to training. Using *in situ* hybridization of a new molecular marker identified to be preferentially upregulated in early differentiating OLs, Enpp6, a choline-specific ectonucleotide pyrophosphatase/phosphodiesterase, learning on the complex wheel task was shown to induce new OL differentiation in the subcortical WM within just 2.5 h and at 4 h in the motor cortex (Xiao et al., 2016). Differences in the generation of new OLs increased further over 24 h, and were seen even 8 days later, suggesting sustained differences in OL number during motor learning. Environmental enrichment also affects the populations of OLs, increasing proliferation of primarily Olig2+ cells in the amygdala (Okuda et al., 2009) and the number of CNP+ cells counted in the corpus callosum (Zhao et al., 2011). Future research should investigate the bases for the differences in responses of myelinating glia depending upon the brain region, developmental age of the animal, and type of experimental paradigm.

NEURON-GLIAL SIGNALING FOR MYELIN PLASTICITY

Since myelination can be influenced by neuronal activity, it follows that neurons and myelinating glia must somehow communicate with each other. It was previously suggested that axonal activity leading to the accumulation of signaling molecules and ions in the extracellular space could be sensed by glia (Ransom and Orkand, 1996). A number of studies show that OPCs and perhaps OLs express various glutamatergic receptors, including α-amino-3-hydroxy-5-methyl-4-isoxazolepropionic acid receptors (AMPAR) and N-methyl-D-aspartate receptors (NMDAR) (**Figures 1A,B**). Metabotropic glutamate receptors and other neurotransmitter receptors may also be involved (see review by Bakiri et al., 2009). For example, currents recorded in hippocampal OPCs include both a fast AMPAR-mediated component, and a slower component, mediated by GABA (Lin and Bergles, 2004). Purinergic receptors participate in myelination: in dorsal root ganglion and OPC cocultures, the inhibition of OPC proliferation, and the promotion of differentiation and myelination in response to action potential firing is prevented by blocking adenosine receptors, and adenosine application mimics the effect of action potentials (Stevens et al., 2002). NG2+ OPCs express voltage-gated ion channels, including for Na^+, K^+, Cl^-, and Ca^{2+} ions, hyperpolarization-activated cyclic nucleotide-gated (HCN) channels, and transient receptor potential (TRP) channels (see review by Larson et al., 2016). Electrical activity could also directly stimulate the release of factors or exosomes from neurons or glia (see review by Wang and Young, 2014). These factors may include platelet-derived growth factor, basic fibroblast growth factor, and other pro-myelinating factors. Exosomes may contain proteins important for myelination, as well as microRNAs that act as epigenetic regulators of OPC differentiation. While previous reviews have examined the evidence for glutamatergic receptors on myelinating glia (Káradóttir and Attwell, 2007; Bakiri et al., 2009; Spitzer et al., 2016), here, we focus on ionotropic glutamatergic transmission as a mechanism of myelin plasticity.

The "axomyelinic synapse" (Stys, 2011) has been suggested as a potential cellular structure where important neuron-glia signaling would occur (**Figure 1B**). This model requires that myelinating glia express neurotransmitter receptors, form synapses with neurons, and exhibit electrical responses. Morphologically defined synaptic junctions between unmyelinated axons and OPCs in the rat corpus callosum were observed by immunofluorescence and electron microscopy (Kukley et al., 2007; Ziskin et al., 2007). They appeared to be the sites of neurotransmitter release from unmyelinated axons onto Ca^{2+}-permeable AMPARs on postsynaptic-like densities of OPCs, However, investigations in DRG and OPC cocultures implicated glutamate and ATP release directly from axon varicosities to nearby OPC processes at axoglial contact sites, which lacked the characteristic features of synapses and likely arose from spontaneous vesicular release (Wake et al., 2015). This suggests that axonal exocytosis promoting myelination is not necessarily restricted to a synaptic structure, although some alternative explanations for these contradictory observations may include differences in cerebral versus spinal cord neuron–glia communication, timing of observation at day 1 upon addition of OPCs rather than waiting for 12 h or more for synapses to form, as well as potential artifacts of the coculture system.

Crucial to understanding the neuron-glial signaling that underlies myelin plasticity are observations of electrical responses in cells of the OL lineage, including excitatory postsynaptic currents (EPSCs) elicited by glutamate, and even action potentials. Action potentials were observed in a subset of NG2+ OPCs in cerebellar slices expressing voltage-gated Na^+ and K^+ channels (Káradóttir et al., 2008), and in a subset of pre-myelinating OLs in the auditory brainstem following glutamate stimulation (Berret et al., 2017). These action potentials are then thought to trigger Ca^{2+} influx in OLs and myelin sheaths. Following an induction of vesicular glutamate release in the optic nerve by electrical stimulation or sucrose application, *ex vivo* Ca^{2+} imaging showed Ca^{2+} influx from axonal stores into the myelin (Micu et al., 2016). In hindbrain neurons projecting to the zebrafish spinal cord, electrical stimulation increased Ca^{2+} in OL processes and sheaths, and led to sheath elongation, while TTX injection had the opposite effect (Krasnow et al., 2018). Interestingly, calcium imaging of GCaMP6s-expressing OLs revealed Ca^{2+} signatures for sheath retraction versus extension: high-amplitude, long-duration Ca^{2+} transients precede sheath retractions, while higher- frequency transients that are smaller and shorter are associated with sheath elongation (Baraban et al., 2018; Krasnow et al., 2018).

Roles of AMPARs on Myelinating Glia

AMPARs have been observed on OPCs (see reviews by Káradóttir and Attwell, 2007; Bakiri et al., 2009). Pharmacological AMPAR activation decreases OPC proliferation and differentiation in culture (Gallo et al., 1996), on cells isolated from cerebellar slices (Yuan et al., 1998), and in cerebellar slices *in situ* (Fannon et al., 2015). Correspondingly, administration of TTX and the AMPAR non-competitive antagonist GYKI, also reduced MBP expression and the elongation and branching of OPC processes, thus decreasing overall myelination (Fannon et al., 2015). In mouse subcortical WM, knocking out AMPAR subunits increased the number of apoptotic OLs at P14, and consequently, reduced the number of myelin sheaths, but did not appear to affect OPC differentiation and proliferation, or other properties of myelin, such as sheath length (i.e., internode length of the axon) or thickness (Kougioumtzidou et al., 2017). The seemingly contradictory effects of decreased OPC proliferation and differentiation, and myelination, following AMPAR activation, but no effect with AMPAR knockout, may be reconciled in light of the limitations to current approaches. First, AMPAR agonists and antagonists may work on cells beyond the intended targets, especially with prolonged drug exposure. On the other hand, with a genetic approach, most knockout studies affect AMPARs from embryogenesis instead of at a developmentally relevant timepoint, allowing for significant alterations in the signaling cascades or in the microenvironment, which together prevent an accurate recapitulation of the baseline, physiological condition. Better insight into the complexity of AMPAR-mediated effects requires the continued development and utilization of experimental manipulations that are more temporally and spatially selective, involving inducible and reversible cell-specific targeting of AMPARs.

In OPCs and immature OLs, glutamate application evokes AMPAR currents in culture (Barres et al., 1990; Borges et al., 1994; Patneau et al., 1994; Borges and Kettenmann, 1995; Gallo et al., 1996; Yuan et al., 1998) and *ex vivo* in slices (Berger et al., 1992). Electrical stimulation of the hippocampus also elicited glutamatergic currents in NG2+ OPCs, characterized as small inward currents, which could be abolished by blocking AMPARs, and specifically by blocking Ca^{2+}-permeable AMPARs (Bergles et al., 2000). Tetanic stimulation of axons in hippocampal slices led to permanent enhancement of EPSCs in NG2+ cells, mediated by Ca^{2+}-permeable AMPARs (Ge et al., 2006). Similarly, in thalamocortical slices, stimulation of the ventrobasal nucleus evoked EPSCs in CNP+ NG2+ cells, which could be inhibited by AMPAR antagonist 6-cyano-7-nitroquinoxaline-2,3-dione (CNQX) (Mangin et al., 2012). Moreover, within the CNS WM, synaptic inputs are detected on OPCs (Kukley et al., 2007; Ziskin et al., 2007; Káradóttir et al., 2008, 2005). These morphologically defined synaptic junctions between unmyelinated axons and OPCs in the rat corpus callosum, observed by immunofluorescence and electron microscopy, appeared to be the sites of neurotransmitter release from unmyelinated axons onto Ca^{2+}-permeable AMPARs on postsynaptic-like densities on the OPCs (Kukley et al., 2007; Ziskin et al., 2007). However, investigations in DRG and OPC cocultures instead implicated glutamate and ATP release directly from axon varicosities onto nearby OPC processes at axoglial contact sites that lacked the characteristic features of synapses (Wake et al., 2015). This suggests that the promotion of myelination by axonal transmitter exocytosis is not necessarily restricted to a synaptic structure, although some alternative explanations should also be considered, including differences in spinal cord versus cerebral neuron–glia communication, timing of observation at day 1 upon addition of OPCs rather than waiting for 12 h or more for synapses to form, as well as potential artifacts of the coculture system.

NMDARs on Myelinating Glia

NMDAR activation was reported on OPCs in voltage-clamp recordings. NMDA application on O2A+ cells, which are progenitors of the OL and astroglial lineages, activated an inward current with properties similar to neuronal NMDA currents, including current amplitudes in the range of 20–100 pA, Mg^{2+}-dependent rectification at hyperpolarized potentials, and blockade by MK-801 (Wang et al., 1996). In cerebellar slices, a subset of NG2+ OPCs were found to express voltage-gated Na^{+} and K^{+} channels (Káradóttir et al., 2008). From these cells, action potentials could be recorded, and were prevented by blocking AMPAR- or NMDAR-mediated transmission with NBQX or D(−)-2-amino-5-phosphonovaleric acid (D-AP5), respectively. Similarly, in the auditory brainstem, in a subset of pre-myelinating OLs, glutamate stimulation induced firing of action potentials (Berret et al., 2017). *In vitro*, NMDA application appears to specifically regulate OPC differentiation, rather than survival and proliferation, contributing to increased levels of myelination in cocultures of DRGs with OPCs and leading to remyelination in a rodent model of demyelination (Li et al., 2013; Lundgaard et al., 2013).

The effect of NMDAR activity on OPCs is controversial. NMDA application regulated OPC differentiation, rather than survival and proliferation, contributing to increased levels of myelination in cocultures of DRG with OPCs from the cerebellum (Li et al., 2013) or forebrain (Lundgaard et al., 2013). However, application of NMDAR antagonists AP5 and MK-801 to cerebellar slice cultures did not change OPC proliferation, differentiation, branching or extension of their processes, despite observed effects of TTX and GYKI (Fannon et al., 2015). GluN1 deletion from OPCs *in vivo* also had no detectable effect on OPC morphology, basic membrane properties, differentiation, proliferation, or myelination (De Biase et al., 2011; Guo et al., 2012). This finding should be interpreted with caution, however, as GluN1 deletion did lead to an up-regulation in Ca^{2+}-permeable AMPARs (De Biase et al., 2011), perhaps compensating for the loss of NMDARs. Second, these studies only looked at earlier time points (no later than P60) but at 10–12 months, mice with OL-targeted GluN1 knockout exhibited neuroinflammation, neurodegeneration, and corresponding severe neurological phenotypes, including hindlimb clasping, hunchback, and ataxia (Saab et al., 2016), indicating different short-term versus long-term actions of oligodendrocytic NMDARs. In line with this reasoning, blocking NMDARs with MK-801 prevented remyelination in rodent demyelination models, including following a cuprizone diet (Li et al., 2013) and ethidium bromide-induced lesion in the cerebellar peduncle (Lundgaard et al., 2013). Taken together, a plausible explanation is that NMDARs do play a role in the differentiation of OPCs into myelinating OLs but this role may be masked by redundancy in the system during development or the roles of NMDARs on both OPCs and neurons.

NMDARs have also been detected on OLs. Pharmacological evidence suggests subcellular targeting of glutamatergic receptors on OLs, with AMPARs enriched on somata and NMDARs on processes (Salter and Fern, 2005). The presence of NMDARs on OLs, including the subunits GluN1, GluN2A,-B,-C,-D, and GluN3A, have been confirmed by RT-PCR, Western blot analysis, and immunostaining (Salter and Fern, 2005; Micu et al., 2006; Li et al., 2013). OLs showed currents evoked by the application of glutamate or NMDA, with partial Mg^{2+} sensitivity, suggesting the presence of functional NMDARs (Káradóttir et al., 2005) with different subunit compositions as compared to neurons, most likely a mixed GluN1/GluN2C/D/GluN3 combination (Káradóttir et al., 2005; Burzomato et al., 2010). Using an array of pharmacological agents, these studies make a strong case for NMDAR-dependent electrical activity in OLs, especially evident following ischaemia induction.

Ex vivo Ca^{2+} imaging showed myelinic Ca^{2+} influx following optic nerve stimulation at 50 Hz or following sucrose application to induce vesicular glutamate release, which could be prevented by blocking NMDARs with the glycine site antagonist 5,7-dichlorokynurenic acid (Micu et al., 2016). Genetic ablation of the GluN2D, GluN3A, or both NMDAR subtypes attenuated most of the myelinic Ca^{2+} influx. However, in cerebellar slices under ischaemic conditions, Ca^{2+}-sensitive dye-loaded

OLs exhibited no change in Ca^{2+} currents in response to activation or inhibition of NMDARs, despite the presence of spontaneous Ca^{2+} currents (Hamilton et al., 2016). Rather than NMDARs, the authors suggested that Ca^{2+} entry into the OLs may be induced by a reduction in cytoplasmic pH until H^+-gated TRPA1 channels become activated, but this may be a mechanism specific to ischaemia and may not reflect myelinic Ca^{2+} changes following NMDAR activity under normal conditions. Interestingly, glutamatergic receptors are not only expressed on OL lineage cell somata but also on the myelin sheaths (**Figure 1D**), with sheaths expressing a unique NMDAR consisting of the GluN1 subunit with GluN3, but lacking glutamate-binding GluN2 subunits (Piña-Crespo et al., 2010). This subunit combination renders this myelinic NMDAR insensitive to glutamate, while permitting Ca^{2+} influx into the axon upon activation with glycine or D-serine. Live Ca^{2+} imaging of the optic nerve revealed that this novel receptor had lower Ca^{2+} permeability than other NMDAR subtypes, which may be helpful in preventing Ca^{2+} overload within the relatively small space of the myelinated regions around axons while enabling Ca^{2+} activation even in the absence of glutamate.

NMDAR Involvement in Myelin Plasticity

Just as potentiation at a classical neuronal synapse enables synaptic plasticity in learning and memory, a mechanism involving axonal activity and NMDAR activation may underlie myelin plasticity. Furthering their observations of decreased myelination following blocked vesicular release, Wake et al. (2011) saw that local MBP translation in response to 10 Hz stimulation was suppressed when axons were pretreated with botulinum toxin or stimulated in the presence of the NMDAR antagonist AP5, whereas AMPAR blockade did not prevent MBP translation. Taken together, these findings suggest that axonal activity may trigger a signaling cascade that acts to target MBP to discrete regions of OPC processes, thus enabling formation and wrapping of myelin around the axon in that discrete region.

The breadth of observations about neuron–glia communication and myelin suggest that myelination may be influenced or regulated by a number of mechanisms. For example, Lundgaard et al. (2013) suggest that neuregulin acts as a myelin "switch": TTX and MK-801 reduced myelination if exogenous neuregulin was applied, but otherwise showed no effect. Hence, they proposed that neuregulin expression may switch myelination between an activity-independent mode and a NMDAR-sensitive, activity-dependent mode. The latter neuregulin mode is also a faster mode of myelination, which is perhaps why it developed in the CNS to quickly respond to changes and is more prominent during particular developmental time points. Interestingly, neuregulin-1 signaling with its receptor, ErbB, has been previously implicated in myelination: increased type III neuregulin-1 signaling led to thicker myelin sheaths in mice, although normal myelin assembly was observed in conditional NRG1 null mutants until adulthood, and in ErbB3/4 double null mutants until P11 (Brinkmann et al., 2008). Additionally, in conditional ErbB3 mutants, tamoxifen-induced loss of ErbB3 later in life at P19 led to hypomyelination in the medial PFC (Makinodan et al., 2012). For a detailed review of neuregulin-ErbB signaling in nervous system function including myelination, see Mei and Nave (2014).

A different kind of switch has also been proposed, emphasizing the role of OLs in metabolic support (**Figure 1F**). This switch is thought to developmentally regulate the energy consumption by OLs, initially favoring lipid production and myelination, but later providing glycolytic metabolites like lactate to axons to help support energetically-demanding firing of action potentials (Fünfschilling et al., 2011). Compelling evidence comes from transgenic mouse lines engineered to induce loss of mitochondrial cytochrome C oxidase (COX) function specifically in OLs and at different developmental timepoints. COX is the terminal complex, complex IV, of the electron transport chain in the mitochondria, which produces most of the ATP needed to meet cellular energy demands. Since full loss of mitochondrial function in these animals required several weeks, it is not surprising that initial myelin formation remained unaffected. Based on this study, the authors suggested a model involving OLs switching from an earlier mode of initial myelin formation that utilizes mitochondrial-dependent aerobic respiration to a later mode wherein glycolysis is sufficient for OL survival and provides metabolites, such as lactate, for surrounding axons. Thus, reliance on glycolysis does not appear to have a detrimental effect on OL survival or myelin morphology in the CNS, despite severe consequences in the PNS, raising the possibility that mature OLs may normally provide glycolytic metabolites as a source of energy for axons, similar to the astroglial lactate shuttle at synapses. In a later study, OL NMDAR activation increased the trafficking of the glucose transporter 1 (GLUT1) to OL membranes, an increase in cytoplasmic glucose in OLs, and the concentration of lactate in the culture media (Saab et al., 2016). GluN1 knockouts had reduced myelinic GLUT1, thinner myelin and fewer myelinated axons in the optic nerve from P18 to P21 although this difference was no longer seen at P70. Reduced compound action potential profiles and limited recovery of axonal function following oxygen-glucose deprivation were also observed in GluN1 knockout mice from P19–P21. Taken together, these experiments suggest that once myelin has been formed, OLs switch from a mode of aerobic respiration and myelin formation to a glycolysis-dependent mode that provides metabolic support to axons. It is in the latter mode where NMDAR activation may signal to OLs that a particular axon is firing, and this increased energy demand may recruit increased exchange of metabolites from OLs.

While there is converging evidence that myelinating glia engage in glutamatergic signaling, there are many questions that would benefit from further investigation: How do OLs and OPCs respond differently to glutamate, and what implication does this have for their differentiation, proliferation, and migration? What is the temporal and spatial specificity of the communication between neurons and glia, and what regulates this specificity? And finally, what are the precise signaling pathways following glutamate binding at its receptors – are they similar to neuronal pathways or do glia have their own downstream pathways? Understanding these precise mechanisms will allow for more specific investigations of glutamatergic-dependent myelin plasticity, and ultimately reveal targets for preventing demyelination and promoting repair in myelin-related pathologies.

DOES MYELIN PLASTICITY HAVE A CRITICAL PERIOD?

Developmental plasticity of circuits is often subject to a "critical period," a particular time in the organism's lifetime during which the system is highly adaptable, preceding a period of relative stability or a lack of change in the system. Is myelin plasticity subject to a critical period?

Critical periods for myelination have been observed during development. In the zebrafish spinal cord, OLs form new myelin sheaths during a period of just 5 h, and subsequently, sheaths can only be retracted, with no new sheaths being extended (Czopka et al., 2013). In rodents, early social isolation from P21 to P35 leads to deficits in PFC-dependent behavior and PFC changes including simplified OL morphology, reduced MBP and MAG mRNA, and reduced myelin thickness. These myelin-related and behavioral deficits showed equal severity regardless of whether the social isolation lasted from P21 to P35 or until P65, suggesting a critical period ending after the first postnatal month (Makinodan et al., 2012). Furthermore, rats that were socially isolated as adults (4 months old) did not show changes in the myelin content of the corpus callosum, either in the size of the genu or the number of myelinated axons in the splenium at 6 months (Markham et al., 2009). The inability of later social experiences to have an effect that overrides earlier experiences suggests that mice may have a critical period for myelin regulation of social behaviors.

However, not all brain regions necessarily demonstrate critical periods. The effects of TTX administration on OL number fail to persist by about P30 in rats (Barres and Raff, 1993; Demerens et al., 1996). The thinner myelin and fewer myelinated axons in the optic nerve, as compared to controls, observed in GluN1 knockouts at P18–P21, are no longer seen by P70 (Saab et al., 2016). If early activity-dependent changes in myelination can be mitigated with time, it is possible that myelination remains open to ongoing changes in regions like the optic nerve.

There is also evidence that myelin plasticity continues into adulthood, at least in certain domains. In cell fate mapping experiments, Young et al. (2013) measured the rate of oligodendrogenesis in different regions of the CNS, and saw that new OLs are observed at P21, P60, and in 4 months old adult mice, suggesting that adult-born OLs are involved in continued myelin remodeling. However, these adult-born OLs produced more but shorter myelin sheaths than their earlier-born counterparts. In older rats housed in environmentally enriched conditions from 14 months of age and tested on the Morris water maze, there was increased corpus callosum volume, myelinated fiber and sheath volume, and myelinated fiber length, particularly of smaller axons that were less than 1 μm wide (Zhao et al., 2012). The beginning of this review also enumerated several studies of FA changes in healthy human adults, suggesting training-related myelin plasticity in WM. Looking specifically at older adults (mean age of 61 years), 8 weeks of memory training was still able to drive significant FA changes in certain WM association tracts (Engvig et al., 2012). These studies show that learning-induced WM plasticity can continue to occur into late adulthood. Moreover, changes in connectivity do not appear to occur uniformly across the brain. Rather, it has been observed that distinct networks tend to covary with respect to myelin changes with age (Evans, 2013). Interestingly, these network correlations in myelination changes were shown to potentially increase the resilience of covarying networks to damage, using simulations in which network hubs were deleted (Melie-Garcia et al., 2018). Thus, the specific changes in connectivity that occur in the aging brain may confer improved resistance to increasingly probable network damage as individuals age.

The question of critical periods in myelin plasticity is complex, since it appears to vary depending on the developmental age, neurocognitive domain, and neuroanatomical correlate. Further investigation may resolve questions about which brain networks, if any, are under the regulation of critical periods for myelination.

CONCLUSION

Myelin plays an important role in the control of timing in functional circuits, but we are only recently beginning to elucidate how it may interact with neuronal activity to facilitate experience-dependent plasticity. Myelin plasticity is a challenging phenomenon to study, as it is difficult to discriminate from neuronal mechanisms, and myelination varies based on developmental age, anatomical region, and neuronal identity. We have reviewed evidence of how neuronal activity alters myelination from gross WM changes to cellular and molecular changes involving glial proliferation, differentiation, morphology, and the features of myelin. This neuron–glia interaction has been shown to be mediated in part through glutamatergic signaling, but it is yet to be determined exactly how this signal may manifest changes in myelination. For example, it may enable axo-glial potentiation driving local myelin synthesis, or it may identify the cells in need of metabolic support. Continued investigations that will elucidate more specific mechanisms, critical periods, and functional outcomes of myelin plasticity will be critical in advancing our understanding of myelinated circuitry in experience-dependent plasticity.

AUTHOR CONTRIBUTIONS

This review was written by ZC with feedback and editing by RTK and ESR.

FUNDING

This work was supported by NSERC CGS-M, Douglas Avrith Graduate Studentship, and McGill IPN Returning Student Award to ZC and a MNI-Cambridge Joint Research Partnership Grant to ESR and RTK.

REFERENCES

Ackerman, S. D., and Monk, K. R. (2016). The scales and tales of myelination: using zebrafish and mouse to study myelinating glia. *Brain Res.* 1641, 79–91. doi: 10.1016/j.brainres.2015.10.011

Anatürk, M., Demnitz, N., Ebmeier, K. P., and Sexton, C. E. (2018). A systematic review and meta-analysis of structural magnetic resonance imaging studies investigating cognitive and social activity levels in older adults. *Neurosci. Biobehav. Rev.* 93, 71–84. doi: 10.1016/j.neubiorev.2018.06.012

Arancibia-Cárcamo, I. L., Ford, M. C., Cossell, L., Ishida, K., Tohyama, K., and Attwell, D. (2017). Node of Ranvier length as a potential regulator of myelinated axon conduction speed. *eLife* 6:e23329. doi: 10.7554/eLife.23329

Baker, G. E., and Stryker, M. P. (1990). Retinofugal fibres change conduction velocity and diameter between the optic nerve and tract in ferrets. *Nature* 344, 342–345. doi: 10.1038/344342a0

Bakiri, Y., Burzomato, V., Frugier, G., Hamilton, N. B., Káradóttir, R. T., and Attwell, D. (2009). Glutamatergic signalling in the brain's white matter. *Neuroscience* 158, 266–274. doi: 10.1016/j.neuroscience.2008.01.015

Baraban, M., Koudelka, S., and Lyons, D. A. (2018). Ca^{2+} activity signatures of myelin sheath formation and growth in vitro. *Nat. Neurosci.* 21, 19–23. doi: 10.1038/s41593-017-0040-x

Barres, B. A., Koroshetz, W. J., Swartz, K. J., Chun, L. L. Y., and Corey, D. P. (1990). Ion channel expression by white matter glia: the O-2A glial progenitor cell. *Neuron* 4, 507–524. doi: 10.1016/0896-6273(90)90109-S

Barres, B. A., and Raff, M. C. (1993). Proliferation of oligodendrocyte precursor cells depends on electrical activity in axons. *Nature* 361, 258–260. doi: 10.1038/361258a0

Beaulieu, C. (2002). The basis of anisotropic water diffusion in the nervous system – a technical review. *NMR Biomed.* 15, 435–455. doi: 10.1002/nbm.782

Bechler, M. E., Byrne, L., and Ffrench-Constant, C. (2015). CNS myelin sheath lengths are an intrinsic property of oligodendrocytes. *Curr. Biol.* 25, 2411–2416. doi: 10.1016/j.cub.2015.07.056

Bechler, M. E., Swire, M., and Ffrench-Constant, C. (2018). Intrinsic and adaptive myelination – A sequential mechanism for smart wiring in the brain. *Dev. Neurobiol.* 78, 68–79. doi: 10.1002/dneu.22518

Bengtsson, S. L., Nagy, Z., Skare, S., Forsman, L., Forssberg, H., and Ullen, F. (2005). Extensive piano practicing has regionally specific effects on white matter development. *Nat. Neurosci.* 8, 1148–1150. doi: 10.1038/nn1516

Berger, T., Walz, W., Schnitzer, J., and Kettenmann, H. (1992). GABA- and glutamate-activated currents in glial cells of the mouse corpus callosum slice. *J. Neurosci. Res.* 31, 21–27. doi: 10.1002/jnr.490310104

Bergles, D. E., Roberts, J. D. B., Somogyi, P., and Jahr, C. E. (2000). Glutamatergic synapses on oligodendrocyte precursor cells in the hippocampus. *Nature* 405, 187–191. doi: 10.1038/35012083

Berret, E., Barron, T., Xu, J., Debner, E., Kim, E. J., and Kim, J. H. (2017). Oligodendroglial excitability mediated by glutamatergic inputs and Nav1.2 activation. *Nat. Commun.* 8:557. doi: 10.1038/s41467-017-00688-0

Bin, J. M., Harris, S. N., and Kennedy, T. E. (2016). The oligodendrocyte-specific antibody 'CC1' binds Quaking 7. *J. Neurochem.* 139, 181–186. doi: 10.1111/jnc.13745

Blumenfeld-Katzir, T., Pasternak, O., Dagan, M., and Assaf, Y. (2011). Diffusion MRI of structural brain plasticity induced by a learning and memory task. *PLoS One* 6:e20678. doi: 10.1371/journal.pone.0020678

Borges, K., and Kettenmann, H. (1995). Blockade of K^+ channels induced by AMPA/kainate receptor activation in mouse oligodendrocyte precursor cells is mediated by Na^+ entry. *J. Neurosci. Res.* 42, 579–593. doi: 10.1002/jnr.490420416

Borges, K., Ohlemeyer, C., Trotter, J., and Kettenmann, H. (1994). AMPA/kainate receptor activation in murine oligodendrocyte precursor cells leads to activation of a cation conductance, calcium influx and blockade of delayed rectifying K^+ channels. *Neuroscience* 63, 135–149. doi: 10.1016/0306-4522(94)90012-4

Borra, E., and Luppino, G. (2016). Functional anatomy of the macaque temporo-parieto-frontal connectivity. *Cortex* 97, 306–326. doi: 10.1016/j.cortex.2016.12.007

Brill, M. H., Waxman, S. G., Moore, J. W., and Joyner, R. W. (1977). Conduction velocity and spike configuration in myelinated fibres: computed dependence on internode distance. *J. Neurol. Neurosurg. Psychiatry* 40, 769–774. doi: 10.1136/jnnp.40.8.769

Brinkmann, B. G., Agarwal, A., Sereda, M. W., Garratt, A. N., Müller, T., Wende, H., et al. (2008). Neuregulin-1/ErbB signaling serves distinct functions in myelination of the peripheral and central nervous system. *Neuron* 59, 581–595. doi: 10.1016/j.neuron.2008.06.028

Burzomato, V., Frugier, G., Pérez-Otaño, I., Kittler, J. T., and Attwell, D. (2010). The receptor subunits generating NMDA receptor mediated currents in oligodendrocytes. *J. Physiol.* 588, 3403–3414. doi: 10.1113/jphysiol.2010.195503

Butts, D. A., and Kanold, P. O. (2010). The applicability of spike time dependent plasticity to development. *Front. Synaptic Neurosci.* 2:30. doi: 10.3389/fnsyn.2010.00030

Campbell, J. S. W., Leppert, I. R., Narayanan, S., Boudreau, M., Duval, T., Cohen-Adad, J., et al. (2017). Promise and pitfalls of g-ratio estimation with MRI. *Neuroimage* 182, 80–96. doi: 10.1016/j.neuroimage.2017.08.038

Caporale, N., and Dan, Y. (2008). Spike timing–dependent plasticity: a Hebbian learning rule. *Ann. Rev. Neurosci.* 31, 25–46. doi: 10.1146/annurev.neuro.31.060407.125639

Carreiras, M., Seghier, M. L., Baquero, S., Estevez, A., Lozano, A., Devlin, J. T., et al. (2009). An anatomical signature for literacy. *Nature* 461, 983–986. doi: 10.1038/nature08461

Chang, E. H., Argyelan, M., Aggarwal, M., Chandon, T.-S. S., Karlsgodt, K. H., Mori, S., et al. (2017). Diffusion tensor imaging measures of white matter compared to myelin basic protein immunofluorescence in tissue cleared intact brains. *Data Brief* 10, 438–443. doi: 10.1016/j.dib.2016.12.018

Czopka, T., Ffrench-Constant, C., and Lyons, D. A. (2013). Individual oligodendrocytes have only a few hours in which to generate new myelin sheaths in vivo. *Dev. Cell* 25, 599–609. doi: 10.1016/j.devcel.2013.05.013

Dan, Y., and Poo, M. M. (2004). Spike timing-dependent plasticity of neural circuits. *Neuron* 44, 23–30. doi: 10.1016/j.neuron.2004.09.007

De Biase, L. M., Kang, S. H., Baxi, E. G., Fukaya, M., Pucak, M. L., Mishina, M., et al. (2011). NMDA receptor signaling in oligodendrocyte progenitors is not required for oligodendrogenesis and myelination. *J. Neurosci.* 31, 12650–12662. doi: 10.1523/JNEUROSCI.2455-11.2011

De Faria, O. Jr., Pama, E. A. C., Evans, K., Luzhynskaya, A., and Káradóttir, R. T. (2017). Neuroglial interactions underpinning myelin plasticity. *Dev. Neurobiol.* 78, 93–107. doi: 10.1002/dneu.22539

Demerens, C., Stankoff, B., Logak, M., Anglade, P., Allinquant, B., Couraud, F., et al. (1996). Induction of myelination in the central nervous system by electrical activity. *Proc. Natl. Acad. Sci. U.S.A.* 93, 9887–9892. doi: 10.1073/pnas.93.18.9887

Dong, W., Lee, R. H., Xu, H., Yang, S., Pratt, K. G., Cao, V., et al. (2009). Visual avoidance in *Xenopus* tadpoles is correlated with the maturation of visual responses in the optic tectum. *J. Neurophysiol.* 101, 803–815. doi: 10.1152/jn.90848.2008

Engert, F., Tao, H. W., Zhang, L. I., and Poo, M. (2002). Moving visual stimuli rapidly induce direction sensitivity of developing tectal neurons. *Nature* 419, 470–475. doi: 10.1038/nature00988

Engvig, A., Fjell, A. M., Westlye, L. T., Moberget, T., Sundseth, Ø., Larsen, V. A., et al. (2012). Memory training impacts short-term changes in aging white matter: a longitudinal diffusion tensor imaging study. *Hum. Brain Mapp.* 33, 2390–2406. doi: 10.1002/hbm.21370

Etxeberria, A., Hokanson, K. C., Dao, D. Q., Mayoral, S. R., Mei, F., Redmond, S. A., et al. (2016). Dynamic modulation of myelination in response to visual stimuli alters optic nerve conduction velocity. *J. Neurosci.* 36, 6937–6948. doi: 10.1523/JNEUROSCI.0908-16.2016

Evans, A. C. (2013). Networks of anatomical covariance. *Neuroimage* 80, 489–504. doi: 10.1016/j.neuroimage.2013.05.054

Fannon, J., Tamriel, W., and Fulton, D. (2015). Neuronal activity and AMPA-type glutamate receptor activation regulates the morphological development of oligodendrocyte precursor cells. *Glia* 63, 1021–1035. doi: 10.1002/glia.22799

Feldman, D. E. (2000). Timing-based LTP and LTD at vertical inputs to layer II/III pyramidal cells in rat barrel cortex. *Neuron* 27, 45–56. doi: 10.1016/S0896-6273(00)00008-8

Fields, R. D. (2015). A new mechanism of nervous system plasticity: activity-dependent myelination. *Nat. Rev. Neurosci.* 16, 757–767. doi: 10.1038/nrn4023

Ford, M. C., Alexandrova, O., Cossell, L., Stange-Marten, A., Sinclair, J., Kopp-Scheinpflug, C., et al. (2015). Tuning of Ranvier node and internode properties in myelinated axons to adjust action potential timing. *Nat. Commun.* 6:8073. doi: 10.1038/ncomms9073

Fünfschilling, U., Supplie, L. M., Mahad, D., Boretius, S., Saab, A. I., Edgar, J., et al. (2011). Glycolytic oligodendrocytes maintain myelin and long-term axonal integrity. *Nature* 485, 517–521. doi: 10.1038/nature11007

Gallo, V., Zhou, J. M., McBain, C. J., Wright, P., Knutson, P. L., and Armstrong, R. C. (1996). Oligodendrocyte progenitor cell proliferation and lineage progression are regulated by glutamate receptor-mediated K^+ channel block. *J. Neurosci.* 16, 2659–2670. doi: 10.1523/JNEUROSCI.16-08-02659.1996

Gautier, H. B., Evans, K. A., Volbracht, K., James, R., Sitnikov, S., Lundgaard, I., et al. (2015). Neuronal activity regulates remyelination via glutamate signalling to oligodendrocyte progenitors. *Nat. Commun.* 6:8518. doi: 10.1038/ncomms9518

Ge, W., Yang, X., Zhang, Z., Wang, H., Shen, W., Deng, Q., et al. (2006). Long-term potentiation of neuron-glia synapses mediated by Ca^{2+}-permeable AMPA receptors. *Science* 312, 1533–1537. doi: 10.1126/science.1124669

Giacosa, C., Karpati, F. J., Foster, N. E. V., Penhune, V. B., and Hyde, K. L. (2016). Dance and music training have different effects on white matter diffusivity in sensorimotor pathways. *Neuroimage* 135, 273–286. doi: 10.1016/j.neuroimage.2016.04.048

Gibson, E. M., Wood, L. S., Inema, I., Miller, S. E., Bieri, G., Zuchero, B., et al. (2014). Neuronal activity promotes oligodendrogenesis and adaptive myelination in the mammalian brain. *Science* 344:1252304. doi: 10.1126/science.1252304

Guo, F., Maeda, Y., Ko, E. M., Delgado, M., Horiuchi, M., Soulika, A., et al. (2012). Disruption of NMDA receptors in oligodendroglial lineage cells does not alter their susceptibility to experimental autoimmune encephalomyelitis or their normal development. *J. Neurosci.* 32, 639–645. doi: 10.1523/JNEUROSCI.4073-11.2012

Gyllensten, L., and Malmfors, T. (1963). Myelinization of the optic nerve and its dependence on visual function-a quantitative investigation in mice. *J. Embryol. Exp. Morphol.* 11, 255–266.

Hamilton, N. B., Kolodziejczyk, K., Kougioumtzidou, E., and Attwell, D. (2016). Proton-gated Ca^{2+}-permeable TRP channels damage myelin in conditions mimicking ischaemia. *Nature* 529, 523–527. doi: 10.1038/nature16519

Hebb, D. O. (1949). *The Organization of Behavior: a Neuropsychological Theory.* New York, NY: Wiley.

Herholz, S. C., and Zatorre, R. J. (2012). Musical training as a framework for brain plasticity: behavior, function, and structure. *Neuron* 76, 486–502. doi: 10.1016/j.neuron.2012.10.011

Hill, R. A., Patel, K. D., Goncalves, C. M., Grutzendler, J., and Nishiyama, A. (2014). Modulation of oligodendrocyte generation during a critical temporal window after NG2 cell division. *Nat. Neurosci.* 17, 1518–1527. doi: 10.1038/nn.3815

Hines, J. H., Ravanelli, A. M., Schwindt, R., Scott, E. K., and Appel, B. (2015). Neuronal activity biases axon selection for myelination in vivo. *Nat. Neurosci.* 18, 683–689. doi: 10.1038/nn.3992

Hofstetter, S., Tavor, I., Moryosef, S. T., and Assaf, Y. (2013). Short-term learning induces white matter plasticity in the fornix. *J. Neurosci.* 33, 12844–12850. doi: 10.1523/JNEUROSCI.4520-12.2013

Jeffress, L. A. (1948). A place theory of sound localization. *J. Comp. Physiol. Psychol.* 41, 35–39. doi: 10.1037/h0061495

Káradóttir, R. T., and Attwell, D. (2007). Neurotransmitter receptors in the life and death of oligodendrocytes. *Neuroscience* 145, 1426–1438. doi: 10.1016/j.neuroscience.2006.08.070

Káradóttir, R. T., Cavelier, P., Bergersen, L. H., and Attwell, D. (2005). NMDA receptors are expressed in oligodendrocytes and activated in ischaemia. *Nature* 438, 1162–1166. doi: 10.1038/nature04302

Káradóttir, R. T., Hamilton, N. B., Bakiri, Y., and Attwell, D. (2008). Spiking and nonspiking classes of oligodendrocyte precursor glia in CNS white matter. *Nat. Neurosci.* 11, 450–456. doi: 10.1038/nn2060

Koudelka, S., Voas, M. G., Almeida, R. G., Baraban, M., Soetaert, J., Meyer, M. P., et al. (2016). Individual neuronal subtypes exhibit diversity in CNS myelination mediated by synaptic vesicle release. *Curr. Biol.* 26, 1447–1455. doi: 10.1016/j.cub.2016.03.070

Kougioumtzidou, E., Shimizu, T., Hamilton, S. B., Tohyama, K., Sprengel, R., Monyer, H., et al. (2017). Signalling through AMPA receptors on oligodendrocyte precursors promotes myelination by enhancing oligodendrocyte survival. *eLife* 6:e28080. doi: 10.7554/eLife.28080

Krasnow, A. M., Ford, M. C., Valdivia, L. E., Wilson, S. W., and Attwell, D. (2018). Regulation of developing myelin sheath elongation by oligodendrocyte calcium transients in vivo. *Nat. Neurosci.* 21, 24–28. doi: 10.1038/s41593-017-0031-y

Kukley, M., Capetillo-Zarate, E., and Dietrich, D. (2007). Vesicular glutamate release from axons in white matter. *Nat. Neurosci.* 10, 311–320. doi: 10.1038/nn1850

Larson, V. A., Zhang, Y., and Bergles, D. E. (2016). Electrophysiological properties of NG^{2+} cells: matching physiological studies with gene expression profiles. *Brain Res.* 1638, 138–160. doi: 10.1016/j.brainres.2015.09.010

Li, C., Xiao, L., Liu, X., Yang, W., Shen, W., Hu, C., et al. (2013). A functional role of NMDA receptor in regulating the differentiation of oligodendrocyte precursor cells and remyelination. *Glia* 61, 732–749. doi: 10.1002/glia.22469

Li, Q., Brus-Ramer, M., Martin, J. H., and McDonald, J. W. (2010). Electrical stimulation of the medullary pyramid promotes proliferation and differentiation of oligodendrocyte progenitor cells in the corticospinal tract of the adult rat. *Neurosci. Lett.* 479, 128–133. doi: 10.1016/j.neulet.2010.05.043

Lin, S., and Bergles, D. E. (2004). Synaptic signaling between GABAergic interneurons and oligodendrocyte precursor cells in the hippocampus. *Nat. Neurosci.* 7, 24–32. doi: 10.1038/nn1162

Lundgaard, I., Swire, M., Ffrench-Constant, C., Luzhynskaya, A., Stockley, J. H., Wang, Z., et al. (2013). Neuregulin and BDNF induce a switch to NMDA receptor-dependent myelination by oligodendrocytes. *PLoS Biol.* 11:e1001743. doi: 10.1371/journal.pbio.1001743

Makinodan, M., Rosen, K. M., Ito, S., and Corfas, G. (2012). A critical period for social experience–dependent oligodendrocyte maturation and myelination. *Science* 337, 1357–1360. doi: 10.1126/science.1220845

Mangin, J. M., Li, P., Scafidi, J., and Gallo, V. (2012). Experience-dependent regulation of NG2 progenitors in the developing barrel cortex. *Nat. Neurosci.* 15, 1192–1194. doi: 10.1038/nn.3190

Markham, J. A., Herting, M. M., Luszpak, A. E., Juraska, J. M., and Greenough, W. T. (2009). Myelination of corpus callosum in male and female rats following complex environment housing during adulthood. *Brain Res.* 1288, 9–17. doi: 10.1016/j.brainres.2009.06.087

Markram, H., Gerstner, W., and Sjöström, P. J. (eds). (2012). *Spike-Timing Dependent Plasticity: A Comprehensive Overview.* Lausanne: Frontiers Media SA, doi: 10.3389/978-2-88919-043-0

Marques, S., Zeisel, A., Codeluppi, S., van Bruggen, D., Mendanha Falcão, A., Xiao, L., et al. (2016). Oligodendrocyte heterogeneity in the mouse juvenile and adult central nervous system. *Science* 352, 1326–1329. doi: 10.1126/science.aaf6463

McKenzie, I. A., Ohayon, D., Li, H., de Faria, P. S., Emery, B., Tohyama, K., et al. (2014). Motor skill learning requires central myelination. *Science* 346, 318–322. doi: 10.1126/science.1254960

Mei, L., and Nave, K. (2014). Neuregulin-ERBB signaling in nervous system development and neuropsychiatric diseases. *Neuron* 83, 27–49. doi: 10.1016/j.neuron.2014.06.007

Melie-Garcia, L., Slater, D., Ruef, A., Sanabria-Diaz, G., Preisig, M., Kherif, F., et al. (2018). Networks of myelin covariance. *Hum. Brain Mapp.* 39, 1532–1554. doi: 10.1002/hbm.23929

Mensch, S., Baraban, M., Almeida, R., Czopka, T., Ausborn, J., El Manira, A., et al. (2015). Synaptic vesicle release regulates myelin sheath number of individual oligodendrocytes in vivo. *Nat. Neurosci.* 18, 628–630. doi: 10.1038/nn.3991

Micu, I., Jiang, Q., Zamponi, G. W., Coderre, E., Wang, W., Stys, P. K., et al. (2006). NMDA receptors mediate calcium accumulation in myelin during chemical ischaemia. *Nature* 439, 988–992. doi: 10.1038/nature04474

Micu, I., Plemel, J. R., Lachance, C., Proft, J., Jansen, A. J., Cummins, K., et al. (2016). The molecular physiology of the axo-myelinic synapse. *Exp. Neurol.* 276, 41–50. doi: 10.1016/j.expneurol.2015.10.006

Mitew, S., Gobius, I., Fenlon, L. R., McDougall, S. J., Hawkes, D., Xing, Y. L., et al. (2018). Pharmacogenetic stimulation of neuronal activity increases myelination in an axon-specific manner. *Nat. Commun.* 9:306. doi: 10.1038/s41467-017-02719-2

Mitew, S., Hay, C. M., Peckham, H., Xiao, J., Koenning, M., and Emery, B. (2014). Mechanisms regulating the development of oligodendrocytes and central nervous system myelin. *Neuroscience* 276, 29–47. doi: 10.1016/j.neuroscience.2013.11.029

Mount, C. W., and Monje, M. (2017). Wrapped to adapt: experience-dependent myelination. *Neuron* 95, 743–756. doi: 10.1016/j.neuron.2017.07.009

Mu, Y., and Poo, M. (2006). Spike timing-dependent LTP/LTD mediates visual experience-dependent plasticity in a developing retinotectal system. *Neuron* 50, 115–125. doi: 10.1016/j.neuron.2006.03.009

Okuda, H., Tatsumi, K., Makinodan, M., Yamauchi, T., Kishimoto, T., and Wanaka, A. (2009). Environmental enrichment stimulates progenitor cell proliferation in the amygdala. *J. Neurosci. Res.* 87, 3546–3553. doi: 10.1002/jnr.22160

Overholt, E. M., Rubel, E. W., and Hyson, R. L. (1992). A circuit for coding interaural time differences in the chick brainstem. *J. Neurosci.* 12, 1698–1708. doi: 10.1523/JNEUROSCI.12-05-01698.1992

Pajevic, S., Basser, P. J., and Fields, R. D. (2014). Role of myelin plasticity in oscillations and synchrony of neuronal activity. *Neuroscience* 276, 135–147. doi: 10.1016/j.neuroscience.2013.11.007

Patneau, D. K., Wright, P. W., Winters, C., Mayer, M. L., and Gallo, V. (1994). Glial cells of the oligodendrocyte lineage express both kainate- and AMPA-preferring subtypes of glutamate receptor. *Neuron* 12, 357–371. doi: 10.1016/0896-6273(94)90277-1

Piña-Crespo, J. C., Talantova, M., Micu, I., States, B., Chen, H., Tu, S., et al. (2010). Excitatory glycine responses of CNS myelin mediated by NR1/NR3 "NMDA" receptor subunits. *J. Neurosci.* 34, 11501–11505. doi: 10.1523/JNEUROSCI.1593-10.2010

Pratt, K. G., Dong, W., and Aizenman, C. D. (2008). Development and spike timing-dependent plasticity of recur- rent excitation in the *Xenopus* optic tectum. *Nat. Neurosci.* 11, 467–475. doi: 10.1038/nn2076

Purger, D., Gibson, E. M., and Monje, M. (2016). Myelin plasticity in the central nervous system. *Neuropharmacology* 110, 563–573. doi: 10.1016/j.neuropharm.2015.08.001

Ransom, B. R., and Orkand, R. K. (1996). Glial-neuronal interactions in non-synaptic areas of the brain: studies in the optic nerve. *Trends Neurosci.* 19, 352–358. doi: 10.1016/0166-2236(96)10045-X

Richards, B. A., Aizenman, C. D., and Akerman, C. J. (2010). *In vivo* spike-timing-dependent plasticity in the optic tectum of *Xenopus laevis*. *Front. Synaptic Neurosci.* 2:7. doi: 10.3389/fnsyn.2010.00007

Rushton, W. A. H. (1951). A theory of the effects of fibre size in medullated nerve. *J. Physiol.* 115, 101–122. doi: 10.1113/jphysiol.1951.sp004655

Saab, A. S., Tzvetavona, I. D., Trevisiol, A., Baltan, S., Dibaj, P., Kusch, K., et al. (2016). Oligodendroglial NMDA receptors regulate glucose import and axonal energy metabolism. *Neuron* 91, 119–132. doi: 10.1016/j.neuron.2016.05.016

Salami, M., Itami, C., Tsumoto, T., and Kimura, F. (2003). Change of conduction velocity by regional myelination yields constant latency irrespective of distance between thalamus and cortex. *Proc. Natl. Acad. Sci. U.S.A.* 100, 6174–6179. doi: 10.1073/pnas.0937380100

Salter, M. G., and Fern, R. (2005). NMDA receptors are expressed in developing oligodendrocyte processes and mediate injury. *Nature* 438, 1167–1171. doi: 10.1038/nature04301

Sampaio-Baptista, C., and Johansen-Berg, H. (2017). White matter plasticity in the adult brain. *Neuron* 96, 1239–1251. doi: 10.1016/j.neuron.2017.11.026

Sampaio-Baptista, C., Khrapitchev, A. A., Foxley, S., Schlagheck, T., Scholz, J., Jbabdi, S., et al. (2013). Motor skill learning induces changes in white matter microstructure and myelination. *J. Neurosci.* 33, 19499–19503. doi: 10.1523/JNEUROSCI.3048-13.2013

Scholz, J., Klein, M. C., Behrens, T. E. J., and Johansen-Berg, H. (2009). Training induces changes in white-matter architecture. *Nat. Neurosci.* 12, 1370–1371. doi: 10.1038/nn.2412

Seidl, A. H. (2014). Regulation of conduction time along axons. *Neuroscience* 276, 126–134. doi: 10.1016/j.neuroscience.2013.06.047

Seidl, A. H., Rubel, E. W., and Harris, D. M. (2010). Mechanisms for adjusting interaural time differences to achieve binaural coincidence detection. *J. Neurosci.* 30, 70–80. doi: 10.1523/JNEUROSCI.3464-09.2010

Simon, C., Gotz, M., and Dimou, L. (2011). Progenitors in adult cerebral cortex: cell cycle properties and regulation by physiological stimuli and injury. *Glia* 59, 869–881. doi: 10.1002/glia.21156

Sinclair, J. L., Fischl, M. J., Alexandrova, O., Heβ, M., Grothe, B., Leibold, C., et al. (2017). Sound-evoked activity influences myelination of brainstem axons in the trapezoid body. *J. Neurosci.* 37, 8239–8255. doi: 10.1523/JNEUROSCI.3728-16.2017

Sjöström, P. J., and Gerstner, W. (2010). Spike-timing dependent plasticity. *Scholarpedia J.* 5:1362. doi: 10.4249/scholarpedia.1362

Sjöström, P. J., Turrigiano, G. G., and Nelson, S. B. (2003). Neocortical LTD via coincident activation of presynaptic NMDA and cannabinoid receptors. *Neuron* 39, 641–654. doi: 10.1016/S0896-6273(03)00476-8

Spitzer, S., Volbracht, K., Lundgaard, I., and Káradóttir, R. T. (2016). Glutamate signalling: a multifaceted modulator of oligodendrocyte lineage cells in health and disease. *Neuropharmacology* 110, 574–585. doi: 10.1016/j.neuropharm.2016.06.014

Steele, C. J., Bailey, J. A., Zatorre, R. J., and Penhune, V. B. (2013). Early musical training and white-matter plasticity in the corpus callosum: evidence for a sensitive period. *J. Neurosci.* 33, 1282–1290. doi: 10.1523/JNEUROSCI.3578-12.2013

Stent, G. S. (1973). A physiological mechanism for Hebb's postulate of learning. *Proc. Natl. Acad. Sci. U.S.A.* 70, 997–1001. doi: 10.1073/pnas.70.4.997

Stevens, B., Porta, S., Haak, L. L., Gallo, V., and Fields, R. D. (2002). Adenosine: a neuron-glial transmitter promoting myelination in the CNS in response to action potentials. *Neuron* 36, 855–868. doi: 10.1016/S0896-6273(02)01067-X

Stys, P. K. (2011). The axo-myelinic synapse. *Trends Neurosci.* 34, 393–400. doi: 10.1016/j.tins.2011.06.004

Sullivan, W. E., and Konishi, M. (1986). Neural map of interaural phase difference in the owl's brainstem. *Proc. Natl. Acad. Sci. U.S.A.* 83, 8400–8404. doi: 10.1073/pnas.83.21.8400

Takahashi, N., Kitamura, K., Matsuo, N., Mayford, M., Kano, M., Matsuki, N., et al. (2012). Locally synchronized synaptic inputs. *Science* 335, 353–356. doi: 10.1126/science.1210362

Takeuchi, H., Sekiguchi, A., Taki, Y., Yokoyoma, S., Yomogida, Y., Komuro, N., et al. (2010). Training of working memory impacts structural connectivity. *J. Neurosci.* 30, 3297–3303. doi: 10.1523/JNEUROSCI.4611-09.2010

Tao, H. W., and Poo, M. (2005). Activity-dependent matching of excitatory and inhibitory inputs during refinement of visual receptive fields. *Neuron* 45, 829–836. doi: 10.1016/j.neuron.2005.01.046

Tao, H. W., Zhang, L. I., Engert, F., and Poo, M. (2001). Emergence of input specificity of LTP during development of retinotectal connections in vivo. *Neuron* 31, 569–580. doi: 10.1016/S0896-6273(01)00393-2

Tasaki, I. (1939). The electro-saltatory transmission of the nerve impulse and the effect of narcosis upon the nerve fiber. *Am. J. Physiol.* 127, 211–227. doi: 10.1152/ajplegacy.1939.127.2.211

Tauber, H., Waehneldt, T. V., and Neuhoff, V. (1980). Myelination in rabbit optic nerves is accelerated by artificial eye opening. *Neurosci. Lett.* 16, 235–238. doi: 10.1016/0304-3940(80)90003-8

Taubert, M., Draganski, B., Anwander, A., Müller, K., Horstmann, A., Villringer, A., et al. (2010). Dynamic properties of human brain structure: learning-related changes in cortical areas and associated fiber connections. *J. Neurosci.* 30, 11670–11677. doi: 10.1523/JNEUROSCI.2567-10.2010

Tort, A. B. L., Komorowski, R. W., Manns, J. R., Kopell, N. J., and Eichenbaum, H. (2009). Theta–gamma coupling increases during the learning of item–context associations. *Proc. Natl. Acad. Sci. U.S.A.* 106, 20942–20947. doi: 10.1073/pnas.0911331106

Vislay-Meltzer, R. L., Kampff, A. R., and Engert, F. (2006). Spatiotemporal specificity of neuronal activity directs the modification of receptive fields in the developing retinotectal system. *Neuron* 50, 101–114. doi: 10.1016/j.neuron.2006.02.016

Wake, H., Lee, P. R., and Fields, R. D. (2011). Control of local protein synthesis and initial events in myelination by action potentials. *Science* 333, 1647–1651. doi: 10.1126/science.1206998

Wake, H., Ortiz, F. C., Woo, D. H., Lee, P. R., Angulo, M. C., and Fields, R. D. (2015). Nonsynaptic junctions on myelinating glia promote preferential myelination of electrically active axons. *Nat. Commun.* 6:7844. doi: 10.1038/ncomms8844

Wang, C., Pralong, W., Schulz, M., Rougon, G., Aubry, J., Pagliusi, S., et al. (1996). Functional N-methyl-D-aspartate receptors in O-2A glial precursor cells: a critical role in regulating polysialic acid-neural cell adhesion molecule expression and cell migration. *J. Cell Biol.* 135, 1565–1581. doi: 10.1083/jcb.135.6.1565

Wang, S., and Young, K. M. (2014). White matter plasticity in adulthood. *Neuroscience* 276, 148–160. doi: 10.1016/j.neuroscience.2013.10.018

Waxman, S. G. (1975). Electron-microscopic observations on preterminal fibers in the oculomotor nucleus of the cat. With special reference to the relation between axon diameter and myelin thickness in mammalian gray matter. *J. Neurol. Sci.* 26, 395–400. doi: 10.1016/0022-510X(75)90210-5

Xiao, L., Ohayon, D., McKenzie, I. A., Sinclair-Wilson, A., Wright, J. L., Fudge, A. D., et al. (2016). Rapid production of new oligodendrocytes is required in the earliest stages of motor-skill learning. *Nat. Neurosci.* 19, 1210–1217. doi: 10.1038/nn.4351

Yamazaki, Y., Hozumi, Y., Kaneko, K., Sugihara, T., Fujii, S., Goto, K., et al. (2007). Modulatory effects of oligodendrocytes on the conduction velocity of action potentials along axons in the alveus of the rat hippocampal CA1 region. *Neuron Glia Biol.* 3, 325–334. doi: 10.1017/S1740925X08000070

Yao, H., and Dan, Y. (2001). Stimulus timing-dependent plasticity in cortical processing of orientation. *Neuron* 32, 315–323. doi: 10.1016/S0896-6273(01) 00460-3

Young, K. M., Psachoulia, K., Tripathi, R. B., Dunn, S. J., Cossell, L., Attwell, D., et al. (2013). Oligodendrocyte dynamics in the healthy adult CNS: evidence for myelin remodeling. *Neuron* 77, 873–885. doi: 10.1016/j.neuron.2013.01.006

Yuan, X., Eisen, A. M., McBain, C. J., and Gallo, V. (1998). A role for glutamate and its receptors in the regulation of oligodendrocyte development in cerebellar tissue slices. *Development* 125, 2901–2914.

Zatorre, R. J., Fields, R. D., and Johansen-Berg, H. (2012). Plasticity in gray and white: neuroimaging changes in brain structure during learning. *Nat. Neurosci.* 15, 528–536. doi: 10.1038/nn.3045

Zeisel, A., Hochgerner, H., Lönnerberg, P., Johnsson, A., Memic, F., van der Zwan, J., et al. (2018). Molecular architecture of the mouse nervous system. *Cell* 174, 999–1014. doi: 10.1016/j.cell.2018.06.021

Zhang, L. I., Tao, H. W., Holt, C. E., Harris, W. A., and Poo, M. (1998). A critical window for cooperation and competition among developing retinotectal synapses. *Nature* 395, 37–44. doi: 10.1038/25665

Zhao, Y., Shi, X., Qiu, X., Lu, W., Yang, S., Li, C., et al. (2012). Enriched environment increases the myelinated nerve fibers of aged rat corpus callosum. *Anat. Rec.* 295, 999–1005. doi: 10.1002/ar.22446

Zhao, Y., Shi, X., Qiu, X., Zhang, L., Lu, W., Yang, S., et al. (2011). Enriched environment increases the total number of CNPase positive cells in the corpus callosum of middle-aged rats. *Acta Neurobiol. Exp.* 71, 322–330.

Ziskin, J. L., Nishiyama, A., Rubio, M., Fukaya, M., and Bergles, D. E. (2007). Vesicular release of glutamate from unmyelinated axons in white matter. *Nat. Neurosci.* 10, 321–330. doi: 10.1038/nn1854

11

Morphological and Functional Differences between Athletes and Novices in Cortical Neuronal Networks

Xiao-Ying Tan[1†], Yan-Ling Pi[2†], Jue Wang[3], Xue-Pei Li[4], Lan-Lan Zhang[4], Wen Dai[4], Hua Zhu[4], Zhen Ni[5], Jian Zhang[4] and Yin Wu[6]*

[1] School of Physical Education and Coaching, Shanghai University of Sport, Shanghai, China, [2] Shanghai Punan Hospital of Pudong New District, Shanghai, China, [3] Institutes of Psychological Sciences, HangZhou Normal University, Hangzhou, China, [4] School of Kinesiology, Shanghai University of Sport, Shanghai, China, [5] Division of Neurology, Krembil Neuroscience Centre and Toronto Western Research Institute, University Health Network, University of Toronto, Toronto, ON, Canada, [6] School of Economics and Management, Shanghai University of Sport, Shanghai, China

Edited by:
Louis Bherer, Université de Montréal, Canada

Reviewed by:
Arun Bokde, Trinity College, Dublin, Ireland
Betty M. Tijms, VU University Medical Center, Netherlands
Teresa Liu-Ambrose, University of British Columbia, Canada

***Correspondence:**
Yin Wu
wuyin@sus.edu.cn

† These authors have contributed equally to this work.

The cortical structural and functional differences in athletes and novices were investigated with a cross-sectional paradigm. We measured the gray matter volumes and resting-state functional connectivity in 21 basketball players and 21 novices with magnetic resonance imaging (MRI) techniques. It was found that gray matter volume in the left anterior insula (AI), inferior frontal gyrus (IFG), inferior parietal lobule (IPL) and right anterior cingulate cortex (ACC), precuneus is greater in basketball players than that in novices. These five brain regions were selected as the seed regions for testing the resting-state functional connectivity in the second experiment. We found higher functional connectivity in default mode network, salience network and executive control network in basketball players compared to novices. We conclude that the morphology and functional connectivity in cortical neuronal networks in athletes and novices are different.

Keywords: basketball player, motor expertise, magnetic resonance imaging, plasticity, resting state functional connectivity

INTRODUCTION

Cortical plasticity is an intrinsic property of the human brain and occurs after long-term training under various conditions (Blakemore and Frith, 2005; Pascual-Leone et al., 2005). Structural differences were found in regional cortical morphology between musicians and non-musicians (Gaser and Schlaug, 2003). Interestingly, London taxi drivers have larger gray matter volume than that in healthy controls or even non-taxi drivers in posterior hippocampi where information of spatial representation is stored (Maguire et al., 2000). However, it is not clear whether long-term training may have effects on cortical morphology with plasticity in motor related cortical areas and whether these effects may contribute to the improvement in motor functions. Elite athletes in the confrontational sports (e.g., basketball etc.) start training since childhood. The sophisticated skills in confrontational sports are likely due to the involvement of different brain areas related to various cortical networks (di Pellegrino et al., 1992; Gallese et al., 1996). These elite athletes offer a special model for studying the long-term training related cortical plasticity with changes in multiple brain areas. In contrast to the long time period required for the longitudinal studies (or often nearly impossible due to extremely long time consumption), a cross-sectional paradigm (cohort paradigm) with a comparison between highly skilled elite athletes and novices was widely used recently (Imfeld et al., 2009; Jäncke et al., 2009; Wei et al., 2011; Fauvel et al., 2014). Although the cross-sectional paradigm may not be more sufficient than the longitudinal paradigm, the study using cross-sectional paradigm is more practicable and the results obtained from a cross-sectional designed study also provide an important indication of the presence of plasticity effects with long-term training. Voxel-based morphometry (VBM) is a neuroimaging analysis technique that allows investigation of focal differences in brain anatomy (Ashburner and Friston, 2000). In the present study, we compared the gray matter volumes in various brain areas in basketball players with those in novices in a cross-sectional paradigm by measuring the structural variation in cortical morphology with VBM. We hypothesize that the gray matter volumes in motor related cortical areas are different between basketball players and novices. In addition, since long-term training process leads to refined cognitive functions such as visual search (Williams et al., 1999; McRobert et al., 2007) and sensory perceptions (Aglioti et al., 2008; Wu et al., 2013) in elite athletes, we also expect that the morphological difference between basketball player and novices may be present in cortical areas responsible for cognitive functions.

Motor expertise involves several internal processes requiring organization and integration of sensory and motor information in different cortical areas (Lisberger, 1988). Neuroimaging studies have showed that the human brain is intrinsically organized into a set of spatially distributed, functionally specific networks (Damoiseaux et al., 2006; Bressler and Menon, 2010). Cortical plasticity with long-term training to gain motor expertise is complex. The interaction of cortical activation among different brain areas at the network level may be associated with multi-factorial process of cortical plasticity (Dosenbach et al., 2008). In particular, default mode network, salience network and executive control network are major functional networks relevant to motor and cognitive functions (Bressler and Menon, 2010; Cocchi et al., 2014). Default mode network is activated during motor related spontaneous cognition (Buckner et al., 2008; Mantini and Vanduffel, 2013). The salience network plays an important role in guiding orientation of attention and monitoring of errors during events with internal and external activities (Eckert et al., 2009). The executive control network is responsible for high-level cognitive functions during motor behaviors (Alvarez and Emory, 2006; Fox et al., 2006). Our second hypothesis is that the resting-state functional connectivity in basketball players and novices are different, as relatively less evidence was found in functional brain network in top athletes. We selected the cortical areas with larger gray matter volumes in basketball players (compared to novices, defined in the VBM analysis) as the seed regions and used a seed-based approach to test the functional connectivity in two subject groups. We predicted that the different resting-state functional connectivity between basketball players and novices will be related to the cortical areas located in default mode network, salience network and executive control network which are relevant to the motor and cognitive functions in the basketball players.

MATERIALS AND METHODS

Participants

Twenty-one basketball players (mean age 21.3 $\pm$ 1.3 years, age range 18–23 years) and 21 novices (mean age 21.9 $\pm$ 0.8 years, age range 19–24 years) were studied. All subjects were male (Shanghai University of Sport is one of the major training centers for men's basketball in China). The basketball players were national first-class athletes and were trained five sessions per week (each daily session about 3 h) for 10–15 years (mean duration, 11.4 $\pm$ 2.3 years). The novices were university students without professional training in basketball or any other sports. Basketball players were taller (190.6 $\pm$ 3.4 cm) than healthy controls (176.8 $\pm$ 2.9 cm; $t = 14.1$, $p < 0.001$). The experimental protocol was approved by the regional ethics committee of the Shanghai University of Sport. All subjects gave written informed consent in accordance with the Declaration of Helsinki.

Magnetic Resonance Imaging

Imaging scanning was performed using a 3T Siemens scanner in the functional magnetic resonance imaging (fMRI) center at the East China Normal University. The anatomical difference in gray matter volume between basketball players and novices was tested using the T1-weighted structural image scanning. A high-resolution image with 192 slices was acquired using a 3-dimension fast-field echo sequence (echo time (TE) = 2.34 ms, repetition time (TR) = 2530 ms, flip angle (FA) = 7°, field of view (FOV) = 256 mm^2 × 256 mm^2, slice thickness = 1 mm, inversion time (TI) = 1100 ms). The resting-state fMRI scanning was performed with a gradient echo planar imaging sequence (TE = 30 ms, TR = 2000 ms, FA = 90°, FOV = 240 mm^2 × 240 mm^2, slice thickness = 3 mm). A total of 210 scans were obtained from each subject. Subjects were instructed to keep themselves relaxed while lying still in the scanner with their eyes closed.

Optimized Voxel-Based Morphometry Analysis

The imaging data analysis was performed using Statistical Parametric Mapping version 8 software[1] implemented in MATLAB 7.4. As the basketball players were taller than novices and the brain volume varied with the height in individuals, we applied the optimized VBM approach (Good et al., 2001) to compare the gray matter volumes in two groups by creating a study-specific template. In the pre-processing step, each reoriented image was segmented (unified segmentation) into gray matter, white matter and cerebrospinal fluid (Ashburner and Friston, 2005). Segmented gray matter images of all subjects were rigidly transformed and averaged to create the study-specific template. The aligned gray matter images in each subject were normalized with the study-specific template. Modulation

[1] http://www.fil.ion.ucl.ac.uk/spm/

with Jacobian determinant was used to correct volume changes caused by spatial normalization. The modulated images were finally transformed into the Montreal Neurological Institute space and smoothed with a 6-mm full-width at half maximum Gaussian kernel.

Pre-processed gray matter images in basketball players and novices were compared with a two-sample t-test (second-level) run at the whole brain level. The height of subject was set as a covariate to exclude the potential contamination caused by different sizes of brain in two groups. The t-map was set at a corrected significance level of $p < 0.05$. AlphaSim correction (REST_V1.8) with Monte Carlo simulation was used to correct for multiple comparisons (Poline et al., 1997; Song et al., 2011) with consideration both for the individual voxel probability and cluster size threshold. Based on the results of optimized VBM analysis, brain areas with larger gray matter volume in basketball players were identified (**Figure 1**). We also tested the correlation between gray matter volumes in these areas and training time in basketball players with the Pearson correlation coefficient. These areas were further selected as the seeds for the subsequent functional connectivity analyses. The seed was defined as a 6 mm radius sphere.

Functional Connectivity Analysis

We defined five seeds (**Figure 1**) for the resting-state functional imaging analysis. The pre-processing for the resting-state functional imaging analysis included slice time correction, rigid body movement correction, normalization of the functional images by directly registering onto the Montreal Neurological Institute echo planar imaging template (interpolated spatial resolution 3 mm^3 × 3 mm^3 × 3 mm^3) and spatially smoothing (6 mm full-width at half maximum). The voxel-wise correlation analysis was conducted after the initial imaging data were temporally filtered (0.01–0.08 Hz). The resting-state time series of the five selected seed regions were extracted using MarsBaR toolbox (Brett et al., 2002). The correlation coefficient (r-value) between the seed region (6 mm radius sphere) and other voxels of the whole brain (excluding those in the seed region) was computed. The correlation coefficient was converted into a z score by Fisher's r-to-z transformation to generate a contrast matrix for each seed region in each subject. For the group data analysis, we used a two-sample t-test to compare the difference between basketball players and novices (**Figure 2**). The t-test was repeated five times (one t-test for each seed region). AlphaSim correction with Monte Carlo simulation was used to correct for multiple comparisons. The t-map was set at a corrected significance level of $p < 0.05$.

One purpose of our study was to investigate the differences in functional connectivity between two groups as they were applied to the cortical networks with potential interests. We predicted the differences in functional connectivity between two subject groups would be due to different motor and cognitive functions in them which were likely related to different cortical networks. We specifically focused on three cortical networks, including the default mode network, salience network and executive control network. Therefore, we illustrated the data with functional connectivity from five seed regions (superimposed results of 5 t-tests) and projected the data onto a network brain template (Brain NetViewer[2]; Xia et al., 2013; **Figure 3**). The clusters of involved brain areas were extracted separately for each seed region and an ICBM152 brain template was used (REST_V1.8; Song et al., 2011). This three-dimensional volume-to-surface mapping provided more intuitive information about the seed regions and other functionally connected brain areas within three cortical networks and exhibited the spatial distribution of these cortical networks in the brain (Margulies et al., 2013).

RESULTS

Gray Matter Volume

We used an optimized VBM technique to analyze T1-weighted anatomical scanning and set height as a covariate to correct

[2]http://www.nitrc.org/projects/bnv/

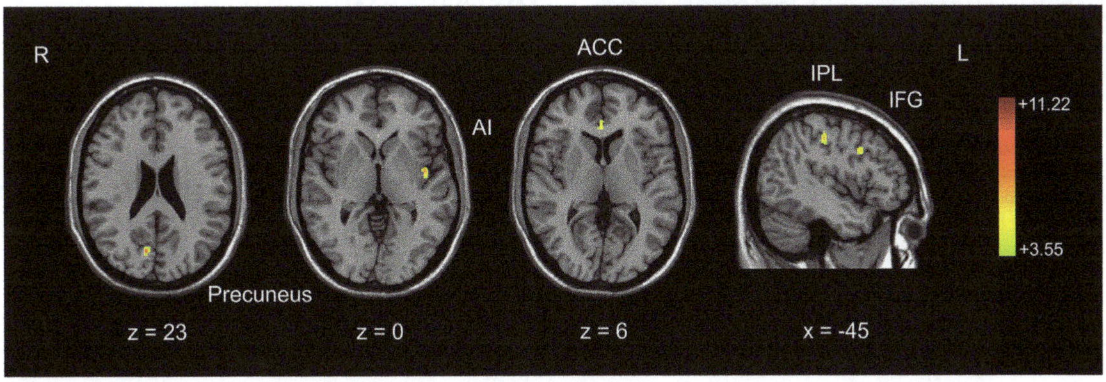

FIGURE 1 | Comparison of gray matter volume between basketball players and novices. Cortical areas with more gray matter volume in basketball players compared to novices was shown. Color scale represents the significant t-values (corrected $p < 0.05$). L = left; R = right. Abbreviations for brain areas: ACC, anterior cingulate cortex; AI, anterior insula; IFG, inferior frontal gyrus; IPL, inferior parietal lobule.

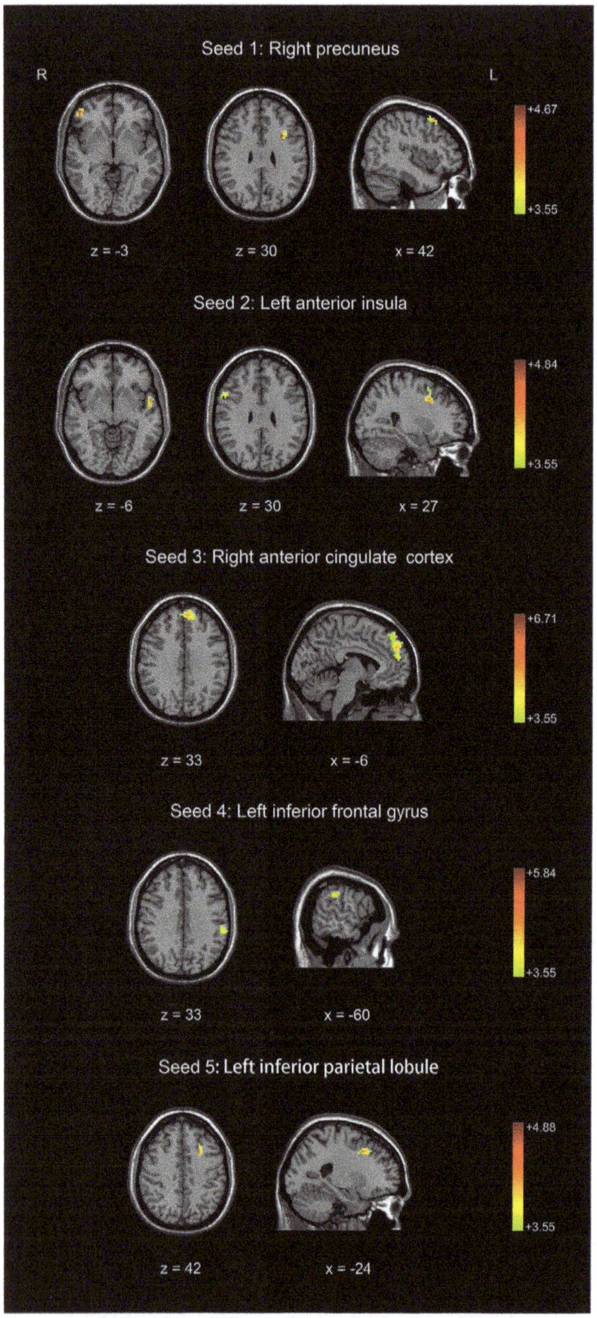

FIGURE 2 | Comparison of resting-state functional connectivity between basketball players and novices. Higher resting-state functional connectivity in basketball players compared to novices was shown. Five seed regions (three in the left brain and two in the right brain) were extracted. Color scale represents the significant *t*-values (corrected $p < 0.05$).

for the potential effect of contamination caused by different brain sizes in two subject groups. It was found that basketball players had larger gray matter volumes than novices in multiple brain areas. These areas included right precuneus, left anterior insula (AI), right anterior cingulate cortex (ACC), left inferior frontal gyrus (IFG) and left inferior parietal lobule (IPL; **Figure 1**; **Table 1**). These areas were selected as the seeds for the functional connectivity analyses. The inverse contrast analysis did not show larger volumes in novices compared to players in any brain areas. No significant correlation was found between the gray matter volume and training time in five seed regions in basketball players.

Resting-State Functional Connectivity

Five seed regions were connected with multiple brain areas at resting state both in basketball players and novices. Importantly, we found resting-state functional connectivity is different for basketball players and healthy controls in functional networks related to various brain areas (**Figure 2**; **Table 2**). Specifically, the right precuneus showed more resting connectivity with right inferior orbitofrontal gyrus (IOG), left pars opercularis (POP) of the IFG and right middle frontal gyrus (MFG) in the basketball players group. The connectivity between left AI and right MFG, right IFG, left superior temporal poles (STP) was stronger in the player group than that in the novice group. Right ACC was more functionally connected with left medial superior frontal gyrus (MSFG) in the basketball player group. Left IFG was more functionally connected with the left IPL while the left IPL was more functionally connected with the left MFG in the basketball player group compared to the novice group. On the other hand, the reversed comparison did not find stronger connectivity between seed region and any other cortical areas in novices compared to basketball players.

Furthermore, we projected the data onto a network brain template. It was confirmed that right precuneus had stronger connectivity with left POP of the IFG and right IOG, MFG in default mode network in basketball players compared to that in novices (**Figure 3A**). For the salience network (**Figure 3B**), left AI had stronger connectivity with left STP and right IFG while right ACC was more functionally connected with left MSFG in basketball players than novices. For the executive control network (**Figure 3C**), functional connectivity between left IFG and IPL and that between IPL and MFG was stronger in basketball players than that in novices.

DISCUSSION

We investigated the difference in brain structure and resting-state functional connectivity between basketball players and novices. The novel finding was that basketball players showed greater gray matter volume in five brain areas (**Figure 1**). Furthermore, basketball players displayed higher resting-state functional connectivity between these five seed regions and other cortical areas compared to novices. These cortical areas are located in default mode network, salience network and executive control network which are related to motor and cognitive functions in basketball players (**Figures 2, 3**).

Gray Matter Volume

We found larger volume of gray matter in right precuneus, left AI, right ACC, left IFG and left IPL in basketball players compared to novices. Precuneus is associated with processing

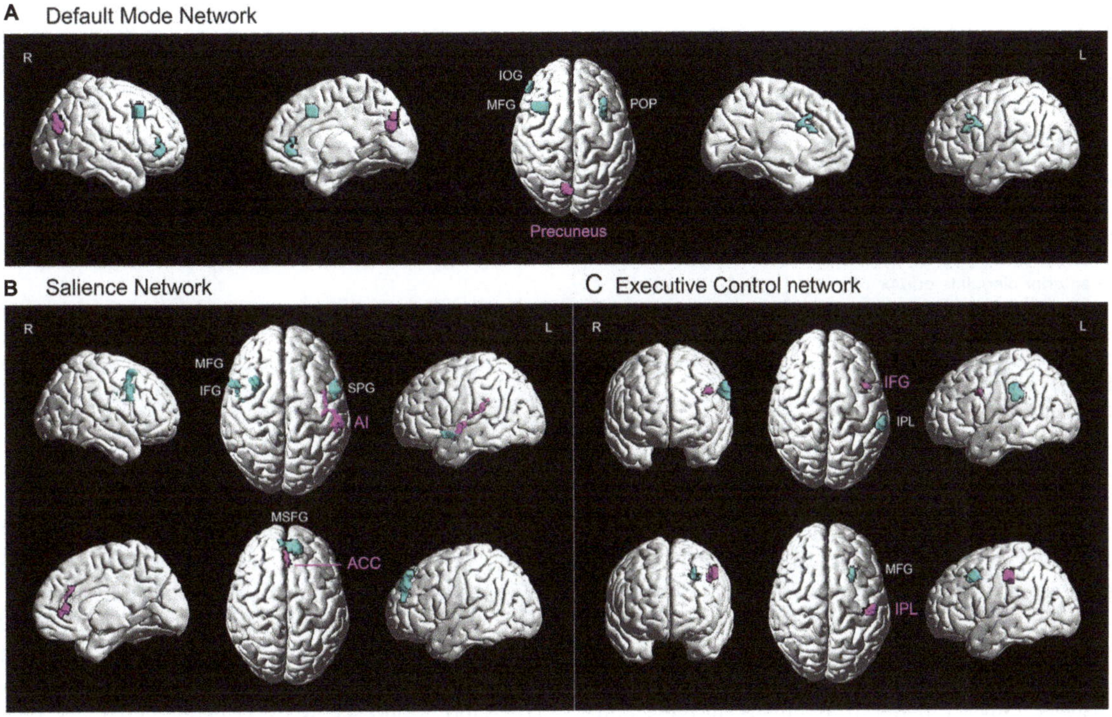

FIGURE 3 | Higher resting-state functional connectivity in basketball players related to three cortical networks. Five seed regions (purple) with enhanced gray matter volume showed stronger functional connectivity with several brain areas (green) in the basketball players compared to novices. These functionally connected brain areas are parts of default mode network **(A)**, executive control network **(B)** and attention network **(C)**. L = left; R = right. Abbreviations for brain areas: ACC, anterior cingulate cortex; AI, anterior insula; IFG, inferior frontal gyrus; IOG, inferior orbitofrontal gyrus; IPL, inferior parietal lobule; MFG, middle frontal gyrus; MSFG, medial superior frontal gyrus; POP, pars opercularis (of the inferior frontal gyrus); STP, superior temporal pole.

spatial information during motor execution and preparation (Kawashima et al., 1995; Cavanna and Trimble, 2006). In particular, precuneus was involved in target tracking tasks with special requirement for attention to spatial information (Wenderoth et al., 2005; Cavanna and Trimble, 2006). Regular practicing skill of tracking the frequently moving targets in basketball may explain the volume increase in precuneus in basketball players compared to novices. Insula shows high activation during complex behavioral tasks (Craig, 2009) and plays an important role in making a rapid decision in a risky situation (Craig, 2002; Singer et al., 2009). Such ability with superior motor related perceptual functions is required in basketball because the players often perceive their self-positioning in the court and make decision in offending/defending strategy (Bar-Eli and Tractinsky, 2000; Llorca-Miralles et al., 2013; Kinrade et al., 2015). Our results also confirmed that physical exercise induces volume increase in the ACC (Flöel et al., 2010; Prakash et al., 2010) and supported the opinion that ACC is the major neuronal substrate for attention (Osaka et al., 2007) and action selection (Rushworth, 2008). The IFG is related to the action observation and imitation (Buccino et al., 2004; Calvo-Merino et al., 2005, 2006; Iseki et al., 2008; Caspers et al., 2010), which may be essential in basketball because the programming and execution of motor plan in basketball highly relies on the action observation of the opponent players (Fujii et al., 2014a,b). The IPL is important for complex cognitive functions, including visual perception, spatial perception and visuomotor integration (Anderson, 2011). The present finding of more gray matter volume in IPL in basketball players was consistent with previous evidence from neuroimaging studies that IPL was activated during action observation (Grèzes and Decety, 2001; Buccino et al., 2004; Hamilton and Grafton, 2006; Chong et al., 2008) and anticipation with correct understanding of the movement (Rizzolatti et al., 2006).

TABLE 1 | Gray matter volumes in five seed areas in basketball players and novices (players > novices).

Brain region	Side	*x*	*y*	*z*	Voxels	*t*-value
Precuneus (BA 31)	R	11	−74	23	52	8.52
Anterior insula (BA 13)	L	−42	−6	−0	136	7.88
Anterior cingulate cortex (BA 32)	R	2	32	6	35	6.32
Inferior frontal gyrus (BA 9)	L	−45	11	33	48	6.75
Inferior parietal lobule (BA 3)	L	−45	−24	44	75	7.50

BA, Brodmann's area; L, left; R, right. Coordinates refer to Talairach space. Brain areas with corrected $p < 0.05$ were listed.

The basketball players in the present study are top athletes in China. The expertise in basketball skill largely varies

TABLE 2 | Resting-state functional connectivity between seed regions and other brain areas in basketball players and novices (players > novices).

Brain region	Side	*x*	*y*	*z*	Voxels	*t*-value
Seed 1: Right precuneus						
Inferior orbitofrontal gyrus (BA 47)	R	51	45	−3	53	4.43
Inferior frontal gyrus (pars opercularis, BA 47)	L	−30	12	30	58	4.52
Middle frontal gyrus (BA 8)	R	42	18	57	49	3.89
Seed 2: Left anterior insula						
Superior temporal pole (BA 38)	L	−57	3	−6	34	4.05
Middle frontal gyrus (BA 6/BA 8)	R	27	12	39	84	4.39
Inferior frontal gyrus (BA 9)	R	54	12	30	48	3.82
Seed 3: Right anterior cingulate cortex						
Medial superior frontal gyrus (BA 9)	L	−6	51	33	167	4.96
Seed 4: Left inferior frontal gyrus						
Inferior parietal lobule (BA 40)	L	−60	−33	33	31	4.15
Seed 5: Left inferior parietal lobule						
Middle frontal gyrus (BA 8)	L	−24	15	42	25	3.78

BA, Brodmann's area; L, left; R, right. Coordinates refer to Talairach space. Brain areas with corrected $p < 0.05$ were listed.

depending on the special role that the athlete plays on the court (e.g., point guard and center have completely different playing styles) although our subjects have a similar duration in basketball training. The diversity in playing style with similar training duration might explain why we did not find significant correlation between gray matter volume and training duration in basketball players. This is different from our recent transcranial magnetic stimulation study in badminton players whose motor cortical excitation and inhibition are correlated to training years (Dai et al., 2016).

Functional Connectivity in Cortical Neuronal Networks

Independent component analysis and seed-based correlation analysis are two most common techniques used in functional connectivity data analysis (Biswal et al., 1995; Fox et al., 2005). Although network map obtained from the independent component analysis may be used as a reference to interpret the results from seed-based correlation analysis, two data analysis techniques are based on different mathematical models (Calhoun et al., 2001; van de Ven et al., 2004; Joel et al., 2011). Independent component analysis provides a means to test several spatially separated cortical networks at once. However, the value of a voxel being tested with the independent component analysis represents the correlation between the time series of this voxel and the mean time series of a particular cortical network. The interpretation for these data-driven networks largely depends on the predetermined number of components for production which changes the patterns of spatially separated cortical networks. The interpretation is further challenged by the complexity of noise identification process which is often determined with system selection by the user. On the other hand, seed-based correlation analysis requires the selection of the seed regions. Voxel value from seed-based correlation analysis reflects the degree to which the time series of a tested voxel is correlated with the time series of the seed region. Owing to inherent simplicity, high sensitivity and ease of interpretation, seed-based correlation analysis is widely used to test the functional connectivity between a given seed region and the other cortical areas. We defined five seed regions with larger gray matter volumes in basketball players through VBM analysis at the first step in our study. Therefore, we specifically tested whether the correlations of time series between the seed regions and other cortical areas were different in basketball players and novices. A seed-based correlation approach is likely better and more practicable to identify the difference between two groups in our study. In addition, it may be worth mentioning that previous studies reported similar results when same resting-state fMRI data set was processed by independent component analysis and seed-based correlation analysis techniques (Damoiseaux et al., 2006).

Default mode network includes precuneus, posterior cingulate, medial prefrontal cortex and inferior parietal cortex (Raichle et al., 2001; Fox et al., 2005). We found greater connectivity between precuneus and medial prefrontal cortex in basketball players, supporting the functions of precuneus and the medial prefrontal cortex as the core nodes in default mode network (Martinelli et al., 2013). Our results were consistent with previous study performed in musicians that long-term motor learning and expertise experience lead to resting-state functional connectivity changes in the default mode network (Fauvel et al., 2014). As precuneus and medial prefrontal cortex highly involve in self-related episodic memory (Dörfel et al., 2009), it may be explained that higher activity in the default mode network is caused by frequently processed self-related episodic memory in basketball playing.

Salience network is composed of AI, dorsal ACC (dACC) and ventrolateral prefrontal cortex (Seeley et al., 2007; Chan et al., 2008). We found high connectivity between AI, frontal cortex and STP in basketball players. The result may be consistent with the notion that AI is highly involved in extracting key salient stimuli from multiple inputs (Menon and Uddin, 2010). Our previous study also reported greater AI activity when basketball players noticed incorrect anticipation during observation of a basketball free throw (Wu et al., 2013). Frontal cortex is responsible for the episodic memory extraction

(McDermott et al., 1999; Wagner, 1999; Lepage et al., 2000; Cabeza et al., 2002) while STP is related to the storage of semantic memory (Markowitsch, 1995; Simmons and Martin, 2009). Our results support the idea that memory extraction and storage are essential in basketball. We also found strong connectivity between ACC and MSFG (one part of frontal cortex) in basketball players. As ACC is related to the detection and processing of salient information and monitoring of errors (Kiehl et al., 2000; Hester et al., 2005; Etkin et al., 2011), our results may suggest that the process of semantic memory with interaction between ACC and frontal cortical area is important to maintain the high performance for the basketball players.

Executive control network is distributed in the frontoparietal system which comprises the dorsolateral prefrontal cortex and posterior parietal cortex. Particularly, frontal cortex is a primary region in modulating regular allocation of spatial attention (Schafer and Moore, 2011) and parietal cortex is heavily involved in spatial awareness (Behrmann et al., 2004). Our results that connectivity between the IFG, MFG and IPL is stronger in basketball players compared to novices may verify the idea that executive control network is the key structure for converting selective and spatial attention (Wu et al., 2007) in athletes with high motor expertise.

Motor and Cognitive Functions in Basketball Players

Basketball is a confrontational sport with open motor skill in which movements and actions of the players largely depend on the understanding of the environment and actions of other players (both the team mates and the players on the opposite side; Schmidt and Wrisberg, 2008). Our results with larger gray matter volume and higher functional connectivity in basketball players involved in multiple cortical areas and various cortical networks suggest that complex motor and cognitive functions combining visual search, perceptual anticipation and action execution are required in the development of motor expertise (Abernethy, 1996; Vickers, 2004). It is not surprising that the gray matter volumes in motor related cortical areas increase and show enhanced connectivity with other cortical areas as frequent engagement of these cortical areas during long-term training induces the cortical plasticity in the underlying neuronal components and facilitates the communication of these components within the networks (Fries, 2005; Lewis et al., 2009; Duan et al., 2012). Interestingly, we found gray matter volume increases and functional connectivity enhanced in a wide range of cortical areas among three different functional networks in basketball players. Structural and functional changes in these areas largely contribute to the improvement of cognitive functions including temporal and spatial attention (Wright et al., 2013; Wu et al., 2013), memory processing (Wan et al., 2011; Wang et al., 2013), decision making and error correction (Koelewijn et al., 2008; Cocchi et al., 2013) in the population with professional experience. Our results are consistent with previous studies performed in other sports players (Di et al., 2012; Wang et al., 2013) and support the view that development of motor expertise relies on the improvement both in motor and cognitive functions (Aglioti et al., 2008). Future studies with further consideration about the interaction and mutual advantage between motor and cognitive components may help elucidate the mechanisms of cortical plasticity during the acquisition of high-level motor expertise.

We did not find increase in gray matter volume and functional connectivity related to primary motor cortex in basketball players compared to novices. This is consistent with previous studies in cohorts with other motor expertise, such as musicians (Fauvel et al., 2014), taxi drivers (Maguire et al., 2000) and athletes (Wei et al., 2011; Di et al., 2012; Wang et al., 2013). Interestingly, our previous studies with transcranial magnetic stimulation found increased motor cortical excitability during different motor tasks in athletes (Wang et al., 2014; Dai et al., 2016). It may be inferred that changes (both gray matter volume and functional connectivity) in other motor and cognitive related brain areas alter the cortico-cortical projections to the primary motor cortex and eventually lead to the increased output from the motor cortex in athletes. However, we cannot exclude the possibility that functional or even structural changes occur in the primary motor cortex itself after different courses of long-term motor training (Gaser and Schlaug, 2003; Draganski et al., 2004).

Limitations

We investigated the morphological and functional differences between athletes and novices with a cross-sectional paradigm. It may be argued that larger gray matter volume and stronger functional connectivity observed in basketball players are not induced by long-term training but simply due to the natural property in this cohort which potentially leads to an "expert" brain with better structure and functions during development. Although our optimized VBM analysis partly ruled out the effect caused by inherent brain size difference in two groups, the question how cortical plasticity with long-term training is related to the structural and functional changes in the brain should be further addressed by longitudinal studies performed along the whole career of the athletes.

In addition, stronger connectivity in three functional networks was identified in the basketball players. It has long been controversial whether and how the resting-state functional connectivity represents the anatomical and biological connections in the brain (Raichle et al., 2001; Fox et al., 2005, 2006). Our study does not directly approach the question how the strong functional connectivity in the basketball players is related to the biological changes after the long-term training. However, our findings that functional connectivity was relevant to the seed region where structural (gray matter volume) difference was found between two groups and that we did not perform any pre-selection in determination of the seed region might suggest the potential biological changes with cortical plasticity after long-term training in athletes. The opinion is also consistent with the evidence obtained from neuroimaging studies performed in musicians that changes in functional map are often accompanied with structural changes during acquisition of motor expertise (Schlaug, 2001).

A reversed question is whether the result of functional connectivity analysis is affected by the difference in seed regions determined in the VBM approach. The findings that higher resting-state functional connectivity seen in basketball players compared to novices in the present study was based on the whole brain wide correlation analysis and that the cortical areas where higher functional connectivity were found (except for the seed regions) did not show greater gray matter volumes might partly deny the cause of increase in functional connectivity with simple changes in seed sizes. Similar increases both in gray matter volumes in seed regions and functional connectivity with the seed regions were also found in musicians (Fauvel et al., 2014). In addition, the reference time series in two subject groups are likely slightly different due to more gray matter volume in basketball players compared to novices when parametric approach is used in our time domain analysis (Friston et al., 1994). The comparison for functional connectivity between two groups may further be confounded by the partial volume effect around the seed regions (Müller-Gärtner et al., 1992). Although we performed additional masks in the seed regions by excluding voxels with low gray matter density (value below 0.3) to minimize partial volume effect, it may still be argued that the functional connectivity in novices is potentially underestimated with the fact that the selected seeds in the novices are contaminated by gray matter in other adjacent cortical areas or even white matter. The interaction between structural and functional changes during the long-term course of motor training is complex and the answer to this complex question again requires future work with longitudinal studies performed in the training course.

CONCLUSION

Using structural and resting-state functional imaging techniques, the present study revealed larger volumes of gray matter in five seed regions and higher functional connectivity in default mode network, salience network and executive control network in basketball players compared to novices. We conclude that the morphology and functional connectivity in cortical neuronal networks in athletes and novices are different, and the differences may be related to higher level of motor expertise in athletes with better motor and cognitive functions.

AUTHOR CONTRIBUTIONS

X-YT and Y-LP conceived, designed and conducted experiments. YW analyzed data, interpreted results and wrote the manuscript. X-PL, L-LZ, WD and HZ helped conduct experiments and edited the manuscript. ZN, JW and JZ revised the manuscript. All authors approved the submitted version.

ACKNOWLEDGMENTS

We thank collaborators in East China Normal University for data acquisition.

REFERENCES

Abernethy, B. (1996). Training the visual-perceptual skills of athletes. Insights from the study of motor expertise. *Am. J. Sports Med.* 24,S89–S92.

Aglioti, S. M., Cesari, P., Romani, M., and Urgesi, C. (2008). Action anticipation and motor resonance in elite basketball players. *Nat. Neurosci.* 11, 1109–1116. doi: 10.1038/nn.2182

Alvarez, J. A., and Emory, E. (2006). Executive function and the frontal lobes: a meta-analytic review. *Neuropsychol. Rev.* 16, 17–42. doi: 10.1007/s11065-006-9002-x

Anderson, R. A. (2011). "Inferior parietal lobule function in spatial perception and visuomotor integration," in *Comprehensive Physiology*, ed. D. M. Pollock 483–518.

Ashburner, J., and Friston, K. J. (2000). Voxel-based morphometry—the methods. *Neuroimage* 11, 805–821. doi: 10.1006/nimg.2000.0582

Ashburner, J., and Friston, K. J. (2005). Unified segmentation. *Neuroimage* 26, 839–851. doi: 10.1016/j.neuroimage.2005.02.018

Bar-Eli, M., and Tractinsky, N. (2000). Criticality of game situations and decision making in basketball: an application of performance crisis perspective. *Psychol. Sport Exerc.* 1, 27–39. doi: 10.1016/s1469-0292(00) 00005-4

Behrmann, M., Geng, J. J., and Shomstein, S. (2004). Parietal cortex and attention. *Curr. Opin. Neurobiol.* 14, 212–217. doi: 10.1016/j.conb.2004.03.012

Biswal, B., Yetkin, F. Z., Haughton, V. M., and Hyde, J. S. (1995). Functional connectivity in the motor cortex of resting human brain using echo-planar MRI. *Magn. Reson. Med.* 34, 537–541. doi: 10.1002/mrm.1910340409

Blakemore, S. J., and Frith, U. (2005). The learning brain: lessons for education: a précis. *Dev. Sci.* 8, 459–465. doi: 10.1111/j.1467-7687.2005.00434.x

Bressler, S. L., and Menon, V. (2010). Large-scale brain networks in cognition: emerging methods and principles. *Trends Cogn. Sci.* 14, 277–290. doi: 10.1016/j.tics.2010.04.004

Brett, M. A. J., Anton, J. L., Valabregue, R., and Poline, J. B. (2002). Region of interest analysis using an spm toolbox. *Neuroimage* 13, 210–217.

Buccino, G., Lui, F., Canessa, N., Patteri, I., Lagravinese, G., Benuzzi, F., et al. (2004). Neural circuits involved in the recognition of actions performed by nonconspecifics: an fMRI study. *J. Cogn. Neurosci.* 16, 114–126. doi: 10.1162/089892904322755601

Buckner, R. L., Andrews-Hanna, J. R., and Schacter, D. L. (2008). The brain's default network: anatomy, function and relevance to disease. *Ann. N Y Acad. Sci.* 1124, 1–38. doi: 10.1196/annals.1440.011

Cabeza, R., Dolcos, F., Graham, R., and Nyberg, L. (2002). Similarities and differences in the neural correlates of episodic memory retrieval and working memory. *Neuroimage* 16, 317–330. doi: 10.1006/nimg.2002.1063

Calhoun, V. D., Adali, T., Pearlson, G. D., and Pekar, J. J. (2001). A method for making group inferences from functional MRI data using independent component analysis. *Hum. Brain Mapp.* 14, 140–151. doi: 10.1002/hbm.1048

Calvo-Merino, B., Glaser, D. E., Grèzes, J., Passingham, R. E., and Haggard, P. (2005). Action observation and acquired motor skills: an fMRI study with expert dancers. *Cereb. Cortex* 15, 1243–1249. doi: 10.1093/cercor/bhi007

Calvo-Merino, B., Grèzes, J., Glaser, D. E., Passingham, R. E., and Haggard, P. (2006). Seeing or doing? Influence of visual and motor familiarity in action observation. *Curr. Biol.* 16, 1905–1910. doi: 10.1016/j.cub.2006.07.065

Caspers, S., Zilles, K., Laird, A. R., and Eickhoff, S. B. (2010). ALE meta-analysis of action observation and imitation in the human brain. *Neuroimage* 50, 1148–1167. doi: 10.1016/j.neuroimage.2009.12.112

Cavanna, A. E., and Trimble, M. R. (2006). The precuneus: a review of its functional anatomy and behavioural correlates. *Brain* 129, 564–583. doi: 10.1093/brain/awl004

Chan, R. C., Shum, D., Toulopoulou, T., and Chen, E. Y. H. (2008). Assessment of executive functions: review of instruments and identification of critical issues. *Arch. Clin. Neuropsychol.* 23, 201–216. doi: 10.1016/j.acn.2007.08.010

Chong, T. T., Williams, M. A., Cunnington, R., and Mattingley, J. B. (2008). Selective attention modulates inferior frontal gyrus activity during action observation. *Neuroimage* 40, 298–307. doi: 10.1016/j.neuroimage.2007.11.030

Cocchi, L., Halford, G. S., Zalesky, A., Harding, I. H., Ramm, B. J., Cutmore, T., et al. (2014). Complexity in relational processing predicts changes in functional brain network dynamics. *Cereb. Cortex* 24, 2283–2296. doi: 10.1093/cercor/bht075

Cocchi, L., Zalesky, A., Fornito, A., and Mattingley, J. B. (2013). Dynamic cooperation and competition between brain systems during cognitive control. *Trends Cogn. Sci.* 17, 493–501. doi: 10.1016/j.tics.2013.08.006

Craig, A. D. (2002). How do you feel? Interoception: the sense of the physiological condition of the body. *Nat. Rev. Neurosci.* 3, 655–666. doi: 10.1038/nrn894

Craig, A. D. (2009). How do you feel—now? The anterior insula and human awareness. *Nat. Rev. Neurosci.* 10, 59–70. doi: 10.1038/nrn2555

Dai, W., Pi, Y., Ni, Z., Tan, X., Zhang, J., and Wu, Y. (2016). Maintenance of balance between motor cortical excitability and inhibition after long-term training. *Neuroscience* 336, 114–122. doi: 10.1016/j.neuroscience.2016.08.053

Damoiseaux, J. S., Rombouts, S. A., Barkhof, F., Scheltens, P., Stam, C. J., Smith, S. M., et al. (2006). Consistent resting-state networks across healthy subjects. *Proc. Natl. Acad. Sci. U S A* 103, 13848–13853. doi: 10.1073/pnas.0601417103

Di, X., Zhu, S., Jin, H., Wang, P., Ye, Z., Zhou, K., et al. (2012). Altered resting brain function and structure in professional badminton players. *Brain Connect.* 2, 225–233. doi: 10.1089/brain.2011.0050

di Pellegrino, G., Fadiga, L., Fogassi, L., Gallese, V., and Rizzolatti, G. (1992). Understanding motor events: a neurophysiological study. *Exp. Brain Res.* 91, 176–180. doi: 10.1007/bf00230027

Dörfel, D., Werner, A., Schaefer, M., von Kummer, R., and Karl, A. (2009). Distinct brain networks in recognition memory share a defined region in the precuneus. *Eur. J. Neurosci.* 30, 1947–1959. doi: 10.1111/j.1460-9568.2009.06973.x

Dosenbach, N. U., Fair, D. A., Cohen, A. L., Schlaggar, B. L., and Petersen, S. E. (2008). A dual-networks architecture of top-down control. *Trends Cogn. Sci.* 12, 99–105. doi: 10.1016/j.tics.2008.01.001

Draganski, B., Gaser, C., Busch, V., Schuierer, G., Bogdahn, U., and May, A. (2004). Neuroplasticity: changes in grey matter induced by training. *Nature* 427, 311–312. doi: 10.1038/427311a

Duan, X., He, S., Liao, W., Liang, D., Qiu, L., Wei, L., et al. (2012). Reduced caudate volume and enhanced striatal-DMN integration in chess experts. *Neuroimage* 60, 1280–1286. doi: 10.1016/j.neuroimage.2012.01.047

Eckert, M. A., Menon, V., Walczak, A., Ahlstrom, J., Denslow, S., Horwitz, A., et al. (2009). At the heart of the ventral attention system: the right anterior insula. *Hum. Brain Mapp.* 30, 2530–2541. doi: 10.1002/hbm.20688

Etkin, A., Egner, T., and Kalisch, R. (2011). Emotional processing in anterior cingulate and medial prefrontal cortex. *Trends Cogn. Sci.* 15, 85–93. doi: 10.1016/j.tics.2010.11.004

Fauvel, B., Groussard, M., Chételat, G., Fouquet, M., Landeau, B., Eustache, F., et al. (2014). Morphological brain plasticity induced by musical expertise is accompanied by modulation of functional connectivity at rest. *Neuroimage* 90, 179–188. doi: 10.1016/j.neuroimage.2013.12.065

Flöel, A., Ruscheweyh, R., Krüger, K., Willemer, C., Winter, B., Völker, K., et al. (2010). Physical activity and memory functions: Are neurotrophins and cerebral gray matter volume the missing link? *Neuroimage* 49, 2756–2763. doi: 10.1016/j.neuroimage.2009.10.043

Fox, M. D., Corbetta, M., Snyder, A. Z., Vincent, J. L., and Raichle, M. E. (2006). Spontaneous neuronal activity distinguishes human dorsal and ventral attention systems. *Proc. Natl. Acad. Sci. U S A* 103, 10046–10051. doi: 10.1073/pnas.0604187103

Fox, M. D., Snyder, A. Z., Vincent, J. L., Corbetta, M., Van Essen, D. C., and Raichle, M. E. (2005). The human brain is intrinsically organized into dynamic, anticorrelated functional networks. *Proc. Natl. Acad. Sci. U S A* 102, 9673–9678. doi: 10.1073/pnas.0504136102

Fries, P. (2005). A mechanism for cognitive dynamics: neuronal communication through neuronal coherence. *Trends Cogn. Sci.* 9, 474–480. doi: 10.1016/j.tics.2005.08.011

Friston, K. J., Worsley, K. J, Frackowiak, R. S., Mazziotta, J. C., and Evans, A. C (1994). Assessing the significance of focal activations using their spatial extent. *Hum. Brain Mapp.* 1, 210–220. doi: 10.1002/hbm.460010306

Fujii, K., Shinya, M., Yamashita, D., Kouzaki, M., and Oda, S. (2014a). Anticipation by basketball defenders: an explanation based on the three-dimensional inverted pendulum model. *Eur. J. Sport Sci.* 14, 538–546. doi: 10.1080/17461391.2013.876104

Fujii, K., Shinya, M., Yamashita, D., Oda, S., and Kouzaki, M. (2014b). Superior reaction to changing directions for skilled basketball defenders but not linked with specialised anticipation. *Eur. J. Sport Sci.* 14, 209–216. doi: 10.1080/17461391.2013.780098

Gallese, V., Fadiga, L., Fogassi, L., and Rizzolatti, G. (1996). Action recognition in the premotor cortex. *Brain* 119, 593–609. doi: 10.1093/brain/119.2.593

Gaser, C., and Schlaug, G. (2003). Brain structures differ between musicians and non-musicians. *J. Neurosci.* 23, 9240–9245.

Good, C. D., Johnsrude, I. S., Ashburner, J., Henson, R. N., Friston, K. J., and Frackowiak, R. S. (2001). A voxel-based morphometric study of ageing in 465 normal adult human brains. *Neuroimage* 14, 21–36. doi: 10.1006/nimg.2001.0786

Grèzes, J., and Decety, J. (2001). Functional anatomy of execution, mental simulation, observation and verb generation of actions: a meta-analysis. *Hum. Brain Mapp.* 12, 1–19. doi: 10.1002/1097-0193(200101)12:1<1::AID-HBM10>3.0.CO;2-V

Hamilton, A. F., and Grafton, S. T. (2006). Goal representation in human anterior intraparietal sulcus. *J. Neurosci.* 26, 1133–1137. doi: 10.1523/JNEUROSCI.4551-05.2006

Hester, R., Foxe, J. J., Molholm, S., Shpaner, M., and Garavan, H. (2005). Neural mechanisms involved in error processing: a comparison of errors made with and without awareness. *Neuroimage* 27, 602–608. doi: 10.1016/j.neuroimage.2005.04.035

Imfeld, A., Oechslin, M. S., Meyer, M., Loenneker, T., and Jancke, L. (2009). White matter plasticity in the corticospinal tract of musicians: a diffusion tensor imaging study. *Neuroimage* 46, 600–607. doi: 10.1016/j.neuroimage.2009.02.025

Iseki, K., Hanakawa, T., Shinozaki, J., Nankaku, M., and Fukuyama, H. (2008). Neural mechanisms involved in mental imagery and observation of gait. *Neuroimage* 41, 1021–1031. doi: 10.1016/j.neuroimage.2008.03.010

Jäncke, L., Koeneke, S., Hoppe, A., Rominger, C., and Hanggi, J. (2009). The architecture of the golfer's brain. *PLoS One* 4:e4785. doi: 10.1371/journal.pone.0004785

Joel, S. E., Caffo, B. S., van Zijl, P. C., and Pekar, J. J. (2011). On the relationship between seed-based and ICA-based measures of functional connectivity. *Magn. Reson. Med.* 66, 644–657. doi: 10.1002/mrm.22818

Kawashima, R., Roland, P. E., and O'Sullivan, B. T. (1995). Functional anatomy of reaching and visuomotor learning: a positron emission tomography study. *Cereb. Cortex* 5, 111–122. doi: 10.1093/cercor/5.2.111

Kiehl, K. A., Liddle, P. F., and Hopfinger, J. B. (2000). Error processing and the rostral anterior cingulate: an event-related fMRI study. *Psychophysiology* 37, 216–223. doi: 10.1111/1469-8986.3720216

Kinrade, N. P., Jackson, R. C., and Ashford, K. J. (2015). Reinvestment, task complexity and decision making under pressure in basketball. *Psychol. Sport Exerc.* 20, 11–19. doi: 10.1016/j.psychsport.2015.03.007

Koelewijn, T., van Schie, H. T., Bekkering, H., Oostenveld, R., and Jensen, O. (2008). Motor-cortical beta oscillations are modulated by correctness of observed action. *Neuroimage* 40, 767–775. doi: 10.1016/j.neuroimage.2007.12.018

Lepage, M., Ghaffar, O., Nyberg, L., and Tulving, E. (2000). Prefrontal cortex and episodic memory retrieval mode. *Proc. Natl. Acad. Sci. U S A* 97, 506–511. doi: 10.1073/pnas.97.1.506

Lewis, C. M., Baldassarre, A., Committeri, G., Romani, G. L., and Corbetta, M. (2009). Learning sculpts the spontaneous activity of the resting human brain. *Proc. Natl. Acad. Sci. U S A* 106, 17558–17563. doi: 10.1073/pnas.0902455106

Lisberger, S. G. (1988). The neural basis for learning of simple motor skills. *Science* 242, 728–735. doi: 10.1126/science.3055293

Llorca-Miralles, J., Sanchez-Delgado, G., Pinar, M. I., Cardenas, D., and Perales, J. C. (2013). Basketball training influences shot selection assessment: a multi-attribute decision-making approach. *Rev. Psicol. Deporte* 22, 223–226.

Maguire, E. A., Gadian, D. G., Johnsrude, I. S., Good, C. D., Ashburner, J., Frackowiak, R. S., et al. (2000). Navigation-related structural change in the hippocampi of taxi drivers. *Proc. Natl. Acad. Sci. U S A* 97, 4398–4403. doi: 10.1073/pnas.070039597

Mantini, D., and Vanduffel, W. (2013). Emerging roles of the brain's default network. *Neuroscientist* 19, 76–87. doi: 10.1177/1073858412446202

Margulies, D. S., Böttger, J., Watanabe, A., and Gorgolewski, K. J. (2013). Visualizing the human connectome. *Neuroimage* 80, 445–461. doi: 10.1016/j.neuroimage.2013.04.111

Markowitsch, H. J. (1995). Which brain regions are critically involved in the retrieval of old episodic memory? *Brain Res. Rev.* 21, 117–127. doi: 10.1016/0165-0173(95)00007-0

Martinelli, P., Sperduti, M., and Piolino, P. (2013). Neural substrates of the self-memory system: new insights from a meta-analysis. *Hum. Brain Mapp.* 34, 1515–1529. doi: 10.1002/hbm.22008

McDermott, K. B., Buckner, R. L., Petersen, S. E., Kelley, W. M., and Sanders, A. L. (1999). Set- and code-specific activation in frontal cortex: an fMRI study of encoding and retrieval of faces and words. *J. Cogn. Neurosci.* 11, 631–640. doi: 10.1162/089892999563698

McRobert, A. P., Williams, A. M., Ward, P., Eccles, D. W., and Ericsson, K. A. (2007). Contextual information and anticipation skill in cricket batting. *J. Sport Exerc. Psychol.* 29:S187.

Menon, V., and Uddin, L. Q. (2010). Saliency, switching, attention and control: a network model of insula function. *Brain Struct. Funct.* 214, 655–667. doi: 10.1007/s00429-010-0262-0

Müller-Gärtner, H. W., Links, J. M., Prince, J. L., Bryan, R. N., McVeigh, E. and Leal, J. P. (1992). Measurement of radiotracer concentration in brain gray matter using positron emission tomography: MRI-based correction for partial volume effects. *J. Cereb. Blood Flow Metab.* 12, 571–583. doi: 10.1038/jcbfm.1992.81

Osaka, M., Komori, M., Morishita, M., and Osaka, N. (2007). Neural bases of focusing attention in working memory: an fMRI study based on group differences. *Cogn. Affect. Behav. Neurosci.* 7, 130–139. doi: 10.3758/cabn.7.2.130

Pascual-Leone, A., Amedi, A., Fregni, F., and Merabet, L. B. (2005). The plastic human brain cortex. *Annu. Rev. Neurosci.* 28, 377–401. doi: 10.1146/annurev.neuro.27.070203.144216

Poline, J. B., Worsley, K. J., Evans, A. C., and Friston, K. J. (1997). Combining spatial extent and peak intensity to test for activations in functional imaging. *Neuroimage* 5, 83–96. doi: 10.1006/nimg.1996.0248

Prakash, R. S., Snook, E. M., Motl, R. W., and Kramer, A. F. (2010). Aerobic fitness is associated with gray matter volume and white matter integrity in multiple sclerosis. *Brain Res.* 1341, 41–51. doi: 10.1016/j.brainres.2009.06.063

Raichle, M. E., MacLeod, A. M., Snyder, A. Z., Powers, W. J., Gusnard, D. A., and Shulman, G. L. (2001). A default mode of brain function. *Proc. Natl. Acad. Sci. U S A* 98, 676–682. doi: 10.1073/pnas.98.2.676

Rizzolatti, G., Ferrari, P. F., Rozzi, S., and Fogassi, L. (2006). The inferior parietal lobule: where action becomes perception. *Novartis Found. Symp.* 270, 129–140; discussion 140–145, 164–169. doi: 10.1002/9780470034989.ch11

Rushworth, M. F. (2008). Intention, choice and the medial frontal cortex. *Ann. N Y Acad. Sci.* 1124, 181–207. doi: 10.1196/annals.1440.014

Schafer, R. J., and Moore, T. (2011). Selective attention from voluntary control of neurons in prefrontal cortex. *Science* 332, 1568–1571. doi: 10.1126/science.1199892

Schlaug, G. (2001). The brain of musicians. a model for functional and structural adaptation. *Ann. N Y Acad. Sci.* 930, 281–299. doi: 10.1111/j.1749-6632.2001.tb05739.x

Schmidt, R. A., and Wrisberg, C. A. (2008). *Motor Learning and Performance (Fourth Edn.)* Champaign, IL: Human Kinetics.

Seeley, W. W., Menon, V., Schatzberg, A. F., Keller, J., Glover, G. H., Kenna, H., et al. (2007). Dissociable intrinsic connectivity networks for salience processing and executive control. *J. Neurosci.* 27, 2349–2356. doi: 10.1523/JNEUROSCI.5587-06.2007

Simmons, W. K., and Martin, A. (2009). The anterior temporal lobes and the functional architecture of semantic memory. *J. Int. Neuropsychol. Soc.* 15, 645–649. doi: 10.1017/s1355617709990348

Singer, T., Critchley, H. D., and Preuschoff, K. (2009). A common role of insula in feelings, empathy and uncertainty. *Trends Cogn. Sci.* 13, 334–340. doi: 10.1016/j.tics.2009.05.001

Song, X. W., Dong, Z. Y., Long, X. Y., Li, S. F., Zuo, X. N., Zhu, C. Z., et al. (2011). REST: a toolkit for resting-state functional magnetic resonance imaging data processing. *PLoS One* 6:e25031. doi: 10.1371/journal.pone.0025031

van de Ven, V. G., Formisano, E., Prvulovic, D., Roeder, C. H., and Linden, D. E. (2004). Functional connectivity as revealed by spatial independent component analysis of fmri measurements during rest. *Hum. Brain Mapp.* 22, 165–178. doi: 10.1002/hbm.20022

Vickers, J. N. (2004). Cognitive control in motor expertise. *Int. J. Sport Exerc. Psychol.* 2, 274–300. doi: 10.1080/1612197x.2004.9671746

Wagner, A. D. (1999). Working memory contributions to human learning and remembering. *Neuron* 22, 19–22. doi: 10.1016/s0896-6273(00)80674-1

Wan, X., Nakatani, H., Ueno, K., Asamizuya, T., Cheng, K., and Tanaka, K. (2011). The neural basis of intuitive best next-move generation in board game experts. *Science* 331, 341–346. doi: 10.1126/science.1194732

Wang, B., Fan, Y., Lu, M., Li, S., Song, Z., Peng, X., et al. (2013). Brain anatomical networks in world class gymnasts: a DTI tractography study. *Neuroimage* 65, 476–487. doi: 10.1016/j.neuroimage.2012.10.007

Wang, Z., Wang, S., Shi, F. Y., Guan, Y., Wu, Y., Zhang, L. L., et al. (2014). The effect of motor imagery with specific implement in expert badminton player. *Neuroscience* 275, 102–112. doi: 10.1016/j.neuroscience.2014.06.004

Wei, G., Zhang, Y., Jiang, T., and Luo, J. (2011). Increased cortical thickness in sports experts: a comparison of diving players with the controls. *PLoS One* 6:e17112. doi: 10.1371/journal.pone.0017112

Wenderoth, N., Debaere, F., Sunaert, S., and Swinnen, S. P. (2005). The role of anterior cingulate cortex and precuneus in the coordination of motor behaviour. *Eur. J. Neurosci.* 22, 235–246. doi: 10.1111/j.1460-9568.2005.04176.x

Williams, A. M., Davids, K., and Williams, J. G. (1999). *Visual Perception and Action in Sport.* London: E and FN Spon.

Wright, M. J., Bishop, D. T., Jackson, R. C., and Abernethy, B. (2013). Brain regions concerned with the identification of deceptive soccer moves by higher-skilled and lower-skilled players. *Front. Hum. Neurosci.* 7:851. doi: 10.3389/fnhum.2013.00851

Wu, C. T., Weissman, D. H., Roberts, K. C., and Woldorff, M. G. (2007). The neural circuitry underlying the executive control of auditory spatial attention. *Brain Res.* 1134, 187–198. doi: 10.1016/j.brainres.2006.11.088

Wu, Y., Zeng, Y., Zhang, L., Wang, S., Wang, D., Tan, X., et al. (2013). The role of visual perception in action anticipation in basketball athletes. *Neuroscience* 237, 29–41. doi: 10.1016/j.neuroscience.2013.01.048

Xia, M., Wang, J., and He, Y. (2013). BrainNet Viewer: a network visualization tool for human brain connectomics. *PLoS One* 8:e68910. doi: 10.1371/journal.pone.0068910

12

The Relationship Between Autophagy and Brain Plasticity in Neurological Diseases

*Man-Man Wang[1], Ya-Shuo Feng[1], Si-Dong Yang[2], Ying Xing[1], Jing Zhang[1], Fang Dong[3] and Feng Zhang[1,4]**

[1] Department of Rehabilitation Medicine, The Third Hospital of Hebei Medical University, Shijiazhuang, China, [2] Department of Spine Surgery, The Third Hospital of Hebei Medical University, Shijiazhuang, China, [3] Department of Clinical Laboratory Medicine, The Third Hospital of Hebei Medical University, Shijiazhuang, China, [4] Hebei Provincial Orthopedic Biomechanics Key Laboratory, The Third Hospital of Hebei Medical University, Shijiazhuang, China

Edited by:
Zhang Pengyue,
Yunnan University of Traditional Chinese Medicine, China

Reviewed by:
Yuchuan Ding,
Wayne State University, United States
Yulong Bai,
Huashan Hospital Affiliated to Fudan University, China
Qiang Wang,
The Affiliated Hospital of Qingdao University, China
Long Yu Wei,
Beijing University of Chinese Medicine, China

***Correspondence:**
Feng Zhang
zjk20019@126.com

Autophagy, a catabolic degradation system, is utilized for destroying and recycling the damaged or unnecessary cellular components. Brain plasticity refers to the remarkable characteristics of brain neurons that change their structure and function according to previous experience. This review was performed by searching the relevant articles in databases of SCIENCEDIRECT, PUBMED, and Web of Science, from respective inception to January 2019. Here, we review the neuroprotective effect of autophagy in neurological diseases and the mechanism of autophagy in brain plasticity. Moreover, the mechanism of autophagy in the process of brain plasticity can provide the possibility for the development of new treatment methods in the future, thus benefiting patients with neurological diseases. In summary, autophagy and brain plasticity play important roles in neurological diseases.

Keywords: autophagy, brain plasticity, neuroprotective effect, signal pathway, neurological disease

INTRODUCTION

Autophagy is a lysosome-reliant degradation mechanism that regulate many biological courses, such as neuroprotection and cellular stress reactions (Shen and Ganetzky, 2009). There are different kinds of autophagy in most mammalian cells, and each type of autophagy performs very specific tasks in the course of intracellular degradation (Tasset and Cuervo, 2016). The autophagy-lysosomal pathway is a main proteolytic pathway, which mainly embraces chaperone-mediated autophagy and macroautophagy in mammalian systems (Xilouri and Stefanis, 2010). Macroautophagy, as a lysosomal pathway in charge of the circulation of long-lived proteins and organelles, is mainly considered as the inducible course in neurons, which is activated in conditions of injury and stress (Boland and Nixon, 2006). Coupled with macro-autophagy, chaperone-mediated autophagy (CMA) is crucial for maintaining intracellular survival and homeostasis via selectively reducing oxidized, misfolded, or degraded cytoplasmic proteins (Cai et al., 2015).

The plasticity of the central nervous system(CNS) can be regarded as changes of functional interaction between different types of cells, astrocytes, neurons, and oligodendrocytes (Aberg et al., 2006). The mature brain, as a highly dynamic organ, constantly alters its structure via eliminating and forming new connections. In general, these changes are known as brain plasticity and are related to functional changes (Viscomi and D'Amelio, 2012). Brain plasticity can be divided into structure plasticity and function plasticity. The structural plasticity of the brain refers to the fact that the connections between synapses and neurons in the brain can be established due to the influence of learning and experience. It includes the plasticity of synapses and neurons. Synaptic plasticity refers to the changes of pre-existing relationship between two neurons including structure and function alteration (De Pitta et al., 2016). Synaptic plasticity is considered as the representative of cellular mechanisms of memory and learning. Mitochondria are related to the modulation of complicated course of synaptic plasticity (Todorova and Blokland, 2017). For a long period, synaptic plasticity has been considered as a neuronal mechanism under the regulation of neural network action (Ronzano, 2017). Recent data indicate that autophagy is a homeostatic mechanism which is compatible with the microenvironment of the synapse, with the purpose of serving local functions linked with synaptic transmission (Todorova and Blokland, 2017). Neuronal plasticity is maintained by the fine modulation of organelle biogenesis and degradation and protein synthesis and degradation to assure high-efficiency turnover (Viscomi and D'Amelio, 2012). Protein degradation plays an important role in the course of synaptic plasticity, but the involved molecular mechanisms are unclear (Haynes et al., 2015). Therefore, Autophagy is a quality control mechanism of organelles and proteins in neurons, which plays a crucial role in their physiology and pathology (Viscomi and D'Amelio, 2012). In a word, there is a close relationship between autophagy and brain plasticity, and the related mechanisms are summarized in this review paper (as **Table 1** and **Figure 1** demonstrate).

THE NEUROPROTECTIVE EFFECT OF AUTOPHAGY IN NEUROLOGICAL DISEASES

Autophagy is involved in the occurrence and treatment for a series of neurological diseases. However, there are only sporadic reports for the relationship between autophagy and some types of the neurological diseases, which have not been accumulated enough to be reviewed. Therefore, in this review, we summarize the relationship between autophagy and brain plasticity in stroke, traumatic brain injury, cerebral tumor, and neurodegenerative diseases.

Autophagy and Stroke

Autophagy plays different roles in various conditions, and both autophagy activation and autophagy inhibition could exert neuroprotective effects in the process of stroke.

The Neuroprotective Effect of Autophagy Activation in Stroke

The co-modulation of autophagy and apoptosis is involved in ischemic stroke (IS)-induced injuries, and apoptosis and mitochondrial autophagy play an important role in this process (Guo Y. et al., 2017). RIPer (Remote ischemic perconditioning) has obvious neuroprotective effect on cerebral ischemia reperfusion injury in rats, and the autophagic lysosomal pathway is activated by RIPer. Autophagy activation promotes the neuroprotective effect of RIPer on focal cerebral ischemia in rats (Su et al., 2014). Liu et al. (2018b) report that activation of autophagy flux in astrocytes might conduce to neural recovery mechanisms and endogenous neuroprotective following stroke. Nampt promotes neuronal survival via inducing autophagy by modulating the TSC2-mTOR-S6K1 signaling pathway in a SIRT1-reliant manner during cerebral ischemia (Wang et al., 2012).

The Neuroprotective Effect of Autophagy Inhibition in Stroke

There is increasing evidence that autophagy dysfunction leads to the accumulation of damaged organelles and/or abnormal proteins. This accumulation is associated with synaptic functional disorder, neuronal death, and cellular stress (Xilouri and Stefanis, 2010). RIPreC (Remote ischemic preconditioning) + IPOC(ischemic post-conditioning) reduced the plasma HMGB1 level to exert its neuroprotective effect on cerebral ischemia reperfusion injury by suppressing the autophagy process (Wang et al., 2016a). SMXZF, which is a kind of compound extracted from Chinese traditional medicine, plays a neuroprotective part in focal ischemia-reperfusion injury, which might be related to the autophagy inactivation via AMPK/mTOR and JNK pathways (Guo et al., 2014).

TABLE 1 | The summary for involved signal pathways for the neuroprotective effect via regulating autophagy.

References	Pathway	Neuroprotective effect via activating / inhibiting autophagy	Diseases
Wang et al., 2012	TSC2-mTOR-S6K1	Activating	Cerebral ischemia.
Guo et al., 2014	AMPK/mTOR and JNK pathways	Inhibiting	Ischemia-reperfusion injury
Chen et al., 2018	mTOR/p70S6K	Inhibiting	Ischemia/ reperfusion injury
Jiang J. et al., 2018	mTOR/Ulk1	Inhibiting	Ischemic stroke
He et al., 2018	PI3K/AKT	Activating	Traumatic Brain Injury
Feng et al., 2017	PERK and IRE1	Inhibiting	Ischemic stroke
Shen et al., 2017	AMPK	Activating	Stroke
Wang et al., 2014	MiRNA-30a	Activating	Ischemic stroke
Zhou et al., 2011	Gsk-3	Activating	Ischemic brain injury
Zhang Y. et al., 2016	MiR-214-3p	Inhibiting	Sporadic Alzheimer's disease
Hu et al., 2017	ATG5	Activating	Parkinson's Disease

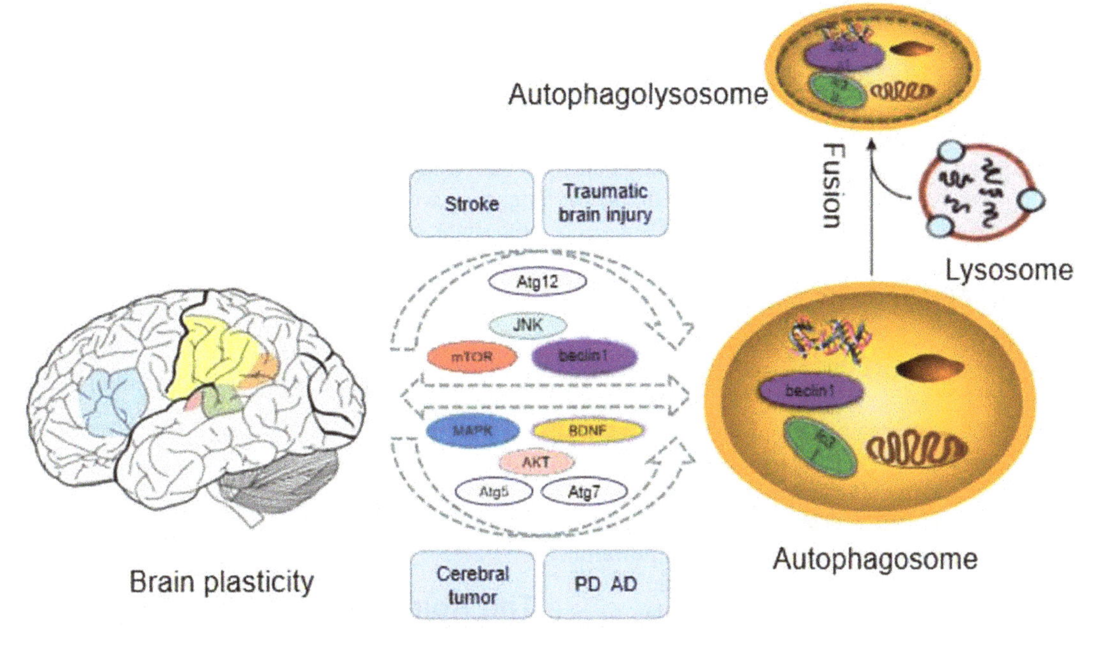

FIGURE 1 | The related important factors of autophagy and brain plasticity.

Guo D. et al. (2017) demonstrate for the first time that suppression of MALAT1 reduces beclin1-reliant autophagy via regulating the expression of mir-30a in cerebral IS, thereby reducing neuron cell death. Moreover, autophagy is regulated by mammalian target proteins in the PI3K/AKT/mTOR/p70S6K signaling pathway (Fan et al., 2015). RIPostC could suppress autophagy via activating the mTOR/p70S6K signaling pathway, thus reducing the brain I/R damage (Chen et al., 2018). Vitexin regulated autophagy dysfunction to alleviate MCAO-induced cerebral IS through mTOR/Ulk1 pathway (Jiang J. et al., 2018). The increasing evidence indicates that the AMPK-mTOR signaling pathway mediates the autophagy activity by the coordinated phosphorylation of ULK1 (Wang et al., 2018). Zheng et al. (2012) have demonstrated that NAD(+) administration reduced ischemic brain injury at least partly via inhibiting autophagy. LncRNA H19 inhibits autophagy through dusp5-erk1/2 axis. Blood samples from patients with IS showed that H19 gene mutation increased the risk of IS. LncRNA H19 could be a novel therapeutic target for IS (Wang et al., 2017a).

In summary, different studies obtained various results for the role of autophagy in the process of stroke, and further studies are required to explore the relationship between autophagy and stroke.

Autophagy and Traumatic Brain Injury

Similar to the relationship between autophagy and stroke, the relationship between autophagy and traumatic brain injury is also not simple. Both inhibition and activation of autophagy could exert neuroprotective effects following the occurrence of traumatic brain injury.

The Neuroprotective Effect of Autophagy Activation in Traumatic Brain Injury (TBI)

The promotion of autophagy and neuronal apoptosis are related to the secondary neural injury after Traumatic Brain Injury (TBI). Sevoflurane post-conditioning regulates autophagy through PI3K/AKT signaling, which alleviates the TBI-triggered neuronal apoptosis (He et al., 2018). Zhang L. et al. (2016) for the first time reveal that FTY720 plays a neuroprotective role following TBI, at least partially through the activation of the PI3K/AKT pathway and autophagy. In addition, Melatonin promotes autophagy, and suppresses mitochondrial apoptosis pathway, thus alleviating secondary brain injury of mice following traumatic brain injury (Ding et al., 2015). RIPoC alleviates brain IR injury via activating AMPK-reliant autophagy (Guo et al., 2018). Calcitriol treatment promotes the expression of VDR protein and alleviated the neural defect in the TBI model of rats. Its protective effect might be related to the decrease of apoptosis and the recovery of autophagy flux in the cortex area of rat brain (Cui et al., 2017). HS (heat stroke) can lead to brain injury via impaired autophagy flux and lysosomal dysfunction, and HA (heat acclimation) has a protective exerts neuroprotection on HS-induced brain injury through the mechanism of autophagy - lysosomal pathway (Yi et al., 2017).

The Neuroprotective Effect of Autophagy Inhibition in Traumatic Brain Injury

The autophagy pathway is associated with the pathophysiological reactions following TBI, and suppression of this pathway might contribute to the alleviation of traumatic injury and functional outcome defects (Luo et al., 2011). Melatonin administration before ischemia could notably alleviate brain IR damage by suppressing ER stress-reliant autophagy (Feng et al., 2017). The over-expression of mir-27a may mitigate brain injury by inhibiting Foxo3a-regulated neuronal autophagy after TBI (Sun et al., 2017). Jiang H. et al. (2018) report that the down-regulation of TLR4 improves the neuroinflammatory response and brain injury following TBI by inhibiting astrocyte activation and autophagy induction. Therefore, the effect of activation and inhibition of autophagy on traumatic brain injury should be further clarified before future clinical applications.

Autophagy and Neurodegenerative Disease

Autophagy is the core regulator of central nervous system senescence and neurodegeneration. The delivery of organelles and toxic molecules to lysosomes by autophagy is critical for the health and survival of neurons (Plaza-Zabala et al., 2017). Most of the neurodegenerative diseases that perplex humans are related to the intracytoplasmic deposition of proteins that tend to accumulate in neurons, and autophagy is a powerful process for removing these proteins (Frake et al., 2015). Autophagy up-regulation is a promising treatment due to its potential to protect cells from the toxicity of accumulated proteins in neurodegenerative diseases (Karabiyik et al., 2017). Autophagy-regulated degradation of synaptic elements sustains synaptic homeostasis but also involves in a mechanism of neurodegeneration (Luningschror et al., 2017). Autophagy is vital for neuronal integrity, and the reduction of important autophagic components results in the structural defects and progressive neurodegenerative changes in pre- and post-synaptic morphologies (Nikoletopoulou et al., 2017). It is demonstrated that autophagy defects arise in the early stage of Alzheimer's disease (AD) (Li et al., 2017). A considerable amount of evidence indicates that the p38-mitogen-activated protein kinase (MAPK) signaling pathway plays an important part in neurodegenerative diseases and synaptic plasticity (Correa and Eales, 2012). MiR-181a regulates apoptosis and autophagy in PD(Parkinson's Disease) by inhibiting the p38 MAPK/JNK pathway (Liu Y. et al., 2017). In addition, RhEPO may alleviate hippocampal injury in epileptic seizure rats via regulating autophagy in a time-reliant manner through the S6 protein (Li et al., 2018).

In summary, autophagy has a close relationship with neurodegenerative disease, and activation of autophagy could improve the neurodegenerative changes, which might be a novel target in clinical treatment for such diseases.

Autophagy and Cerebral Tumor

The role of autophagy in tumor cell survival and death has attracted much attention in recent years (Noonan et al., 2016). As for glioblastoma (GBM), the most lethal tumor of the CNS, there is increasing evidence that the autophagy process is closely related to the tumorigenesis of GBM (Jawhari et al., 2017). Glioblastoma multiform is the most common and invasive primary brain tumor. Due to its adaptive ability of autophagy, it is highly resistant to various treatments (Jawhari et al., 2017). (Gammoh et al. (2016) elucidate that autophagy is the key to the occurrence and growth of GBM, which is an important therapeutic target for the treatment of GBM. The inhibition of autophagy is a promising strategy against GBM, and ATG9 is identified as a new target for hypoxic-induced autophagy (Abdul Rahim et al., 2017). Autophagy played a critical role in the formation of vasculogenic mimicry(VM) via Glioma stem cells (GSCs), which could be used as a therapeutic target for drug-resistant gliomas (Wu et al., 2017). The inhibition of autophagy promotes the anti-tumor activity of ibrutinib in GBM. Wang et al. (2017b) provides important insights into the role of anticancer drugs combined with autophagy inhibitors in the treatment of GBM.

In summary, autophagy provides new therapeutic expectations for cerebral tumor which is a big challenging for human. Therefore, the application of novel therapy for cerebral tumor on the basis of autophagy mechanisms elucidation should be explored in depth.

THE MECHANISM OF AUTOPHAGY IN BRAIN PLASTICITY

The Role of Mammalian Target of Rapamycin (mTOR) in the Relationship Between Autophagy and Brain Plasticity

Brain Plasticity and mTOR

The mTOR-controlled signaling pathways regulate many integrated physiological functions of the nervous system including neuronal development, synaptic plasticity, memory storage, and cognition (Bockaert and Marin, 2015). Mammalian target of rapamycin, as a protein kinase, is implicated in long-lasting synaptic plasticity and translation control of synapse (Hoeffer and Klann, 2010). It is reported that mTOR modulates many functions in the process of brain development, including proliferation, differentiation, migration, and dendrite formation. Moreover, mTOR plays an important role in the formation and plasticity of synapses (LiCausi and Hartman, 2018). Moreover, the mammalian target of rapamycin complex 1 (mTORC1) is a key modulator for cap-dependent protein synthesis, which is necessary for many forms of long-lasting memory and long-term synaptic plasticity (Santini et al., 2014). Therefore, it is demonstrated that mTOR plays a key role in the process of brain plasticity.

Autophagy and mTOR

As a key regulator of autophagy, the mTOR plays an important role in autophagy, translation, cell growth and survival (Hwang et al., 2017). Mammalian target of rapamycin and autophagy are tightly bound within cells, and defects of mTOR and autophagy process might lead to a variety of human diseases (Hoeffer and Klann, 2010). Studies have shown that mTOR is widely involved in autophagy activation and synaptic plasticity (Ryskalin et al., 2018). The mTOR modulates long-lasting synaptic plasticity, memory and learning via regulating the synthesis of dendritic proteins (Liu et al., 2018a). Macroautophagy can degrade organelles and long-lived proteins in case of mTOR inactivation. Synaptic plasticity is further modulated by mTOR and neurodegeneration occurs when macroautophagy is absent (Hernandez et al., 2012). Therefore, macroautophagy following mTOR inactivation at the presynaptic terminal rapidly changes the neural transmission and presynaptic structure (Hernandez et al., 2012). The mechanisms for the target of rapamycin have been involved in modulating neurodegeneration and synaptic plasticity, but the role of mTOR in regulating presynaptic function via autophagy has not been clarified clearly (Torres and Sulzer, 2012).

In summary, there is a close relationship among mTOR, brain plasticity and autophagy. The mTOR related pathways play important role in regulating the process of autophagy and brain plasticity.

The Related Signaling Pathways of Autophagy and Brain Plasticity

The PI3K/Akt Pathway

Autophagy acts as a central mediator of cellular disease and health, and this self-balancing process seems to affect synaptic growth and plasticity in the CNS (Alirezaei et al., 2011). The inhibition of autophagy was necessary for memory improvement and for brain-derived neurotrophic factor (BDNF)-caused synaptic plasticity under the circumstances of nutritional stress, indicating that autophagy was a key component of BDNF signaling pathway, which was critical to BDNF-induced synaptic plasticity (Nikoletopoulou et al., 2017). The BDNF-activated ILK-Akt and PI3K-Akt signaling pathway play an important role in structural synaptic plasticity (Li et al., 2012). The activation of PI3K/Akt pathway might conduce to the memory consolidation and mechanisms of synaptic plasticity via increasing protein synthesis via mTOR pathway and promoting cell survival through FKHR pathway (Horwood et al., 2006). (Xu et al. (2017) reported that the neuroprotection of L-3-n-Butylphthalide (L-NBP) in attenuating learning and memory deficits in mice after repeated cerebral ischemia-reperfusion (RCIR) might be associated with the modulation of the expressions of proteins involved in apoptosis and autophagy and the promotion of Akt/mTOR signaling pathway. Moreover, the activation of PI3 kinase-Akt signaling pathway played an important role in promoting the survival of newly generated granule cells originated during exercise and the related increase of synaptic plasticity of dentate gyrus through an anti-apoptosis function (Bruel-Jungerman et al., 2009). Tetrahydrocurcumin alleviated the damage on neurons against TBI-induced apoptotic neuronal death, possibly through regulating autophagy and the PI3K/AKT pathway (Gao et al., 2016).

Moreover, neuronal stimulation led to NMDA receptor (NMDAR)-dependent autophagy via PI3K-Akt-mTOR pathway suppression, which might work in AMPA receptor (AMPAR) degradation, thus showing autophagy as a promoting factor to brain functions and NMDAR-reliant synaptic plasticity (Shehata et al., 2012). Curcumin exerts neuroprotective role through regulating the PI3K/Akt/mTOR pathway and down-regulating the autophagy activities (Huang et al., 2018). However, the interaction between the PI3K/AKT/mTOR pathway and the autophagy process is complicated, more detailed studies on the mechanism of disease as well as animal and cell models is needed.

The MAPK/Erk Pathway

There is increasing evidence that MAPKs can regulate autophagy/macroautophagy (Wang et al., 2016b). MAPK/ErK and p38 play key roles in the strict control of the autophagy process during maturation (Corcelle et al., 2007). In addition, some studies have shown that mitophagy requires MAPKs MAPK1/ERK2 and MAPK14/p38 (Hirota et al., 2015). As a protein kinase, MAPK/Erk is mobilized by neurotrophic factors involved in synaptic plasticity and formation, acting at both the cytoplasmic and nuclear levels (Giachello et al., 2010). The activity-reliant short-term plasticity and formation of these synapses are relied on the MAPK/Erk pathway (Giachello et al., 2010). Recently, there is increasing evidence that Ras and MAPK signaling plays a key role in neuronal function related to synaptic plasticity (Mazzucchelli and Brambilla, 2000).

In summary, the related signaling pathways of autophagy and brain plasticity has not be well clarified, which is worthy of further exploration.

THE ROLE OF AUTOPHAGY MECHANISM IN THE TREATMENT OF NERVOUS SYSTEM DISEASES

The dysfunction of autophagy pathway is related to a variety of neuropathologic conditions, and numerous studies have demonstrated that autophagy is a potential target for pharmacological regulation of neuroprotection (Russo et al., 2015). Autophagy and AMPK play a key role in CSD-induced ischemic tolerance. AMPK-regulated autophagy might be a novel target for stroke (Shen et al., 2017). Wang et al. (2014) report that the suppression of mirna-30a ameliorates ischemic injury by enhancing beclin1-regulated autophagy, which represents a possible therapeutic target for IS. Gsk-3 depressor hinders neuroinflammation following ischemic brain injury via activating autophagy, thereby providing a novel target for the prevention of ischemic brain damage (Zhou et al., 2011). (Peng et al. (2018) definitely indicates that mitofusin 2 mitigates I/R injury primarily by promoting autophagy, providing a potential new strategy for the neuroprotection of brain I/R injury. In addition, miR-214-3p inhibits autophagy and reduces the apoptosis of hippocampal neurons, suggesting that miR-214-3p is a new potential target for sporadic Alzheimer's disease (SAD) (Zhang Y. et al., 2016). The effect of autophagy related gene 5 (ATG5) in protecting dopaminergic neurons in zebrafish PD model is induced by 1-methyl-4-phenyl-1,2,3, 6-tetrahydropyridine (MPTP) (Hu et al., 2017). Autophagy is closely related to the occurrence and development of various neurological diseases in humans. Therefore, the study of autophagy mechanism has important clinical significance for the diagnosis of diseases and the search for new drug targets.

CONCLUSION

Brain plasticity is one of the most fundamental mechanism for neural function recovery following neurological diseases.

Autophagy is a crucial lysosome-reliant degradation process that controls various physiological and pathological courses in the brain. The summary for the interaction of autophagy and brain plasticity might provide novel therapy targets for neurological diseases, thus benefiting the patients in clinic.

AUTHOR CONTRIBUTIONS

M-MW and FZ conceived the main ideas and wrote the manuscript. Y-SF, JZ, FD, S-DY, and YX searched the references and designed the framework.

REFERENCES

Abdul Rahim, S. A., Dirkse, A., Oudin, A., Schuster, A., Bohler, J., Barthelemy, V., et al. (2017). Regulation of hypoxia-induced autophagy in glioblastoma involves ATG9A. *Br. J. Cancer* 117, 813–825. doi: 10.1038/bjc.2017.263

Aberg, N. D., Brywe, K. G., and Isgaard, J. (2006). Aspects of growth hormone and insulin-like growth factor-I related to neuroprotection, regeneration, and functional plasticity in the adult brain. *ScientificWorldJournal* 6, 53–80. doi: 10.1100/tsw.2006.22

Alirezaei, M., Kemball, C. C., and Whitton, J. L. (2011). Autophagy, inflammation and neurodegenerative disease. *Eur. J. Neurosci.* 33, 197–204. doi: 10.1111/j.1460-9568.2010.07500.x

Bockaert, J., and Marin, P. (2015). mTOR in brain physiology and pathologies. *Physiol. Rev.* 95, 1157–1187. doi: 10.1152/physrev.00038.2014

Boland, B., and Nixon, R. A. (2006). Neuronal macroautophagy: from development to degeneration. *Mol. Aspects Med.* 27, 503–519. doi: 10.1016/j.mam.2006.08.009

Bruel-Jungerman, E., Veyrac, A., Dufour, F., Horwood, J., Laroche, S., Davis, S., et al. (2009). Inhibition of PI3K-Akt signaling blocks exercise-mediated enhancement of adult neurogenesis and synaptic plasticity in the dentate gyrus. *PLoS One* 4:e7901. doi: 10.1371/journal.pone.0007901

Cai, Z., Zeng, W., Tao, K., Wang, Z. E. B., and Yang, Q. (2015). Chaperone-mediated autophagy: roles in neuroprotection. *Neurosci. Bull.* 31, 452–458. doi: 10.1007/s12264-015-1540-x

Chen, G. Z., Shan, X. Y., Li, X. S., and Tao, H. M. (2018). Remote ischemic postconditioning protects the brain from focal ischemia/reperfusion injury by inhibiting autophagy through the mTOR/p70S6K pathway. *Neurol. Res.* 40, 182–188. doi: 10.1080/01616412.2018.1424696

Corcelle, E., Djerbi, N., Mari, M., Nebout, M., Fiorini, C., Fenichel, P., et al. (2007). Control of the autophagy maturation step by the MAPK ERK and p38: lessons from environmental carcinogens. *Autophagy* 3, 57–59. doi: 10.4161/auto.3424

Correa, S. A., and Eales, K. L. (2012). The role of p38 Mapk and its substrates in neuronal plasticity and neurodegenerative disease. *J. Signal. Transduct.* 2012:649079. doi: 10.1155/2012/649079

Cui, C., Cui, J., Jin, F., Cui, Y., Li, R., Jiang, X., et al. (2017). Induction of the vitamin D receptor attenuates autophagy dysfunction-mediated cell death following traumatic brain injury. *Cell Physiol. Biochem* 42, 1888–1896. doi: 10.1159/000479571

De Pitta, M., Brunel, N., and Volterra, A. (2016). Astrocytes: orchestrating synaptic plasticity? *Neuroscience* 323, 43–61. doi: 10.1016/j.neuroscience.2015.04.001

Ding, K., Xu, J., Wang, H., Zhang, L., Wu, Y., and Li, T. (2015). Melatonin protects the brain from apoptosis by enhancement of autophagy after traumatic brain injury in mice. *Neurochem. Int.* 91, 46–54. doi: 10.1016/j.neuint.2015.10.008

Fan, S., Zhang, B., Luan, P., Gu, B., Wan, Q., Huang, X., et al. (2015). PI3K/AKT/mTOR/p70S6K pathway is involved in Abeta25-35-induced autophagy. *Biomed. Res. Int.* 2015:161020. doi: 10.1155/2015/161020

Feng, D., Wang, B., Wang, L., Abraham, N., Tao, K., Huang, L., et al. (2017). Pre-ischemia melatonin treatment alleviated acute neuronal injury after ischemic stroke by inhibiting endoplasmic reticulum stress-dependent autophagy via PERK and IRE1 signalings. *J. Pineal Res.* 62:e12395. doi: 10.1111/jpi.12395

Frake, R. A., Ricketts, T., Menzies, F. M., and Rubinsztein, D. C. (2015). Autophagy and neurodegeneration. *J. Clin. Invest.* 125, 65–74.

Gammoh, N., Fraser, J., Puente, C., Syred, H. M., Kang, H., Ozawa, T., et al. (2016). Suppression of autophagy impedes glioblastoma development and induces senescence. *Autophagy* 12, 1431–1439. doi: 10.1080/15548627.2016.1190053

Gao, Y., Li, J., Wu, L., Zhou, C., Wang, Q., Li, X., et al. (2016). Tetrahydrocurcumin provides neuroprotection in rats after traumatic brain injury: autophagy and the PI3K/AKT pathways as a potential mechanism. *J. Surg. Res.* 206, 67–76. doi: 10.1016/j.jss.2016.07.014

Giachello, C. N., Fiumara, F., Giacomini, C., Corradi, A., Milanese, C., Ghirardi, M., et al. (2010). MAPK/Erk-dependent phosphorylation of synapsin mediates formation of functional synapses and short-term homosynaptic plasticity. *J. Cell Sci.* 123, 881–893. doi: 10.1242/jcs.056846

Guo, D., Ma, J., Yan, L., Li, T., Li, Z., Han, X., et al. (2017). Down-regulation of lncrna MALAT1 attenuates neuronal cell death through suppressing beclin1-dependent autophagy by regulating mir-30a in cerebral ischemic stroke. *Cell Physiol. Biochem.* 43, 182–194. doi: 10.1159/000480337

Guo, H., Zhao, L., Wang, B., Li, X., Bai, H., Liu, H., et al. (2018). Remote limb ischemic postconditioning protects against cerebral ischemia-reperfusion injury by activating AMPK-dependent autophagy. *Brain Res. Bull.* 139, 105–113. doi: 10.1016/j.brainresbull.2018.02.013

Guo, Y., Ma, Y., Zhang, Y., Zhou, L., Huang, S., Wen, Y., et al. (2017). Autophagy-related gene microarray and bioinformatics analysis for ischemic stroke detection. *Biochem. Biophys. Res. Commun.* 489, 48–55. doi: 10.1016/j.bbrc.2017.05.099

Guo, Z., Cao, G., Yang, H., Zhou, H., Li, L., Cao, Z., et al. (2014). A combination of four active compounds alleviates cerebral ischemia-reperfusion injury in correlation with inhibition of autophagy and modulation of AMPK/mTOR and JNK pathways. *J. Neurosci. Res.* 92, 1295–1306. doi: 10.1002/jnr.23400

Haynes, K. A., Smith, T. K., Preston, C. J., and Hegde, A. N. (2015). Proteasome inhibition augments new protein accumulation early in long-term synaptic plasticity and rescues adverse Abeta effects on protein synthesis. *ACS Chem. Neurosci.* 6, 695–700. doi: 10.1021/acschemneuro.5b00068

He, H., Liu, W., Zhou, Y., Liu, Y., Weng, P., Li, Y., et al. (2018). Sevoflurane post-conditioning attenuates traumatic brain injury-induced neuronal apoptosis by promoting autophagy via the PI3K/AKT signaling pathway. *Drug Des. Devel. Ther.* 12, 629–638. doi: 10.2147/DDDT.S158313

Hernandez, D., Torres, C. A., Setlik, W., Cebrian, C., Mosharov, E. V., Tang, G., et al. (2012). Regulation of presynaptic neurotransmission by macroautophagy. *Neuron* 74, 277–284. doi: 10.1016/j.neuron.2012.02.020

Hirota, Y., Yamashita, S., Kurihara, Y., Jin, X., Aihara, M., Saigusa, T., et al. (2015). Mitophagy is primarily due to alternative autophagy and requires the MAPK1 and MAPK14 signaling pathways. *Autophagy* 11, 332–343. doi: 10.1080/15548627.2015.1023047

Hoeffer, C. A., and Klann, E. (2010). mTOR signaling: at the crossroads of plasticity, memory and disease. *Trends Neurosci.* 33, 67–75. doi: 10.1016/j.tins.2009.11.003

Horwood, J. M., Dufour, F., Laroche, S., and Davis, S. (2006). Signalling mechanisms mediated by the phosphoinositide 3-kinase/Akt cascade in synaptic plasticity and memory in the rat. *Eur. J. Neurosci.* 23, 3375–3384. doi: 10.1111/j.1460-9568.2006.04859.x

Hu, Z. Y., Chen, B., Zhang, J. P., and Ma, Y. Y. (2017). Up-regulation of autophagy-related gene 5 (ATG5) protects dopaminergic neurons in a zebrafish model of Parkinson's disease. *J. Biol. Chem.* 292, 18062–18074. doi: 10.1074/jbc.M116.764795

Huang, L., Chen, C., Zhang, X., Li, X., Chen, Z., Yang, C., et al. (2018). Neuroprotective effect of curcumin against cerebral ischemia-reperfusion via mediating autophagy and inflammation. *J. Mol. Neurosci.* 64, 129–139. doi: 10.1007/s12031-017-1006-x

Hwang, J. Y., Gertner, M., Pontarelli, F., Court-Vazquez, B., Bennett, M. V., Ofengeim, D., et al. (2017). Global ischemia induces lysosomal-mediated degradation of mTOR and activation of autophagy in hippocampal neurons destined to die. *Cell Death. Differ.* 24, 317–329. doi: 10.1038/cdd.2016.140

Jawhari, S., Bessette, B., Hombourger, S., Durand, K., Lacroix, A., Labrousse, F., et al. (2017). Autophagy and TrkC/NT-3 signaling joined forces boost the hypoxic glioblastoma cell survival. *Carcinogenesis* 38, 592–603. doi: 10.1093/carcin/bgx029

Jiang, H., Wang, Y., Liang, X., Xing, X., Xu, X., and Zhou, C. (2018). Toll-Like Receptor 4 knockdown attenuates brain damage and neuroinflammation after traumatic brain injury via inhibiting neuronal autophagy and astrocyte activation. *Cell Mol. Neurobiol.* 38, 1009–1019. doi: 10.1007/s10571-017-0570-5

Jiang, J., Dai, J., and Cui, H. (2018). Vitexin reverses the autophagy dysfunction to attenuate MCAO-induced cerebral ischemic stroke via mTOR/Ulk1 pathway. *Biomed. Pharmacother.* 99, 583–590. doi: 10.1016/j.biopha.2018.01.067

Karabiyik, C., Lee, M. J., and Rubinsztein, D. C. (2017). Autophagy impairment in Parkinson's disease. *Essays Biochem.* 61, 711–720. doi: 10.1042/EBC20170023

Li, M., Dai, F. R., Du, X. P., Yang, Q. D., Zhang, X., Chen, Y., et al. (2012). Infusion of BDNF into the nucleus accumbens of aged rats improves cognition and structural synaptic plasticity through PI3K-ILK-Akt signaling. *Behav. Brain Res.* 231, 146–153. doi: 10.1016/j.bbr.2012.03.010

Li, Q., Han, Y., Du, J., Jin, H., Zhang, J., Niu, M., et al. (2018). Recombinant human erythropoietin protects against hippocampal damage in developing rats with seizures by modulating autophagy via the s6 protein in a time-dependent manner. *Neurochem. Res.* 43, 465–476. doi: 10.1007/s11064-017-2443-1

Li, Q., Liu, Y., and Sun, M. (2017). Autophagy and alzheimer's disease. *Cell Mol. Neurobiol* 37, 377–388.

LiCausi, F., and Hartman, N. W. (2018). Role of mTOR Complexes in Neurogenesis. *Int. J. Mol. Sci.* 19:1544. doi: 10.3390/ijms19051544

Liu, X., Li, Y., Yu, L., Vickstrom, C. R., and Liu, Q. S. (2018a). VTA mTOR signaling regulates dopamine dynamics, cocaine-induced synaptic alterations, and reward. *Neuropsychopharmacology* 43, 1066–1077. doi: 10.1038/npp.2017.247

Liu, X., Tian, F., Wang, S., Wang, F., and Xiong, L. (2018b). Astrocyte autophagy flux protects neurons against oxygen-glucose deprivation and ischemic/reperfusion injury. *Rejuven. Res.* 21, 405–415. doi: 10.1089/rej.2017.1999

Liu, Y., Song, Y., and Zhu, X. (2017). MicroRNA-181a regulates apoptosis and autophagy process in parkinson's disease by inhibiting p38 mitogen-activated protein kinase (MAPK)/c-Jun N-terminal kinases (JNK) signaling pathways. *Med. Sci. Monit.* 23, 1597–1606. doi: 10.12659/msm.900218

Luningschror, P., Binotti, B., Dombert, B., Heimann, P., Perez-Lara, A., Slotta, C., et al. (2017). Plekhg5-regulated autophagy of synaptic vesicles reveals a pathogenic mechanism in motoneuron disease. *Nat. Commun.* 8:678. doi: 10.1038/s41467-017-00689-z

Luo, C. L., Li, B. X., Li, Q. Q., Chen, X. P., Sun, Y. X., Bao, H. J., et al. (2011). Autophagy is involved in traumatic brain injury-induced cell death and contributes to functional outcome deficits in mice. *Neuroscience* 184, 54–63. doi: 10.1016/j.neuroscience.2011.03.021

Mazzucchelli, C., and Brambilla, R. (2000). Ras-related and MAPK signalling in neuronal plasticity and memory formation. *Cell Mol. Life Sci.* 57, 604–611. doi: 10.1007/pl00000722

Nikoletopoulou, V., Sidiropoulou, K., Kallergi, E., Dalezios, Y., and Tavernarakis, N. (2017). Modulation of autophagy by BDNF underlies synaptic plasticity. *Cell Metab.* 26, 230.e5–242.e5. doi: 10.1016/j.cmet.2017.06.005

Noonan, J., Zarrer, J., and Murphy, B. M. (2016). Targeting autophagy in glioblastoma. *Crit. Rev. Oncog.* 21, 241–252. doi: 10.1615/critrevoncog.2016017008

Peng, C., Rao, W., Zhang, L., Gao, F., Hui, H., Wang, K., et al. (2018). Mitofusin 2 exerts a protective role in ischemia reperfusion injury through increasing autophagy. *Cell Physiol. Biochem.* 46, 2311–2324. doi: 10.1159/000489621

Plaza-Zabala, A., Sierra-Torre, V., and Sierra, A. (2017). Autophagy and microglia: novel partners in neurodegeneration and aging. *Int. J. Mol. Sci.* 18:E598. doi: 10.3390/ijms18030598

Ronzano, R. (2017). Astrocytes and microglia: active players in synaptic plasticity. *Med. Sci.* 33, 1071–1078. doi: 10.1051/medsci/20173312014

Russo, R., Nucci, C., Corasaniti, M. T., Bagetta, G., and Morrone, L. A. (2015). Autophagy. dysregulation and the fate of retinal ganglion cells in glaucomatous optic neuropathy. *Prog. Brain Res.* 220, 87–105. doi: 10.1016/bs.pbr.2015.04.009

Ryskalin, L., Limanaqi, F., Frati, A., Busceti, C. L., and Fornai, F. (2018). mTOR-related brain dysfunctions in neuropsychiatric disorders. *Int. J. Mol. Sci.* 19:E2226. doi: 10.3390/ijms19082226

Santini, E., Huynh, T. N., and Klann, E. (2014). Mechanisms of translation control underlying long-lasting synaptic plasticity and the consolidation of long-term memory. *Prog. Mol. Biol. Transl. Sci.* 122, 131–167. doi: 10.1016/B978-0-12-420170-5.00005-2

Shehata, M., Matsumura, H., Okubo-Suzuki, R., Ohkawa, N., and Inokuchi, K. (2012). Neuronal stimulation induces autophagy in hippocampal neurons that is involved in AMPA receptor degradation after chemical long-term depression. *J. Neurosci.* 32, 10413–10422. doi: 10.1523/JNEUROSCI.4533-11.2012

Shen, P., Hou, S., Zhu, M., Zhao, M., Ouyang, Y., and Feng, J. (2017). Cortical spreading depression preconditioning mediates neuroprotection against ischemic stroke by inducing AMP-activated protein kinase-dependent autophagy in a rat cerebral ischemic/reperfusion injury model. *J. Neurochem.* 140, 799–813. doi: 10.1111/jnc.13922

Shen, W., and Ganetzky, B. (2009). Autophagy promotes synapse development in *Drosophila*. *J. Cell Biol.* 187, 71–79. doi: 10.1083/jcb.200907109

Su, J., Zhang, T., Wang, K., Zhu, T., and Li, X. (2014). Autophagy activation contributes to the neuroprotection of remote ischemic perconditioning against focal cerebral ischemia in rats. *Neurochem. Res.* 39, 2068–2077. doi: 10.1007/s11064-014-1396-x

Sun, L., Zhao, M., Wang, Y., Liu, A., Lv, M., Li, Y., et al. (2017). Neuroprotective effects of miR-27a against traumatic brain injury via suppressing FoxO3a-mediated neuronal autophagy. *Biochem. Biophys. Res. Commun.* 482, 1141–1147. doi: 10.1016/j.bbrc.2016.12.001

Tasset, I., and Cuervo, A. M. (2016). Role of chaperone-mediated autophagy in metabolism. *FEBS J.* 283, 2403–2413. doi: 10.1111/febs.13677

Todorova, V., and Blokland, A. (2017). Mitochondria and synaptic plasticity in the mature and aging nervous system. *Curr. Neuropharmacol.* 15, 166–173. doi: 10.2174/1570159x14666160414111821

Torres, C. A., and Sulzer, D. (2012). Macroautophagy can press a brake on presynaptic neurotransmission. *Autophagy* 8, 1540–1541. doi: 10.4161/auto.21330

Viscomi, M. T., and D'Amelio, M. (2012). The "Janus-faced role" of autophagy in neuronal sickness: focus on neurodegeneration. *Mol. Neurobiol.* 46, 513–521. doi: 10.1007/s12035-012-8296-3

Wang, J., Cao, B., Han, D., Sun, M., and Feng, J. (2017a). Long non-coding RNA H19 induces cerebral ischemia reperfusion injury via activation of autophagy. *Aging Dis.* 8, 71–84. doi: 10.14336/AD.2016.0530

Wang, J., Han, D., Sun, M., and Feng, J. (2016a). A combination of remote ischemic perconditioning and cerebral ischemic postconditioning inhibits autophagy to attenuate plasma HMGB1 and induce neuroprotection against stroke in rat. *J. Mol. Neurosci.* 58, 424–431. doi: 10.1007/s12031-016-0724-9

Wang, J., Liu, X., Hong, Y., Wang, S., Chen, P., Gu, A., et al. (2017b). Ibrutinib, a Bruton's tyrosine kinase inhibitor, exhibits antitumoral activity and induces autophagy in glioblastoma. *J. Exp. Clin. Cancer Res.* 36:96. doi: 10.1186/s13046-017-0549-6

Wang, J., Zhou, J. Y., Kho, D., Reiners, J. J. Jr., and Wu, G. S. (2016b). Role for DUSP1 (dual-specificity protein phosphatase 1) in the regulation of autophagy. *Autophagy* 12, 1791–1803. doi: 10.1080/15548627.2016.1203483

Wang, J. F., Mei, Z. G., Fu, Y., Yang, S. B., Zhang, S. Z., Huang, W. F., et al. (2018). Puerarin protects rat brain against ischemia/reperfusion injury by suppressing autophagy via the AMPK-mTOR-ULK1 signaling pathway. *Neural Regen. Res.* 13, 989–998. doi: 10.4103/1673-5374.233441

Wang, P., Guan, Y. F., Du, H., Zhai, Q. W., Su, D. F., Miao, C. Y., et al. (2012). Induction of autophagy contributes to the neuroprotection of nicotinamide phosphoribosyltransferase in cerebral ischemia. *Autophagy* 8, 77–87. doi: 10.4161/auto.8.1.18274

Wang, P., Liang, J., Li, Y., Li, J., Yang, X., Zhang, X., et al. (2014). Down-regulation of miRNA-30a alleviates cerebral ischemic injury through enhancing beclin 1-mediated autophagy. *Neurochem. Res.* 39, 1279–1291. doi: 10.1007/s11064-014-1310-6

Wu, H. B., Yang, S., Weng, H. Y., Chen, Q., Zhao, X. L., Fu, W. J., et al. (2017). Autophagy-induced KDR/VEGFR-2 activation promotes the formation of vasculogenic mimicry by glioma stem cells. *Autophagy* 13, 1528–1542. doi: 10.1080/15548627.2017.1336277

Xilouri, M., and Stefanis, L. (2010). Autophagy in the central nervous system: implications for neurodegenerative disorders. *CNS Neurol Disord. Drug Targets* 9, 701–719. doi: 10.2174/187152710793237421

Xu, J., Huai, Y., Meng, N., Dong, Y., Liu, Z., Qi, Q., et al. (2017). L-3-n-butylphthalide activates Akt/mTOR signaling, inhibits neuronal apoptosis and autophagy and improves cognitive impairment in mice with repeated cerebral ischemia-reperfusion injury. *Neurochem. Res.* 42, 2968–2981. doi: 10.1007/s11064-017-2328-3

Yi, J., He, G., Yang, J., Luo, Z., Yang, X., and Luo, X. (2017). Heat acclimation regulates the autophagy-lysosome function to protect against heat stroke-induced brain injury in mice. *Cell Physiol. Biochem.* 41, 101–114. doi: 10.1159/000455979

Zhang, L., Ding, K., Wang, H., Wu, Y., and Xu, J. (2016). Traumatic brain injury-induced neuronal apoptosis is reduced through modulation of PI3K and autophagy pathways in mouse by FTY720. *Cell Mol. Neurobiol.* 36, 131–142. doi: 10.1007/s10571-015-0227-1

Zhang, Y., Li, Q., Liu, C., Gao, S., Ping, H., Wang, J., et al. (2016). MiR-214-3p attenuates cognition defects via the inhibition of autophagy in SAMP8 mouse model of sporadic Alzheimer's disease. *Neurotoxicology* 56, 139–149. doi: 10.1016/j.neuro.2016.07.004

Zheng, C., Han, J., Xia, W., Shi, S., Liu, J., Ying, W., et al. (2012). NAD(+) administration decreases ischemic brain damage partially by blocking autophagy in a mouse model of brain ischemia. *Neurosci. Lett.* 512, 67–71. doi: 10.1016/j.neulet.2012.01.007

Zhou, X., Zhou, J., Li, X., Guo, C., Fang, T., Chen, Z., et al. (2011). GSK-3beta inhibitors suppressed neuroinflammation in rat cortex by activating autophagy in ischemic brain injury. *Biochem. Biophys. Res. Commun.* 411, 271–275. doi: 10.1016/j.bbrc.2011.06.117

13

Motor-Enriched Learning Activities Can Improve Mathematical Performance in Preadolescent Children

Mikkel M. Beck[1,2†], *Rune R. Lind*[1,2†], *Svend S. Geertsen*[1,2], *Christian Ritz*[1], *Jesper Lundbye-Jensen*[1,2] *and Jacob Wienecke*[1,2*]

[1] *Department of Nutrition, Exercise and Sports, University of Copenhagen, Copenhagen, Denmark,* [2] *Department of Neuroscience and Pharmacology, University of Copenhagen, Copenhagen, Denmark*

Edited by:
Claudia Voelcker-Rehage, Chemnitz University of Technology, Germany

Reviewed by:
Jascha Ruesseler, University of Bamberg, Germany
Caterina Pesce, Italian University Sport and Movement "Foro Italico", Italy

***Correspondence:**
Jacob Wienecke
wienecke@nexs.ku.dk

[†] *These authors have contributed equally to this work.*

Objective: An emerging field of research indicates that physical activity can benefit cognitive functions and academic achievements in children. However, less is known about how academic achievements can benefit from specific types of motor activities (e.g., fine and gross) integrated into learning activities. Thus, the aim of this study was to investigate whether fine or gross motor activity integrated into math lessons (i.e., motor-enrichment) could improve children's mathematical performance.

Methods: A 6-week within school cluster-randomized intervention study investigated the effects of motor-enriched mathematical teaching in Danish preadolescent children ($n = 165$, age $= 7.5 \pm 0.02$ years). Three groups were included: a control group (CON), which received non-motor enriched conventional mathematical teaching, a fine motor math group (FMM) and a gross motor math group (GMM), which received mathematical teaching enriched with fine and gross motor activity, respectively. The children were tested before (T0), immediately after (T1) and 8 weeks after the intervention (T2). A standardized mathematical test (50 tasks) was used to evaluate mathematical performance. Furthermore, it was investigated whether motor-enriched math was accompanied by different effects in low and normal math performers. Additionally, the study investigated the potential contribution of cognitive functions and motor skills on mathematical performance.

Results: All groups improved their mathematical performance from T0 to T1. However, from T0 to T1, the improvement was significantly greater in GMM compared to FMM (1.87 ± 0.71 correct answers) ($p = 0.02$). At T2 no significant differences in mathematical performance were observed. A subgroup analysis revealed that normal math-performers benefitted from GMM compared to both CON 1.78 ± 0.73 correct answers ($p = 0.04$) and FMM 2.14 ± 0.72 correct answers ($p = 0.008$). These effects were not observed in low math-performers. The effects were partly accounted for by visuo-spatial short-term memory and gross motor skills.

Conclusion: The study demonstrates that motor enriched learning activities can improve mathematical performance. In normal math performers GMM led to larger improvements than FMM and CON. This was not the case for the low math performers. Future studies should further elucidate the neurophysiological mechanisms underlying the observed behavioral effects.

Keywords: children, motor skills, exercise, integrated physical activity, academic achievement, cognition, learning

INTRODUCTION

The acquisition and development of mathematical skills can be seen as a central cognitive attribute in a modern technological society. Successful acquisition of basic mathematical skills early in life provides a framework which later academic achievements are based upon (Duncan et al., 2007), and is a predictor of future academic and professional success (Butterworth, 2005; Parsons and Bynner, 2005). Consequently, it is an important area for researchers in the field of behavioral neuroscience to identify strategies to improve mathematical skill acquisition in children and to explore the mechanisms involved in the acquisition of academic skills.

An emerging line of research has focused on investigating the relationships between physical activity, cognitive functions and academic achievements in children (Hillman et al., 2008; Diamond and Ling, 2016; Donnelly et al., 2016; Pesce and Ben-Soussan, 2016; Vazou et al., 2016; Tomporowski et al., 2015). The term physical activity is a comprehensive concept covering various activities. These activities cover cardiovascular exercise focusing on the quantitative characteristics of the activity (e.g., intensity and duration) aiming at improving the cardiovascular fitness, in addition to activities concerned with the qualitative characteristics of the physical activity (e.g., the coordinative demands and cognitive engagement) leading, for instance, to improved motor skills (Pesce, 2012; Diamond, 2015). Currently, the majority of the performed studies have been concerned with linking cognitive functions (Hillman et al., 2005; Voss et al., 2011) and academic achievements (Castelli et al., 2007; Chaddock-Heyman et al., 2015) to cardiovascular fitness in cross-sectional designs. Recent cross-sectional studies have positively linked motor skills to cognitive and academic measures (Kantomaa et al., 2013; Lopes et al., 2013; Haapala et al., 2014; Geertsen et al., 2016) and recent reviews have stressed the importance of the qualitative characteristics of the performed physical activity as compared to the quantitative characteristics of the physical activity (Best, 2010; Pesce, 2012; Diamond, 2015). In general, however, less focus has been paid to the qualitative characteristics of physical activity, and the relation of these to cognitive functions and academic achievements.

In addition to cross-sectional findings, interventional studies have also focused on the potential of cardiovascular exercise to facilitate cognitive performance and academic achievements (for reviews, see Hillman et al., 2008; Pesce and Ben-Soussan, 2016; Vazou et al., 2016; Donnelly et al., 2016). The theoretical framework for these effects are related to the structural and functional differences and adaptations associated with or resulting from the increased cardiovascular fitness or exercise (Hillman et al., 2008). Indeed, higher-fit preadolescent children display greater gray matter hippocampal volumes (Chaddock et al., 2010), lower gray matter thickness in the frontal cortex (Chaddock-Heyman et al., 2015) and greater white matter integrity (Chaddock-Heyman et al., 2014) which altogether might translate into superior cognitive and academic performance (Chaddock et al., 2010; Chaddock-Heyman et al., 2015). Moreover, interventions focusing on various cardiovascular engaging activities result in brain electrophysiological adaptations, including an increased amplitude of the P3 component of the event-related potentials (ERPs), indicating a more efficient allocation of attentional resources (Polich, 2007). These effects are speculatively based upon neurobiological and molecular events related to cardiovascular exercise which positively affect neuroplastic processes within the central nervous system (Gomez-Pinilla and Hillman, 2013). Again, less focus has been paid to the qualitative characteristics of the physical activity. However, Schmidt et al. (2016) highlighted the promising effects of a cognitively engaging 6-week physical activity intervention in promoting executive functions independently of the exercise intensity. Furthermore, Chang et al. (2013) found a positive effect on measures of cognitive functioning of an 8-week intervention focusing on coordinative demanding intensity-independent physical activity. This positive effect was related to brain electrophysiological measures, including both increased amplitudes and shorter latencies of the P3 ERP component, reflecting more efficient and faster cognitive processing (Polich, 2007).

Altogether, these studies highlight two different approaches of physical activity to facilitate cognitive functions, and suggest differential, but beneficial, mechanisms for the observed behavioral effects (Voelcker-Rehage and Niemann, 2013). This has led to research conducted to investigate the effects of including both quantitatively and qualitatively approaches of physical activity as interventions in ecologically valid school settings to promote cognition and academic achievements. One way of investigating the impact of physical activity on cognition in school settings is to include classroom-based physical activity, prescribed either as physical activity breaks ("energizers") or physical activity integrated into the academic curriculum. Ahamed et al. (2007) implemented quantitative, cardiovascular "energizers" of 15 min in a 16-month intervention, but did not see any positive effects for the intervention group. Conversely, Mullender-Wijnsma et al. (2016) found that 15-min of classroom-based integrated cardiovascular exercise improved the mathematical and spelling performance to a greater extent than conventional teaching. A paucity of literature exists investigating classroom-based qualitatively focused physical activity. However, a newly published study by Vazou et al. (2016) employed classroom-based integrated multi-faceted physical activity into the taught academic content and found greater improvements in mathematical performance for the intervention group compared to a control group.

Collectively, studies evaluating the effects of classroom-based physical activity (prescribed as breaks or integrated into the curriculum), whether focusing on quantitative or qualitative characteristics, yield inconsistent results. In line with this, Donnelly et al. (2016) recently proposed the need for further research in this specific field to delineate the potential effects. Furthermore, no previous studies have investigated the effects of different qualitatively focused motor enriching interventions (fine vs. gross motor skill) on cognitive and academic performance in children. Recently published cross-sectional study have indeed indicated that different coordinative motor skills, including both gross and fine motor skills, are associated with objective measures of cognitive functions and academic achievement, including mathematical performance, in children (Kantomaa et al., 2013; Haapala et al., 2014; Geertsen et al., 2016). While these associations are intriguing, they are correlational in nature. Therefore, longitudinal interventional studies investigating potential causal effects of integrating different types of qualitative motor activities, including both gross and fine classroom-based motor activities on measures of academic achievements are needed.

Furthermore, a number of studies have aimed at investigating the differential effects of physical activity on cognitive functioning and academic achievement related to the baseline performance of the children (high and low performers). These studies have primarily employed interventions focusing on the quantitative characteristics of the physical activity. Acute cardiovascular exercise interventions have yielded the strongest effects in individuals with the lowest cognitive baseline performance (Mahar et al., 2006; Pontifex et al., 2013; Drollette et al., 2014), highlighting an interesting possibility of using physical activity to support those individuals who need it the most. Yet, the literature regarding the effects of chronic physical activity interventions are sparse. One study that investigated this found that typically developing children benefitted the greatest from a physical education based intervention with additional cognitive demands (cognitive enrichment), while children with coordinative impairments did not (Pesce et al., 2013). This points to the need of optimally challenging every individual. Whether this is the case for classroom-based physical activity interventions is currently unknown. Indeed, studies evaluating classroom-based integrated qualitative physical activity in relation to the children's cognitive and academic baseline performance are lacking.

Additionally, previous studies evaluating the effects of classroom-based physical activity interventions have not accounted for cognitive and motor covariates related to academic achievements, including executive functions (St. Clair-Thompson and Gathercole, 2006; Bull et al., 2008), short-term memory (Raghubar et al., 2010) and motor skills (e.g., Geertsen et al., 2016). Importantly, theoretical models have been proposed, suggesting a mediating role for cognitive efficiency, and particularly executive and metacognitive functions, in the relationship between physical activity and academic achievements (Howie and Pate, 2012; Tomporowski et al., 2015). In line with this, Pesce et al. (2016) recently proposed that improvements in children's ball skills mediated the effects of a coordinative and cognitively demanding physical activity intervention on measures of executive functioning. Moreover, as indicated in a review by Tomporowski et al. (2015) the number of studies investigating the stability and maintenance of the effects resulting from physical activity interventions on measures of cognitive functioning and academic achievement is sparse.

Taken together, the present study has three primary aims: (1) to investigate the immediate and maintained causal effects of classroom-based integrated gross and fine motor activity on mathematical performance in preadolescent children, (2) to investigate whether differences exist in the intervention effects between children characterized as normal and low mathematical performers, and (3) to investigate whether, and to what extent, different cognitive functions and motor skills contribute to the physical activity-academic achievement relationship.

We hypothesize that classroom-based gross and fine motor activity will result in an increased mathematical performance following a 6-week intervention compared to a conventional teaching strategy. We further hypothesize that the addition of extra coordinative demands will primarily benefit normal performing children, in relation to the optimal challenge point theory (Pesce et al., 2013). Finally, based on prior studies highlighting cognitive and motor skills as potential mediators of the effects of physical activity, we hypothesize that both cognitive and motor performance will account for some of the interventional effects on mathematical performance.

MATERIALS AND METHODS

Participants

We invited 186 children from the 1st grade level from three different Danish public schools, containing 9 different school classes, in the Copenhagen area. The schools were selected based on similar demographic profiles (determined by the placement of the schools) and on grade-based graduation performance (included schools ranked 48, 56, 57, of 59 public schools in Copenhagen). One-hundred-sixty-five children (77 girls, mean age = 7.5, SEM = 0.02) were included in the study after obtaining written consent, corresponding to 89% of the invited children (see **Table 1** for demographic characteristics within each intervention group). School classes were stratified based on baseline mathematical performance, and cluster-randomly allocated to one of three groups, explained in detail below (**Figure 1**). The study was approved by the Ethical Committee of Copenhagen, Denmark (protocol: H-15009418), and was carried out in accordance with the Helsinki Declaration II.

Intervention Groups

The three groups were gross motor math (GMM), fine motor math (FMM) and control (CON). The groups mainly

TABLE 1 | Demographic characteristics of two intervention groups (FMM, Fine motor math; GMM, Gross motor math) and the control (CON) group.

	CON	FMM	GMM
Participants (n)	57	53	55
Age (Years)	7.5 ± 0.02	7.5 ± 0.03	7.5 ± 0.02
Gender (% Boys)	49.1 ± 3.8	56.6 ± 3.9	54.5 ± 3.9
Bilingualism (% Bilingual)	36.8 ± 3.7	35.8 ± 3.8	34.5 ± 3.7
BMI (Weight/Height^2)	16.5 ± 0.3	15.8 ± 0.3	16.5 ± 0.3
Cardiovascular fitness (Distance covered, m)	878 ± 17	866 ± 18	894 ± 12

Data reported as mean ± SEM. Estimate of cardiovascular fitness obtained using the Andersen test (Andersen et al., 2008). No significant between-group differences were observed for any of the measures. BMI, body mass index.

differed in the applied teaching methods. GMM focused on integrating gross motor movements into the learning activities covering the mathematical curriculum (gross motor enrichment), using different gross motor movements supporting the mathematical principles and procedures to be acquired. Desks and chairs were moved to the sides in the classroom ensuring adequate space for performing gross motor movements. Children in the GMM group performed inter-limb gross motor movements that alternated between dynamic and static movements and involved a large range of movement (e.g., skipping, crawling, hopscotching, throwing, one-legged balance). The gross motor movements were performed while solving mathematical problems throughout all lessons (lasting approximately 60 min each). FMM focused on integrating fine motor movements into the learning activities covering the mathematical curriculum (fine motor enrichment). The learning activities involved a modified version of the LEGO MoreToMath® concept. The children used fine motor activity to manipulate LEGO® bricks supporting the mathematical principles and procedures to be acquired. The children were primarily sitting at their desks throughout the lesson. The children bimanually selected, moved and modeled the bricks using both hands and fingers while solving mathematical problems throughout all lessons (lasting approximately 60 min each). CON employed conventional math teaching, and was restricted to not make use of additional motor activity or cardiovascular exercise during the math lessons. In all three groups (i.e., CON, FMM, GMM), the children worked individually or in small groups during the lessons. During the intervention, the learning activities in the three groups were matched on content, i.e., the mathematical principles and procedures to be acquired, and time of the day of the math lessons. The standardization within and between the intervention groups was ensured through three workshops of 3 h for the involved teachers hosted by the experimental staff. The workshops were conducted prior to the allocation of classes into groups. In addition to thorough instructions, teachers received thoroughly designed teaching manuals, describing what, when and how the teaching should be conducted during the intervention period. Furthermore, the experimental supervisors were in ongoing dialogue with the teachers of all three intervention groups to ensure the intended intervention, however no quantitative measures were obtained during this process.

Procedure

The children had their mathematical achievement, cognitive functions and motor skills tested at three time-points. Testing took place before (T0), immediately (T1), and 8 weeks (T2) after the intervention. Substantial effort was paid to ensure that the children were tested at the same time of the day ± 1 h, in the same sequence of testing, and by the same experimental supervisor at all three time-points. At T0, the children's cardiovascular fitness was also tested. The intervention lasted 6 continuous weeks, and included 3 weekly math lessons of approximately 60-min duration. During the intervention, the amount and intensity of the physical activity (or load) during the math lessons was evaluated through spot tests involving accelerometers and heart rate monitoring.

Measures

Mathematical Test

The children's mathematical achievement was tested through a paper-and-pencil, standardized, diagnostic test developed by experts within the neuropsychological field of mathematical testing in Denmark (Hogrefe Psykologiske Forlag A/S, Virum, Denmark). Specifically, the test consisted of 50 mathematical tasks to be solved, including 39 1st grade tasks and 11 2nd grade tasks. The tasks covered different age-related mathematical themes, including arithmetic and geometry. The test was conducted individually in a classroom with 15–20 children completing it simultaneously under supervision from two experimental supervisors and the teacher of the class. The children were thoroughly instructed prior to the test. During the test, each problem was presented verbally in a standardized format by an experimental supervisor. Next, the children were to solve the presented problems. When the entire classroom had answered, the test proceeded in a similar fashion. Halfway through the test, the children had a 10 min mandatory break. The entire testing session lasted between 60 and 90 min. The tests were reviewed offline by a single experimental supervisor using standardized guidelines provided by the authors of the test.

Cognitive Tests

Three standardized cognitive tests were applied to estimate the capacity of the children in different domains of cognitive functions, including executive functions and short-term memory. The cognitive tests were completed on a computer in a one-to-one session between a child and an experimental supervisor.

Executive functions

The children's executive functions were assessed using a computer-based modified Eriksen Flanker Task (Eriksen and Eriksen, 1974). Since the test was carried out in young children, the stimuli consisted of fish requiring feeding (e.g., Hillman

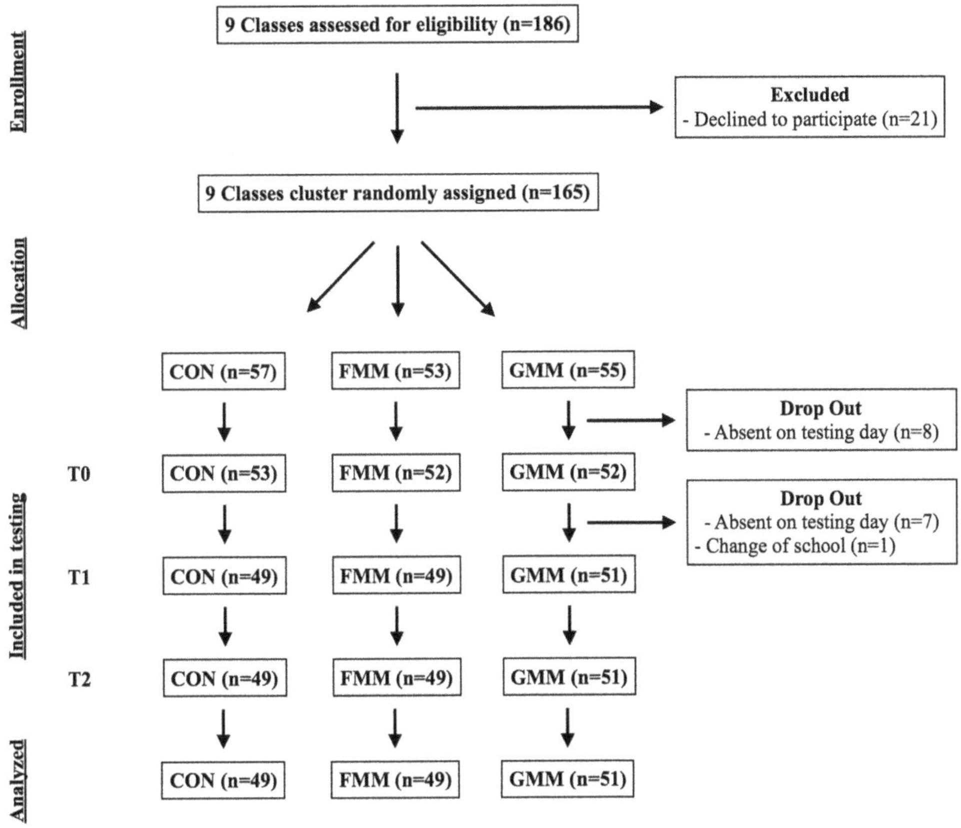

FIGURE 1 | Flow diagram for the study.

et al., 2014; Schonert-Reichl et al., 2015; Vazou and Smiley-Oyen, 2014). The children were comfortably placed in front of a 15.4″ laptop placed at a distance that allowed them to press the response buttons with their index fingers, with their elbows resting on the edge of the table. The laptop presented the stimuli using Presentation (Neurobehavioral Systems Inc., California, USA). Stimuli (90 × 10 mm) were placed in the center of the screen on a white background. The children were presented with congruent (compatible) stimuli (i.e., > > > > >) and incongruent (incompatible) stimuli (i.e., > > < > >) in a pseudo-randomized sequence with an equi-probable (0.5) frequency of congruent and incongruent stimuli. The children completed a single block of 60 trials, preceded by four familiarization trials, ensuring task compliance. The children were instructed to respond to the inside stimulus, while ignoring the flanking stimuli as fast and accurate as possible. The children's response latency and accuracy were logged for both congruent and incongruent trials. Responses faster than 200 ms were considered as an anticipatory response and were excluded from the analyses. From the congruent and incongruent trials, interference effects (i.e., flanker effects) were computed as the difference between incongruent trials and congruent trials. These measures were used as an estimate of the children's inhibitory control (e.g., Hillman et al., 2009).

Visuo-spatial short-term memory

The children's visuo-spatial short-term memory was assessed using a spatial span test from the Cambridge Neuropsychological Test Automated Battery (CANTAB) (Cambridge Cognition Ltd, Cambridge, UK). The spatial span test is a neuropsychological test specifically assessing the memory for sequentially presented visuo-spatial information, and it has been used in previous studies assessing visuo-spatial short-term memory in children aged 4–12 (Luciana and Nelson, 2002). The children were comfortably placed in front of a 23″ touchscreen and equipped with headphones. The touchscreen was placed approximately 30 cm from the edge of the table. During the test, nine white squares (43 × 43 mm each) were presented on a black background on the touch-screen, and the squares changed color one by one. After the presentation, the participants were to replicate the sequence by touching the squares with the index finger of their dominant hand. If correct, an additional color-changing square was added to the sequence in a progressive manner (from 2 to a total of 9 squares). The longest completed sequence, the span length, was logged and used as a measure of the visuo-spatial short-term memory.

Phonological short-term memory

The children's phonological (semantic) short-term memory was assessed using a free-recall wordlist memory task inspired by

Pesce et al. (2009). Specifically, the test evaluated the children's ability to remember as many words as possible out of 20. The words were all age-appropriate nouns. The children were comfortably placed in front of a 13.3″ laptop and equipped with headphones. During the test, 20 words were visually displayed and presented orally in a standardized and timed sequence for 5-s each using a Microsoft PowerPoint presentation yielding a 100-s presentation time. After the presentation, the children were exposed to a 120-s period in which they were to sit with their eyes closed and remember the words. Then, the children had an additional 120-s period to verbally recall as many words as possible in a free-recall manner. The number of correctly recalled words were logged and used as a measure of the phonological short-term memory.

Motor Tests

Two motor tasks were applied estimating the children's gross and fine motor skills. The tasks were completed in a one-to-one session between a child and an experimental supervisor.

Gross motor skills

To evaluate gross motor skills, the children completed a coordination wall, which has previously been used to assess gross motor coordinative skills in preadolescent children (Geertsen et al., 2016; Larsen et al., 2016). The children were standing facing the coordination wall, which consisted of an upright rectangular 9 × 8 grid, with the numbers 1–10 distributed on the grid. Half of the numbers were blue, half red. Red and blue numbers appeared on both sides of the vertical midline. The coordination wall was split in two by a horizontal dividing line, yielding an upper section (top seven rows), and a lower section (bottom two rows). The children were equipped with a red dot on their right hand and a blue dot on the left hand and foot. The children were instructed to touch the numbers in the correct order, from one to ten, with their hands (upper section) or feet (lower section), according to the color of the number. The movements performed required crossing of the vertical midline. They had to complete the task as fast and accurate as possible. If a mistake was made, the children were immediately instructed to correct it, and proceed. Prior to the test the children were thoroughly instructed. Next, the children had three attempts on the coordination wall, and the shortest time (best time) of completion (in sec) was used as a measure of the children's bimanual, inter-limb coordinative gross motor skills.

Fine motor skills

The children's fine motor skills were evaluated using the Perdue Pegboard test (US Neurologicals LLC, Washington, USA). Specifically, the Perdue Pegboard (Tiffin and Asher, 1948) assesses manual dexterity and bimanual fine motor coordination, and has previously been used testing preadolescent children (Gardner and Broman, 1979). The children were comfortably placed on a chair in front of the Purdue Pegboard. Prior to test, the children's handedness were assessed using a name-writing test supplemented with self-report (Scharoun and Bryden, 2014), and the children were thoroughly instructed in the test. The test consisted of four sessions: 30-s uni-manual placement of pins using the dominant hand (i) and the non-dominant hand (ii). Thirteen-seconds bimanual placement of pins using both hands (iii), and 60-s bimanual assembly, consisting of three parts assembled in a specific sequence (iv). The latter served as a measure of the children's fine motor skills, expressed as the number of correctly assembled parts.

Cardiovascular Fitness

The children's cardiovascular fitness was estimated using the Andersen test (Andersen et al., 2008), which is a validated measure of cardiovascular fitness in 6–9 year old children (Ahler et al., 2012). The test was modified to fit the available space in the gyms of the involved schools. Prior to test, the participants completed a 5-min warm-up and were thoroughly instructed in the test protocol. In the test, the children ran between cones placed diagonally across each other in a distance of 17 m in 15-s intervals interspersed by 15-s mandatory breaks. The test was completed in 10 min. The children ran as fast as they could during the running intervals to cover the greatest distance possible. Heart rate was monitored (Polar Team 2 System, Polar, Finland), and the test was videotaped using a GoPro HERO4 camera (GoPro Inc., California, USA), to ensure that the performance of each child was logged. The videos were inspected offline and the total running distance was registered as a measure of cardiovascular fitness.

Physical Load during the Intervention

In a subsample of the children, covering all three intervention groups ($n = 49$), the physical load during the math lessons was estimated combining time-synced heart rate monitoring (Polar Team 2 System, Polar, Finland) and accelerometers (MinimaxX S4, Catapult Innovations, Canberra, Australia) on 6 occasions. Individual heart rate during the lessons was compared to each participant's maximum heart rate (HRmax) collected during the Andersen test, yielding an individual percent of HRmax. Time spent in low (0–60% of HRmax), moderate-to-vigorous (60–90% of HRmax) and high (90–100% of HRmax) heart rate zones during the lessons were used as outcome measures. The accelerometers sampled tri-axially [forward (fwd), sideways (side), upwards (up)] with a sampling-rate of 100 Hz. Based on the MinimaxX proprietary software (Sprint, Catapult Sports, Canberra, Australia) the physical load (i.e., player load) was computed by the software using the following formula:

$$\text{Player load} = \sqrt{\left(fwd_{y1} - fwd_{y-1}\right)^2 + \left(side_{x1} - side_{x-1}\right)^2 + \left(up_{z1} - up_{z-1}\right)^2}$$

where fwd_y, $side_x$, *and* up_z indicate the accelerations in the forward, sideways and upwards plane, respectively. The player load is an arbitrary unit correlated with subjective perceived exertion measures of physical exhaustion (Casamichana et al., 2013), and the measure has previously been used to assess the intensity of various physical activities in preadolescent children (Larsen et al., 2016).

Statistical Analysis

The statistical analyses were performed in the open-access software R Studio (R Core Team, Vienna, Austria). The analyses were carried out on complete datasets (complete-case analysis). Baseline characteristics were compared between groups using one-way analysis of variance or chi-square tests for continuous (age, BMI, cardiovascular fitness) and categorical (gender, bilingualism) measures, respectively. Data from the mathematical, cognitive and motor tests were analyzed using linear mixed models with group-time interactions as fixed effects, using R package *lme4* (Bates et al., 2014). Random effects were included in the models to account for dependencies between measurements on the same subjects, school classes, and schools. Model validation was based upon visual inspection of residual plots and normal probability plots. To accommodate the specific hypotheses of this study, specific sets of contrasts between intervention groups across the included time-points were evaluated using global F-tests. Subsequently, model-based t-tests were used to identify the significant differences, using the R-package *multcomp* (Hothorn et al., 2008). These pairwise comparisons were adjusted for multiplicity using the 'single-step' adjustment, which is a recently developed procedure providing a less conservative adjustment of p-values as compared to Bonferroni adjustment and related adjustments, by utilizing the correlations between tests. Additionally, between-group differences and within-group differences at, and between, specific time-points were compared using model-based t-tests. An explorative analysis sought to examine whether differences between intervention groups were related to the baseline mathematical performance level of the children. The authors of the standardized and validated math test describe that an individual performance at 75% correct answers, or lower, might reflect difficulties acquiring mathematical content. This subgroup was termed *low performers* (n = 49, based on the math performance at T0). The other subgroup (i.e., >75% c.a.) was termed *normal performers* (n = 116) and was characterized by not having difficulties acquiring mathematical content. Moreover, to gauge the tentative contribution or mediating effect of cognitive and motor performance on mathematical achievement, each cognitive and motor measure was added one by one, using an univariate approach, to the overall linear mixed model as an additional covariate, and differences in estimates between models with and without the covariate were reported. Data are reported as mean ± SEM unless otherwise stated. A significance level of 0.05 was applied.

RESULTS

Baseline Mathematical, Cognitive, and Motor Performance

At T0, the groups performed equally well in the measures of mathematical and visuo-spatial short-term memory performance, in addition to gross and fine motor performance. This is presented in **Table 2**. Indeed, model-based t-tests revealed no significant between-group differences in these measures ($p > 0.05$). However, significant between-group differences at T0 were found in measures of inhibitory control and phonological short-term memory (**Table 2**). FMM performed significantly better in the accuracy interference score compared to GMM ($p = 0.01$), and CON performed significantly worse than FMM ($p = 0.049$) and GMM ($p = 0.03$) at T0 in phonological short-term memory.

Physical Load and Attendance during the Intervention

To evaluate the physical load of the math lessons during the intervention we applied combined accelerometer and heart rate measures at 6 randomly selected math lessons. Furthermore, we recorded the attendance in the math lessons during the intervention. Group means of the physical load during the math lessons as well as the attendance during the intervention are presented in **Table 3**. No between-group difference was found in the measure of attendance [$F_{(2, 161)} = 0.51$; $p = 0.60$], indicating homogeneity in the attendance between groups during the intervention. An overall significant between-group difference was found for player load [$F_{(2, 48)} = 27.2, p < 0.001$], and revealed that GMM displayed a higher player load during the math lessons compared to both FMM ($t = 6.33$, $p < 0.001$) and CON ($t = 6.13$, $p < 0.001$). A significant group-zone interaction was found for time spent in different heart rate zones [$F_{(2, 138)} = 4.58, p = 0.002$], and revealed that GMM spent more time in the moderate-to-vigorous heart rate zone (60–90% of HRmax) compared to both FMM 10.0 ± 4.0% ($p = 0.03$) and CON 10.6 ± 4.1 % ($p = 0.03$). These results indicate that GMM performed significantly more accelerations during the math lessons in the intervention, and spent more time in the moderate-to-vigorous heart rate zone compared to both FMM and CON.

Performance in the Mathematical Test

All groups improved their performance within the mathematical task from T0 to T1 and T0 to T2, as can be seen in **Table 2**. A significant group-time interaction was found from T0 to T1 [$F_{(2, 288)} = 3.49$, $p = 0.03$]. As summarized in **Figure 2A**, the changes in mean mathematical performance were significantly greater from T0 to T1 for GMM compared to FMM 1.87 ± 0.71 correct answers (c.a.) ($p = 0.02$). This effect was not evident from T0 to T2 [$F_{(2, 434)} = 1.89$, $p = 0.15$]. This indicated that GMM transiently improved children's performance in the mathematical task more than FMM.

Performance in the Mathematical Test in Normal and Low Performers

To assess whether differences existed between children characterized as normal and low mathematical performers we performed a subgroup analysis. Within the normal performers, the improvements in mean mathematical performance were significantly greater for GMM compared to both CON 1.78 ± 0.73 c.a. ($p = 0.04$) and FMM 2.14 ± 0.72 c.a. ($p = 0.008$) from T0 to T1 (**Figure 2B**). Additionally, the improvements in mean mathematical performance were significantly greater for GMM compared to CON 2.67 ± 0.71 c.a. ($p < 0.001$) from T0 to T2 (**Figure 2B**). No significant differences between groups were observed within the low performing individuals from T0 to T1 or T0 to T2 (all $p > 0.05$) (**Figure 2C**). This indicates that the normal performers benefitted from GMM compared to both FMM and CON, whereas the low performers did not.

TABLE 2 | Mathematical, cognitive and motor performance at T0, T1 and T2 for the two intervention groups (FMM, Fine motor math; GMM, Gross motor math) and the control (CON) group.

Measure	CON			FMM			GMM		
	T0	T1	T2	T0	T1	T2	T0	T1	T2
MATHEMATICAL PERFORMANCE (N = 149)									
Math score (No. correct answers)	36.1 ± 1.3	38.9 ± 1.3*	39.2 ± 1.2*	37.3 ± 1.2	39.1 ± 1.2*	40.4 ± 1.1*§	36.8 ± 1.2	40.6 ± 1.2*	41.1 ± 1.1*
VISUO-SPATIAL SHORT-TERM MEMORY (N = 139)									
Span length (No. boxes)	5.0 ± 0.2	5.1 ± 0.2	5.6 ± 0.2*§	4.8 ± 0.2	5.2 ± 0.2	5.9 ± 0.2*§	4.8 ± 0.2	5.5 ± 0.2*	5.8 ± 0.2*
PHONOLOGICAL SHORT-TERM MEMORY (N = 136)									
Words recalled (No. words)	5.4 ± 0.5[b,c]	5.7 ± 0.5	5.4 ± 0.5	6.4 ± 0.5	5.7 ± 0.5	6.6 ± 0.4§	6.3 ± 0.4	5.1 ± 0.4*	6.3 ± 0.4§
EXECUTIVE FUNCTIONS (N = 134)									
Accuracy (% correct): congruent trials	94.6 ± 0.8	96.6 ± 0.8	97.2 ± 0.7*	97.1 ± 0.8[a]	98.9 ± 0.8	98.1 ± 0.7	96.5 ± 0.8	97.7 ± 0.8	97.7 ± 0.7
Accuracy (% correct): incongruent trials	93.4 ± 1.1	95.0 ± 1.1	95.0 ± 1.0	96.3 ± 1.0[c]	97.6 ± 1.0	96.9 ± 1.0	92.6 ± 1.0	95.7 ± 1.0*	94.4 ± 1.0
Response latency (ms): congruent trials	802 ± 44	733 ± 44*	707 ± 33*	861 ± 43	704 ± 43*	657 ± 33*	851 ± 42	723 ± 42*	692 ± 32*
Response latency (ms): incongruent trials	863 ± 61	763 ± 61*	743 ± 48*	927 ± 61	753 ± 61*	700 ± 48*	943 ± 60	800 ± 60*	756 ± 47*
Interference effect: accuracy (% correct)	−1.3 ± 0.9	−1.6 ± 0.9	−2.2 ± 0.8	−0.7 ± 0.9[c]	−1.3 ± 0.9	−1.2 ± 0.9	−3.9 ± 0.9	−2.0 ± 0.9	−3.2 ± 0.8
Interference effect: response latency (ms)	62 ± 23	31 ± 23	38 ± 21	66 ± 23	49 ± 23	43 ± 21	92 ± 23	78 ± 23	66 ± 21
GROSS MOTOR PERFORMANCE (N = 136)									
Best time (s)	20.9 ± 0.7	17.6 ± 0.7*	15.7 ± 0.9*§	20.0 ± 0.7	17.9 ± 0.7*	14.7 ± 0.8*§	21.5 ± 0.7	17.7 ± 0.7*	15.2 ± 0.8*§
FINE MOTOR PERFORMANCE (N = 126)									
Assembly (No. of parts)	20.1 ± 1.7	21.5 ± 1.7*	24.9 ± 1.6*§	21.6 ± 2.0	22.7 ± 2.0	27.9 ± 1.9*§	21.3 ± 1.6	22.8 ± 1.6*	25.6 ± 1.6*§

*Data reported as means ± SEM. Mathematical performance estimated by standardized, diagnostic Danish test. Visuo-spatial and phonological memory estimated using a spatial span and a word-recall task. Executive functions estimated using a modified Eriksen Flanker Task. Interference effect is the difference between incongruent and congruent trials. Gross and fine motor performance evaluated through a coordination wall task and the Perdue Pegboard, respectively. *Indicates a significant within-group difference from T0. §Indicates a significant within-group difference from T1.*

[a]Indicates a significant between-group difference from CON at T0.

[b]Indicates a significant between-group difference from FMM at T0.

[c]Indicates a significant between-group difference from GMM at T0 ($p < 0.05$).

Contribution of Cognitive and Motor Covariates to Changes in Mathematical Performance

Additionally, we investigated whether, and to what extent, potential covariates contributed to the results observed for the mathematical performance, by using an univariate analysis. Group means of the cognitive and motor performance measures can be seen in **Table 2**. The results of the univariate analysis are presented in **Table 4**. When controlling for visuo-spatial short-term memory the difference in mathematical performance between GMM and FMM was reduced to 1.22 ± 0.8 (p = 0.40). Changes in visuo-spatial short-term memory accounted for approximately 35% of the effects of the intervention on mathematical performance. Similar results were not found for any other measure of cognitive performance (see **Table 4**). When controlling for gross motor skills the difference in mathematical performance between GMM and FMM was reduced to 1.41 ± 0.77 (p = 0.16). Changes in gross motor skill performance accounted for approximately 25% of the effects of the intervention on mathematical performance (see **Table 4**).

DISCUSSION

The aims of this study were 3-fold. First, we sought to investigate the immediate and longer-term effects of classroom-based integrated gross and fine motor activities on mathematical achievement in preadolescent children. Secondly, it was investigated whether the intervention elicited different effects in normal and low math performers. Thirdly, we sought to investigate the potential role of cognitive functions and motor skills in the physical activity-academic achievement relationship.

The main findings of the study were that motor enriched learning activities can improve mathematical achievement. Indeed, in normal performers, applying gross motor enriched

TABLE 3 | Attendance and physical load during the intervention for the two intervention groups (FMM, Fine motor math; GMM, Gross motor math) and the control (CON) group.

	CON	FMM	GMM
ATTENDANCE ($N = 165$)			
Attended math lessons (%)	90.9 ± 1.4	92.7 ± 1.2	91.3 ± 1.3
PHYSICAL LOAD ($N = 49$)			
Time spend in low HR zone (%)	88.8 ± 3.1[c]	87.9 ± 2.9[c]	77.9 ± 2.7[a,b]
Time spend in MVPA HR zone (%)	11.1 ± 3.1[c]	11.7 ± 2.9[c]	21.6 ± 2.7[a,b]
Time spend in high HR zone (%)	0.2 ± 3.1	0.4 ± 2.9	0.4 ± 2.7
Player Load/min (a.u.)	0.07 ± 0.006[c]	0.07 ± 0.006[c]	0.12 ± 0.007[a,b]

Data reported as means ± SEM. Physical load obtained through six spot tests using time-synced heart rate measures and accelerometers. MVPA, moderate-to-vigorous physical activity; HR, Heart rate. Low HR zone corresponds to 0–60% of HR_{max}, MVPA HR zone corresponds to 60–90% of HR_{max} and high HR zone corresponds to 90–100% of HRmax.
[a]Indicates a significant between-group difference from CON at T0.
[b]Indicates a significant between-group difference from FMM at T0.
[c]Indicates a significant between-group difference from GMM ($p < 0.05$).

math lessons resulted in a greater improvement in mathematical performance compared to fine motor enriched math and conventional math lessons after a 6-week intervention. The effects on mathematical performance were maintained between gross motor enriched and conventional teaching in the normal performers 8 weeks after the cessation of the intervention. In all children, these positive effects were observed between gross motor enriched learning and fine motor enriched learning. These effects seem to be partly accounted for by changes in the visuo-spatial short-term memory, gross motor skills and, to a minor degree, fine motor skills. These results add to the emerging literature, consolidating the positive effects of integrating classroom-based motor activity to improve cognitive and academic performance in children (Donnelly et al., 2016). Interestingly, our results specify that only normal achieving children benefit from adding motor activity to the classroom curriculum, and that cognitive and motor abilities could contribute to the observed positive effects of the motor enriched learning activities.

Effects of Gross Motor-Enriched Learning Activities on Mathematical Performance

The observed behavioral effects might be the result of a combination of different mechanisms. Indeed, a recently published review proposed that classroom-based integrated physical activity could influence learning through various processes (Chandler and Tricot, 2015), including acute and chronic effects of the physiological response to exercise on the central nervous system (CNS) (Hillman et al., 2008). For example, physical exercise causes a release of a plethora of neurobiological substances, including brain-derived neurotrophic factor (BDNF), lactate and insulin-like-growth factor (IGF-1) (Skriver et al., 2014). Animal studies suggest that these neurotrophic agents might benefit neuroplastic processes, acutely related to memory formation (e.g., Cotman and Berchtold, 2002; Cotman et al., 2007). However, previous studies have demonstrated an intensity-dependent dose-response relationship of exercise on the neurotrophic response (Ferris et al., 2007; Winter et al., 2007), leading to the greatest physiological response at intensities higher than the one experienced in the gross motor enriched learning activities in the current study (22% in moderate-to-vigorous heart rate zone). Additionally, a direct transfer of the animal-based molecular findings to human behavioral outcomes is irrefutably challenging (Voss et al., 2013). Indeed, while some human studies have found associations between blood concentrations of a number of neurotrophic agents and behavioral outcomes (Winter et al., 2007; Skriver et al., 2014), others have failed (Ferris et al., 2007; Schmidt-Kassow et al., 2013).

At a functional and behavioral level in children, single bouts of moderate-to-vigorous physical activity have been related to efficient and rapid allocation of attentional resources (Hillman et al., 2009) and improved classroom behavior (Mullender-Wijnsma et al., 2015). Results from chronic intervention studies focusing on moderate-to-vigorous physical activity have also pinpointed these positive effects (e.g., Hillman et al., 2014). Moreover, single bouts of coordinatively demanding physical activity have been found to improve attention in adolescents (Budde et al., 2008), and chronic interventions employing coordinatively demanding physical activity have successfully improved children's attention (Chang et al., 2013; Gallotta et al., 2015). Attention is a key mediator of hippocampal-related declarative memory formation (Aly and Turk-Browne, 2016), probably related to schema-dependent academic learning and performance (van Kesteren et al., 2014).

We hypothesized a general effect of motor enriched learning strategies. Yet, the gross motor learning activities were the single effective strategy in promoting mathematical performance. Arguably, the greater time spent in moderate-to-vigorous physical activity during the gross motor enriched learning activities, working in conjunction with greater coordinative demands, could have favored brain processes positively contributing to the effects of gross motor enriched learning activities on both an acute (during the lessons) and chronic (throughout the entire intervention) temporal scale.

Additionally, based on theories of embodied cognition (e.g., that cognitive knowledge is based on bodily experiences) (Barsalou, 2008), learning could be influenced by integrating task-related motor activity, bridging the content to be acquired to the performed motor activity. Indeed, procedural sensorimotor experiences might contribute to declarative knowledge acquisition (Koziol et al., 2012). Moreover, neuroanatomical structures, including the cerebellum, previously thought to be primarily motor related might also be critically involved in controlling higher-order cognitive functions (Diamond, 2000; Koziol et al., 2012). Previous studies have indeed found a positive effect of performing movements related to the content to be acquired in academically related domains in both adults (Macedonia et al., 2011; Mayer et al., 2015) and young children (Mavilidi et al., 2015). Collectively, these studies demonstrate the positive effects of performing congruent motor activity to improve learning. Theoretically, it could be speculated that the gross motor enriched learning activities involved motor activity

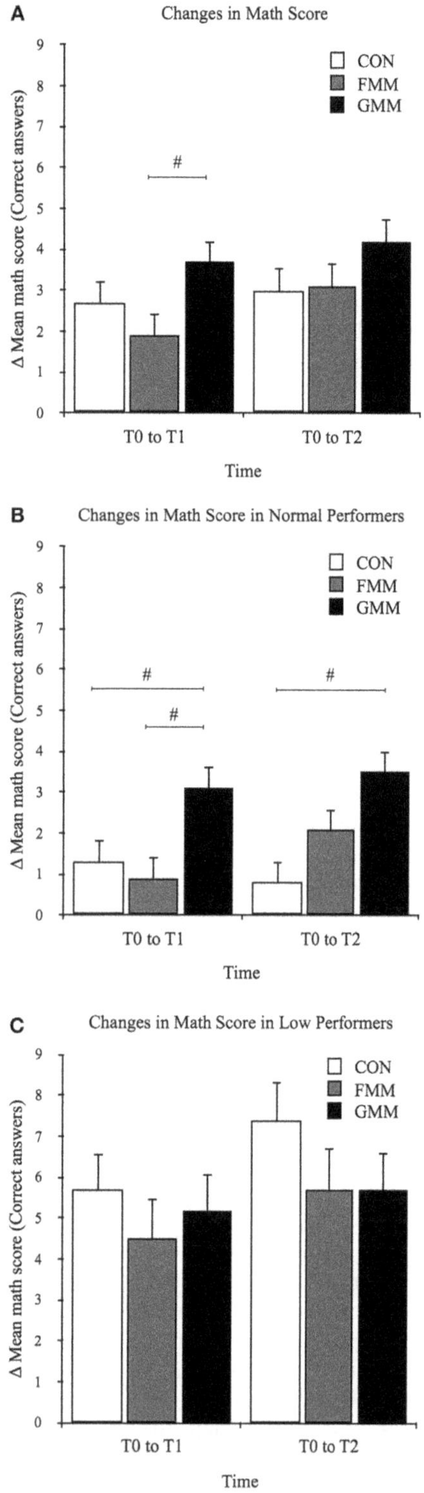

FIGURE 2 | Changes in mathematical performance. Displays changes in mathematical performance expressed as means ± SEM from T0-T1 and T0-T2 in **(A)** all children, **(B)** normal performers ($\geq$75% c.a. in 1st grade tasks at T0), **(C)** low performers ($\geq$75% c.a. in 1st grade tasks at T0). CON, Control; FMM, Fine motor math; GMM, Gross motor math. # indicates a significant between-group difference in the improvements in mathematical performance between time points ($p < 0.05$).

TABLE 4 | Estimated between-group differences (GMM vs. FMM) with cognitive and motor covariates.

	Estimated between-group difference	Percent contribution
Without covariate	1.87 ± 0.7	
Phonological short-term memory (No. words)	1.81 ± 0.7	3.2
Visuo-spatial short-term memory (No. boxes)	1.22 ± 0.8	34.8
Executive functions (Interference effect, accuracy %)	1.94 ± 1.0	−3.7
Executive functions (Interference effect, RT in ms)	1.99 ± 1.0	−6.4
Fine motor skills (No. of parts)	1.67 ± 0.9	10.7
Gross motor skills (Best time, in sec)	1.41 ± 0.8	24.6

Data reported as means ± SEM. Different covariates added to the statistical model explaining intervention effects in mathematical performance. Percent contribution displays percent accounted for by a single covariate. The intervention effects are primarily accounted for by visuo-spatial short-term memory and gross motor skills.

more likely to be subjectively perceived as more figuratively meaningful and congruent, compared to the motor activity performed during the fine motor enriched learning activities. This was, however, not assessed during the study.

Taken together, while both the quantitative (e.g., exercise intensity), qualitative (e.g., coordinative demands) and embodied (e.g., congruency) characteristics of the physical activity might explain the behavioral differences observed, more research is needed to pinpoint the exact mechanisms underlying the effects.

Differential Effects of Interventions on Mathematical Performance Related to the Baseline Level of the Children

The results obtained in our subgroup analyses showed that the benefits of gross motor enriched learning activities were confined to the normal performing individuals. The low-performing children generally improved their mathematical performance more. However, no differences were observed in the improvements between groups. This was in contrast to the normal performing individuals, where benefits of gross motor enriched learning activities were present. Previous research have, on the other hand, shown that the effects of physical activity on cognition and academic involvement were greatest for low-performing children (Mahar et al., 2006; Drollette et al., 2014). However, whereas this study included measures of mathematical performance in a longitudinal interventional perspective, previous studies have used measures of executive functioning (Drollette et al., 2014) and class-room behavior (Mahar et al., 2006) in acute study designs. Furthermore, these studies all employed physical activity interventions centered around the quantitative characteristics of the performed activity. Moreover, the results of the abovementioned studies might be partially biased by the statistical phenomenon of regression toward the mean, explaining the tendency for an "extreme" measure to be closer to the mean when measured the second time (e.g., Moreau et al., 2016). In contrast, the results of the current study do not seem to be biased by this statistically observable phenomenon, as it was within the normal performing subgroup that the benefits of gross motor learning activities were observed. Taken together, the parameters mentioned above complicate direct comparisons to the results of the current study.

Importantly, however, our results contribute with novel knowledge clarifying who benefits from classroom-based integrated motor activity. It seems that the combined cognitive and motor demands of the gross motor enriched teaching strategies result in positive effects uniquely for normal performers, and not for the low performers. These findings support the notion of an optimal challenge point, as initially proposed by Pesce and colleagues (Pesce et al., 2013). Specifically, Pesce et al. (2013) found that enriching a physical activity intervention with additional cognitive demands specifically centered around the executive functions of the participants, resulted in greater improvements in measures of flexible attention for typically developing children, but not for children with developmental coordinative motor deficits. The authors argued that children with motor deficits required a higher amount of cognitive control merely performing the physical activity, leaving less cognitive resources available to deal with additional cognitive challenges (Pesce et al., 2013). In line with this, one could speculate that the low-performing individuals were sufficiently challenged by the cognitive demands of the mathematical content to be acquired during the lessons, due to their initial lower mathematical skill proficiency, leaving fewer mental resources available to benefit from the additional motor activity posed by the gross motor enrichment. Collectively, enriching mathematical lessons with gross motor activity seems to be optimal for normal performing individuals, but not for low performing individuals.

Despite these interesting findings, the current evidence in the field does not allow for clear conclusions regarding the responsiveness of physical activity interventions in individuals achieving at different levels at baseline. Future research is needed to investigate the potential inter-individual differences in the effectiveness of interventions aiming at improving academic achievements in children, using studies specifically designed for evaluating this question.

Visuo-Spatial Short-Term Memory and Gross Motor Skill Performance Accounts for Mathematical Improvements

The performed univariate covariation analysis arguably provides novel, interesting perspectives on the effects of physical activity on academic achievement, by showing that changes in visuo-spatial short-term memory in addition to gross motor skill performance partially accounted for the effects of the intervention on mathematical performance. This was not the case, to the same extent, for the other included cognitive or motor measures, indicating specific associations between physical activity, visuo-spatial memory, gross motor skills and mathematical achievement. In support of this, visuo-spatial memory has previously been related to mathematical achievements (Bull et al., 2008), especially in young children (Holmes and Adams, 2006). Moreover, previous cross-sectional findings have supported a relationship between measures of fine and gross motor proficiency and cognitive functions in both elderly (Voelcker-Rehage et al., 2010) and children (Geertsen et al., 2016). A non-interventional longitudinal study also found that motor skills in kindergarten predicted academic achievement in 1st grade children (Roebers et al., 2014). The results of the current study add longitudinal and interventional evidence to the current knowledge, suggesting that gross motor enriched learning activities might improve mathematical performance through improved gross motor skills and visuo-spatial short-term memory. These results fit nicely with the only other developmental study addressing the potential mediating role of gross motor skills, but not fine motor skills, on executive functioning (Pesce et al., 2016), which is closely related to mathematical performance in children (St. Clair-Thompson and Gathercole, 2006). However, the causal interactions between the performance measures included in the current study are difficult to infer from these results, and the results should be seen as an initial exploration of possible mediating effects. Previous studies applying classroom-based interventions to improve academic achievements through physical activity have not controlled for the contribution of covariates to the same extent as in the current study. Thus, the novelty of the current findings warrants the need for investigating the contribution of cognitive and motor covariates when evaluating the effects of physical activity on academic achievements in future studies.

Strengths and Limitations

This study was strengthened by the ecological value of the design including school classes as the level of randomization in the cluster-randomized controlled trial. In addition, by controlling what, when and how the participants were taught while still keeping their regular teachers and framework, we ensured that these factors did not influence our results substantially. Moreover, we evaluated the long-term effects caused by the intervention, which adds extremely important knowledge about the stability of the intervention. However, some limitations should also be kept in mind when interpreting the results of the study. First, the combination of a relatively small sample size and a substantial intra- and inter-individual variability might have influenced the power of the study. A larger sample size could strengthen the effects of the intervention (Gelman and Carlin, 2014; Moreau et al., 2016). Additionally, we acknowledge that the test measures included in the study are subject to practice-effects (i.e., test-retest effects). However, these would expectedly affect the included groups equally, and hence would not bias the inter-group comparisons on which our conclusions are based. Even though we included various objective measures of motor skills and cognitive functions as potential covariates affecting the effects of the intervention on mathematical performance, our study could also have included measures of motivation, social interactions during the lessons and mental well-being as recently pointed out in the review by Diamond and Ling (2016) to strengthen the interpretation of the results. Indeed, integrating physical activity into the classroom have been found to influence motivational aspects (e.g., Vazou and Smiley-Oyen, 2014; Vazou and Skrade, 2016). Moreover, the results of our univariate approach did not account for collinearity between predictors and, with this shortcoming in mind, they should be seen as an initial exploration of possible mediating effects. However, more sophisticated techniques for mediation analysis, beyond the scope of the present study, such as the one applied by Pesce et al. (2016), would allow a more comprehensive exploration while accommodating for collinearity. Inferring the exact mechanisms underlying the observed behavioral effects in the current study design is challenging. Future studies should investigate these. Structural and functional imaging techniques could prove a valuable tool to widen our understanding of the underlying mechanisms.

CONCLUSION

Participation in math lessons focusing on integrating gross motor activity can positively contribute to mathematical achievements in preadolescent children. In normal math performers, gross motor enrichment led to larger improvements than fine motor enrichment and conventional teaching. Across all children gross motor enrichment resulted in greater mathematical achievement compared to fine motor enrichment. From a practical perspective, teachers and related personnel should consider integrating gross motor activity in learning activities relevant to the academic curriculum as a promising way to engage children and improve academic achievement. The subgroup differences suggest the need of individually tailored teaching activities, specifically related to the individuals' optimal challenge point, to enhance learning in academic domains in children.

AUTHOR CONTRIBUTIONS

MB, RL, JW, SG, and JL designed the experiment. MB, RL, and JW collected the data. MB, RL, JW, SG, and CR conducted the required data analysis. All authors contributed to drafting the manuscript, and all authors approved the final version of the manuscript.

ACKNOWLEDGMENTS

We would like to thank Lasse Rehné Jensen, Laurits Munk Højberg, Christian Lillelund Jacobsen, Stefan Madsen, Hanna Wårfors, Meaghan Spedden, Andreas Blaaholm Nielsen, Sisse Kofoed Seide, Sofie Rejkjær Elleby for their help with data collection. We would like to thank Richard Thomas for valuable feedback on a previous version of this manuscript. We would like to thank the included schools and their teachers, and most importantly the children for participating in the study.

REFERENCES

Ahamed, Y., MacDonald, H., Reed, K., Naylor, P.-J., Liu-Ambrose, T., and McKay, H. (2007). School-based physical activity does not compromise children's academic performance. *Med. Sci. Sports Exerc.* 39, 371–376. doi: 10.1249/01.mss.0000241654.45500.8e

Ahler, T., Bendiksen, M., Krustrup, P., and Wedderkopp, N. (2012). Aerobic fitness testing in 6- to 9-year-old children: reliability and validity of a modified Yo-Yo IR1 test and the Andersen test. *Eur. J. Appl. Physiol.* 112, 871–876. doi: 10.1007/s00421-011-2039-4

Aly, M., and Turk-Browne, N. B. (2016). Attention promotes episodic encoding by stabilizing hippocampal representations. *Proc. Natl. Acad. Sci. U.S.A.* 113, E420–E429. doi: 10.1073/pnas.1518931113

Andersen, L. B., Andersen, T. E., Andersen, E., and Anderssen, S. A. (2008). An intermittent running test to estimate maximal oxygen uptake: the Andersen test. *J. Sports Med. Phys. Fitness* 48, 434–437.

Barsalou, L. W. (2008). Grounded cognition. *Annu. Rev. Psychol.* 59, 617–645. doi: 10.1146/annurev.psych.59.103006.093639

Bates, D., Mächler, M., Bolker, B. M., and Walker, S. C. (2014). Fitting linear mixed-effects models using lme4. *arXiv:1406.5823v1[stat.CO]23*, 1–51.

Best, J. R. (2010). Effects of physical activity on children's executive function: contributions of experimental research on aerobic exercise. *Dev. Rev.* 30, 331–351. doi: 10.1016/j.dr.2010.08.001

Budde, H., Voelcker-Rehage, C., Pietrabyk-Kendziorra, S., Ribeiro, P., and Tidow, G. (2008). Acute coordinative exercise improves attentional performance in adolescents. *Neurosci. Lett.* 441, 219–223. doi: 10.1016/j.neulet.2008.06.024

Bull, R., Espy, K. A., and Wiebe, S. A. (2008). Short-term memory, working memory, and executive functioning in preschoolers: longitudinal predictors of mathematical achievement at age 7 years. *Dev. Neuropsychol.* 33, 205–228. doi: 10.1080/87565640801982312

Butterworth, B. (2005). The development of arithmetical abilities. *J. Child Psychol. Psychiatry* 46, 3–18. doi: 10.1111/j.1469-7610.2004.00374.x

Casamichana, D., Castellano, J., Calleja-Gonzalez, J., San Román, J., and Castagna, C. (2013). Relationship between indicators of training load in soccer players. *J. Strength Cond. Res.* 27, 369–374. doi: 10.1519/JSC.0b013e3182548af1

Castelli, D. M., Hillman, C. H., Buck, S. M., and Erwin, H. E. (2007). Physical fitness and academic achievement in third- and fifth-grade students. *J. Sport Exerc. Psychol.* 29, 239–52. doi: 10.1123/jsep.29.2.239

Chaddock, L., Erickson, K. I., Prakash, R. S., Kim, J. S., Voss, M. W., Vanpatter, M., et al. (2010). A neuroimaging investigation of the association between aerobic fitness, hippocampal volume, and memory performance in preadolescent children. *Brain Res.* 1358, 172–183. doi: 10.1016/j.brainres.2010.08.049

Chaddock-Heyman, L., Erickson, K. I., Holtrop, J. L., Voss, M. W., Pontifex, M. B., Raine, L. B., et al. (2014). Aerobic fitness is associated with greater white matter integrity in children. *Front. Hum. Neurosci.* 8:584. doi: 10.3389/fnhum.2014.00584

Chaddock-Heyman, L., Erickson, K. I., Kienzler, C., King, M., Pontifex, M. B., Raine, L. B., et al. (2015). The role of aerobic fitness in cortical thickness and mathematics achievement in preadolescent children. *PLoS ONE* 10:e0134115. doi: 10.1371/journal.pone.0134115

Chandler, P., and Tricot, A. (2015). Mind your body: the essential role of body movements in children's learning. *Educ. Psychol. Rev.* 27, 365–370. doi: 10.1007/s10648-015-9333-3

Chang, Y. K., Tsai, Y. J., Chen, T. T., and Hung, T. M. (2013). The impacts of coordinative exercise on executive function in kindergarten children: An ERP study. *Exp. Brain Res.* 225, 187–196. doi: 10.1007/s00221-012-3360-9

Cotman, C. W., and Berchtold, N. C. (2002). Exercise: a behavioral intervention to enhance brain health and plasticity. *Trends Neurosci.* 25, 295–301. doi: 10.1016/S0166-2236(02)02143-4

Cotman, C. W., Berchtold, N. C., and Christie, L.-A. (2007). Exercise builds brain health: key roles of growth factor cascades and inflammation. *Trends Neurosci.* 30, 464–472. doi: 10.1016/j.tins.2007.06.011

Diamond, A. (2000). Close interrelation of motor development and cognitive development and of the cerebellum and prefrontal cortex. *Child Dev.* 71, 44–56. doi: 10.1111/1467-8624.00117

Diamond, A. (2015). Effects of physical exercise on executive functions: going beyond simply moving to moving with thought. *Ann. Sports Med. Res.* 2, 1011–1015.

Diamond, A., and Ling, D. S. (2016). Conclusions about interventions, programs, and approaches for improving executive functions that appear justified and those that, despite much hype, do not. *Dev. Cogn. Neurosci.* 18, 34–48. doi: 10.1016/j.dcn.2015.11.005

Donnelly, J. E., Hillman, C. H., Castelli, D., Etnier, J. L., Lee, S., Tomporowski, P., et al. (2016). Physical activity, fitness, cognitive function, and academic achievement in children. *Med. Sci. Sports Exerc.* 48, 1197–1222. doi: 10.1249/MSS.0000000000000901

Drollette, E. S., Scudder, M. R., Raine, L. B., Moore, R. D., Saliba, B. J., Pontifex, M. B., et al. (2014). Acute exercise facilitates brain function and cognition in children who need it most: an ERP study of individual differences in inhibitory control capacity. *Dev. Cogn. Neurosci.* 7, 53–64. doi: 10.1016/j.dcn.2013.1 1.001

Duncan, G. J., Claessens, A., Magnuson, K., Klebanov, P., Pagani, L. S., Feinstein, L., et al. (2007). School readiness and later achievement. *Dev. Psychol.* 43, 1428–1446. doi: 10.1037/0012-1649.43.6.1428

Eriksen, B. A., and Eriksen, C. W. (1974). Effects of noise letters upon the identification of a target letter in a nonsearch task. *Percept. Psychophys.* 16, 143–149. doi: 10.3758/BF03203267

Ferris, L. T., Williams, J. S., and Shen, C.-L. (2007). The effect of acute exercise on serum brain-derived neurotrophic factor levels and cognitive function. *Med. Sci. Sports Exerc.* 39, 728–734. doi: 10.1249/mss.0b013e31802f04c7

Gallotta, M. C., Emerenziani, G. P., Iazzoni, S., Meucci, M., Baldari, C., and Guidetti, L. (2015). Impacts of coordinative training on normal weight and overweight/obese children's attentional performance. *Front. Hum. Neurosci.* 9:577. doi: 10.3389/fnhum.2015.00577

Gardner, R. A., and Broman, M. (1979). The Purdue pegboard: normative data on 1334 school children. *J. Clin. Child Psychol.* 8, 156–162. doi: 10.1080/15374417909532912

Geertsen, S. S., Thomas, R., Larsen, M. N., Dahn, I. M., Andersen, J. N., Krause-Jensen, M., et al. (2016). Motor skills and exercise capacity are associated with objective measures of cognitive functions and academic performance in preadolescent children. *PLoS ONE* 11:e0161960. doi: 10.1371/journal.pone.0161960

Gelman, A., and Carlin, J. (2014). Beyond power calculations: assessing Type S (Sign) and Type M (Magnitude) errors. *Perspect. Psychol. Sci.* 9, 641–651. doi: 10.1177/1745691614551642

Gomez-Pinilla, F., and Hillman, C. (2013). The influence of exercise on cognitive abilities. *Compr. Physiol.* 3, 403–428. doi: 10.1002/cphy.c110063

Haapala, E. A., Poikkeus, A. M., Tompuri, T., Kukkonen-Harjula, K., Leppänen, P. H., Lindi, V., et al. (2014). Associations of motor and cardiovascular performance with academic skills in children. *Med. Sci. Sports Exerc.* 46, 1016–1024. doi: 10.1249/MSS.0000000000000186

Hillman, C. H., Castelli, D. M., and Buck, S. M. (2005). Aerobic fitness and neurocognitive function in healthy preadolescent children. *Med. Sci. Sports Exerc.* 37, 1967–1974. doi: 10.1249/01.mss.0000176680.79702.ce

Hillman, C. H., Erickson, K. I., and Kramer, A. F. (2008). Be smart, exercise your heart: exercise effects on brain and cognition. *Nat. Rev. Neurosci.* 9, 58–65. doi: 10.1038/nrn2298

Hillman, C. H., Pontifex, M. B., Castelli, D. M., Khan, N. A., Raine, L. B., Scudder, M. R., et al. (2014). Effects of the FITKids randomized controlled trial on executive control and brain function. *Pediatrics* 134, e1063–e1071. doi: 10.1542/peds.2013-3219

Hillman, C. H., Pontifex, M. B., Raine, L. B., Castelli, D. M., Hall, E. E., and Kramer, A. F. (2009). The effect of acute treadmill walking on cognitive control and academic achievement in preadolescent children. *Neuroscience* 159, 1044–1054. doi: 10.1016/j.neuroscience.2009.01.057

Holmes, J., and Adams, J. W. (2006). Working memory and children's mathematical skills: implications for mathematical development and mathematics curricula. *Educ. Psychol.* 26, 339–366. doi: 10.1080/0144341 0500341056

Hothorn, T., Bretz, F., and Westfall, P. (2008). Simultaneous inference in general parametric models. *Biom. J.* 50, 346–363. doi: 10.1002/bimj.200810425

Howie, E. K., and Pate, R. R. (2012). Physical activity and academic achievement in children: a historical perspective. *J. Sport Health Sci.* 1, 160–169. doi: 10.1016/j.jshs.2012.09.003

Kantomaa, M. T., Stamatakis, E., Kankaanpää, A., Kaakinen, M., Rodriguez, A., Taanila, A., et al. (2013). Physical activity and obesity mediate the association between childhood motor function and adolescents' academic achievement. *Proc. Natl. Acad. Sci. U.S.A.* 110, 1917–1922. doi: 10.1073/pnas. 1214574110

Koziol, L. F., Budding, D. E., and Chidekel, D. (2012). From movement to thought: executive function, embodied cognition, and the cerebellum. *Cerebellum* 11, 505–525. doi: 10.1007/s12311-011-0321-y

Larsen, M. N., Helge, E. W., Madsen, M., Manniche, V., Hansen, L., Hansen, P. R., et al. (2016). Positive effects on bone mineralisation and muscular fitness after 10 months of intense school-based physical training for children aged 8–10 years: the FIT FIRST randomised controlled trial. *Br. J. Sports Med.* doi: 10.1136/bjsports-2016-096219. [Epub ahead of print].

Lopes, L., Santos, R., Pereira, B., and Lopes, V. P. (2013). Associations between gross motor coordination and academic achievement in elementary school children. *Hum. Mov. Sci.* 32, 9–20. doi: 10.1016/j.humov.2012.05.005

Luciana, M., and Nelson, C. A. (2002). Assessment of neuropsychological function through use of the Cambridge neuropsychological testing automated battery: performance in 4- to 12-Year- old children. *Dev. Neuropsychol.* 22, 595–624. doi: 10.1207/S15326942DN2203_3

Macedonia, M., Müller, K., and Friederici, A. D. (2011). The impact of iconic gestures on foreign language word learning and its neural substrate. *Hum. Brain Mapp.* 32, 982–998. doi: 10.1002/hbm.21084

Mahar, M. T., Murphy, S. K., Rowe, D. A., Golden, J., Shields, A. T., and Raedeke, T. D. (2006). Effects of a classroom-based program on physical activity and on-task behavior. *Med. Sci. Sports Exerc.* 38, 2086–2094. doi: 10.1249/01.mss.0000235359.16685.a3

Mavilidi, M. F., Okely, A. D., Chandler, P., Cliff, D. P., and Paas, F. (2015). Effects of integrated physical exercises and gestures on preschool children's foreign language vocabulary learning. *Educ. Psychol. Rev.* 27, 413–426. doi: 10.1007/s10648-015-9337-z

Mayer, K. M., Yildiz, I. B., Macedonia, M., and von Kriegstein, K. (2015). Visual and motor cortices support the translation of foreign language words. *Curr. Biol.* 25, 530–535. doi: 10.1016/j.cub.2014.11.068

Moreau, D., Kirk, I. J., and Waldie, K. E. (2016). Seven pervasive statistical flaws in cognitive training interventions. *Front. Hum. Neurosci.* 10:153. doi: 10.3389/fnhum.2016.00153

Mullender-Wijnsma, M. J., Hartman, E., de Greeff, J. W., Bosker, R. J., Doolaard, S., and Visscher, C. (2015). Moderate-to-vigorous physically active academic lessons and academic engagement in children with and without a social disadvantage: a within subject experimental design. *BMC Public Health* 15:404. doi: 10.1186/s12889-015-1745-y

Mullender-Wijnsma, M. J., Hartman, E., de Greeff, J. W., Doolaard, S., Bosker, R. J., and Visscher, C. (2016). Physically active math and language lessons improve scademic schievement: a cluster randomized controlled trial. *Pediatrics* 137, e20152743. doi: 10.1542/peds.2015-2743

Parsons, S., and Bynner, J. (2005). *Does Numeracy Matter More?* London: National Research and Development Centre for Adult Literacy and Numeracy.

Pesce, C. (2012). Shifting the focus from quantitative to qualitative exercise characteristics in exercise and cognition research. *J. Sport Exerc. Psychol.* 34, 766–786. doi: 10.1123/jsep.34.6.766

Pesce, C., and Ben-Soussan, T. D. (2016). "Cogito ergo sum or "ambulo ergo sum?" New perspectives in developmental exercise and cognition research," in *Exercise-Cognition Interaction*, ed T. McMorris (London: Elsevier Inc.), 251.

Pesce, C., Crova, C., Cereatti, L., Casella, R., and Bellucci, M. (2009). Physical activity and mental performance in preadolescents: Effects of acute exercise on free-recall memory. *Ment. Health Phys. Act.* 2, 16–22. doi: 10.1016/j.mhpa.2009.02.001

Pesce, C., Crova, C., Marchetti, R., Struzzolino, I., Masci, I., Vannozzi, G., et al. (2013). Searching for cognitively optimal challenge point in physical activity for children with typical and atypical motor development. *Ment. Health Phys. Act.* 6, 172–180. doi: 10.1016/j.mhpa.2013.07.001

Pesce, C., Masci, I., Marchetti, R., Vazou, S., Sääkslahti, A., and Tomporowski, P. D. (2016). Deliberate play and preparation jointly benefit motor and cognitive development: mediated and moderated effects. *Front. Psychol.* 7:349. doi: 10.3389/fpsyg.2016.00349

Polich, J. (2007). Updating P300: an integrative theory of P3a and P3b. *Clin. Neurophysiol.* 118, 2128–2148. doi: 10.1016/j.clinph.2007.04.019

Pontifex, M. B., Saliba, B. J., Raine, L. B., Picchietti, D. L., and Hillman, C. H. (2013). Exercise improves behavioral, neurocognitive and scholastic performance in children with ADHD. *J. Pediatr.* 162, 543–551. doi: 10.1016/j.jpeds.2012.08.036

Raghubar, K. P., Barnes, M. A., and Hecht, S. A. (2010). Working memory and mathematics: a review of developmental, individual difference, and cognitive approaches. *Learn. Individ. Differ.* 20, 110–122. doi: 10.1016/j.lindif.2009.10.005

Roebers, C. M., Röthlisberger, M., Neuenschwander, R., Cimeli, P., Michel, E., and Jäger, K. (2014). The relation between cognitive and motor performance and their relevance for children's transition to school: a latent variable approach. *Hum. Mov. Sci.* 33, 284–297. doi: 10.1016/j.humov.2013.08.011

Scharoun, S. M., and Bryden, P. J. (2014). Hand preference, performance abilities, and hand selection in children. *Front. Psychol.* 5:82. doi: 10.3389/fpsyg.2014.00082

Schmidt-Kassow, M., Deusser, M., Thiel, C., Otterbein, S., Montag, C., Reuter, M., et al. (2013). Physical exercise during encoding improves vocabulary learning in young female adults: a neuroendocrinological study. *PLoS ONE* 8:e64172. doi: 10.1371/journal.pone.0064172

Schmidt, M., Benzing, V., and Kamer, M. (2016). Classroom-based physical activity breaks and children's attention: cognitive engagement works! *Front. Psychol.* 7:1474. doi: 10.3389/fpsyg.2016.01474

Schonert-Reichl, K. A., Oberle, E., Lawlor, M. S., Abbott, D., Thomson, K., Oberlander, T. F., et al. (2015). Enhancing cognitive and social-emotional development through a simple-to-administer mindfullness-based school program for elementary school children: a randomized controlled trial. *Dev. Psychol.* 51, 52–66. doi: 10.1037/a0038454

Skriver, K., Roig, M., Lundbye-Jensen, J., Pingel, J., Helge, J. W., Kiens, B., et al. (2014). Acute exercise improves motor memory: exploring potential biomarkers. *Neurobiol. Learn. Mem.* 116, 46–58. doi: 10.1016/j.nlm.2014.08.004

St. Clair-Thompson, H. L., and Gathercole, S. E. (2006). Executive functions and achievements in school: shifting, updating, inhibition, and working memory. *Q. J. Exp. Psychol. (Hove).* 59, 745–759. doi: 10.1080/17470210500162854

Tiffin, J., and Asher, E. J. (1948). The Purdue pegboard; norms and studies of reliability and validity. *J. Appl. Psychol.* 32, 234–247. doi: 10.1037/h0061266

Tomporowski, P. D., McCullick, B., Pendleton, D. M., and Pesce, C. (2015). Exercise and children's cognition: the role of exercise characteristics and a place for metacognition. *J. Sport Health Sci.* 4, 47–55. doi: 10.1016/j.jshs.2014.09.003

van Kesteren, M. T., Rijpkema, M., Ruiter, D. J., Morris, R. G., and Fernández, G. (2014). Building on prior knowledge: schema-dependent encoding processes relate to academic performance. *J. Cogn. Neurosci.* 26, 2250–2261. doi: 10.1162/jocn_a_00630

Vazou, S., and Smiley-Oyen, A. (2014). Moving and academic learning are not antagonists: acute effects on executive function and enjoyment. *J. Sport Exerc. Psychol.* 36, 474–485. doi: 10.1123/jsep.2014-0035

Vazou, S., Pesce, C., Lakes, K., and Smiley-Oyen, A. (2016). More than one road leads to Rome: a narrative review and meta-analysis of physical activity intervention effects on cognition in youth. *Int. J. Sport Exerc. Psychol.* doi: 10.1080/1612197X.2016.1223423. [Epub ahead of print].

Vazou, S., and Skrade, M. A. B. (2016). Intervention integrating physical activity with math: math performance, perceived competence, and need satisfaction. *Int. J. Sport Exerc. Psychol.* doi: 10.1080/1612197x.2016.1164226. [Epub ahead of print].

Voelcker-Rehage, C., Godde, B., and Staudinger, U. M. (2010). Physical and motor fitness are both related to cognition in old age. *Eur. J. Neurosci.* 31, 167–176. doi: 10.1111/j.1460-9568.2009.07014.x

Voelcker-Rehage, C., and Niemann, C. (2013). Structural and functional brain changes related to different types of physical activity across the life span. *Neurosci. Biobehav. Rev.* 37, 2268–2295. doi: 10.1016/j.neubiorev.2013.01.028

Voss, M. W., Chaddock, L., Kim, J. S., Vanpatter, M., Pontifex, M. B., Raine, L. B., et al. (2011). Aerobic fitness is associated with greater efficiency of the network underlying cognitive control in preadolescent children. *Neuroscience* 199, 166–176. doi: 10.1016/j.neuroscience.2011.10.009

Voss, M. W., Vivar, C., Kramer, A. F., and van Praag, H. (2013). Bridging animal and human models of exercise-induced brain plasticity. *Trends Cogn. Sci.* 17, 525–544. doi: 10.1016/j.tics.2013.08.001

Winter, B., Breitenstein, C., Mooren, F. C., Voelker, K., Fobker, M., Lechtermann, A., et al. (2007). High impact running improves learning. *Neurobiol. Learn. Mem.* 87, 597–609. doi: 10.1016/j.nlm.2006.11.003

14

Enhancing Brain Plasticity to Promote Stroke Recovery

*Fan Su and Wendong Xu**

Department of Hand Surgery, Huashan Hospital, Shanghai Medical College, Fudan University, Shanghai, China

Edited by:
Rick M. Dijkhuizen, University Medical Center Utrecht, Netherlands

Reviewed by:
Eduardo Candelario-Jalil, University of Florida, United States
Natasha A. Lannin, Monash University, Australia

***Correspondence:**
Wendong Xu
wendongxu@fudan.edu.cn

Stroke disturbs both the structural and functional integrity of the brain. The understanding of stroke pathophysiology has improved greatly in the past several decades. However, effective therapy is still limited, especially for patients who are in the subacute or chronic phase. Multiple novel therapies have been developed to improve clinical outcomes by improving brain plasticity. These approaches either focus on improving brain remodeling and restoration or on constructing a neural bypass to avoid brain injury. This review describes emerging therapies, including modern rehabilitation, brain stimulation, cell therapy, brain-computer interfaces, and peripheral nervous transfer, and highlights treatment-induced plasticity. Key evidence from basic studies on the underlying mechanisms is also briefly discussed. These insights should lead to a deeper understanding of the overall neural circuit changes, the clinical relevance of these changes in stroke, and stroke treatment progress, which will assist in the development of future approaches to enhance brain function after stroke.

Keywords: brain restoration, plasticity, stroke, neural bypass, brain remodeling

INTRODUCTION

Stroke represents the leading cause of long-term disability and causes substantial medical and financial burdens. Even with standard rehabilitation after stroke, the majority of stroke patients are disabled when they enter the chronic phase (1). The lack of effective neurorepair and limitations of functional recovery have led researchers to consider other approaches that improve the scope for recovery by enhancing brain plasticity.

Brain plasticity is defined as the intrinsic ability of the brain to reorganize its function and structure in response to stimuli and injuries. After stroke, the plasticity process is initiated in an attempt to compensate for both the lesion itself and its remote effects. Changed neural activity and connectivity in terms of function and structure could be detected in the perilesional and remote regions and even in the contralateral hemisphere, which were assumed to be the mechanisms underlying spontaneous recovery (2, 3). Generally, increased neural activity and connectivity in the ipsilesional hemisphere were reported as indicators of better functional recovery (4). However, the roles of the recruitment of the contralateral hemisphere seem to be mixed, as both supportive and inhibitory influences of the unaffected hemisphere were detected during recovery. Compensatory or maladaptive processes may contribute to the inconsistency; these processes were attributed to, at least partially, the time since stroke, location and size of the lesion, and other biological factors (e.g., age of the patient) (5, 6).

Various post-stroke interventions have been developed to improve recovery, which either intentionally or not promote the plasticity of the remaining neural circuit. In addition to conventional therapies (i.e., physical, occupational, and speech), novel approaches have shown promising effects in clinical trials. Many of the approaches were designed to enhance plasticity in the ipsilesional hemisphere, in which increased activity/connectivity was related to better functional performance. However, the results obtained thus far are complicated, and even when significant improvements were made, the effect sizes were not satisfactory in most cases.

As mentioned above, stroke leads to disturbances across the brain, and interhemispheric interactions have complex influences on functional recovery (6, 7). Accordingly, strategies for recovery may include modulation of the intact hemisphere, and work related to this approach has been performed. In this review, we summarize post-stroke interventions that enhance brain plasticity and functional recovery, placing emphasis on modulation of the intact hemisphere. Acute revascularization and neuroprotection are not included, and approaches that were only utilized in basic researches were also excluded. We searched the PubMed from January 1990 to May 2020. Search key words were combinations of "stroke" and "plasticity or neural plasticity or neuroplasticity or brain remodeling or brain rewire." The article type was limited to Clinical trial. The final list of references is based on the relevance of the articles to the scope of this review. We did not intend to provide a comprehensive analysis but instead aimed to highlight novel evidence from well-designed trials. In the next section, we discuss the selected examples of promising approaches listed in **Figure 1**, including modern rehabilitation, brain stimulation, cell therapy, brain-computer interfaces (BCIs), and peripheral nerve transfer. The representative trails that evaluated each intervention were listed in **Table 1**.

MAIN TEXT

Modern Rehabilitation

Conventional rehabilitation approaches, such as physical therapy for motor disability and speech and language therapy for aphasia, have been widely practiced. Meta-analyses and recent large-scale randomized controlled clinical trials suggested that therapy is beneficial if it has a high intensity, involves a high dose or occurs over a long period of time (45, 46). Therapy-induced plasticity was suggested to mediate recovery. Generally, increased structural connectivity in both hemispheres correlated with better performance, and functional reactivation on the affected side promoted recovery (2, 47, 48). Two forms of rehabilitation are expected to exceed the efficacy of conventional approaches, i.e., constraint-induced movement therapy (CIMT) and mirror therapy/action observation therapy (49–51). In CIMT, the constraint of the unaffected limb relieved the learned disuse and modified the amendment of maladaptive plasticity across the brain (52). Mirror therapy improved post-stroke recovery on the basis of enhancing the mirror neuron system, which refers to the neurons that are involved in the performance of the observed actions (53). In addition to physiotherapy, advances in modern technology have enriched the means of promoting post-stroke recovery. The combinations of physiotherapy and new technologies have been extensively tested in clinical trials. For example, telerehabilitation is an emerging field owing to the advancement of telehealth, which enables patients to receive home-based, high-dose supervised practice. The field is still emerging, and meta-analysis has suggested that telerehabilitation may be a promising intervention aimed at improving multiple functional deficits after stroke; however, more studies are needed to draw definitive conclusions (54, 55).

Robot-Assisted Training

Electromechanical and robot-assisted training are of particular interest, and studies have been performed to explore their efficiency. According to a recent Cochrane review, high-quality evidence supports that robot-assisted arm training improves activities of daily living, arm function, and muscle strength in stroke survivors (56). For lower limbs, patients receiving electromechanical-assisted gait training combined with physiotherapy were more likely to walk independently (57). The main reason for the robot-induced improvements was speculated to be the motivation due to the feedback of the device, the novelty of a robotic device, or both. Although concern remains as to whether robot-assisted therapy is more beneficial than traditional interventions at the same intensity, specific brain plasticity was found during robot-assisted therapy. For patients with stroke, increased ipsilateral sensorimotor cortex activation was detected when performing the practiced task delivered by a robot (8), and ipsilateral somatosensory integration strongly modified hand function gains after robot-assisted training (9). Furthermore, interhemispheric plasticity was also shown to be involved in the recovery process. For instance, a relationship was reported between motor recovery and the normalization of the interhemispheric connectivity between bilateral primary somatosensory areas (10). Further, in stroke models, the combination of robot-assisted training and inactivation of the unaffected hemisphere contributed to significantly improved motor function compared to that achieved with robot-assisted training alone, and functional recovery was accompanied by significantly reduced interhemispheric inhibition (IHI) (58). In brief, robot-assisted therapy appears to be effective for patients with stroke, and the modification of plasticity in both hemispheres seems to mediate functional recovery. Nevertheless, it should be noted that the absolute improvements of robotic therapy were small in some investigations, which limits its clinical promotion (11).

Virtual Reality

In addition to robotic therapy, virtual reality (VR) technology has also been widely tested in post-stroke therapy. Numerous clinical studies have been conducted in the field, and the latest meta-analysis suggests that when combined with traditional therapy, VR technology can further improve the prognosis of patients, especially in regards to the dimensions of their upper limb motor function and daily living ability (59). Favorable results were also reported in improving post-stroke balance, gait and neglect (12, 60). At the mechanistic level, VR-induced neuroplasticity has also been confirmed. Similarly, increased recruitment of the ipsilesional hemisphere may mediate functional recovery. For instance, enhanced activation in the ipsilesional sensorimotor

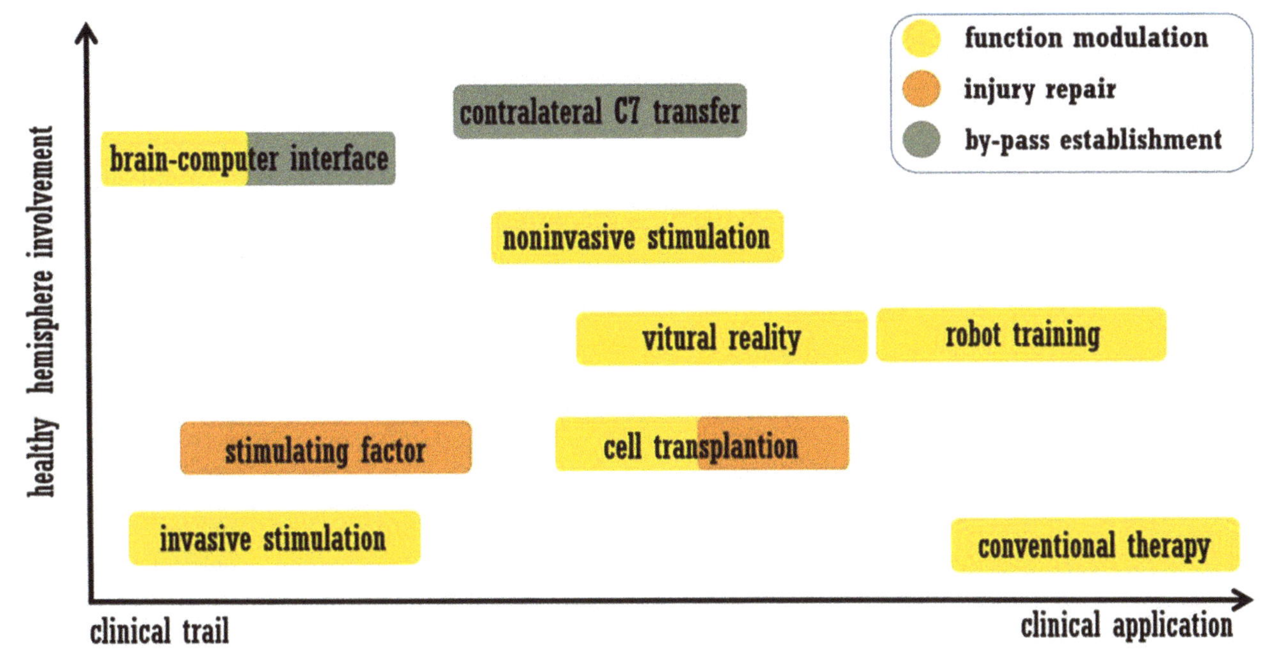

FIGURE 1 | Summary of treatment approaches discussed in this review. The abscissa indicates the readiness of clinical application, and the ordinate indicates the involvement of the healthy hemisphere.

cortex correlates with motor improvement (13), and increases in frontal neuronal activity may reflect the plasticity processes underlying positive rehabilitation effects for chronic neglect (12, 61). VR treatment can also induce plasticity in the contralateral hemisphere and cerebellum. On the one hand, functional relateralization to the ipsilesional side was reported to support recovery (14, 62), while on the other hand, improved overall brain activity (including that in the contralateral cortex and cerebellum) was also suggested to drive recovery (15, 16). Although specific neural patterns of reorganization were highlighted by the above trials, there was insufficient evidence to reach definitive conclusions about VR-induced plasticity. Additional studies should address specific questions about the type, timing, frequency, and duration of modern tech-assisted therapy. A deeper understanding of the treatment-related mechanisms and large, definitive and pragmatic phase III trials should be encouraged. Individualized treatment and the use of multiple techniques in combination (such as VR and BCI) (63) are also worth investigating.

Compared with conventional rehabilitation, VR and robot-assisted therapy may advantageously increase the frequency and motivation of rehabilitation training and independent exercise (64, 65). Furthermore, it also enables the participants to practice everyday activities that are not available in the hospital (59). However, a decline in the participant's medical condition (e.g., treatment-unrelated infection), private reasons (e.g., difficulty traveling) and absence of a physiotherapist may limit access to therapy. Although no serious side effects related to treatment have been reported thus far, participants may experience pain, dizziness, headache and high tension after therapy (56, 57, 59).

Brain Stimulation

Brain stimulation represents a promising area of research because it allows the excitability of the target area to be manipulated directly; pertinently, techniques including transcranial magnetic stimulation (TMS), transcranial direct current stimulation (tDCS), cortical microelectrode stimulation and deep brain stimulation (DBS) have been utilized in this field. Compared to non-invasive stimulation approaches, invasive approaches can deliver stimulation for longer periods at more precise locations. Pilot clinical studies have demonstrated safety and feasibility for implanted cortical electrical stimulation in the ipsilesional M1 region, and improved arm function has also been suggested (66). Evidence has suggested that DBS can help manage various post-stroke maladaptive disorders, especially reducing pain (67).

TMS/tDCS in Stroke Treatment

Non-invasive stimulations have been more widely used, and the stimulation parameters determine whether the stimulation increases or decreases brain activity. Generally, anodal tDCS (A-tDCS) has been shown to enhance cortical activity, whereas cathodal tDCS (C-tDCS) usually has the opposite effect. Depending on the frequency, repetitive TMS (rTMS) can reduce [low frequency (LF): ~1 Hz] or increase [high frequency (HF): 5~20 Hz] corticospinal excitability. Both tDCS and rTMS have been used to treat various post-stroke deficits, particularly motor impairment and aphasia. Meta-analyses may imply the effectiveness of non-invasive stimulations, and recent trials with randomized, blind and controlled designs have encouraged further investigation in this field (68–70). For

TABLE 1 | Representative clinical trials evaluating novel interventions for stroke recovery.

Trial	Stroke phrase	No. of subjects	Intervention	Main outcome	Others
Takahashi et al. (8)	Chronic	13	Robot	Safety, improved arm motor	fMRI: Increased sensorimotor cortex activation after therapy
Ingemanson et al. (9)	Chronic	30	Robot	Safety, improved arm motor	fMRI: Somatosensory system integrity predicts recovery
Pellegrino et al. (10)	Chronic	7	Robot	Improved arm motor	EEG: Modulation of the interhemispheric coherence correlated with recovery
Klamroth-Marganska et al. (11)	Chronic	73	Robot	Safety, improved arm motor	-
Ekman et al. (12)	Chronic	12	VR	Improvement in chronic neglect	fMRI: increased activation in prefrontal and temporal cortex
Xiao et al. (13)	Subacute	8	VR	Improved walking	fMRI: Increased activation in primary sensorimotor cortex correlated with recovery
Saleh et al. (14)	Chronic	19	Robot-Assisted VR	Improved arm motor	fMRI: Brain activity re-lateralized to the ipsilesional side, which correlated with recovery
Orihuela-Espina et al. (15)	Chronic	8	VR	Improved arm motor	fMRI: Increased contralesional activation correlated with recovery
Wang et al. (16)	Subacute	26	VR	Safety and feasibility	fMRI: Increased activation intensity and the laterality index of the contralateral primary sensorimotor cortex
Saposnik et al. (17)	Subacute	141	VR	Safety and improved arm motor	No superiority over recreational activity interventions
Jang et al. (18)	Chronic	5	VR	Improved arm motor	fMRI: Decreased ipsilateral activation and increased contralateral activation
Kim et al. (19)	Chronic	24	VR	Improved balance and walking	-
Stagg et al. (20)	Chronic	24*	A-tDCS over affected hemisphere or C-tDCS over unaffected hemisphere	Improved arm motor in both experiments	fMRI: Increased ipsilesional activation correlated with recovery
Chang et al. (21)	Subacute	24	A-tDCS over affected hemisphere	Better lower limb motor (not significant)	MEP: shorter in latency and higher in amplitude
Darkow et al. (22)	Chronic	16	A-tDCS over left M1	No improvement of naming	fMRI: Reduced activity in regions mediating cognitive control; increased language network activity; increased within-network communication
Meinzer et al. (23)	Chronic	26	A-tDCS over left M1	Improved naming and communication	-
Monti et al. (24)	Chronic	8	C-tDCS over left frontotemporal region	Improved naming	A-tDCS failed to improve aphasia
Au-Yeung et al. (25)	Chronic	10	C-tDCS over unaffected M1	Improved hand dexterity	A-tDCS failed to improve motor
Du et al. (26)	Acute	60	LF-TMS over the unaffected hemisphere	Improved arm motor	fMRI: decreased activity in the unaffected cortex
Au-Yeung et al. (27)	Acute, subacute and chronic	49	LF-TMS over the unaffected hemisphere	Improved arm motor	Effectiveness depends on hemispheric dominance

(Continued)

TABLE 1 | Continued

Trial	Stroke phrase	No. of subjects	Intervention	Main outcome	Others
Nowak et al. (28)	Subacute	15	LF-TMS over the unaffected hemisphere	Improved arm motor	fMRI: Decreased overactivity in the contralesional hemisphere; overactivity of the contralesional hemisphere predicted recovery
Grefkes et al. (29)	Subacute	11	LF-TMS over the unaffected hemisphere	Improved arm motor	fMRI: Reduction of interhemisphere inhibition correlated with motor recovery
Kondziolka et al. (30)	Chronic	18	Intracranial delivery of NT2	Safety, feasibility and improved arm motor	-
Prasad et al. (31)	Subacute	120	Intravenous delivery of BMSCs	Safety and feasibility; no improvement in stroke outcome	-
Friedrich et al. (32)	Acute	20	Intraarterial delivery of BMSCs	Safety and feasibility	Some patients showed good outcome
Savitz et al. (33)	Subacute	100	Intracarotid delivery of ALD-401	Safety and feasibility; no improvement of stroke outcome	Smaller lesions in treatment group (no significant)
Steinberg et al. (34)	Chronic	18	Intracerebral implantation of SB623	Safety; improved stroke outcome	-
Muir et al. (35)	Subacute and chronic	23	intracerebral implantation of CTX0E03	Safety, feasibility, improved arm motor	-
Sharma et al. (36)	Chronic	24	Intrathecal delivery of BMSCs	Safety; improved arm motor and balance	-
Fang et al. (37)	Acute	18	Intravenous delivery of EPCs	Safety and feasibility	No significant improvement of stroke outcome
Ramos-Murguialday et al. (38)	Chronic	30	BCI	Improved arm motor	fMRI: No significant difference
Wu et al. (39)	Subacute	25	BCI	Improved arm motor	fMRI: Increased neural activity across the whole brain; inter-hemispheric connectivity correlated with recovery
Pichiorri et al. (40)	Subacute	28	BCI	Improved arm motor	EEG: Ipsilesional intrahemispheric connectivity correlated with recovery
Carino-Escobar et al. (41)	Subacute and chronic	9	BCI	Improved arm motor	EEG: Longitudinal Trends ERD/ERS correlated with recovery
Hua et al. (42)	Chronic	12	CC7	Safety and improved arm motor	-
Zheng et al. (43)	Chronic	36	CC7	Safety and improved arm motor	TMS and fMRI: Connectivity between the ipsilateral hemisphere and paralyzed arm; establishment of functional regions in ipsilateral hemisphere to control paralyzed arm
Qiu et al. (44)	Chronic	2	Contralateral lumbar-to-sacral nerve rerouting	Safety and improved ambulatory status	-

The trial consisted of two experiments. Experiment 1 enrolled 13 participants and experiment 2 enrolled 11 participants. Seven participants took part in both experiments, which were performed more than 1 year apart.

VR, virtual reality; A-tDCS, anodal transcranial direct current stimulation; C-tDCS, cathodal transcranial direct current stimulation; LF-TMS, low-frequency transcranial magnetic stimulation; BMSCs, bone marrow mononuclear stem cells; SB623, modified bone marrow-derived mesenchymal stem cells; CTX0E03, human neural stem cell line; ALD-401, enriched population of aldehyde dehydrogenase-bright stem cells; EPCs, endothelial progenitor cells; BCI, brain-computer interfaces; CC7, contralateral seventh cervical nerve transfer; ERD/ERS, event-related desynchronization or synchronization.

example, Fridriksson et al. (71) reported that activating the left hemisphere by A-tDCS in chronic stroke patients with aphasia led to a relative 70% increase in correct naming compared to that in the sham tDCS group; this effect lasted for 24 weeks after treatment. For acute stroke patients with motor impairment, enhancing cortical activity via HF-TMS and A-tDCS resulted in improved motor function, and stimulation-induced increased neural activity correlated with recovery (21, 72).

Despite the exciting results described above, the use of TMS/tDCS as a clinical treatment after stroke seems premature (73). As shown in **Figure 2**, A-tDCS and HF-TMS over the injured hemisphere paired with rehabilitation is theoretically assumed to promote post-stroke recovery. However, no definite conclusion has been obtained in regards to aphasia and upper/lower extremity function (68, 74), as more evidence from randomized trials is required. Similarly, the outcomes of stimulating the unaffected hemisphere were also mixed. According to the IHI model, stroke disrupts the interhemispheric balance, and the unaffected hemisphere becomes overactive, which further inhibits the activity of the injured hemisphere (75). Thus, theoretically, suppressing the unaffected hemisphere could also be beneficial for stroke recovery, and evidence supports this concept. For stroke patients in the acute phase, LF-TMS over the unaffected hemisphere in the M1 area led to improved arm function compared to that observed after sham stimulation; this improvement seemed to be mediated by the decreased neural activity in the M1 area of the unaffected hemisphere as measured by fMRI (26). Similar results were also reported in independent participants within 6 months of stroke onset (27, 28). However, inconsistent data were also reported (76), and a reason for the contradiction may be that the inhibitory protocols were effective only for patients with abnormal IHI. As shown by Grefkes et al. rTMS-induced inhibition of the contralesional M1 area showed the greatest therapeutic effects in patients who showed the strongest reduction in IHI as measured by fMRI (29).

The advantage of TMS and tDCS is the non-invasive, precise regulation of excitability within specific brain regions. However, some concerns remain regarding clinical applications that need to be further explored, including the stimulation target, therapeutic time point, and stimulation frequency and parameters (73). Regarding safety, both interventions have been suggested to be safe and well-tolerated. Common adverse effects include dizziness, headache, transient aching and burning sensations. Skin reactions at the electrode contact site are also reported. Serious adverse events, such as epileptic seizures, have rarely been reported in related trials (68, 77).

TMS/tDCS-Induced Plasticity

To conclude, more work is needed to demonstrate the efficiency of brain stimulation in post-stroke recovery. Revealing the

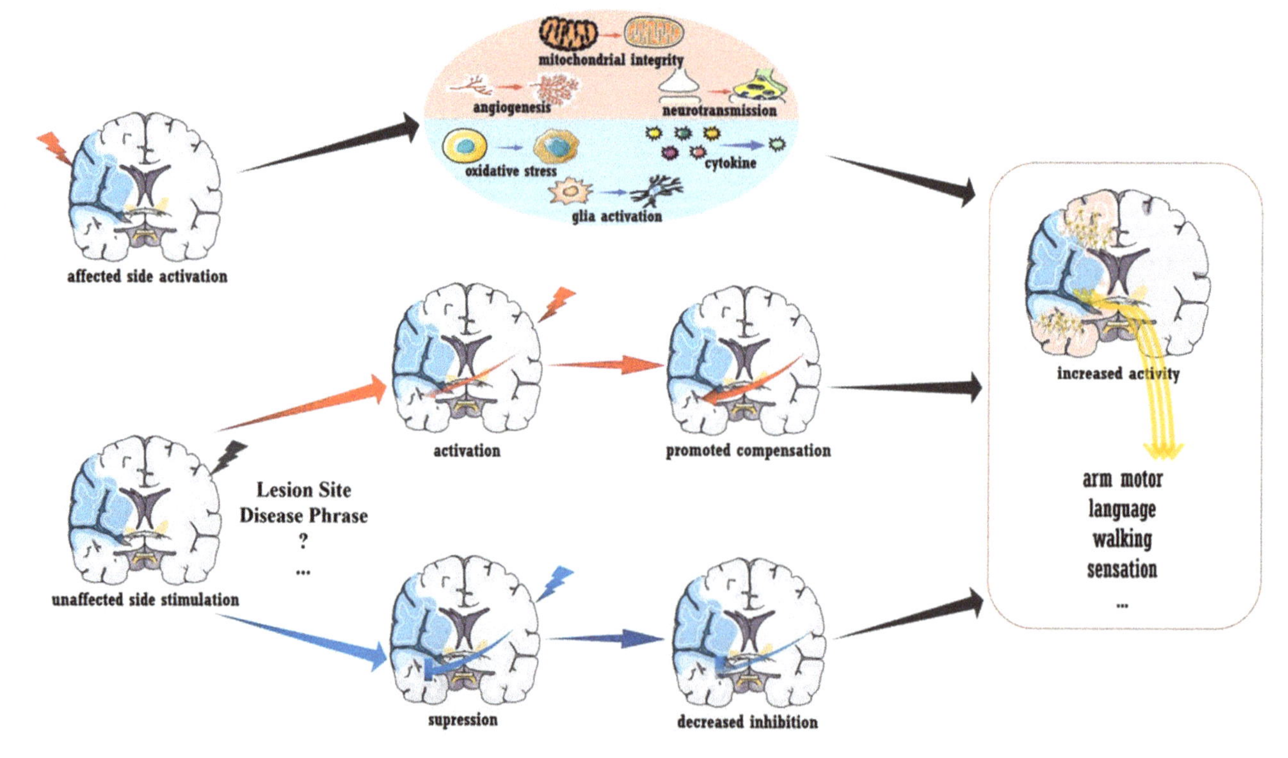

FIGURE 2 | Brain stimulation to promote stroke recovery. Activation of the injured hemisphere can improve prognosis, and the underlying mechanisms may include the promotion of angiogenesis, mitochondrial integrity and neurotransmission and the inhibition of glial activation, pro-inflammatory mediator secretion and oxidative stress. Healthy hemisphere stimulation could have various influences on stroke recovery. Increased interhemispheric compensation (induced by activated stimulation) or reduced interhemispheric suppression (induced by inhibitory stimulation) may mediate clinical recovery.

mechanism underlying plasticity will certainly be advantageous. In addition to the stimulation-induced functional remodeling mentioned above, increased structural connectivity was also detected in a recent preliminary diffusion tensor imaging (DTI) study. As reported, acute patients receiving rTMS showed increased fractional anisotropy (FA) in the contralesional corticospinal tract and bilateral cerebellum (78). In rodent models with acute stroke, stimulation-induced recovery was related to the inhibition of pro-inflammatory cytokines, oxidative stress, and glial activation as well as to the promotion of mitochondrial integrity, angiogenesis, and neurotransmission (shown in **Figure 2**) (79, 80). The modulation of long-term potentiation and long-term depression has been demonstrated *in vitro*, and the brain-derived neurotrophic factor (BDNF)-mediated signaling pathway is involved in this process (81, 82). More importantly, stimulation-induced plasticity should be viewed at the "whole-brain" level rather than at areas of local activation or inhibition. A pilot clinical study reported that activating the premotor cortex and supplementary motor helped the recruitment of the contralesional hemisphere (83). Furthermore, contralesional M1 inhibition could also improve coupling between the premotor cortex and M1 area in the ipsilesional brain (29), and stimulating the left M1 area was reported to enhance language function in chronic stroke patients with aphasia (23). These interactions between different functional areas (i.e., motor-language interaction) and the interhemispheric modulations are believed to mediate functional recovery. Understanding post-stroke and treatment-related plasticity from a holistic and dynamic perspective is key to promoting brain stimulation therapy, and the combination of multiple techniques, such as fMRI, may be an effective approach.

Cell Therapy

Cell therapy is emerging as a viable neurorestorative therapy for stroke, and the number of investigations in this field have surged in recent decades. Stem cells are self-perpetuating and have the ability to transform into multiple cell types. Theoretically, both endogenous and exogenous therapeutic strategies are capable of promoting post-stroke plasticity. The former refers to increasing mobilization, longevity and autologous stem cell production, and the therapeutic targets have focused on neurotrophic and growth factors, inflammatory circumstances, and chemokine receptors (84). Currently, most research in this research has been limited to preclinical studies except for that regarding growth factors. However, according to a recent meta-analysis, there are significant safety concerns regarding the stimulating factors (including erythropoietin, granulocyte colony-stimulating factor and analogs) for patients with acute or subacute stroke (85). Therefore, whether the above treatment can be used in the clinic needs further clarification.

Exogenous Cell Transplantation in Stroke Treatment

In contrast, exogenous cell therapy provides the brain with donor cells, the sources of which are generally divided into three types: immortalized cell lines, neural progenitor or stem cells, and bone marrow-derived progenitor or stem cells (86). Through various administration routes, cells have been assessed in human studies for their ability to improve post-stroke disability. Previous reviews have summarized the evidence to support the safety, feasibility and effectiveness of various cell types, and recent publications have added to our knowledge on this topic (86, 87). The NT2N cell line, derived from teratocarcinoma cells, was first used in clinical trials. By intracerebral administration of the cells into peri-infarct or peri-hemorrhagic regions, safety and functional improvements for patients with chronic stroke were suggested in phase I/II trials (30). Regarding bone marrow mononuclear stem cells (BMSCs), intravenous infusion was tested in a multicenter, randomized trial that included 120 patients with subacute ischemic stroke. Safety was suggested in this trial, but no beneficial effect on stroke outcome was observed (31). Alternative administration (intra-arterial) of BMSCs might be effective, as suggested by a pilot study (88), and the phase II trial is currently ongoing (registered no. NCT02178657 at ClinicalTrials.gov). Furthermore, a recent report showed that intra-arterial BMSC transplantation may modulate circulating miRNA-34a levels; this modulation was related to precursor cell migration and infarct volumes in stroke patients (89). For ALD-401 cells, another type of bone marrow-derived stem cell, intracarotid infusion may be promising for subacute ischemic stroke patients. A recent phase II trial suggested that intracarotid infusion of ALD-401 did not lead to adverse events, and the mean difference in recovery favored the treatment group; however, this difference failed to reach statistical significance (33). The large standard deviation in participants may have contributed to the negative result, and the fact that the trial was terminated when it reached the safety endpoint was also related to the results (90). Phase II trials for bone marrow-derived mesenchymal stem cells (SB623) and human neural stem cells (CTX0E03), which were intravenously and intracellularly implanted, respectively, were completed, and the encouraging results motivated further trials for both cell types (34, 35). Intrathecal injection of bone marrow-derived stem cells was also shown to be safe, and improved functional recovery accompanied by increased brain metabolic activity was suggested by a non-randomized, single-arm trial (36). Further randomized, controlled, blinded trials are in process (registered no. ChiCTR-INR-16008908 at ChiCTR).

In addition to the replacement of dead cells in the infarct area by transplanted cells, the advantages of cell therapy may also be related to the benign regulation of the whole brain microenvironment and plasticity (86, 87) (details in the next section). Regarding safety, despite inconclusiveness between the cell therapy and control groups (91), some potential serious adverse effects should be noted, including neoplastic transformation, worsening of neurological deficit, epilepsy, and even death (91, 92). Moreover, transplantation-related side effects may also include infection, hemorrhage, nausea and vomiting, depression, fatigue and increased blood glucose and CRP levels (93, 94).

Cell Therapy-Induced Plasticity

To conclude, a few questions remain regarding cell therapy for stroke, but the promising results obtained thus far strongly inspire further trials. Several concerns should be carefully addressed in future phase IIb/III investigations, especially regarding the sham procedure and blindness. As illustrated in **Figure 3**, the mechanism underlying cell therapy was originally assumed to be the replacement of injured brain cells by transplanted cells. However, not all evidence supports this concept, especially for cells with a reduced capacity for neural differentiation. It was suggested that ~1/3 of locally injected cells migrate to the focal infarct area (95, 96), while for systematic delivery, <10% exogenous cells arrive at the lesion area (97). Additionally, only a small proportion of migrated cells were shown to differentiate into mature neurons, and the stem cell source dictated the proportion (95, 96, 98). The new neurons were estimated to replace only ~0.2% of the dead neurons due to stroke (99). Furthermore, behavioral improvements were not always related to the number of cells that integrated into the circuit and the timing of synapse formation (100). More importantly, functional recovery independent of integration has also been reported (101). Thus, even though transplanted cells could replace the injured circuit, cell therapy also promoted recovery via other mechanisms. As discussed in other reviews (86, 87), the majority of functional recovery achieved with stem cells was attributed to the enhancement of axonal myelination and synaptic transmission, promotion of neurogenesis and angiogenesis, increased secretion of neurotrophic/growth factors, immunomodulation, reduced apoptosis, maintenance of the blood-brain barrier, and reconstruction of white matter (listed in **Figure 3**). Notably, cell therapy-induced plasticity occurred across the brain. Regarding inflammation and neurotrophic/growth factors, favorable microenvironments were found in both hemispheres and even in the peripheral circulation (86, 102, 103). Landmark evidence was acquired regarding axonal plasticity. For both neural stem cells and bone marrow-derived cells, cell-grafted rats demonstrated increased widespread axonal rewiring from the contralesional side, with transcallosal and corticospinal axonal sprouting correlating with functional recovery (104, 105).

These mechanisms need to be further elucidated. The gap between stroke patients and animal models should be stressed, and it seems that most basic studies focused on acute or subacute stroke. Regarding the different pathophysiological events between acute and chronic stroke, these results may play a limited role in promoting cell therapy for chronic stroke, which has great clinical importance. Furthermore, optimizing the delivery methods and *in vivo* tracking of implanted cells are of great significance.

Brain-Computer Interfaces

Clinical Application of BCI

In contrast to the treatments mentioned above, BCIs constitute a novel idea for functional recovery after stroke, as they avoid the injured area, build a neural bypass based on a healthy brain, and promote dominance in some brain regions. Based on its methodology of measuring brain activity, BCI use can be invasive or non-invasive, and electrical, magnetic or metabolic neuron activity can be recorded. The detected signals are further amplified, filtered, decoded and translated into signals for controlling the external devices or directly

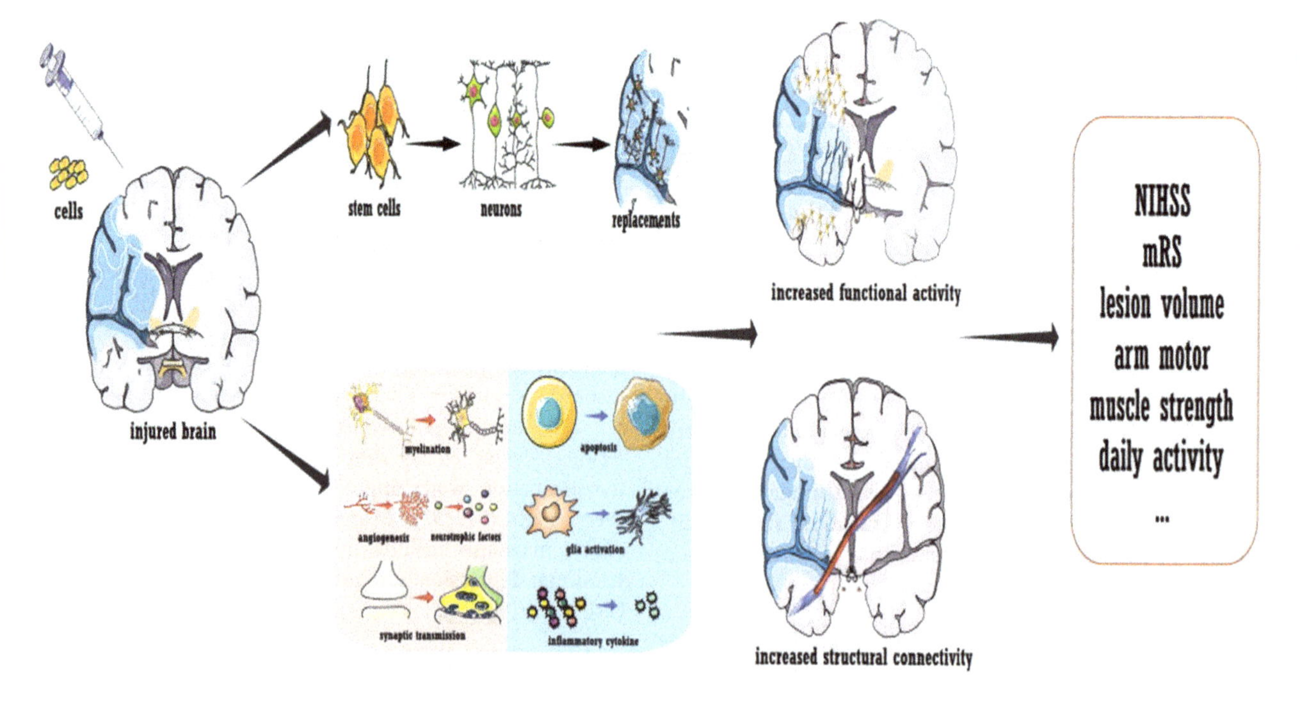

FIGURE 3 | Cell transplantation to promote stroke recovery. Cell therapy was shown to induce the replacement of dead neurons in the infarcted area; more importantly, it ameliorated the microenvironment of the whole brain to promote functional modulation. Treatment not only enhances the neural activity of the injured hemisphere but also improves the structural connection of the whole brain.

stimulating the muscles or the brain (106). The closed-loop system can replace, restore or enhance natural neural output, thereby improving lost function due to brain injury. Although large-scale randomized trials are currently scarce, promising results have been obtained in this field. According to a recent meta-analysis, BCI training was associated with a larger improvement of upper limb motor function (107), which was supported by several other investigations (38, 39). Theoretically, BCI training engages learning and neural adaption processes, and brain remodeling has been detected by posttreatment MRI or electrophysiological tests in stroke patients (108). Overall, increased activity and connectivity in the ipsilesional brain were detected and correlated with behavioral improvements. As suggested by Pichiorri et al. BCIs enhance electroencephalography sensorimotor power spectra and motor improvements associated with increases in ipsilesional intrahemispheric connectivity (40). Furthermore, plasticity may occur in broader brain regions. As determined by both electroencephalography and MRI, increased interhemispheric recruitment correlated with upper limb motor recovery (41). These results may reinforce the hypothesis that broader activation during movement tasks is a form of compensation observed in patients with stroke.

Since BCI was first used in stroke rehabilitation in 2009 (109), evidence supports its safety and effectiveness (106). BCI can be well-integrated with other modern rehabilitation approaches, such as robots, tDCS and motor imagery, providing more feasibility for clinical application (110). However, it should be noted that only a small number of studies explored the long-term effect of BCI in stroke rehabilitation, and this concept needs further validation (110). Moreover, BCI training requires a high degree of concentration and self-regulation; thus, patients with post-stroke emotional or cognitive impairments may not be able to cooperate. To date, no serious BCI-related adverse events have been reported, and common treatment-related side effects include transient nausea, fatigue, and headaches (110, 111).

Basic Research Reveals BCI-Induced Plasticity

Clinical evidence suggests that BCI allowed increased coordination between the multisensory and motor-related cortex and the extrapyramidal system. By inducing neuroplasticity and restoring lost function, BCI represents a feasible option for post-stroke rehabilitation. Exploring BCI-induced plasticity can not only promote post-stroke rehabilitation but also expand our understanding of the mechanisms underlying motor learning. Basic experiments in non-human primates have shed light on this field. As summarized by Shanechi, there may be two neural mechanisms for BCI (108). On the one hand, training directly changed the activity of individual output neurons based on neurofeedback to achieve behavioral goals. Compared with nearby neurons, output neurons exhibited different changes in activity after BCI training. Changes in corticostriatal interactions that are specific to the output neurons were also involved in BCI training (112). On the other hand, training explored an existing pattern of neural activity related to natural movements and then reassociated them, thus serving as a reorganization strategy. This concept was supported by the finding that animals learned to control single-neuron activity by preferentially exploring and exploiting the natural movement repertoire (113). Furthermore, in the population-level changes of neural activity, animals relied on a fixed repertoire of activity patterns and associated those patterns with various movements after learning (114). There was evidence that the seemingly inconsistent processes cooccurred on different time scales in BCI-mediated motor training (108).

The substantial amount of work in preliminary trials and animal models has demonstrated the potential of BCIs to restore upper limb function after stroke. To validate the observed efficiency, more large-scale, randomized, and controlled trials with long-term follow-ups in stroke patients are urgently needed. In addition, BCIs may also play a role in restoring multiple post-stroke functions, such as walking, communication and mood (106, 108, 115). Furthermore, the combination of BCIs and other technologies, such as paired associative stimulation and VR, may represent a feasible approach to optimize BCI treatment (63). The above investigations are still in the initial stage, and only studies in large patient groups can lead to definite conclusions about the value of BCI in specific patient subsets.

Peripheral Nerve Transfer

Contralateral Seventh Cervical Nerve Transfer in the Treatment of Spastic Arm Paralysis

An alternative way to bypass a lesion is contralateral seventh cervical nerve transfer (CC7), a surgical approach developed by our team (43). The principle of the surgery is briefly outlined in **Figure 4**. During the operation, the seventh cervical nerve (C7) from the non-paralyzed side is transferred to the paralyzed side, which enables the development of functional connections between the contralesional hemisphere and the paralyzed arm. This treatment approach has been used for injury to the brachial plexus since the 1980s (116). In addition to the improvement of upper arm function, we also detected post-surgery changes in brain activity (117–119). This phenomenon indicated that rewiring the peripheral nerve connection led to brain plasticity, which supported us in employing surgery to treat spastic arm paralysis (42). As detected by our recent trial enrolling participants with chronic brain injury (25% were stroke patients), CC7 surgery in combination with conventional rehabilitation was associated with a mean increase in the Fugl-Meyer score of 17.7 points (43). The improvement was significantly higher than that of the control group, who received rehabilitation alone, and greatly exceeded the minimal clinically important differences (MCID) for the upper extremity of 5.25 points in chronic stroke cases (120). The surgery induced brain plasticity, mediating functional recovery. The MRI scan showed that at postoperative month 8, voluntary extension of the paralyzed wrist generated neural activation in the contralesional hemisphere. Activation increased in amplitude at postoperative months 10 and 12, while the activation of the ipsilesional hemisphere decreased at postoperative month 12 compared with that at baseline. Furthermore, stimulating the contralesional hemisphere via TMS induced motor-evoked potential in the paralyzed arm at postoperative months 10 and 12. This evidence demonstrates the functional connections between the contralesional hemisphere and the paralyzed arm (indicated in **Figure 4**) (43).

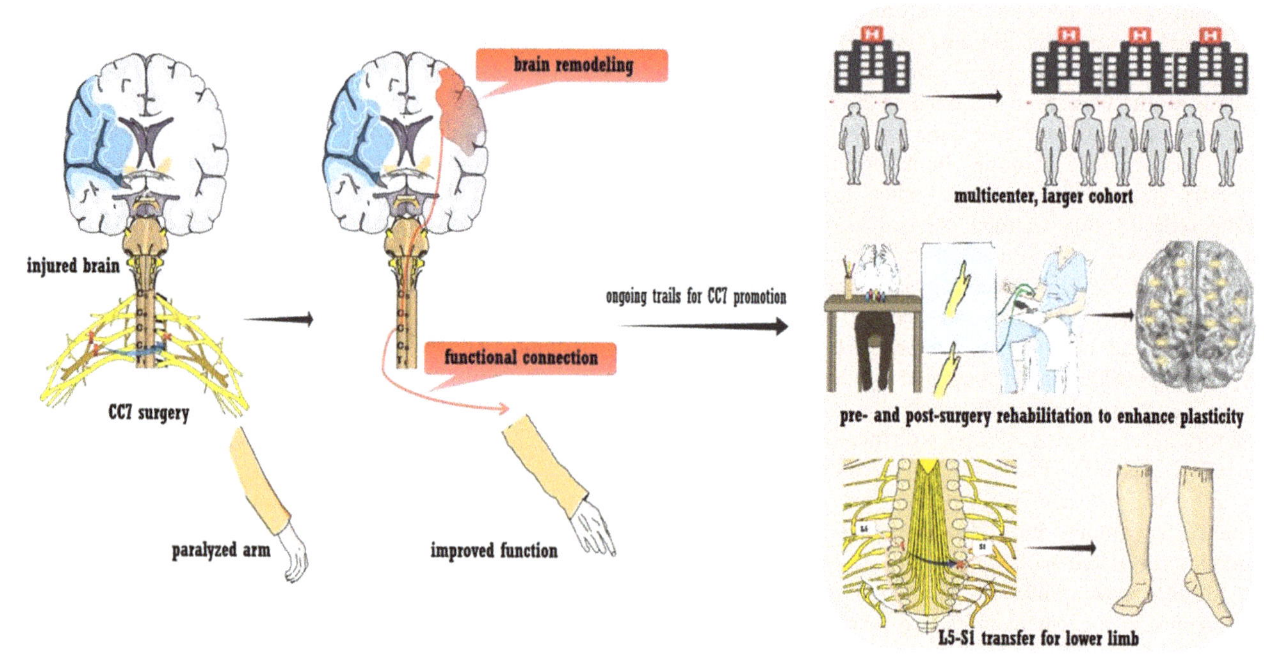

FIGURE 4 | Contralateral seventh cervical nerve transfer (CC7) to promote stroke recovery. A neural bypass was constructed via CC7 surgery to functionally connect the paralyzed hand and healthy hemisphere. Various trials are ongoing regarding CC7 surgery, including a large-sample multicenter trial, L5-S1 transfer to the lower limb, and pre- and post-surgery rehabilitation to facilitate plasticity.

To date, no serious adverse events related to CC7 have occurred. In addition to general surgically related adverse reactions, such as nausea and vomiting, pain in the limb or shoulder, foreign-body sensation while swallowing and fatigue are major adverse events after CC7. Additionally, numbness in the hand, decreased power of elbow/wrist extension and attenuated sensory function occurred on the side of the donor nerve due to neurotomy. All these deficits were almost completely relieved at post-surgery month 3 (43). In the future, we must pay attention to potential risks, including long-term decreases in sensory or motor function, and long-term follow-up is needed to confirm the safety of CC7 surgery.

CC7 in Optimization

Innovative work allows the control of the contralesional hemisphere over the paralyzed arm. In addition to promoting recovery, CC7 surgery also provides opportunities for insights into basic neuroanatomy and neurophysiology. **Figure 4** also shows ongoing trials to promote the treatment approach. First, multicenter trials enrolling larger cohorts with longer follow-ups are in progress to determine whether CC7 results in safe, consistent, and long-term functional improvements. The large sample size will also enable analysis of multidimensional clinical characteristics, exploration of factors that may affect the efficacy of surgery, and provision of a basis for individualized treatment. Second, peripheral nerve transfer has been utilized in treating lower limb dysfunction due to brain injury. Preliminary studies have suggested the feasibility and effectiveness, which needs to be further verified (44). Third, owing to the unique postoperative changes, these traditional rehabilitation approaches may lack a feasible template. The rehabilitation program that targets postoperative dynamic plasticity was assumed to improve efficiency (121). Finally, we hypothesized that intensive preoperative rehabilitation improves brain activity, fully mobilizes brain reserve capacity, and provides a better foundation for postoperative brain remodeling. Thus, a trial testing the effect of preoperative intensive rehabilitation for CC7 is in progress. Last, we are also investigating the mechanisms that underlie brain plasticity in animal models.

Additional evidence will help to confirm the safety and efficiency of CC7, suggest mechanisms underlying brain plasticity, and establish a better CC7 treatment scheme.

CONCLUSIONS

Plasticity is a natural property of the human brain, and its lifelong capacity enables us a much longer therapeutic window for post-stroke neural restoration than previously assumed. As summarized in previous reviews (84, 122, 123), the modulation of plasticity to promote post-stroke recovery has increasingly advanced in recent decades. This current review updates the previous ones by discussing the results from the latest trials. Key evidence from basic studies was also highlighted to provide a more comprehensive overview. Furthermore, stroke is a complicated disease affecting various brain regions, resulting in disruption of entire brain networks and widespread dysfunctions.

A study targeting only certain molecular pathways or areas surrounding the injury may have limited significance. Some innovative ideas, such as BCI and CC7, that induce and employ plasticity in the healthy hemisphere may be of significance, and the promotion and optimization of these novel approaches may contribute to stroke therapy.

Emerging evidence has renewed our knowledge of post-stroke therapy. As discussed in the review, approaches that support injured neural circuits or rewire neural pathways have been developed. Exciting improvements in clinical function were achieved, accompanied by the successful induction of plasticity across the whole brain. Despite the exciting achievements, further investigations are strongly encouraged. The clinical trialists are still looking to test more novel interventions, as the increased understanding of stroke recovery and development of techniques to measure and enhance brain plasticity will continue to promote the interventions. Moreover, the inconsistent results have been constantly reported in trials that evaluating each intervention for stroke recovery. The heterogeneity of participants enrolled and the parameters of treatment may be related to the inconsistency, which should be illustrated in future trial. For instance, the timing for the intervention should be considered. The traditional concept suggests that the degree for improving plasticity is larger in earlier stages than in later stages. Accordingly, many trials tended to enroll patients in the early phase (<6 months) after stroke onset. However, the stressful microenvironment in the early post-stroke stage may inhibit treatment-induced plasticity. Indeed, much evidence has challenged "the earlier the better" principle (123). Additionally, priority should also be given to the individualized treatment, which require a deeper understanding of the pathophysiological process and better measurement of brain activity for participants. The trialists may consider the application of genomics, proteomics, neuroimaging and electrophysiology in future trial. Meanwhile, advancements in basic research will substantially contribute to post-stroke therapy. On one hand, novel therapies are beginning to emerge from the basic research. For example, optogenetics is a revolutionary neuroscience tool that uses bioengineered light-sensitive proteins to selectively activate or inhibit specific cell types and neural circuits, and the optogenetic stimulation to enhance stroke recovery has been widely utilized in animal models (124). There are vast gaps between clinical use and basic research, and the therapy found to be effective in animals may not be efficient in human patients. More work, such as the development of animal model that more accurately reflect the human brain, are needed to overcome the challenge for translating animal study to clinical practice. For example, even with the advanced human brain mapping techniques (such as fMRI and TMS), the microstructural changes at the level of axons and synapses after therapy are still not available. Information from animal models help to provide a comprehensive picture of therapy-induced plasticity, which guides the clinic application of novel intervention. In a word, advancements in both clinical and basic research are required to the development of stroke therapy and the reveal of mechanisms underlying therapy-induced plasticity.

To conclude, the adult brain has strong plasticity potential, which can be exploited by therapeutic approaches in patients with stroke. Various approaches aimed at stimulating or inducing beneficial plasticity have been indicated to be effective. Further progress in this field requires a deeper understanding of the neural circuit changes and their functional implications at the whole-brain level as well as complete elucidation of treatment-induced plasticity.

AUTHOR CONTRIBUTIONS

WX contributed to the concept of this review and revised the manuscript. FS carried out the literature review and drafted the manuscript. Both authors read and approved the final manuscript.

FUNDING

This work was supported by the National Funds for Distinguished Young Scientists (81525009), National Science Foundation of China (81830063 and 81901419), Priority Among Priorities of Shanghai Municipal Clinical Medicine Center (2017ZZ01006), National Key R&D Program of China (2017YFC0840100 and 2017YFC0840106), Technology Innovation Program of Shanghai Science and Technology Committee (18411950100), and China Postdoctoral Science Foundation (2019M661369 and 2020T130110).

REFERENCES

1. Benjamin EJ, Virani SS, Callaway CW, Chamberlain AM, Chang AR, Cheng S, et al. Heart disease and stroke statistics-2018 update: a report from the American Heart Association. *Circulation.* (2018) 137:e67–492. doi: 10.1161/CIR.0000000000000573
2. Dimyan MA, Cohen LG. Neuroplasticity in the context of motor rehabilitation after stroke. *Nat Rev Neurol.* (2011) 7:76–85. doi: 10.1038/nrneurol.2010.200
3. Small SL, Buccino G, Solodkin A. Brain repair after stroke–a novel neurological model. *Nat Rev Neurol.* (2013) 9:698–707. doi: 10.1038/nrneurol.2013.222
4. Crofts A, Kelly ME, Gibson CL. Imaging functional recovery following ischemic stroke: clinical and preclinical fMRI studies. *J Neuroimaging.* (2020) 30:5–14. doi: 10.1111/jon.12668
5. Boddington LJ, Reynolds JNJ. Targeting interhemispheric inhibition with neuromodulation to enhance stroke rehabilitation. *Brain Stimul.* (2017) 10:214–22. doi: 10.1016/j.brs.2017.01.006
6. Grefkes C, Fink GR. Connectivity-based approaches in stroke and recovery of function. *Lancet Neurol.* (2014) 13:206–16. doi: 10.1016/S1474-4422(13)70264-3
7. Silasi G, Murphy TH. Stroke and the connectome: how connectivity guides therapeutic intervention. *Neuron.* (2014) 83:1354–68. doi: 10.1016/j.neuron.2014.08.052
8. Takahashi CD, Der-Yeghiaian L, Le V, Motiwala RR, Cramer SC. Robot-based hand motor therapy after stroke. *Brain.* (2008) 131(Pt 2):425–37. doi: 10.1093/brain/awm311
9. Ingemanson ML, Rowe JR, Chan V, Wolbrecht ET, Reinkensmeyer DJ, Cramer SC. Somatosensory system integrity explains differences

in treatment response after stroke. *Neurology.* (2019) 92:e1098–108. doi: 10.1212/WNL.0000000000007041
10. Pellegrino G, Tomasevic L, Tombini M, Assenza G, Bravi M, Sterzi S, et al. Inter-hemispheric coupling changes associate with motor improvements after robotic stroke rehabilitation. *Restor Neurol Neurosci.* (2012) 30:497–510. doi: 10.3233/RNN-2012-120227
11. Klamroth-Marganska V, Blanco J, Campen K, Curt A, Dietz V, Ettlin T, et al. Three-dimensional, task-specific robot therapy of the arm after stroke: a multicentre, parallel-group randomised trial. *Lancet Neurol.* (2014) 13:159–66. doi: 10.1016/S1474-4422(13)70305-3
12. Ekman U, Fordell H, Eriksson J, Lenfeldt N, Wahlin A, Eklund A, et al. Increase of frontal neuronal activity in chronic neglect after training in virtual reality. *Acta Neurol Scand.* (2018) 138:284–92. doi: 10.1111/ane.12955
13. Xiao X, Lin Q, Lo WL, Mao YR, Shi XC, Cates RS, et al. Cerebral reorganization in subacute stroke survivors after virtual reality-based training: a preliminary study. *Behav Neurol.* (2017) 2017:6261479. doi: 10.1155/2017/6261479
14. Saleh S, Fluet G, Qiu Q, Merians A, Adamovich SV, Tunik E. Neural patterns of reorganization after intensive robot-assisted virtual reality therapy and repetitive task practice in patients with chronic stroke. *Front Neurol.* (2017) 8:452. doi: 10.3389/fneur.2017.00452
15. Orihuela-Espina F, Fernandez del Castillo I, Palafox L, Pasaye E, Sanchez-Villavicencio I, Leder R, et al. Neural reorganization accompanying upper limb motor rehabilitation from stroke with virtual reality-based gesture therapy. *Top Stroke Rehabil.* (2013) 20:197–209. doi: 10.1310/tsr2003-197
16. Wang ZR, Wang P, Xing L, Mei LP, Zhao J, Zhang T. Leap motion-based virtual reality training for improving motor functional recovery of upper limbs and neural reorganization in subacute stroke patients. *Neural Regen Res.* (2017) 12:1823–31. doi: 10.4103/1673-5374.219043
17. Saposnik G, Cohen LG, Mamdani M, Pooyania S, Ploughman M, Cheung D, et al. Efficacy and safety of non-immersive virtual reality exercising in stroke rehabilitation (EVREST): a randomised, multicentre, single-blind, controlled trial. *Lancet Neurol.* (2016) 15:1019–27. doi: 10.1016/S1474-4422(16)30121-1
18. Jang SH, You SH, Hallett M, Cho YW, Park CM, Cho SH, et al. Cortical reorganization and associated functional motor recovery after virtual reality in patients with chronic stroke: an experimenter-blind preliminary study. *Arch Phys Med Rehabil.* (2005) 86:2218–23. doi: 10.1016/j.apmr.2005.04.015
19. Kim JH, Jang SH, Kim CS, Jung JH, You JH. Use of virtual reality to enhance balance and ambulation in chronic stroke: a double-blind, randomized controlled study. *Am J Phys Med Rehabil.* (2009) 88:693–701. doi: 10.1097/PHM.0b013e3181b33350
20. Stagg CJ, Bachtiar V, O'Shea J, Allman C, Bosnell RA, Kischka U, et al. Cortical activation changes underlying stimulation-induced behavioural gains in chronic stroke. *Brain.* (2012) 135(Pt 1):276–84. doi: 10.1093/brain/awr313
21. Chang MC, Kim DY, Park DH. Enhancement of cortical excitability and lower limb motor function in patients with stroke by transcranial direct current stimulation. *Brain Stimul.* (2015) 8:561–6. doi: 10.1016/j.brs.2015.01.411
22. Darkow R, Martin A, Wurtz A, Floel A, Meinzer M. Transcranial direct current stimulation effects on neural processing in post-stroke aphasia. *Hum Brain Mapp.* (2017) 38:1518–31. doi: 10.1002/hbm.23469
23. Meinzer M, Darkow R, Lindenberg R, Floel A. Electrical stimulation of the motor cortex enhances treatment outcome in post-stroke aphasia. *Brain.* (2016) 139(Pt 4):1152–63. doi: 10.1093/brain/aww002
24. Monti A, Cogiamanian F, Marceglia S, Ferrucci R, Mameli F, Mrakic-Sposta S, et al. Improved naming after transcranial direct current stimulation in aphasia. *J Neurol Neurosurg Psychiatry.* (2008) 79:451–3. doi: 10.1136/jnnp.2007.135277
25. Au-Yeung SS, Wang J, Chen Y, Chua E. Transcranial direct current stimulation to primary motor area improves hand dexterity and selective attention in chronic stroke. *Am J Phys Med Rehabil.* (2014) 93:1057–64. doi: 10.1097/PHM.0000000000000127
26. Du J, Yang F, Hu J, Hu J, Xu Q, Cong N, et al. Effects of high- and low-frequency repetitive transcranial magnetic stimulation on motor recovery in early stroke patients: evidence from a randomized controlled trial with clinical, neurophysiological and functional imaging assessments. *Neuroimage Clin.* (2019) 21:101620. doi: 10.1016/j.nicl.2018.101620
27. Ludemann-Podubecka J, Bosl K, Theilig S, Wiederer R, Nowak DA. The effectiveness of 1 Hz rTMS over the primary motor area of the unaffected hemisphere to improve hand function after stroke depends on hemispheric dominance. *Brain Stimul.* (2015) 8:823–30. doi: 10.1016/j.brs.2015.02.004
28. Nowak DA, Grefkes C, Dafotakis M, Eickhoff S, Kust J, Karbe H, et al. Effects of low-frequency repetitive transcranial magnetic stimulation of the contralesional primary motor cortex on movement kinematics and neural activity in subcortical stroke. *Arch Neurol.* (2008) 65:741–7. doi: 10.1001/archneur.65.6.741
29. Grefkes C, Nowak DA, Wang LE, Dafotakis M, Eickhoff SB, Fink GR. Modulating cortical connectivity in stroke patients by rTMS assessed with fMRI and dynamic causal modeling. *Neuroimage.* (2010) 50:233–42. doi: 10.1016/j.neuroimage.2009.12.029
30. Kondziolka D, Steinberg GK, Wechsler L, Meltzer CC, Elder E, Gebel J, et al. Neurotransplantation for patients with subcortical motor stroke: a phase 2 randomized trial. *J Neurosurg.* (2005) 103:38–45. doi: 10.3171/jns.2005.103.1.0038
31. Prasad K, Sharma A, Garg A, Mohanty S, Bhatnagar S, Johri S, et al. Intravenous autologous bone marrow mononuclear stem cell therapy for ischemic stroke: a multicentric, randomized trial. *Stroke.* (2014) 45:3618–24. doi: 10.1161/STROKEAHA.114.007028
32. Friedrich MA, Martins MP, Araujo MD, Klamt C, Vedolin L, Garicochea B, et al. Intra-arterial infusion of autologous bone marrow mononuclear cells in patients with moderate to severe middle cerebral artery acute ischemic stroke. *Cell Transplant.* (2012) 21(Suppl. 1):S13–21. doi: 10.3727/096368912X612512
33. Savitz SI, Yavagal D, Rappard G, Likosky W, Rutledge N, Graffagnino C, et al. A phase 2 randomized, sham-controlled trial of internal carotid artery infusion of autologous bone marrow-derived ALD-401 cells in patients with recent stable ischemic stroke (RECOVER-Stroke). *Circulation.* (2019) 139:192–205. doi: 10.1161/CIRCULATIONAHA.117.030659
34. Steinberg GK, Kondziolka D, Wechsler LR, Lunsford LD, Kim AS, Johnson JN, et al. Two-year safety and clinical outcomes in chronic ischemic stroke patients after implantation of modified bone marrow-derived mesenchymal stem cells (SB623): a phase 1/2a study. *J Neurosurg.* (2018) 131:1462–72. doi: 10.3171/2018.5.JNS173147
35. Muir KW, Bulters D, Willmot M, Sprigg N, Dixit A, Ward N, et al. Intracerebral implantation of human neural stem cells and motor recovery after stroke: multicentre prospective single-arm study (PISCES-2). *J Neurol Neurosurg Psychiatry.* (2020) 91:396–401. doi: 10.1136/jnnp-2019-322515
36. Sharma A, Sane H, Gokulchandran N, Khopkar D, Paranjape A, Sundaram J, et al. Autologous bone marrow mononuclear cells intrathecal transplantation in chronic stroke. *Stroke Res Treat.* (2014) 2014:234095. doi: 10.1155/2014/234095
37. Fang J, Guo Y, Tan S, Li Z, Xie H, Chen P, et al. Autologous endothelial progenitor cells transplantation for acute ischemic stroke: a 4-year follow-up study. *Stem Cells Transl Med.* (2019) 8:14–21. doi: 10.1002/sctm.18-0012
38. Ramos-Murguialday A, Curado MR, Broetz D, Yilmaz O, Brasil FL, Liberati G, et al. Brain-machine interface in chronic stroke: randomized trial long-term follow-up. *Neurorehabil Neural Repair.* (2019) 33:188–98. doi: 10.1177/1545968319827573
39. Wu Q, Yue Z, Ge Y, Ma D, Yin H, Zhao H, et al. Brain functional networks study of subacute stroke patients with upper limb dysfunction after comprehensive rehabilitation including BCI training. *Front Neurol.* (2019) 10:1419. doi: 10.3389/fneur.2019.01419
40. Pichiorri F, Morone G, Petti M, Toppi J, Pisotta I, Molinari M, et al. Brain-computer interface boosts motor imagery practice during stroke recovery. *Ann Neurol.* (2015) 77:851–65. doi: 10.1002/ana.24390
41. Carino-Escobar RI, Carrillo-Mora P, Valdes-Cristerna R, Rodriguez-Barragan MA, Hernandez-Arenas C, Quinzanos-Fresnedo J, et al. Longitudinal analysis of stroke patients' brain rhythms during an intervention with a brain-computer interface. *Neural Plast.* (2019) 2019:7084618. doi: 10.1155/2019/7084618
42. Hua XY, Qiu YQ, Li T, Zheng MX, Shen YD, Jiang S, et al. Contralateral peripheral neurotization for hemiplegic upper extremity after central neurologic injury. *Neurosurgery.* (2015) 76:187–95. doi: 10.1227/NEU.0000000000000590

43. Zheng MX, Hua XY, Feng JT, Li T, Lu YC, Shen YD, et al. Trial of contralateral seventh cervical nerve transfer for spastic arm paralysis. *N Engl J Med.* (2018) 378:22–34. doi: 10.1056/NEJMoa1615208
44. Qiu YQ, Du MX, Yu BF, Jiang S, Feng JT, Shen YD, et al. Contralateral lumbar to sacral nerve rerouting for hemiplegic patients after stroke: a clinical pilot study. *World Neurosurg.* (2019) 121:12–8. doi: 10.1016/j.wneu.2018.09.118
45. Brady MC, Kelly H, Godwin J, Enderby P, Campbell P. Speech and language therapy for aphasia following stroke. *Cochrane Database Syst Rev.* (2010) 5:CD000425. Available online at: https://doi.org/10.1002/14651858.CD000425.pub4
46. Langhorne P, Bernhardt J, Kwakkel G. Stroke rehabilitation. *Lancet.* (2011) 377:1693–702. doi: 10.1016/S0140-6736(11)60325-5
47. McKinnon ET, Fridriksson J, Glenn GR, Jensen JH, Helpern JA, Basilakos A, et al. Structural plasticity of the ventral stream and aphasia recovery. *Ann Neurol.* (2017) 82:147–51. doi: 10.1002/ana.24983
48. Sampaio-Baptista C, Sanders ZB, Johansen-Berg H. Structural plasticity in adulthood with motor learning and stroke rehabilitation. *Annu Rev Neurosci.* (2018) 41:25–40. doi: 10.1146/annurev-neuro-080317-062015
49. Kwakkel G, Veerbeek JM, van Wegen EE, Wolf SL. Constraint-induced movement therapy after stroke. *Lancet Neurol.* (2015) 14:224–34. doi: 10.1016/S1474-4422(14)70160-7
50. Thieme H, Morkisch N, Mehrholz J, Pohl M, Behrens J, Borgetto B, et al. Mirror therapy for improving motor function after stroke. *Cochrane Database Syst Rev.* (2018) 7:CD008449. doi: 10.1002/14651858.CD008449.pub3
51. Borges LR, Fernandes AB, Melo LP, Guerra RO, Campos TF. Action observation for upper limb rehabilitation after stroke. *Cochrane Database Syst Rev.* (2018) 10:CD011887. doi: 10.1002/14651858.CD011887.pub2
52. Fritz SL, Butts RJ, Wolf SL. Constraint-induced movement therapy: from history to plasticity. *Expert Rev Neurother.* (2012) 12:191–8. doi: 10.1586/ern.11.201
53. Chen W, Ye Q, Ji X, Zhang S, Yang X, Zhou Q, et al. Mirror neuron system based therapy for aphasia rehabilitation. *Front Psychol.* (2015) 6:1665. doi: 10.3389/fpsyg.2015.01665
54. Sarfo FS, Ulasavets U, Opare-Sem OK, Ovbiagele B. Tele-rehabilitation after stroke: an updated systematic review of the literature. *J Stroke Cerebrovasc Dis.* (2018) 27:2306–18. doi: 10.1016/j.jstrokecerebrovasdis.2018.05.013
55. Laver KE, Schoene D, Crotty M, George S, Lannin NA, Sherrington C. Telerehabilitation services for stroke. *Cochrane Database Syst Rev.* (2013) 2013:CD010255. doi: 10.1002/14651858.CD010255.pub2
56. Mehrholz J, Pohl M, Platz T, Kugler J, Elsner B. Electromechanical and robot-assisted arm training for improving activities of daily living, arm function, and arm muscle strength after stroke. *Cochrane Database Syst Rev.* (2018) 9:CD006876. doi: 10.1002/14651858.CD006876.pub5
57. Mehrholz J, Thomas S, Werner C, Kugler J, Pohl M, Elsner B. Electromechanical-assisted training for walking after stroke. *Cochrane Database Syst Rev.* (2017) 5:CD006185. doi: 10.1002/14651858.CD006185.pub4
58. Spalletti C, Alia C, Lai S, Panarese A, Conti S, Micera S, et al. Combining robotic training and inactivation of the healthy hemisphere restores pre-stroke motor patterns in mice. *Elife.* (2017) 6:e28662. doi: 10.7554/eLife.28662
59. Laver KE, Lange B, George S, Deutsch JE, Saposnik G, Crotty M. Virtual reality for stroke rehabilitation. *Cochrane Database Syst Rev.* (2017) 11:CD008349. doi: 10.1002/14651858.CD008349.pub4
60. Dominguez-Tellez P, Moral-Munoz JA, Casado-Fernandez E, Salazar A, Lucena-Anton D. [Effects of virtual reality on balance and gait in stroke: a systematic review and meta-analysis]. *Rev Neurol.* (2019) 69:223–34. doi: 10.33588/rn.6906.2019063
61. Wahlin A, Fordell H, Ekman U, Lenfeldt N, Malm J. Rehabilitation in chronic spatial neglect strengthens resting-state connectivity. *Acta Neurol Scand.* (2019) 139:254–9. doi: 10.1111/ane.13048
62. Saleh S, Bagce H, Qiu Q, Fluet G, Merians A, Adamovich S, et al. Mechanisms of neural reorganization in chronic stroke subjects after virtual reality training. *Conf Proc IEEE Eng Med Biol Soc.* (2011) 2011:8118–21. doi: 10.1109/IEMBS.2011.6092002
63. Vourvopoulos A, Pardo OM, Lefebvre S, Neureither M, Saldana D, Jahng E, et al. Effects of a brain-computer interface with Virtual Reality (VR) neurofeedback: a pilot study in chronic stroke patients. *Front Hum Neurosci.* (2019) 13:210. doi: 10.3389/fnhum.2019.00210
64. Kwakkel G, Kollen BJ, Krebs HI. Effects of robot-assisted therapy on upper limb recovery after stroke: a systematic review. *Neurorehabil Neural Repair.* (2008) 22:111–21. doi: 10.1177/1545968307305457
65. Prange GB, Jannink MJ, Groothuis-Oudshoorn CG, Hermens HJ, Ijzerman MJ. Systematic review of the effect of robot-aided therapy on recovery of the hemiparetic arm after stroke. *J Rehabil Res Dev.* (2006) 43:171–84. doi: 10.1682/JRRD.2005.04.0076
66. Levy R, Ruland S, Weinand M, Lowry D, Dafer R, Bakay R. Cortical stimulation for the rehabilitation of patients with hemiparetic stroke: a multicenter feasibility study of safety and efficacy. *J Neurosurg.* (2008) 108:707–14. doi: 10.3171/JNS/2008/108/4/0707
67. Lempka SF, Malone DA Jr, Hu B, Baker KB, Wyant A, et al. Randomized clinical trial of deep brain stimulation for poststroke pain. *Ann Neurol.* (2017) 81:653–63. doi: 10.1002/ana.24927
68. Elsner B, Kugler J, Pohl M, Mehrholz J. Transcranial direct current stimulation (tDCS) for improving activities of daily living, and physical and cognitive functioning, in people after stroke. *Cochrane Database Syst Rev.* (2016) 3:CD009645. doi: 10.1002/14651858.CD009645.pub3
69. Kang N, Summers JJ, Cauraugh JH. Non-invasive brain stimulation improves paretic limb force production: a systematic review and meta-analysis. *Brain Stimul.* (2016) 9:662–70. doi: 10.1016/j.brs.2016.05.005
70. Le Q, Qu Y, Tao Y, Zhu S. Effects of repetitive transcranial magnetic stimulation on hand function recovery and excitability of the motor cortex after stroke: a meta-analysis. *Am J Phys Med Rehabil.* (2014) 93:422–30. doi: 10.1097/PHM.0000000000000027
71. Fridriksson J, Rorden C, Elm J, Sen S, George MS, Bonilha L. Transcranial Direct Current Stimulation vs. Sham Stimulation to Treat Aphasia After Stroke: A Randomized Clinical Trial. *JAMA Neurol.* (2018) 12:1470–76. doi: 10.1001/jamaneurol.2018.2287
72. Svanstrom H, Ueda P, Melbye M, Eliasson B, Svensson AM, Franzen S, et al. Use of liraglutide and risk of major cardiovascular events: a register-based cohort study in Denmark and Sweden. *Lancet Diabetes Endocrinol.* (2019) 7:106–14. doi: 10.1016/S2213-8587(18)30320-6
73. Smith MC, Stinear CM. Transcranial magnetic stimulation (TMS) in stroke: ready for clinical practice? *J Clin Neurosci.* (2016) 31:10–4. doi: 10.1016/j.jocn.2016.01.034
74. Elsner B, Kugler J, Pohl M, Mehrholz J. Transcranial direct current stimulation (tDCS) for improving aphasia in adults with aphasia after stroke. *Cochrane Database Syst Rev.* (2019) 5:CD009760. doi: 10.1002/14651858.CD009760.pub4
75. Di Pino G, Pellegrino G, Assenza G, Capone F, Ferreri F, Formica D, et al. Modulation of brain plasticity in stroke: a novel model for neurorehabilitation. *Nat Rev Neurol.* (2014) 10:597–608. doi: 10.1038/nrneurol.2014.162
76. Grefkes C, Fink GR. Disruption of motor network connectivity post-stroke and its noninvasive neuromodulation. *Curr Opin Neurol.* (2012) 25:670–5. doi: 10.1097/WCO.0b013e3283598473
77. Zheng Y, Zhong D, Huang Y, He M, Xiao Q, Jin R, et al. Effectiveness and safety of repetitive transcranial magnetic stimulation (rTMS) on aphasia in cerebrovascular accident patients: Protocol of a systematic review and meta-analysis. *Medicine.* (2019) 98:e18561. doi: 10.1097/MD.0000000000018561
78. Li J, Zuo Z, Zhang X, Shao X, Lu J, Xue R, et al. Excitatory repetitive transcranial magnetic stimulation induces contralesional cortico-cerebellar pathways after acute ischemic stroke: a preliminary DTI study. *Front Behav Neurosci.* (2018) 12:160. doi: 10.3389/fnbeh.2018.00160
79. Zong X, Dong Y, Li Y, Yang L, Li Y, Yang B, et al. Beneficial effects of theta-burst transcranial magnetic stimulation on stroke injury via improving neuronal microenvironment and mitochondrial integrity. *Transl Stroke Res.* (2019) 11:450–67. doi: 10.1007/s12975-019-00731-w
80. Guo F, Lou J, Han X, Deng Y, Huang X. Repetitive transcranial magnetic stimulation ameliorates cognitive impairment by enhancing neurogenesis and suppressing apoptosis in the hippocampus in rats with ischemic stroke. *Front Physiol.* (2017) 8:559. doi: 10.3389/fphys.2017.00559
81. Kronberg G, Bridi M, Abel T, Bikson M, Parra LC. Direct current stimulation modulates LTP and LTD: activity dependence and dendritic effects. *Brain Stimul.* (2017) 10:51–8. doi: 10.1016/j.brs.2016.10.001

82. Fritsch B, Reis J, Martinowich K, Schambra HM, Ji Y, Cohen LG, et al. Direct current stimulation promotes BDNF-dependent synaptic plasticity: potential implications for motor learning. *Neuron.* (2010) 66:198–204. doi: 10.1016/j.neuron.2010.03.035
83. Cunningham DA, Varnerin N, Machado A, Bonnett C, Janini D, Roelle S, et al. Stimulation targeting higher motor areas in stroke rehabilitation: A proof-of-concept, randomized, double-blinded placebo-controlled study of effectiveness and underlying mechanisms. *Restor Neurol Neurosci.* (2015) 33:911–26. doi: 10.3233/RNN-150574
84. George PM, Steinberg GK. Novel stroke therapeutics: unraveling stroke pathophysiology and its impact on clinical treatments. *Neuron.* (2015) 87:297–309. doi: 10.1016/j.neuron.2015.05.041
85. Bath PM, Sprigg N, England T. Colony stimulating factors (including erythropoietin, granulocyte colony stimulating factor and analogues) for stroke. *Cochrane Database Syst Rev.* (2006) 18:CD005207. doi: 10.1002/14651858.CD005207.pub2
86. Liu X, Ye R, Yan T, Yu SP, Wei L, Xu G, et al. Cell based therapies for ischemic stroke: from basic science to bedside. *Prog Neurobiol.* (2014) 115:92–115. doi: 10.1016/j.pneurobio.2013.11.007
87. Wechsler LR, Bates D, Stroemer P, Andrews-Zwilling YS, Aizman I. Cell therapy for chronic stroke. *Stroke.* (2018) 49:1066–74. doi: 10.1161/STROKEAHA.117.018290
88. Moniche F, Gonzalez A, Gonzalez-Marcos JR, Carmona M, Pinero P, Espigado I, et al. Intra-arterial bone marrow mononuclear cells in ischemic stroke: a pilot clinical trial. *Stroke.* (2012) 43:2242–4. doi: 10.1161/STROKEAHA.112.659409
89. Mancha F, Escudero-Martinez I, Zapata-Arriaza E, Vega-Salvatierra A, Cabezas JA, Lebrato L, et al. Circulating microRNA after autologous bone marrow mononuclear cell (BM-MNC) injection in patients with ischemic stroke. *J Investig Med.* (2020) 68:807–10. doi: 10.1136/jim-2019-001161
90. Boltze J, Jolkkonen J. Safety evaluation of intra-arterial cell delivery in stroke patients-a framework for future trials. *Ann Transl Med.* (2019) 7(Suppl. 8):S271. doi: 10.21037/atm.2019.12.07
91. Boncoraglio GB, Ranieri M, Bersano A, Parati EA, Del Giovane C. Stem cell transplantation for ischemic stroke. *Cochrane Database Syst Rev.* (2019) 5:CD007231. doi: 10.1002/14651858.CD007231.pub3
92. Savitz SI, Dinsmore J, Wu J, Henderson GV, Stieg P, Caplan LR. Neurotransplantation of fetal porcine cells in patients with basal ganglia infarcts: a preliminary safety and feasibility study. *Cerebrovasc Dis.* (2005) 20:101–7. doi: 10.1159/000086518
93. Steinberg GK, Kondziolka D, Wechsler LR, Lunsford LD, Coburn ML, Billigen JB, et al. Clinical outcomes of transplanted modified bone marrow-derived mesenchymal stem cells in stroke: a phase 1/2a study. *Stroke.* (2016) 47:1817–24. doi: 10.1161/STROKEAHA.116.012995
94. Muir KW, Sinden J, Miljan E, Dunn L. Intracranial delivery of stem cells. *Transl Stroke Res.* (2011) 2:266–71. doi: 10.1007/s12975-011-0095-z
95. Darsalia V, Kallur T, Kokaia Z. Survival, migration and neuronal differentiation of human fetal striatal and cortical neural stem cells grafted in stroke-damaged rat striatum. *Eur J Neurosci.* (2007) 26:605–14. doi: 10.1111/j.1460-9568.2007.05702.x
96. Kelly S, Bliss TM, Shah AK, Sun GH, Ma M, Foo WC, et al. Transplanted human fetal neural stem cells survive, migrate, and differentiate in ischemic rat cerebral cortex. *Proc Natl Acad Sci USA.* (2004) 101:11839–44. doi: 10.1073/pnas.0404474101
97. Li Y, Chen J, Chen XG, Wang L, Gautam SC, Xu YX, et al. Human marrow stromal cell therapy for stroke in rat: neurotrophins and functional recovery. *Neurology.* (2002) 59:514–23. doi: 10.1212/WNL.59.4.514
98. Buhnemann C, Scholz A, Bernreuther C, Malik CY, Braun H, Schachner M, et al. Neuronal differentiation of transplanted embryonic stem cell-derived precursors in stroke lesions of adult rats. *Brain.* (2006) 129(Pt 12):3238–48. doi: 10.1093/brain/awl261
99. Arvidsson A, Collin T, Kirik D, Kokaia Z, Lindvall O. Neuronal replacement from endogenous precursors in the adult brain after stroke. *Nat Med.* (2002) 8:963–70. doi: 10.1038/nm747
100. Englund U, Bjorklund A, Wictorin K, Lindvall O, Kokaia M. Grafted neural stem cells develop into functional pyramidal neurons and integrate into host cortical circuitry. *Proc Natl Acad Sci USA.* (2002) 99:17089–94. doi: 10.1073/pnas.252589099
101. Borlongan CV, Hadman M, Sanberg CD, Sanberg PR. Central nervous system entry of peripherally injected umbilical cord blood cells is not required for neuroprotection in stroke. *Stroke.* (2004) 35:2385–9. doi: 10.1161/01.STR.0000141680.49960.d7
102. Cheng Z, Wang L, Qu M, Liang H, Li W, Li Y, et al. Mesenchymal stem cells attenuate blood-brain barrier leakage after cerebral ischemia in mice. *J Neuroinflammation.* (2018) 15:135. doi: 10.1186/s12974-018-1153-1
103. Kaneko Y, Lee JY, Tajiri N, Tuazon JP, Lippert T, Russo E, et al. Translating intracarotid artery transplantation of bone marrow-derived NCS-01 cells for ischemic stroke: behavioral and histological readouts and mechanistic insights into stem cell therapy. *Stem Cells Transl Med.* (2020) 9:203–20. doi: 10.1002/sctm.19-0229
104. Andres RH, Horie N, Slikker W, Keren-Gill H, Zhan K, Sun G, et al. Human neural stem cells enhance structural plasticity and axonal transport in the ischaemic brain. *Brain.* (2011) 134(Pt 6):1777–89. doi: 10.1093/brain/awr094
105. Andrews EM, Tsai SY, Johnson SC, Farrer JR, Wagner JP, Kopen GC, et al. Human adult bone marrow-derived somatic cell therapy results in functional recovery and axonal plasticity following stroke in the rat. *Exp Neurol.* (2008) 211:588–92. doi: 10.1016/j.expneurol.2008.02.027
106. Chaudhary U, Birbaumer N, Ramos-Murguialday A. Brain-computer interfaces for communication and rehabilitation. *Nat Rev Neurol.* (2016) 12:513–25. doi: 10.1038/nrneurol.2016.113
107. Cervera MA, Soekadar SR, Ushiba J, Millan JDR, Liu M, Birbaumer N, et al. Brain-computer interfaces for post-stroke motor rehabilitation: a meta-analysis. *Ann Clin Transl Neurol.* (2018) 5:651–63. doi: 10.1002/acn3.544
108. Shanechi MM. Brain-machine interfaces from motor to mood. *Nat Neurosci.* (2019) 22:1554–64. doi: 10.1038/s41593-019-0488-y
109. Daly JJ, Cheng R, Rogers J, Litinas K, Hrovat K, Dohring M. Feasibility of a new application of noninvasive Brain Computer Interface (BCI): a case study of training for recovery of volitional motor control after stroke. *J Neurol Phys Ther.* (2009) 33:203–11. doi: 10.1097/NPT.0b013e3181c1fc0b
110. Bai Z, Fong KNK, Zhang JJ, Chan J, Ting KH. Immediate and long-term effects of BCI-based rehabilitation of the upper extremity after stroke: a systematic review and meta-analysis. *J Neuroeng Rehabil.* (2020) 17:57. doi: 10.1186/s12984-020-00686-2
111. Frolov AA, Mokienko O, Lyukmanov R, Biryukova E, Kotov S, Turbina L, et al. Post-stroke rehabilitation training with a motor-imagery-based Brain-Computer Interface (BCI)-controlled hand exoskeleton: a randomized controlled multicenter trial. *Front Neurosci.* (2017) 11:400. doi: 10.3389/fnins.2017.00400
112. Moritz CT, Perlmutter SI, Fetz EE. Direct control of paralysed muscles by cortical neurons. *Nature.* (2008) 456:639–42. doi: 10.1038/nature07418
113. Hwang EJ, Bailey PM, Andersen RA. Volitional control of neural activity relies on the natural motor repertoire. *Curr Biol.* (2013) 23:353–61. doi: 10.1016/j.cub.2013.01.027
114. Golub MD, Sadtler PT, Oby ER, Quick KM, Ryu SI, Tyler-Kabara EC, et al. Learning by neural reassociation. *Nat Neurosci.* (2018) 21:607–16. doi: 10.1038/s41593-018-0095-3
115. Xu R, Jiang N, Mrachacz-Kersting N, Lin C, Asin Prieto G, Moreno JC, et al. A closed-loop brain-computer interface triggering an active ankle-foot orthosis for inducing cortical neural plasticity. *IEEE Trans Biomed Eng.* (2014) 61:2092–101. doi: 10.1109/TBME.2014.2313867
116. Gu YD, Zhang GM, Chen DS, Yan JG, Cheng XM, Chen L. Seventh cervical nerve root transfer from the contralateral healthy side for treatment of brachial plexus root avulsion. *J Hand Surg Br.* (1992) 17:518–21. doi: 10.1016/S0266-7681(05)80235-9
117. Hua XY, Liu B, Qiu YQ, Tang WJ, Xu WD, Liu HQ, et al. Long-term ongoing cortical remodeling after contralateral C-7 nerve transfer. *J Neurosurg.* (2013) 118:725–9. doi: 10.3171/2012.12.JNS 12207
118. Liu B, Li T, Tang WJ, Zhang JH, Sun HP, Xu WD, et al. Changes of inter-hemispheric functional connectivity between motor cortices after brachial plexuses injury: a resting-state fMRI study. *Neuroscience.* (2013) 243:33–9. doi: 10.1016/j.neuroscience.2013.03.048
119. Lu Y, Liu H, Hua X, Xu WD, Xu JG, Gu YD. Supplementary motor cortical changes explored by resting-state functional connectivity in brachial plexus injury. *World Neurosurg.* (2016) 88:300–5. doi: 10.1016/j.wneu.2015.12.036

120. Page SJ, Fulk GD, Boyne P. Clinically important differences for the upper-extremity Fugl-Meyer scale in people with minimal to moderate impairment due to chronic stroke. *Phys Ther.* (2012) 92:791–8. doi: 10.2522/ptj.20110009
121. Li J, Ying Y, Su F, Chen L, Yang J, Jia J, et al. The Hua-Shan rehabilitation program after contralateral seventh cervical nerve transfer for spastic arm paralysis. *Disabil Rehabil.* (2020). doi: 10.1080/09638288.2020.1768597
122. Lin DJ, Finklestein SP, Cramer SC. New directions in treatments targeting stroke recovery. *Stroke.* (2018) 49:3107–14. doi: 10.1161/STROKEAHA.118.021359
123. Zhao LR, Willing A. Enhancing endogenous capacity to repair a stroke-damaged brain: an evolving field for stroke research. *Prog Neurobiol.* (2018) 163–164:5–26. doi: 10.1016/j.pneurobio.2018.01.004
124. Cheng MY, Aswendt M, Steinberg GK. Optogenetic approaches to target specific neural circuits in post-stroke recovery. *Neurotherapeutics.* (2016) 13:325–40. doi: 10.1007/s13311-015-0411-5

15

The Effects of Modified Constraint-Induced Movement Therapy in Acute Subcortical Cerebral Infarction

Changshen Yu[1†], Wanjun Wang[1†], Yue Zhang[2], Yizhao Wang[2], Weijia Hou[2], Shoufeng Liu[1], Chunlin Gao[1], Chen Wang[3], Lidong Mo[3] and Jialing Wu[1]*

[1]Department of Neurorehabilitation, Department of Neurology, Tianjin Huanhu Hospital, Tianjin Key Laboratory of Cerebrovascular and Neurodegenerative Diseases, Tianjin, China, [2]Department of Rehabilitation Medicine, Tianjin Huanhu Hospital, Tianjin Key Laboratory of Cerebrovascular and Neurodegenerative Diseases, Tianjin, China, [3]Neurological Disease Biobank, Tianjin Neurosurgical Institute, Tianjin Huanhu Hospital, Tianjin Key Laboratory of Cerebrovascular and Neurodegenerative Diseases, Tianjin, China

Edited by:
Srikantan S. Nagarajan,
University of California,
San Francisco, United States

Reviewed by:
Sandro M. Krieg,
Technische Universität München,
Germany
Filippo Brighina,
University of Palermo, Italy

***Correspondence:**
Jialing Wu
wywjl2009@hotmail.com

†These authors have contributed equally to this work.

Background: Constraint-induced movement therapy (CIMT) promotes upper extremity recovery post stroke, however, it is difficult to implement clinically due to its high resource demand and safety of the restraint. Therefore, we propose that modified CIMT (mCIMT) be used to treat individuals with acute subcortical infarction.

Objective: To evaluate the therapeutic effects of mCIMT in patients with acute subcortical infarction, and investigate the possible mechanisms underlying the effect.

Methods: The role of mCIMT was investigated in 26 individuals experiencing subcortical infarction in the preceding 14 days. Patients were randomly assigned to either mCIMT or standard therapy. mCIMT group was treated daily for 3 h over 10 consecutive working days, using a mitt on the unaffected arm for up to 30% of waking hours. The control group was treated with an equal dose of occupational therapy and physical therapy. During the 3-month follow-up, the motor functions of the affected limb were assessed by the Wolf Motor Function Test (WMFT) and Motor Activity Log (MAL). Altered cortical excitability was assessed via transcranial magnetic stimulation (TMS).

Results: Treatment significantly improved the movement in the mCIMT group compared with the control group. The mean WMF score was significantly higher in the mCIMT group compared with the control group. Further, the appearance of motor-evoked potentials (MEPs) were significantly higher in the mCIMT group compared with the baseline data. A significant change in ipsilesional silent period (SP) occurred in the mCIMT group compared with the control group. However, we found no difference between two groups in motor function or electrophysiological parameters after 3 months of follow-up.

Conclusions: mCIMT resulted in significant functional changes in timed movement immediately following treatment in patients with acute subcortical infarction. Further, early mCIMT improved ipsilesional cortical excitability. However, no long-term effects were seen.

Keywords: constraint-induced movement therapy, rehabilitation, motor evoked potentials, cortical reorganization, acute subcortical stroke

INTRODUCTION

Stroke significantly increases the mortality and morbidity in the developed as well as developing world (Sudlow and Warlow, 1997; Terént, 2003; Truelsen et al., 2003; Mehndiratta et al., 2015). Despite varying levels of functional recovery, substantial sensorimotor and cognitive deficits persist in more than 50% of survivors, resulting in significant socioeconomic burden (Hendricks et al., 2002; Kim, 2014). Approximately 80% of stroke survivors manifest motor impairments associated with the upper limb (Langhorne et al., 2009; Momosaki et al., 2016). The degree of upper limb paresis is correlated with the basic activities of daily living (ADL) after stroke (Veerbeek et al., 2011; van Mierlo et al., 2016).

Constraint-induced movement therapy (CIMT) promotes movement of upper extremities affected by paralytic stroke. The major components of CIMT include intense repetitive (task-oriented) training and behavioral sharping of the impaired limb with immobilization of the unimpaired arm. Animal studies suggest that increased use of the affected limb overcame the reduced motor activity associated with cortical lesions (Nudo et al., 1996; Kleim et al., 1998). Evidence supports the effectiveness of CIMT in improving dexterity and motor function in individuals with chronic hemiplegia (Wolf et al., 1989; van der Lee et al., 1999; Taub, 2000). There are some limitations to widespread use of CIMT in stroke rehabilitation: first, original CIMT protocol requires constant supervision, therefore, it is more expensive than customary care. Second, original CIMT protocol need constraint of the unaffected hand for approximately 90% of waking hours, but some individuals with hemiplegia cannot tolerate this long limit, and there are also some security issues, especially in acute stroke patients. Compared with original CIMT protocol, the modified CIMT (mCIMT) protocols were feasible and well tolerated in acute stroke patients (Souza et al., 2015).

Although stroke damage can be devastating, many patients survive the initial event and undergo some spontaneous recovery, which can be further augmented by rehabilitative therapy. The first few weeks after stroke are vital for neuroplasticity and relearning of impaired activities (Dobkin, 2004; Kwakkel et al., 2006). Randomized controlled studies have demonstrated mCIMT could improve more affected limb use and function in acute or sub-acute cerebrovascular accident (Page et al., 2005; Singh and Pradhan, 2013).

The recovery of motor function in cortical injury varies from that of subcortical injury (Liu et al., 2015) and the effects of mCIMT in early subcortical ischemic stroke is not established. This study is undertaken to determine if mCIMT is effective in the early phase of subcortical ischemic stroke, and investigate the possible mechanisms underlying the effect. We hypothesized that mCIMT could improve functional outcomes of hemiplegic upper limb in patients with acute subcortical ischemic stroke compared with conventional occupational and physical therapy, and increase ipsilateral cortical excitability.

MATERIALS AND METHODS

Study Setting and Trial Registration

In this single-center randomized controlled clinical trial, patients were recruited from November 2013 to January 2016. This study was approved by the ethics committee of Tianjin Huanhu Hospital. All the procedures involving human participants were approved by the ethics committee of Tianjin Huanhu Hospital and were in accordance with the 1964 Helsinki Declaration and its later amendments, or comparable ethical standards. All participants provided informed consent. In this single-center randomized clinical trial, we compared the upper extremity function between the group exposed to mCIMT and a dose-equivalent control group immediately after intervention and 3 months later. Transcranial magnetic stimulation (TMS) was used to assess changes in cortical excitability after treatment and follow-up. The study was registered with the Chinese Clinical Trial Registry (Registration number: ChiCTR-IOR-15005770).

Design and Participants

The inclusion criteria were: (1) stroke within 2 weeks of onset; (2) MRI showing subcortical ischemic stroke; (3) ability to raise two fingers with the forearm pronated on the table or lift the wrist 10° or more starting from a fully bent position; (4) respond to a 2-step command; and (5) a Mini Mental State Examination score exceeding 20. The exclusion criteria were: (1) inability to provide informed consent; (2) a history of stroke; (3) deviation greater than 2 cm on the line bisection test; (4) morbidity of the affected upper extremity resulting in functional limitation prior to stroke; (5) life expectancy less than 1 year; or (6) other neurological conditions affecting motor function or assessment (Thrane et al., 2015). Following informed consent, the patients were assigned to mCIMT or the control group using random odd- and even-numbered tickets in sealed envelopes. Patients selected one of the 60 sealed envelopes. Patients who selected tickets with even numbers represented the control group while those with odd numbers were allocated to mCIMT.

Interventions

The hemiplegic upper extremities in the mCIMT group were trained for 10 days by a licensed occupational therapist. All participants underwent 3 h per day of adaptive task practice and task training of the paretic limb (Wolf et al., 1989; van der Lee et al., 1999; Taub, 2000). Behavioral therapy comprised basic ADL together with skilled functional activities under supervision to improve motor performance. Positive feedback and increased gradations of difficulty were provided. Error data were provided after task training. Tasks with increasing levels of difficulty were assigned. In addition, patients carried a constraining mitt on the unaffected arm for nearly a third of their waking hours.

The control group was exposed to equal doses of traditional occupational therapy and physical therapy using a combination of neurodevelopmental techniques: bimanual tasks for the upper limbs, compensatory techniques for ADLs, strength and range of motion, positioning and mobility training.

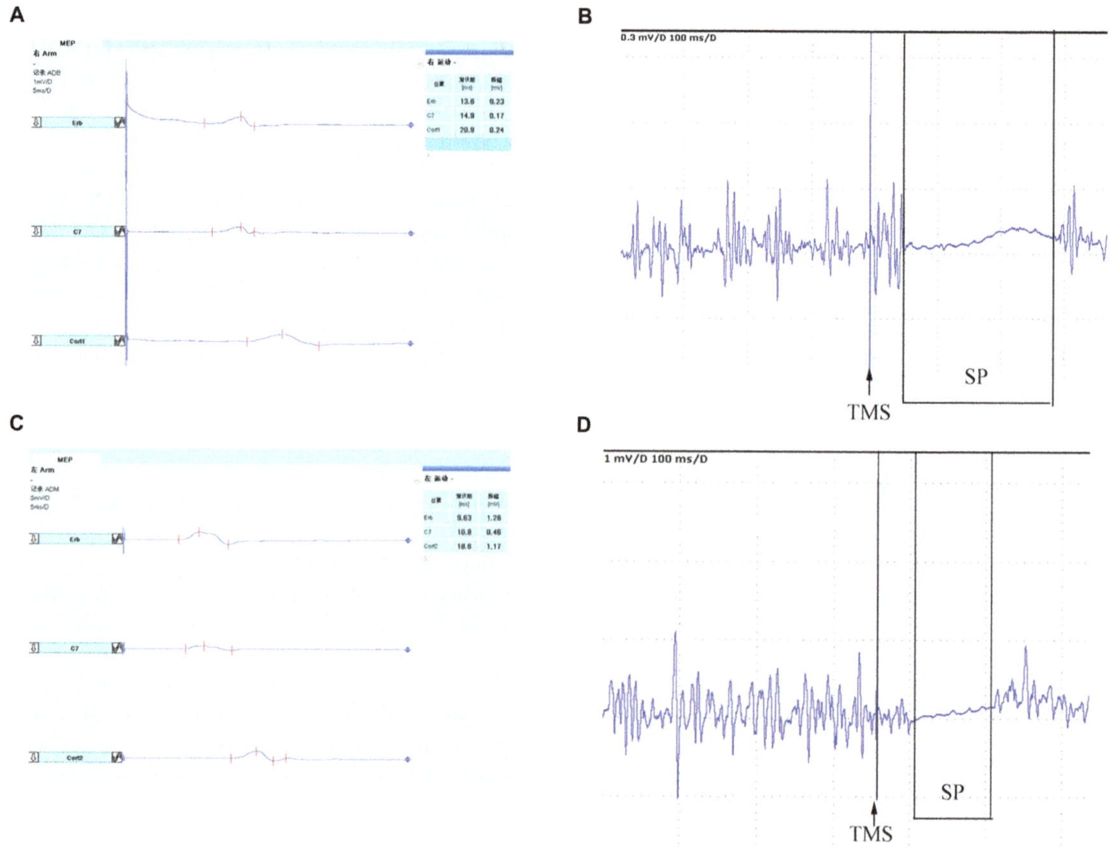

FIGURE 1 | Schematic diagram of TMS-induced MEP. Bilateral MEPs and SP recorded in abductor pollicis brevis. Ipsilesional cortical **(A)** MEP and **(B)** SP, and Contralesional cortical **(C)** MEP and **(D)** SP. TMS, transcranial magnetic stimulation; MEP, motor-evoked potential; SP, silent period.

Outcome Measurements

Primary outcomes included upper extremity motor function (tested with Wolf Motor Function Test (WMFT)) and a structured interview of real-world arm use with Motor Activity Log (MAL). The WMFT comprises 15 timed and two strength tasks (lifting the weighted limb and grip strength). The maximum time to complete a task was 120 s. If a trial was incomplete, the result was recorded as 121 s. The median time of all 15 tasks was used for analysis (Morris et al., 2001). The validity and reliability of the test had been demonstrated in stroke populations (Wolf et al., 2001, 2005; Nijland et al., 2010). The MAL was a structured interview comprising 30 standardized questions encompassing various ADL, which was used to assess the subjects' subjective report of 30 common daily tasks. It included two assessment subscales that rate the more affected upper extremity: an amount of use (AOU) scale and a quality of movement (QOM) scale (Bonifer et al., 2005). The MAL was characterized by stability over a 2-week period with high internal consistency, high inter-rater and test-retest reliability (Taub, 2000). The tool was used extensively in CIMT studies. All participants were assessed after inclusion but before randomization, after 2 weeks and after 3 months.

Secondary outcome was the change of cortical excitability. Motor-evoked potentials (MEPs) and cortical silent period (SP) were examined by Dantec Keypoint 4c eletromyography (EMG; Medtronic A/S, Skovlunde, Denmark) with Danish Medtronic MagPro R30 (Medtronic A/S, Skovlunde, Denmark) magnetic stmulator and a focal figure-eight-shaped coil (outer diameter 4.5 cm). The maximum intensity of the magnetic field was 2.5 tesla. All patients were seated comfortably in the supine position. Surface EMG electrodes (filter bandpass: 20–10 kHz) were attached 3 cm apart over the muscle bellies of the abductor pollicis brevis. The 10–20 International electrode system was used for positioning of the TMS coil which located the electrodes on the scalp using standard cranial landmarks. Five stimulation positions were C4/C3, FC4/FC3, C5/C6, CP4/CP3 and C2/C1 according to the 10–20 International electrode system for measurements of cortical excitability. They were marked with an EEG cap, and stimulated with 90% of maximum stimulator output. The position at which stimuli at slightly suprathreshold intensity consistently yielded maximal MEPs in the contralateral abductor pollicis brevis was defined as "hot spot" (Bergmann et al., 2012). Subsequently, rest motor threshold (RMT) was defined according to the guidelines of

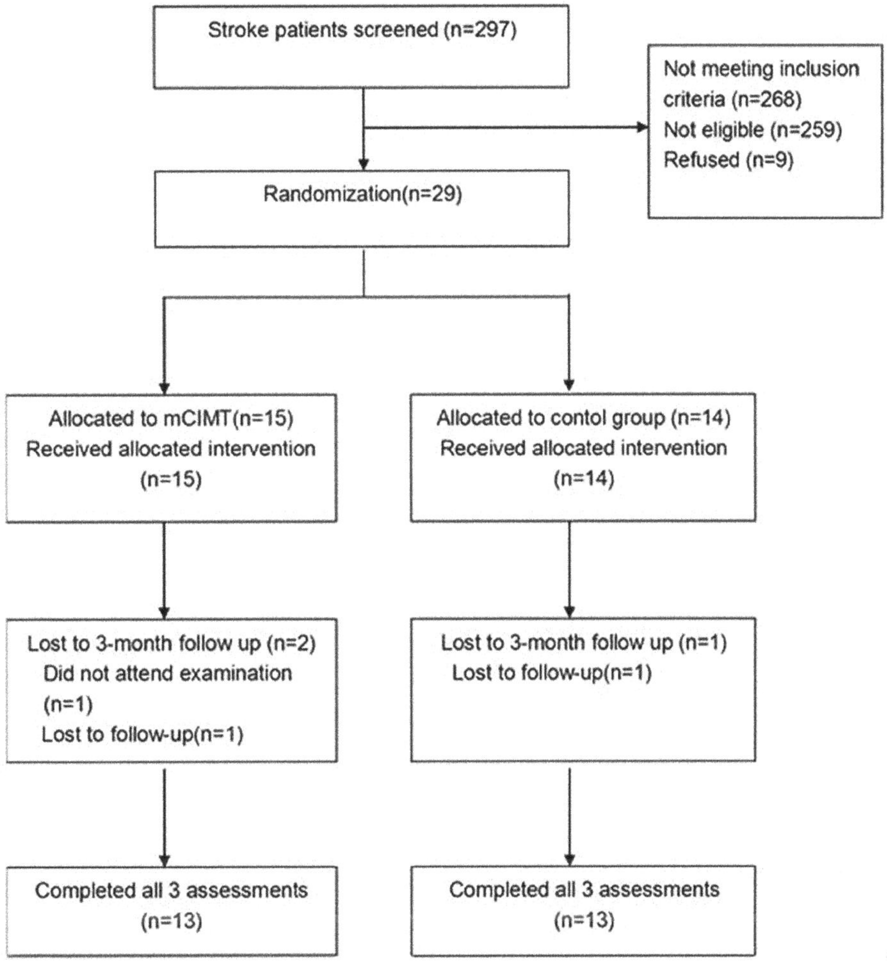

FIGURE 2 | Flowchart outlining participant selection.

the International Federation of Clinical Neurophysiology (IFCN) Committee as the minimum stimulus intensity eliciting MEPs of 0.50 mV in the resting muscle in at least 5 of 10 consecutive trials (Chen et al., 2008). The procedures were performed before the intervention and repeated similarly after the intervention and follow-up. Central motor conduction time (CMCT) was a neurophysiological measure that reflected conduction between the primary motor cortex and spinal cord. CMCT was calculated by subtracting the conduction time from the spinal roots to the muscle from the latency of MEPs evoked magnetically by transcranial cortical stimulation (Heald et al., 1993). In our previous study, cortical SP was an useful tool to predict outcome of acute stroke patients (Zhang et al., 2016). The SP had been proposed as an additional factor to the MEP for predicting motor recovery (van Kuijk et al., 2005). The length of the SP was measured from MEP onset until the return of uninterrupted voluntary EMG activity (Uozumi et al., 1991; Trompetto et al., 2000; **Figure 1**). When TMS was applied during isometric muscle contraction, cortical SP could be evoked following the MEP, which would be lasting up to 100–300 ms (Braune and Fritz, 1995). The intensity of stimulation was 120% RMT. The altered ipsilesional or contralesional MEPs and SPs, were calculated using a change ratio (Δ) as follows:

$$\Delta = \frac{\text{evaluation results post} \mid \text{treatment or follow} \mid \text{up}}{\text{baseline results}}$$

Statistical Analysis

SPSS version 21.0 package for Windows was used for all statistical analyses. Categorical variables were reported as proportions and continuous variables were reported as median values (interquartile range) or means $\pm$ standard deviations (SD). Baseline demographic variables were tested using independent t-test or Chi-square test. Differences between within-group inter-group or within-group analysis were determined by Mann-Whitney U-test or one-way analysis of variance (ANOVA) followed by Bonferroni multiple comparisons test. The level of statistical significance was set at $P = 0.05$.

RESULTS

A total of 297 patients were screened and 29 eligible participants were selected between November 2013 and January 2016. Fifteen patients were assigned to mCIMT and 14 were enrolled in standard therapy. All the participants were inpatients, and no participant dropped out of the post-treatment assessments. One patient refused the 3-month follow-up, and another patient was lost to follow-up in the mCIMT group. Another patient was also lost to follow-up in the standard therapy group after 3 months. The flowchart outlining patient selection is presented in **Figure 2**.

Demographic Data

A total of 26 patients (22 men, 4 women) were enrolled and successfully followed up. No significant differences were seen between groups with medical comorbidities: 22 (88.5%) patients with hypertension, 15 (57.7%) with diabetes, three (11.5%) with atrial fibrillation, six (23.1%) with high homocysteine, and seven (27.9%) cases of stenosis of cerebral artery. The disease in the standard therapy group lasted from 2 days to 14 days with a mean of 6.15 ± 3.98 days. In contrast, the CIMT group lasted from 2 days to 14 days with a mean of 7.31 ± 3.86 days. Patient demographic and baseline data are described in **Table 1**.

Clinical Assessment

No significant differences in baseline data (pretreatment) were observed (**Table 2**). After 2 weeks of intervention, both groups showed an increase in ipsilateral upper limb motor function in the WMFT and MAL compared with baseline. A greater improvement in WMFT scores was observed in the CIMT group than in the standard therapy group ($P < 0.001$), and also in the extent of arm use ($P = 0.038$). However, other items of assessment scales were no different between the two groups. At 3-month follow-up, the scores of the QOM (MAL-QOM) and degree of arm use (MAL-AOU) were no different between mCIMT and standard therapy groups. The WMFT analysis yielded no differences in the functional ability between the groups.

TABLE 1 | Baseline characteristics of study participants shown by group.

	mCIMT	Control group	P value
Age (Years)*	58.54 ± 9.61	56.15 ± 11.91	0.579
Sex (M), *n* (%)	11 (84.6)	11 (84.6)	1.000
Smoking, *n* (%)	8 (61.5)	8 (61.5)	1.000
drinking, *n* (%)	7 (53.8)	5 (38.5)	0.431
Hypertension, *n* (%)	11 (84.6)	12 (92.3)	1.000
CardialDiseases, *n* (%)	1 (7.7)	2 (15.4)	1.000
Diabetes, *n* (%)	9 (69.2)	6 (46.2)	0.234
Hyperlipidemia, *n* (%)	19 (63.3)	13 (76.5)	0.353
High homocysteine, *n* (%)	4 (30.8)	2 (15.4)	0.645
Stenosis of cerebral artery, *n* (%)	4 (30.8)	3 (23.1)	0.534
Dominant side affected, *n* (%)	8 (61.5)	7 (53.8)	0.691
NIHSS at admission*	3.85 ± 1.63	3.77 ± 1.59	0.904
Days from stroke onset*	7.31 ± 3.86	6.15 ± 3.98	0.460

**Represents continuous variable with normal distribution, expressed as mean ± SD; other values are expressed as n (%); mCIMT, modified constraint-induced movement therapy; NIHSS, NIH Stroke Scale.*

TABLE 2 | Effect of mCIMT on primary and secondary outcomes (*N* = 26).

Pre-treatment	Control group	mCIMT group	Value	*p*
WMFT score	2.70 ± 0.87	2.53 ± 1.08	$F = 0.18$	0.674
WMFT time(s)	31.27 ± 18.02	37.23 ± 34.82	$F = 0.30$	0.590
MAL-AOU	0.23 (0.26)	0.27 (0.30)	$U = -0.28$	0.801
MAL-QOM	0.28 (0.34)	0.28 (0.30)	$U = -0.13$	0.897
Post-treatment				
WMFT score	3.29 ± 0.90	4.47 ± 0.24	$F = 20.69$	<0.001
WMFT time(s)	16.08 ± 17.50	12.87 ± 14.12	$F = 0.26$	0.611
MAL-AOU	2.39 (1.10)	2.87 (1.72)	$U = -2.08$	0.038
MAL-QOM	1.42 (0.89)	1.76 (0.61)	$U = -0.90$	0.369
3-month follow-up				
WMFT score	4.61 ± 0.56	4.71 ± 0.12	$F = 0.45$	0.507
WMFT time(s)	4.38 ± 1.90	3.67 ± 1.44	$F = 1.19$	0.286
MAL-AOM	3.20 (1.18)	3.23 (0.67)	$U = -0.23$	0.840
MAL-QOM	3.27 (0.68)	3.44 (1.20)	$U = -0.67$	0.505

Normal distribution variable, expressed as mean ± SD; abnormal distribution variable, expressed as median (inter-quartile range). Normal distribution variables were compared by variance analysis. Abnormal distribution variables were compared by Mann-Whitney U-test. mCIMT, modified constraint-induced movement therapy; WMFT time, Wolf Motor Function Test of Performance Time; WMFT score, Wolf Motor Function Test of Functional Ability; MAL-AOU, Motor Activity Log of Amount Of Arm Usage; MAL-QOM, Motor Activity Log of quality of movement.

Electrophysiology

TMS revealed similarities between the two groups with respect to baseline data (**Table 3**). After 2 weeks of intervention, MEPs were present in 10 (76.9%) patients in the CIMT group, with a significant improvement compared with baseline ($P = 0.047$). In the standard therapy group, the MEPs were observed in seven (53.8%) patients, with no difference compared with baseline ($P = 0.695$). Despite the absence of significant differences between the two groups, the presence of MEPs in mCIMT group were significantly higher than the pre-treatment levels. Concurrently, we found that the ipsilesional SP declined 21% compared with the baseline, which was statistically significant compared with the standard therapy group ($P = 0.029$). Other TMS parameters including contralesional SP and CMCT showed no significant changes from the standard therapy group. At 3 months of follow-up, both groups showed significant changes in ipsilesional SP compared with baseline (mCIMT $p < 0.001$; Control group $P = 0.047$). However, no differences were observed compared with each other.

DISCUSSION

CIMT and mCIMT are most effective improving functional outcomes of the upper paretic limb (Kwakkel et al., 2015). Intermediate level of evidence supports mCIMT as an effective intervention for upper extremity hemiparesis after stroke (Uswatte et al., 2005). A single clinical trial involving hospitalized

TABLE 3 | Effect of mCIMT on cortical excitability.

Pre-treatment	Control group	mCIMT group	Value	p
MEPs, n (%)	5 (38.5)	4 (30.8)		1.000
Ipsilesional SP (ms)	184.7 (164.1)	215.7 (62.6)	U = −0.74	0.462
Ipsilesional CMCT (ms)	8.74 ± 1.96	9.25 ± 2.48	F = −0.12	0.742
Contralesional SP (ms)	104.4 (121.6)	118.9 (68.8)	U = −0.49	0.624
Contralesional CMCT (ms)	8.03 ± 1.47	6.83 ± 2.82	F = 1.02	0.347
Post-treatment				
MEPs, n (%)	7 (53.8)	10 (76.9)		0.411
ΔIpsilesional SP	0.91 ± 0.14	0.69 ± 0.09	F = 7.44	0.029
ΔIpsilesional CMCT	0.74 ± 0.29	0.76 ± 0.15	F = 0.09	0.929
ΔContralesional SP	1.07 ± 0.12	1.06 ± 0.23	F = 0.01	0.948
ΔContralesional CMCT	1.06 ± 0.39	0.77 ± 0.17	F = 1.89	0.968
3-month follow-up				
MEPs, n (%)	10 (76.9)	11 (84.6)		1.000
ΔIpsilesional SP	0.74 ± 0.22	0.65 ± 0.08	F = 0.56	0.479
ΔIpsilesional CMCT	1.06 ± 0.58	0.89 ± 0.29	F = 0.31	0.593
ΔContralesional SP	0.95 ± 0.23	1.03 ± 0.35	F = 0.15	0.710
ΔContralesional CMCT	0.96 ± 0.24	0.83 ± 0.28	F = 0.65	0.447

Δ represents altered ratio of TMS motor evoked potentials (MEPs). Normal distribution variable, expressed as mean ± SD; abnormal distribution variable, expressed as median (interquartile range). Normal distribution variables were compared by one way of variance analysis. abnormal distribution variables were compared by Mann-Whitney U-test.

patients demonstrated significantly a higher total scores of the Action Research Arm Test and pinch subscale scores in the CIMT group immediately after therapy without follow-up assessment (Dromerick et al., 2000).

In this study, we used two standard clinical tests to assess upper motor function in patients with acute subcortical infarction. We observed a significant increase (of 1.18) in mean WMFT score ($P < 0.001$) in the mCIMT group after intervention (post-treatment) compared with the standard therapy, indicating that mCIMT promoted faster recovery. Although the mean WMFT time was not significantly improved in the mCIMT group after treatment, a downward trend was observed in the mean WMFT time. MAL scores below 0.27 in patients before intervention suggested occasional usage of their more affected arms for ADL tasks. Following intervention, subjects in the mCIMT group showed changes exceeding 2.0 points in the amount of use (AOU-MAL). The results suggested increased use of the affected upper limb for ADL tasks. The AOU scale scores were comparable to the results of previous mCIMT studies (Page et al., 2005; Wu et al., 2007). This study demonstrated that CIMT improved immediate motor function in patients with acute subcortical infarction.

After a follow-up of 3 months, no differences were seen in the WMFT and MAL scores between patients receiving mCIMT and standard therapies. Our result was consistent with a randomized controlled trial, which did not find a favorable effect of CIMT during the 6-month follow-up (Thrane et al., 2015). Recently, a home-based CIMT in patients with upper limb dysfunction after stroke showed that patients in both the groups showed improvement in the QOM. The home CIMT group outscored patients in the standard therapy group at 3 months, which was not consistent with our study. The patients in the home-based CIMT were recruited at least 6 months after stroke, and received 5 h of professional therapy in 4 weeks. Our study recruited patients at an earlier phase of stroke and all patients underwent shorter therapy.

TABLE 4 | Within-group changes of electrophysiological parameters.

	Pre-treatment	Post-treatment	Follow-up	P_1	P_2	P_3
Control group						
MEPs, (%)	38.5	53.8	76.9	0.695	0.111	1.000
ΔIpsilesonal SP	1.00	0.92 ± 0.14	0.74 ± 0.22	1.000	0.047	0.244
ΔIpsilesonal CMCT	1.00	0.74 ± 0.29	1.07 ± 0.58	0.892	0.583	1.000
ΔContralesonal SP	1.00	1.07 ± 0.13	0.95 ± 0.23	1.000	1.000	0.732
ΔContralesonal CMCT	1.00	1.06 ± 0.39	0.96 ± 0.24	1.000	1.000	1.000
mCIMT group						
MEPs, (%)	30.8	76.9	84.6	0.047	0.015	0.411
ΔIpsilesonal SP	1.00	0.69 ± 0.09	0.65 ± 0.81	<0.001	<0.001	1.000
ΔIpsilesonal CMCT	1.00	0.76 ± 0.15	0.89 ± 0.29	1.000	1.000	1.000
ΔContralesonal SP	1.00	1.05 ± 0.23	1.03 ± 0.35	0.294	1.000	1.000
ΔContralesonal CMCT	1.00	0.77 ± 0.17	0.82 ± 0.26	0.290	0.569	1.000

Normal distribution variable, expressed as mean ± SD; abnormal distribution variable, expressed as median (interquartile range). Normal distribution variables were compared by variance analysis, and followed by Bonferroni multiple comparisons test. P1 represents statistical difference between Pre-treatment and Post-treatment; P2 represents statistical difference between Pre-treatment and Follow-up; P3 represents statistical difference between Post-treatment and Follow-up.

A series of studies demonstrated increased cortical neuroplasticity in the subacute and chronic post-stroke phases of the brain (Liepert et al., 1998; Ro et al., 2006; Boake et al., 2007; Sawaki et al., 2008; Laible et al., 2012). However, studies conducted on patients with subcortical lesions are rare (Jang, 2007). Our study of patients with subcortical infarction displayed improved MEPs and ipsilesional SP in the mCIMT group after treatment, suggesting significant enhancement in cortical excitability of the lesion side. Studies showed that reduced ipsilesional SP level was a prognostic factor for spasticity in chronic stroke (Uozumi et al., 1992; Cruz Martínez et al., 1998). However, it may play a different role in acute stroke. Our earlier study demonstrated decreased ipsilesional SP levels during the first few days after acute cerebral infarction and significantly predicted the outcome within 3 months (Zhang et al., 2016). Patients with an SP value more than 217.05 showed a 7.69-fold increased risk of unfavorable outcomes compared with patients reporting an SP value less than 217.05. In the present study, we found that ipsilesional SP levels were significantly reduced immediately post-mCIMT compared with the control group. We speculate that reduced SP levels may reflect increased muscle tone and improved functional recovery in the acute phase of cerebral infarction.

Previous studies showed that recruitment of supplementary motor areas on the ipsilesional side enhanced the recovery. However, persistent activation of the contralesional cortex was associated with a slower and less complete recovery (Murphy and Corbett, 2009; Xerri, 2012). The present study found no changes in the SP, and CMCT in the contralesional sides of both groups. Our results suggested that the functional improvement of affected upper limb after treatment were associated with enhanced ipsilesional cortical excitability. At 3 months follow-up, significant change in ipsilesional SP was detected in mCIMT group compared with pre-treatment, and we also the similarly change in standard therapy groups. The reason for those changes may be that patients were not required to adhere to similar training at home (**Table 4**).

Our study limitations are as follows. First, the present study was a single-center clinical trial, and it was difficult to recruit eligible patients. Multi-centered trials are needed to increase the sample size. Second, using non-navigated TMS was a major limitation to the present study. It was well known that navigational systems allow TMS within a spatial deviation of few millimeters to a desired region of the cortex (Rossini and Rossi, 2007; Sparing et al., 2008). Using the International 10–20 electrode system for positioning of the TMS coil was not as accurate as navigational systems, but it was easily applicable in its practicable use. Moreover, using 10–20 electrode system enabled us not only to quickly retrieve the cortical region of interest but also shorten pre-evaluation related time, and avoid some security concerns resulting from navigated TMS in acute stroke patients. Third, we assessed changes of cortical excitability using TMS. However, single TMS pulses were unlikely to distinguish between stimulation of cortico-spinal, intra-cortical and trans-cortical elements, but instead target all three to varying degrees (Bestmann and Krakauer, 2015). We could not determine the contribution of other areas of the brain to the resultant output. Combination of TMS and brain functional imaging or specific stimulation protocols, such as paired-pulse stimulation could facilitate our understanding of neurophysiological mechanisms of stroke recovery.

CONCLUSION

Compared with standard therapy, mCIMT induced significant functional changes in acute subcortical ischemic stroke patients. Early intervention with mCIMT promotes ipsilesional cortical reorganization, without any long-term effect.

AUTHOR CONTRIBUTIONS

JW contributed to the conception and design of the work; contributed in revising the work for important intellectual content. CY, WW, YZ, YW, WH, SL, CG, CW and LM contributed in the data acquisition. CY, WW and JW contributed in the analysis and interpretation of data for the work. CY and WW contributed in drafting the work. All authors approved the final version to be published, and agree to be accountable for all aspects of the work in ensuring that questions related to the accuracy or integrity of any part of the work are appropriately investigated and resolved.

ACKNOWLEDGMENTS

This study was generously supported by Grants from Tianjin Public Health Bureau (2013KG122, to JW), and General Administration of Sport of China (2015B098, to JW), and Program to Establish Scientific Research Resources by Tianjin Municipal Health bureau (Establishment and Quality Control for biobanking of Neurological Diseases).

REFERENCES

Bergmann, T. O., Möle, M., Schmidt, M. A., Lindner, C., Marshall, L., Born, J., et al. (2012). EEG-guided transcranial magnetic stimulation reveals rapid shifts in motor cortical excitability during the human sleep slow oscillation. *J. Neurosci.* 32, 243–253. doi: 10.1523/JNEUROSCI.4792-11.2012

Bestmann, S., and Krakauer, J. W. (2015). The uses and interpretations of the motor-evoked potential for understanding behaviour. *Exp. Brain Res.* 233, 679–689. doi: 10.1007/s00221-014-4183-7

Boake, C., Noser, E. A., Ro, T., Baraniuk, S., Gaber, M., Johnson, R., et al. (2007). Constraint-induced movement therapy during early stroke rehabilitation. *Neurorehabil. Neural Repair* 21, 14–24. doi: 10.1177/1545968306291858

Bonifer, N. M., Anderson, K. M., and Arciniegas, D. B. (2005). Constraint-induced therapy for moderate chronic upper extremity impairment after stroke. *Brain Inj.* 19, 323–330. doi: 10.1080/02699050400004302

Braune, H. J., and Fritz, C. (1995). Transcranial magnetic stimulation-evoked inhibition of voluntary muscle activity (silent period) is impaired in patients with ischemic hemispheric lesion. *Stroke* 26, 550–553. doi: 10.1161/01.str.26.4.550

Chen, R., Cros, D., Curra, A., Di Lazzaro, V., Lefaucheur, J. P., Magistris, M. R., et al. (2008). The clinical diagnostic utility of transcranial magnetic stimulation: report of an IFCN committee. *Clin. Neurophysiol.* 119, 504–532. doi: 10.1016/j.clinph.2007.10.014

Cruz Martínez, A., Muñoz, J., and Palacios, F. (1998). The muscle inhibitory period by transcranial magnetic stimulation. Study in stroke patients. *Electromyogr. Clin. Neurophysiol.* 38, 189–192.

Dobkin, B. H. (2004). Neurobiology of rehabilitation. *Ann. N Y Acad. Sci.* 1038, 148–170. doi: 10.1196/annals.1315.024

Dromerick, A. W., Edwards, D. F., and Hahn, M. (2000). Does the application of constraint-induced movement therapy during acute rehabilitation reduce arm impairment after ischemic stroke? *Stroke* 31, 2984–2988. doi: 10.1161/01.str.31.12.2984

Heald, A., Bates, D., Cartlidge, N. E., French, J. M., and Miller, S. (1993). Longitudinal study of central motor conduction time following stroke. 2. Central motor conduction measured within 72 h after stroke as a predictor of functional outcome at 12 months. *Brain* 116, 1371–1385. doi: 10.1093/brain/116.6.1371

Hendricks, H. T., van Limbeek, J., Geurts, A. C., and Zwarts, M. J. (2002). Motor recovery after stroke: a systematic review of the literature. *Arch. Phys. Med. Rehabil.* 83, 1629–1637. doi: 10.1053/apmr.2002.35473

Jang, S. H. (2007). A review of motor recovery mechanisms in patients with stroke. *NeuroRehabilitation* 22, 253–259.

Kim, J. S. (2014). Stroke in Asia: a global disaster. *Int. J. Stroke* 9, 856–857. doi: 10.1111/ijs.12317

Kleim, J. A., Barbay, S., and Nudo, R. J. (1998). Functional reorganization of the rat motor cortex following motor skill learning. *J. Neurophysiol.* 80, 3321–3325.

Kwakkel, G., Kollen, B., and Twisk, J. (2006). Impact of time on improvement of outcome after stroke. *Stroke* 37, 2348–2353. doi: 10.1161/01.str.0000238594.91938.1e

Kwakkel, G., Veerbeek, J. M., van Wegen, E. E., and Wolf, S. L. (2015). Constraint-induced movement therapy after stroke. *Lancet Neurol.* 14, 224–234. doi: 10.1016/S1474-4422(14)70160-7

Laible, M., Grieshammer, S., Seidel, G., Rijntjes, M., Weiller, C., and Hamzei, F. (2012). Association of activity changes in the primary sensory cortex with successful motor rehabilitation of the hand following stroke. *Neurorehabil. Neural Repair* 26, 881–888. doi: 10.1177/1545968312437939

Langhorne, P., Coupar, F., and Pollock, A. (2009). Motor recovery after stroke: a systematic review. *Lancet Neurol.* 8, 741–754. doi: 10.1016/S1474-4422(09)70150-4

Liepert, J., Miltner, W. H. R., Bauder, H., Sommer, M., Dettmers, C., Taub, E., et al. (1998). Motor cortex plasticity during constraint-induced movement therapy in stroke patients. *Neurosci. Lett.* 250, 5–8. doi: 10.1016/s0304-3940(98)00386-3

Liu, G., Dang, C., Peng, K., Xie, C., Chen, H., Xing, S., et al. (2015). Increased spontaneous neuronal activity in structurally damaged cortex is correlated with early motor recovery in patients with subcortical infarction. *Eur. J. Neurol.* 22, 1540–1547. doi: 10.1111/ene.12780

Mehndiratta, P., Wasay, M., and Mehndiratta, M. M. (2015). Implications of female sex on stroke risk factors, care, outcome and rehabilitation: an Asian perspective. *Cerebrovasc. Dis.* 39, 302–308. doi: 10.1159/000381832

Momosaki, R., Yasunaga, H., Kakuda, W., Matsui, H., Fushimi, K., and Abo, M. (2016). Very early versus delayed rehabilitation for acute ischemic stroke patients with intravenous recombinant tissue plasminogen activator: a nationwide retrospective cohort study. *Cerebrovasc. Dis.* 42, 41–48. doi: 10.1159/000444720

Morris, D. M., Uswatte, G., Crago, J. E., Cook, E. W. III, and Taub, E. (2001). The reliability of the wolf motor function test for assessing upper extremity function after stroke. *Arch. Phys. Med. Rehabil.* 82, 750–755. doi: 10.1053/apmr.2001.23183

Murphy, T. H., and Corbett, D. (2009). Plasticity during stroke recovery: from synapse to behaviour. *Nat. Rev. Neurosci.* 10, 861–872. doi: 10.1038/nrn2735

Nijland, R., van Wegen, E., Verbunt, J., van Wijk, R., van Kordelaar, J., and Kwakkel, G. (2010). A comparison of two validated tests for upper limb function after stroke: the wolf motor function test and the action research arm test. *J. Rehabil. Med.* 42, 694–696. doi: 10.2340/16501977-0560

Nudo, R. J., Wise, B. M., SiFuentes, F., and Milliken, G. W. (1996). Neural substrates for the effects of rehabilitative training on motor recovery after ischemic infarct. *Science* 272, 1791–1794. doi: 10.1126/science.272.5269.1791

Page, S. J., Levine, P., and Leonard, A. C. (2005). Modified constraint-induced therapy in acute stroke: a randomized controlled pilot study. *Neurorehabil. Neural Repair* 19, 27–32. doi: 10.1177/1545968304272701

Ro, T., Noser, E., Boake, C., Johnson, R., Gaber, M., Speroni, A., et al. (2006). Functional reorganization and recovery after constraint-induced movement therapy in subacute stroke: case reports. *Neurocase* 12, 50–60. doi: 10.1080/13554790500493415

Rossini, P. M., and Rossi, S. (2007). Transcranial magnetic stimulation: diagnostic,therapeutic and research potential. *Neurology* 68, 484–488. doi: 10.1212/01.wnl.0000250268.13789.b2

Sawaki, L., Butler, A. J., Leng, X., Wassenaar, P. A., Mohammad, Y. M., Blanton, S., et al. (2008). Constraint-induced movement therapy results in increased motor map area in subjects 3 to 9 months after stroke. *Neurorehabil. Neural Repair* 22, 505–513. doi: 10.1177/1545968308317531

Singh, P., and Pradhan, B. (2013). Study to assess the effectiveness of modified constraint-induced movement therapy in stroke subjects: a randomized controlled trial. *Ann. Indian Acad. Neurol.* 16, 180–184. doi: 10.4103/0972-2327.112461

Souza, W. C., Conforto, A. B., Orsini, M., Stern, A., and André, C. (2015). Similar effects of two modified constraint-induced therapy protocols on motor impairment, motor function and quality of life in patients with chronic stroke. *Neurol. Int.* 7:5430. doi: 10.4081/ni.2015.5430

Sparing, R., Buelte, D., Meister, I. G., Paus, T., and Fink, G. R. (2008). Transcranial magnetic stimulation and the challenge of coil placement: a comparison of conventional and stereotaxic neuronavigational strategies. *Hum. Brain Mapp.* 29, 82–96. doi: 10.1002/hbm.20360

Sudlow, C. L., and Warlow, C. P. (1997). Comparable studies of the incidence of stroke and its pathological types: results from an international collaboration. International Stroke Incidence Collaboration. *Stroke* 28, 491–499. doi: 10.1161/01.str.28.3.491

Taub, E. (2000). Constraint-induced movement therapy and massed practice. *Stroke* 31, 983–991. doi: 10.1161/01.STR.31.4.983-c

Terént, A. (2003). Trends in stroke incidence and 10-year survival in Söderhamn, Sweden, 1975–2001. *Stroke* 34, 1353–1358. doi: 10.1161/01.str.0000074038.71700.1c

Thrane, G., Askim, T., Stock, R., Indredavik, B., Gjone, R., Erichsen, A., et al. (2015). Efficacy of constraint-induced movement therapy in early stroke rehabilitation: a randomized controlled multisite trial. *Neurorehabil. Neural Repair* 29, 517–525. doi: 10.1177/1545968314558599

Trompetto, C., Assini, A., Buccolieri, A., Marchese, R., and Abbruzzese, G. (2000). Motor recovery following stroke: a transcranial magnetic stimulation study. *Clin. Neurophysiol.* 111, 1860–1867. doi: 10.1016/s1388-2457(00)00419-3

Truelsen, T., Mähönen, M., Tolonen, H., Asplund, K., Bonita, R., Vanuzzo, D., et al. (2003). Trends in stroke and coronary heart disease in the WHO MONICA Project. *Stroke* 34, 1346–1352. doi: 10.1161/01.str.0000069724.36173.4d

Uozumi, T., Ito, Y., Tsuji, S., and Murai, Y. (1992). Inhibitory period following motor potentials evoked by magnetic cortical stimulation. *Electroencephalogr. Clin. Neurophysiol.* 85, 273–279. doi: 10.1016/0168-5597(92)90116-s

Uozumi, T., Tsuji, S., and Murai, Y. (1991). Motor potentials evoked by magnetic stimulation of the motor cortex in normal subjects and patients with motor disorders. *Electroencephalogr. Clin. Neurophysiol.* 81, 251–256. doi: 10.1016/0168-5597(91)90010-u

Uswatte, G., Foo, W. L., Olmstead, H., Lopez, K., Holand, A., and Simms, L. B. (2005). Ambulatory monitoring of arm movement using accelerometry: an objective measure of upper-extremity rehabilitation in persons with chronic stroke. *Arch. Phys. Med. Rehabil.* 86, 1498–1501. doi: 10.1016/j.apmr.2005.01.010

van der Lee, J. H., Wagenaar, R. C., Lankhorst, G. J., Vogelaar, T. W., Devillé, W. L., and Bouter, L. M. (1999). Forced use of the upper extremity in chronic stroke patients: results from a single-blind randomized clinical trial. *Stroke* 30, 2369–2375. doi: 10.1161/01.str.30.11.2369 van Kuijk, A. A., Pasman, J. W., Geurts, A. C., and Hendricks, H. T. (2005). How salient is the silent period? The role of the silent period in the prognosis of upper extremity motor recovery after severe stroke. *J. Clin. Neurophysiol.* 22, 10–24. doi: 10.1097/01.WNP.0000150975.83249.71

van Mierlo, M. L., van Heugten, C. M., Post, M. W., Hajós, T. R., Kappelle, L. J., and Visser-Meily, J. M. (2016). Quality of life during the first two years post stroke: the restore 4 stroke cohort study. *Cerebrovasc. Dis.* 41, 19–26. doi: 10.1159/000441197

Veerbeek, J. M., Kwakkel, G., van Wegen, E. E., Ket, J. C., and Heymans, M. W. (2011). Early prediction of outcome of activities of daily living after stroke: a systematic review. *Stroke* 42, 1482–1488. doi: 10.1161/STROKEAHA.110.604090

Wolf, S. L., Catlin, P. A., Ellis, M., Archer, A. L., Morgan, B., and Piacentino, A. (2001). Assessing Wolf motor function test as outcome measure for research in patients after stroke. *Stroke* 32, 1635–1639. doi: 10.1161/01.str.32.7.1635

Wolf, S. L., Lecraw, D. E., Barton, L. A., and Jann, B. B. (1989). Forced use of hemiplegic upper extremities to reverse the effect of learned nonuse among chronic stroke and head-injured patients. *Exp. Neurol.* 104, 125–132. doi: 10.1016/s0014-4886(89)80005-6

Wolf, S. L., Thompson, P. A., Morris, D. M., Rose, D. K., Winstein, C. J., Taub, E., et al. (2005). The EXCITE trial: attributes of the Wolf motor function test in patients with subacute stroke. *Neurorehabil. Neural Repair* 19, 194–205. doi: 10.1177/1545968305276663

Wu, C. Y., Chen, C. L., Tsai, W. C., Lin, K. C., and Chou, S. H. (2007). A randomized controlled trial of modified constraint-induced movement therapy for elderly stroke survivors: changes in motor impairment, daily functioning, and quality of life. *Arch. Phys. Med. Rehabil.* 88, 273–278. doi: 10.1016/j.apmr.2006.11.021

Xerri, C. (2012). Plasticity of cortical maps: multiple triggers for adaptive reorganization following brain damage and spinal cord injury. *Neuroscientist* 18, 133–148. doi: 10.1177/1073858410397894

Zhang, X., Ji, W., Li, L., Yu, C., Wang, W., Liu, S., et al. (2016). The predictive value of motor-evoked potentials and the silent period on patient outcome after acute cerebral infarction. *J. Stroke Cerebrovasc. Dis.* 25, 1713–1720. doi: 10.1016/j.jstrokecerebrovasdis.2016.03.022

16

Adiposity Related Brain Plasticity Induced by Bariatric Surgery

*Michael Rullmann[1,2,3,4], Sven Preusser[3], Sindy Poppitz[1,3], Stefanie Heba[5], Konstantinos Gousias[6], Jana Hoyer[7,8], Tatjana Schütz[1], Arne Dietrich[1,9], Karsten Müller[3], Mohammed K. Hankir[10] and Burkhard Pleger[1,3,4,5]**

[1]IFB Adiposity Diseases, Leipzig University Medical Centre, Leipzig, Germany, [2]Department of Nuclear Medicine, University Hospital Leipzig, Leipzig, Germany, [3]Department of Neurology, Max Planck Institute for Human Cognitive and Brain Sciences, Leipzig, Germany, [4]Collaborative Research Centre 1052 Obesity Mechanisms, University of Leipzig, Leipzig, Germany, [5]Department of Neurology, BG University Hospital Bergmannsheil, Ruhr-University Bochum, Bochum, Germany, [6]Department of Neurosurgery, BG University Hospital Bergmannsheil, Ruhr-University Bochum, Bochum, Germany, [7]Department of Behavioral Epidemiology, Technische Universität Dresden, Dresden, Germany, [8]Department of Psychology, Technische Universität Dresden, Dresden, Germany, [9]Department of Bariatric Surgery, University Hospital Leipzig, Leipzig, Germany, [10]Department of Experimental Surgery, University Hospital Würzburg, Würzburg, Germany

Edited by:
Peter Sörös,
University of Oldenburg, Germany

Reviewed by:
Ilona Dekkers,
Sylvius Laboratory, Leiden University, Netherlands
Alaina Pearce,
Pennsylvania State University, United States

***Correspondence:**
Burkhard Pleger
burkhard.v.pleger@rub.de

Previous magnetic resonance imaging (MRI) studies revealed structural-functional brain reorganization 12 months after gastric-bypass surgery, encompassing cortical and subcortical regions of all brain lobes as well as the cerebellum. Changes in the mean of cluster-wise gray/white matter density (GMD/WMD) were correlated with the individual loss of body mass index (BMI), rendering the BMI a potential marker of widespread surgery-induced brain plasticity. Here, we investigated voxel-by-voxel associations between surgery-induced changes in adiposity, metabolism and inflammation and markers of functional and structural neural plasticity. We re-visited the data of patients who underwent functional and structural MRI, 6 months (n = 27) and 12 months after surgery (n = 22), and computed voxel-wise regression analyses. Only the surgery-induced weight loss was significantly associated with brain plasticity, and this only for GMD changes. After 6 months, weight loss overlapped with altered GMD in the hypothalamus, the brain's homeostatic control site, the lateral orbitofrontal cortex, assumed to host reward and gustatory processes, as well as abdominal representations in somatosensory cortex. After 12 months, weight loss scaled with GMD changes in right cerebellar lobule VII, involved in language-related/cognitive processes, and, by trend, with the striatum, assumed to underpin (food) reward. These findings suggest time-dependent and weight-loss related gray matter plasticity in brain regions involved in the control of eating, sensory processing and cognitive functioning.

Keywords: adiposity, magnetic resonance imaging, brain plasticity, bariatric surgery, gastric-bypass surgery

INTRODUCTION

The incidence of obesity is dramatically increasing worldwide reaching a pandemic level and rendering obesity one of the most challenging health burden of current and future times.

Obese individuals often present comorbidities reaching from cardiovascular and endocrinological diseases to cancer (Dixon, 2010; Ebbert et al., 2014). Impaired cognitive performance and accelerated brain atrophy (Debette et al., 2010; Ho et al., 2010), together with a higher risk of dementia (Knopman et al., 2011; Tosto and Reitz, 2013) indicate negative influences on mental health.

Craving and overconsumption are crucial behavioral features of individuals with obesity. Craving may result from enhanced predictive activity in reward-associated brain regions, whereas during food consumption, reward responses seem to be attenuated probably supporting compensatory overconsumption (Wang et al., 2001; Stice et al., 2008; Johnson and Kenny, 2010). Dysfunctional dopamine release in regions such as the nucleus accumbens, the dorsal striatum and the medial prefrontal cortex seems to have a mediating role in obesogenic effects (Geiger et al., 2008, 2009; Zhang et al., 2015). But dopamine mediates not only food reward suggesting that an aberrant food-related behavior in obese individuals transfers to other reward-related behaviors, such as those associated with monetary incentives (Amlung et al., 2016).

During eating, reward regions permanently interact with the hypothalamus to adjust hedonic responses to current homeostatic demands. In the obese brain, these interactions seem to weaken, and hedonism overpowers homeostasis (Davis et al., 2007; Bryant et al., 2008). Cross-sectional brain imaging studies provide supportive evidence for body weight related functional and structural alteration of hedonic (Wang et al., 2001; Stoeckel et al., 2008; Stice et al., 2010; Mueller et al., 2014) and homeostatic brain regions (Horstmann et al., 2011). But an increased weight also overlapped with executive control regions (e.g., dorsolateral prefrontal cortex, DLPFC) and regions involved in emotional processing (e.g., the amygdala; Jagust et al., 2005; Walther et al., 2010; Debette et al., 2011; Horstmann et al., 2011) suggesting influences on various brain systems guiding everyday eating behavior. An understanding of how this behavior and corresponding brain processes change over time while individuals gain or lose weight may help to develop new therapeutic strategies against obesity.

Bariatric surgery has been established as the gold standard for the treatment of morbid obesity [i.e., body mass index (BMI), BMI $\geq$ 40 kg/m^2]. Over the 1st year after surgery, patients experience the largest weight loss with gastric bypass surgery showing the strongest effect on the BMI (i.e., loss of 32%; Sjöström et al., 2004; Robinson, 2009; Gianos et al., 2012). At the same time, energy balance and hence cardiovascular risk factors, such as diabetes and hypertension are progressively improving (Sjöström, 2013). These positive effects on body weight and health suggest the potential reversibility of central homeostatic and hedonic dysfunctions as well as corresponding adiposity-related structural and functional brain alterations.

Only few brain imaging studies to date investigated the influence of bariatric surgery on brain function and structure. Using magnetic resonance imaging (MRI) together with voxel-based morphometry (VBM), surgery-induced brain plasticity was observed not only in hedonic (e.g., striatum), homeostatic (e.g., hypothalamus) and executive control regions (e.g., DLPFC), but across the entire gray (Rullmann et al., 2018) and white matter compartments (Tuulari et al., 2016). This suggests much more far-reaching behavior adaptations than only those involved in the control of food consumption.

Rullmann et al. (2018) showed that the higher the BMI loss after surgery, the larger MRI-based changes of gray and white matter densities (GMD/WMD) across the entire brain were. No other markers of changes in adiposity, metabolism or inflammation significantly scaled with surgery-induced brain plasticity (Rullmann et al., 2018). These findings render the degree of adiposity (Gurka et al., 2018) a potential marker for surgery-induced widespread white and gray matter plasticity. Significance of this correlation, however, may have been constituted only by some voxels, whereas other voxels may have been less meaningful or even irrelevant. Clusters of significantly correlated voxels may, furthermore, overlap with distinct brain regions providing a more fine-grained picture of adiposity-related influences on the brain induced by bariatric surgery.

To unveil voxel-wise, and potentially region-specific associations with surgery-induced changes in adiposity, metabolism and inflammation, we re-analyzed MRI data from our recent longitudinal study (Rullmann et al., 2018). We computed voxel-by-voxel regression analyses including individual surgery-induced changes in gray matter (i.e., GMD), white matter (i.e., WMD and diffusion tensor imaging, or DTI, to assess fractional anisotropy, FA) and spontaneous neural activity (regional homogeneity, ReHo, and amplitudes of low frequency fluctuation, ALFF). Corresponding surgery-induced improvements in markers of adiposity, metabolism and inflammation [i.e., body weight (kg), fat mass (%), serum high-density lipoproteins (HDL), low-density lipoproteins (LDL), triglyceride, HbA1c, CrP, thyroid-stimulating hormone (TSH)] were included as interacting covariates.

Contrarily to the widespread plasticity, we found in our previous data analyses (Rullmann et al., 2018), we here hypothesized a more detailed picture of surgery-induced clinical improvements and associated structural (i.e., GMD, WMD, FA) and functional plasticity (ALFF, ReHo). We assumed to identify a network consisting of the dorsal striatum, involved in reward processing (Stice et al., 2008), the insular cortex, assumed to host gustatory processes (Tuulari et al., 2016; Rullmann et al., 2018), the hypothalamus, as the main homeostatic control site (van de Sande-Lee et al., 2011; Hollmann et al., 2013; Schlogl et al., 2016), as well as executive control regions in the DLPFC (Hollmann et al., 2013).

MATERIALS AND METHODS

Patients

The data for the present analyses was obtained from the same 27 morbidly obese patients (21 females, age 51.1 $\pm$ 9.6 years, BMI 47.8 $\pm$ 5.5 kg/m^2) who participated in our previous study (Rullmann et al., 2018). Contraindications to MRI were exclusion criteria (see Supplementary Information in Rullmann et al., 2018 for a detailed list). Patients gave written informed consent. **Table 1** lists clinical parameters such as (BMI, kg/m^2), body weight (kg), fat mass (%), cholesterol serum levels (mmol/l), HDL (mmol/l), LDL (mmol/l), triglycerides (mmol/l), as well as glycated hemoglobin (HbA1c, %) which indexes the 3-months

TABLE 1 | The table presents body mass index (BMI), gender, weight, blood parameters [cholesterol, high-density lipoproteins (HDL), low-density lipoproteins (LDL), triglyceride, glycated hemoglobin (HbA1c), C-reactive protein (CrP), thyroid-stimulating hormone (TSH)], and fat mass (%).

Subject	Age	Gender	Weight			BMI			Cholesterol			HDL			LDL			Triglyceride			HbA1c			CrP			TSH			Fat mass		
			pre	½ year	1 year	pre	½ year	1 year	pre	½ year	1 year	pre	½ year	1 year	pre	½ year	1 year	pre	½ year	1 year	pre	½ year	1 year	pre	½ year	1 year	pre	½ year	1 year	pre	½ year	1 year
#1	60	♀	147	105	100	58.7	42.1	40.2	4.84	4.8	4.69	1.61	1.55	1.73	2.58	2.68	2.84	1.33	0.86	1.2	6.46	5.87	5.31	19.5	3.91	2.46	1.04	0.406	0.824	62.2	53.4	48.7
#2	54	♀	123	105	101	44.6	38.1	36.6	4.62	4.29	3.89	1.65	1.55	1.76	2.61	2.38	1.99	1.52	1.19	1.18	4.97	5.1	5.25	8.3	6.18	2.86	2.28	3.18	1.75	N/A	N/A	48.1
#3	49	♂	165	126	113	44.2	33.7	30.4	3.95	3.28	4.35	1.09	1.16	1.31	2.25	1.91	2.96	1.32	0.92	0.82	5.62	5.51	5.3	7.05	1.23	1.48	0.7	0.731	0.64	44.9	33.3	27.3
#4	54	♀	104	79.9	76	44.5	34.1	32.5	4.64	5.09	4.51	1.17	1.44	1.44	3.23	3.19	2.78	1.65	1.48	1.02	5.06	4.83	4.99	5.8	2.61	1.73	0.712	2.63	0.637	49.4	32.9	27.2
#5	59	♀	135	105	95.8	47.3	37.3	33.9	5.99	4.63	5.1	2.27	2.16	2.6	3.35	2.47	2.47	0.8	0.59	0.87	5.28	5.03	5.08	21.4	2.87	1.87	0.787	2.02	1.9	59.9	44.4	39.7
#6	60	♀	120	97.7	96.6	38.7	31.5	31.2	4.95	5.08	4.3	0.98	1.54	1.73	2.96	2.5	1.88	2.92	3.75	1.9	5.6	5.01	5.19	3.77	1.5	0.89	0.65	0.763	0.919	52.8	41.1	N/A
#7	44	♀	143	99.2	87.5	52.3	36.4	32.1	4.53	4.66	4.17	0.83	1.3	1.72	2.95	2.85	2.23	1.42	1.05	0.63	5.45	5.24	5.42	24.7	1.03	0.99	1.22	1.08	0.764	49.0	36.6	38.7
#8	45	♀	161	129	127	47.6	38.1	37.4	3.48	3.52	3.93	1	1.27	1.47	2.03	2	2.39	0.89	1.28	1.19	5.35	4.69	5.07	13.9	8.44	2.26	0.563	1.56	1.09	62.7	39.2	34.0
#9	60	♀	120	103	102	48.1	41.3	40.7	3.72	4.51	5	1.05	1.49	1.26	2.27	2.54	3.04	1.54	1.8	3.05	6.11	5.52	5.66	6.1	2.11	2.05	1.14	0.696	1.24	65.1	54.0	50.5
#10	38	♀	154	123	103	54.0	43.0	36.2	4.98	4.19	3.83	1.03	1.21	1.43	3.51	2.62	2.22	1.83	0.9	1.06	4.97	4.67	5.16	6.53	1.76	0.68	0.75	0.828	0.766	59.4	50.2	38.4
#11	49	♀	138	112	104	52.7	42.6	39.5	4.46	4.15	4.29	1.3	1.81	1.84	2.66	2.03	2.17	1.17	1.44	1.62	5.21	4.85	4.88	9.78	3	1.14	2.22	1.87	2.04	63.1	49.1	43.1
#12	39	♀	121	88	87.5	42.8	31.2	31.0	5.52	3.04	3.47	1.14	1.21	1.08	3.49	1.7	2.18	2.63	0.58	0.7	10.5	5.25	5.73	1.8	0.3	1.71	0.271	0.543	0.598	51.4	22.6	31.7
#13	66	♂	127	96	82.8	40.1	30.3	26.1	4.04	3.6	3.97	1.29	1.4	2.15	2.32	2.06	1.67	0.97	0.74	0.81	7.49	6.18	6.25	0.6	0.45	0.3	0.677	0.543	1	34.4	25.1	17.2
#14	54	♀	116	92.9	89.1	41.0	32.9	31.6	6.01	5.71	5.91	0.99	1.68	1.68	4.4	3.78	4.04	0.98	1.06	0.95	6	5.25	5.62	11.3	6.96	2.28	1.47	1.7	1.6	53.4	39.0	39.9
#15	60	♀	150	130	120	58.7	50.9	46.7	4.88	N/A	3.67	1.17	N/A	0.82	3.17	N/A	2.25	1.28	N/A	1.16	5.59	N/A	5.5	16.2	N/A	30.2	3.73	N/A	2.33	62.1	60.5	57.4
#16	30	♀	120	89.1	80.2	44.2	32.7	29.5	3.2	3.43	2.81	1.13	1.53	1.43	1.72	1.62	1.08	0.94	1.35	0.55	5.19	5.12	5.13	7.84	2.34	47.5	2.55	2.56	0.847	60.5	40.6	36.2
#17	52	♀	138	112	107	45.1	36.6	35.0	4.46	4.01	3.73	1.52	1.56	1.62	2.55	2.11	1.66	1.12	1.36	1.32	5.17	5.27	5.22	4	0.95	1.43	1.33	1.57	1.09	57.2	47.2	38.5
#18	55	♀	115	91.7	101	42.6	34.1	37.5	4.44	3.88	4.74	1.35	1.37	1.37	2.87	2.34	2.96	1.53	1.74	1.42	5.78	5.42	5.75	5.33	1.06	3.06	2.33	1.14	1.16	43.5	30.7	37.5
#19	55	♂	149	105	N/A	46.0	32.5	N/A	2.99	3.21	N/A	0.92	1.05	N/A	1.91	1.98	N/A	0.91	0.95	N/A	6.35	7.03	N/A	0.84	0.3	N/A	1.34	3.25	N/A	41.1	20.1	N/A
#20	54	♀	173	146	133	47.5	40.0	36.6	4.88	N/A	4.52	1.16	N/A	1.35	3.33	N/A	2.75	1.83	N/A	1.5	5.73	5.71	5.96	2.41	2.78	1.12	1.52	0.533	1.08	N/A	N/A	N/A
#21	55	♂	131	109	104	44.7	37.4	35.4	4.72	4.39	5.08	1.02	0.97	1.06	3.2	2.96	3.26	2.03	1.31	0.98	8.21	7.47	7.07	7.79	4.19	4.77	1.75	1.95	1.8	31.5	21.9	25.9
#22	59	♀	112	89.7	88	47.3	37.8	37.1	4.31	3.14	3.25	1.17	1.43	1.49	2.52	1.36	1.45	2.31	0.84	1.09	9.11	7.01	7.07	4.76	0.91	1.27	4.24	2.36	2.63	N/A	N/A	N/A
#23	52	♂	161	127	118	50.8	40.1	37.1	3.82	4.24	3.75	1.03	1.58	1.57	2.42	2.39	2.09	0.76	0.65	0.62	5.34	5.33	5.18	8.93	5.65	3.49	0.956	1.42	1.51	49.2	31.3	27.7
#24	27	♀	166	132	N/A	56.2	44.7	N/A	2.65	2.92	N/A	0.86	1.05	N/A	1.52	1.59	N/A	0.96	0.87	N/A	5.55	5.29	N/A	22.6	14.1	N/A	2.28	1.86	N/A	59.8	47.4	N/A
#25	42	♀	129	87.1	N/A	44.5	30.1	N/A	5.21	4.6	N/A	1.26	1.27	N/A	3.54	2.77	N/A	2.91	0.82	N/A	5.76	5.23	N/A	15.1	2.16	N/A	2.23	2.88	N/A	54.0	30.4	N/A
#26	39	♂	175	130	N/A	55.1	41.2	N/A	5.77	4.46	N/A	1.04	0.85	N/A	4.1	3.12	N/A	1.17	0.96	N/A	5.62	5.22	N/A	5.92	3.65	N/A	2.26	2.75	N/A	52.6	33.2	N/A
#27	57	♀	139	109	N/A	51.7	40.5	N/A	4.95	3.87	N/A	1.27	1.27	N/A	3.2	2.27	N/A	1.31	1.19	N/A	5.91	5.44	N/A	12.5	7.4	N/A	0.579	0.566	N/A	59.7	42.5	N/A

Red indicates outliers (i.e., any changes over time beyond mean plus/minus two times the standard deviation).

average plasma glucose concentration for the three time points (prior to surgery, after 6 and 12 months). C-reactive protein (CrP, mg/l) was used as a measure of peripheral inflammation. As a more global marker of metabolism, we measured blood levels of (TSH, mU/l). Patients were investigated prior to, and 6 months after laparoscopic proximal Roux-en-Y gastric bypass. This procedure involves building a small gastric pouch which is anastomosed to a Roux limb of the jejunum. Twenty-two out of the 27 patients (18 females, age 52.6 ± 8.5 years, BMI 47.6 ± 5.5 kg/m^2) participated in the same experiments 1 year after surgery. The study was carried out in accordance with the recommendation of the ethics guideline, ethics committee of the medical faculty, University of Leipzig. The protocol was approved by the same ethics committee. All patients gave written informed consent in accordance with the Declaration of Helsinki. MRI data was acquired with a 3-Tesla Siemens VERIO system (Siemens, Erlangen, Germany). No hardware or software upgrades were applied during the study. Patients were placed in the scanner in supine position. The MRI data is stored on a computer server located at the Max-Planck-Institute for Human Cognitive and Brain Sciences and the clinical data on a server located at the University Hospital Leipzig, Department of Bariatric Surgery. The data is available on request directed to MR.

MRI Parameters for Voxel-Based Gray Matter Morphometry (GMD/WMD)

We applied a T1-weighted three-dimensional magnetization-prepared rapid gradient echo (MP-RAGE) sequence (Mugler and Brookeman, 1990) in sagittal slice orientation [inversion time (TI) = 900 ms; repetition time (TR) = 1,300 ms; echo time (TE) = 2.98 ms; readout pulse flip angle, α = 9°; bandwidth = 238 Hz/pixel; image matrix = 256 × 240; field of view (FOV) = 256 × 240 mm^2; nominal spatial resolution = 1 × 1 × 1 mm^3; 1 average].

MRI Parameters for Resting-State fMRI (ReHo, ALFF)

Patients were instructed to fixate a cross in the middle of a screen throughout the "resting-state" session. We darkened the MRI cabinet. We assessed 238 echo planar (EPI) images [voxel size of 3 × 3 × 4.8 mm^3, TR of 2,000 ms, TE of 30 ms, slice thickness (ST) of 4 mm]. One patient canceled data acquisition. That is why data of only 26 patients were available for respective ReHo/ALFF analyses.

Parameters for Diffusion-Weighted MRI (FA)

At the end of the session, we acquired whole-brain diffusion-weighted images (twice-refocused spin echo echo-planar-imaging sequence, 64 axial slices, 2-mm thickness, no gap, TE = 88 ms, TR = 12.4 s, α = 90°, bandwidth = 1,684 Hz/pixel, FOV = 220 × 220 mm^2, 110 × 110 image matrix, GRAPPA, acceleration factor 2; Reese et al., 2003). We applied a b-value of 1,000 s/mm^2 and 60 diffusion-encoding gradient directions. As anatomical reference for offline motion correction, we acquired seven images without diffusion weighting (b-value 0 s/mm^2), one at the beginning and one after each block of 10 images.

Data Analyses

Surgery-Induced Changes in Adiposity (Body Weight, Fat Mass)

Since body length did not change over 1 year, we here used body weight (kg) and fat mass (%) instead of the BMI as measures of adiposity. Both measures (weight and fat mass) for each of the three time points were applied to the within-subject two-tailed repeated-measures analysis of variance (ANOVA; significance threshold p = 0.05) followed by Bonferroni-corrected *post hoc* paired t-tests (p adjusted to $p < 0.025$). We also tested for a significant correlation between changes in body weight and fat mass using Pearson's correlation analysis together with Bonferroni-correction ($p < 0.025$ indicated significance).

In the next step, changes in clinical parameters (i.e., deltas), as listed in **Table 1**, including body weight (kg) and fat mass (%) were considered as covariates for one-sample t-tests with functional (ALFF, ReHo) and structural MRI markers (GMD, WMD, FA) of surgery-induced brain plasticity. To rule out, that significant correlations resulted from few outliers, we excluded outliers (i.e., any value beyond mean plus/minus two times the standard deviation, see red-colored data in **Table 1**).

Preprocessing of T1-Weighted MRI Data for VBM

Prior to each processing step, the authors MR and BP visually checked T1-weighted MR images for motion artifacts using the CheckReg option under SPM8 (Wellcome Trust Centre for Neuroimaging, UCL, London, UK) running under Matlab 7 (Mathworks, Sherborn, MA, USA). Anterior/posterior commissure, frontal pole, occipital pole and the cranial peak of the sulcus centralis were used as anatomical landmarks across images. We found no differences in image quality across the three time points and no patient was excluded due to artifacts. We transformed images using the VBM8 toolbox and applied them to the longitudinal approach including segmentation and bias-correction. We used the Diffeomorphic Anatomical RegisTration using Exponentiated Lie algebra (DARTEL) technique (Ashburner, 2007) with a pre-defined tissue probability map registered to the Montreal Neurological Institute (MNI) template to normalize images. Data was then smoothed using a Gaussian filter of 8 mm full width at half maximum (FWHM). In agreement with general practice, we used the term GMD and WMD to describe the normalized gray and white matter probability values, respectively.

Preprocessing of Resting-State fMRI for ReHo and ALFF Analyses

We removed the first four volumes to guarantee steady state of blood oxygenation-level-dependent (BOLD) signals. All other 234 images were applied to SPM8. After each processing step, images were visually checked using SPM's CheckReg function with the same landmarks as for T1-weighted images. Images were slice time corrected and realigned. Averaged scan-to-scan deviations during realignment in all patients indicated appropriately small displacements (x, y, z in mm: pre 0.0003, 0.0002, 0.0001, after 6 months 0.0001, 0.00003,

0.0003, after 12 months 0.006, 0.005, 0.004; pitch, roll, yaw in rad: pre 0.0000005, 0.0000006, 0.000004 after 6 months 0.0000002, 0.00002, 0.000001, after 12 months 0.000002, 0.000007, 0.000006). Finally, images were spatially normalized to the MNI template. We found no differences in image quality across the three time points and no patient was excluded due to artifacts.

ReHo was computed using the REST toolbox for SPM8[1] and for ALFF data was applied to the FMRIB Software Library (FSL[2]).

To assess ReHo, we computed Kendall's coefficient of concordance as a measure of the similarity of a voxel's ranked time series to its nearest 27 neighbor voxels (Zang et al., 2004).

For assessing ALFF, images were spatially smoothed using a Gaussian filter of 8 mm FWHM. ALFF was computed for the low frequency range, from 0.01 Hz to 0.08 Hz. We transformed the voxel-wise time series to the frequency domain and computed the power spectrum. The square of the amplitude of this frequency component is proportional to the power of a given frequency. That is why we computed the square root at each frequency of the power spectrum and obtained the averaged square root across 0.01–0.08 Hz at each voxel (Zou et al., 2008).

Preprocessing of Diffusion Tensor MRI for FA Analyses

We checked the quality of diffusion-weighted images using DTIPrep (Oguz et al., 2014) using the same anatomical landmarks as for the other MRI modalities. We found no differences in image quality across the three time points and no patient was excluded due to artifacts. For further processing we applied images to the FMRIB Software Library (FSL; Smith et al., 2004) and LIPSIA[3] (Lohmann et al., 2001). Images were motion corrected using rigid-body transformation (Jenkinson et al., 2002), based on the anatomical reference images. This was combined with global registration to the T1-weighted images. After skull-stripping images were co-registered to the standard MNI template. We applied rotation parameters to correct gradient direction of each image. We interpolated registered images of individual anisotropy, using an isotropic voxel resolution of 1 mm. The diffusion tensor was fitted to each voxel. FA was calculated from the eigenvalues of the diffusion tensor. Voxel-wise FA using Tract-Based Spatial Statistics (TBSS; Smith et al., 2006) was conducted with FSL (Smith et al., 2004). We applied nonlinearly coregistered to map FA images onto the FMRIB58_FA standard-space skeleton and finally thresholded images at 0.2.

Group-Level Analyses of GMD, WMD, ReHo, ALFF, FA

Voxel-wise one-sample *t*-tests were used to analyze changes of GMD, WMD, ReHo, ALFF, FA in association with clinical improvements (see **Table 1**) including reductions of body weight (kg) and fat mass (%). We subtracted normalized brain images of the pre-session from their corresponding post-session, resulting in brain maps of absolute changes (i.e., 6 months after surgery—pre, 12 months after surgery—pre). Corresponding changes (i.e., deltas) in clinical parameters were inserted as interacting covariates (one model for each parameter). We also included gender, age and global shifts of GM/WM volume over time as nuisance regressors. Significant levels were Bonferroni-corrected to account for repeated measures (i.e., 6 months after surgery—pre, 12 months after surgery—pre). Accordingly, GMD/WMD clusters were assessed by applying a peak-level threshold of $p < 0.0005$ and a cluster-level threshold of $p < 0.025$, family-wise error (FEW)-corrected. Significant changes of FA, ALFF and ReHo were detected with a voxel threshold of $p < 0.025$, FWE-corrected. To assign group effects to the underlying brain anatomy, we used the Anatomy toolbox for SPM (Eickhoff et al., 2005), as well as the WFU_PickAtlas by Joseph Maldjian from the Functional MRI Laboratory at the Wake Forest School of Medicine (see http://www.nitrc.org/projects/wfu_pickatlas).

[1] http://restfmri.net/forum/index.php?q = rest
[2] https://fsl.fmrib.ox.ac.uk/fsl/fslwiki/
[3] https://www.cbs.mpg.de/institute/software/lipsia/download

RESULTS

Changes in Body Weight (kg) and Fat Mass (%) After Surgery

After surgery, patients presented the expected weight/fat loss (**Figure 1A**; repeated measures ANOVA, weight: $p < 2 \times 10^{-16}$, fat mass: $p = 2.54 \times 10^{-16}$), 6 months (weight: 108.2 ± 17.1 kg; fat mass: $39.3 \pm 10.6\%$) as compared to the weight/fat mass assessed prior to surgery ($n = 27$, 138.2 ± 20 kg, $p = 6.4 \times 10^{-12}$, $53.4 \pm 9.3\%$, $p = 9.3 \times 10^{-8}$), as well as 1 year after surgery as compared to prior to surgery ($n = 22$, 100.7 ± 14.9 kg, $p = 0.0002$, $37.5 \pm 10\%$, $p = 0.017$). Loss of body weight (kg) and fat mass (%) were not highly correlated as expected (**Figure 1B**). Six months after surgery, changes in both adiposity measures correlated only by trend ($p = 0.03$, $r = 0.45$), whereas there was no significant correlation after 12 months ($p = 0.23$, $r = 0.31$). Prior to surgery, six patients suffered from diabetes type 2. After surgery, three patients out of these six recovered from diabetes as indicated by normalized glucose and HbA1c blood levels (see **Table 1**).

Weight Loss Associated Alterations of GMD

We only found significant associations between changes in GMD and the surgery-induced weight loss. Other markers of functional (ALFF, ReHo) and structural brain plasticity (FA) remained non-significant. We also found non-significant associations between plasticity markers and fat mass. Also, other possible associations between measures of neural plasticity and any other clinical parameter listed in **Table 1** (i.e., deltas of blood parameters of cholesterol, HDL, LDL, triglyceride, HbA1c, CrP, TSH) remained non-significant.

Analysis of associations between changes in GMD and weight loss across the first two time points (6 months after surgery—pre) revealed Bonferroni and FWE-corrected decreased GMD in the hypothalamus (1st peak-level: 6, 15, −18 in mm, MNI coordinates, $T = 4.95$, $p < 0.0005$; cluster-level: $p = 0.016$ FWE-corrected, $k_E = 461$ voxels; 2nd peak-level: 6, 8, −6, $T = 4.6$;

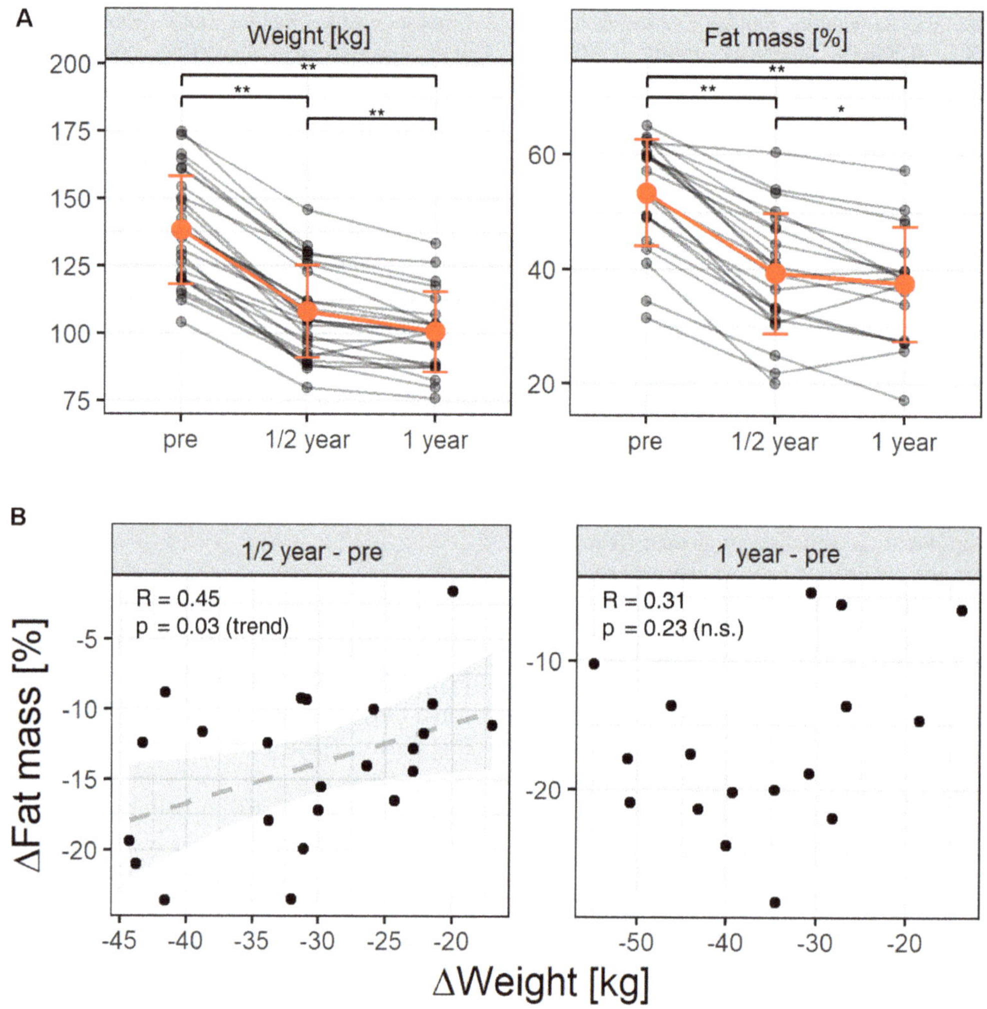

FIGURE 1 | (A) Individual weight and fat loss before and after gastric-bypass surgery (after 6 month and after 1 year). Red color indicates the mean over time. The whiskers the standard deviation. *Indicate a *p*-value of *post hoc t*-tests < 0.025, **indicate *p* < 0.001. **(B)** Pearson-correlation unexpectedly revealed that reductions in fat mass (%) and reductions in body weight (kg) correlated only by trend over the 1st 6 months after surgery, whereas after 12 months we found no correlation between both adiposity measures.

3rd peak-level: −3, 6, −6, $T = 4.41$; **Figure 2**, first row). We identified a second significant cluster of GMD decrease in the left parietal cortex around the central sulcus also consisting of three peaks [1st peak-level: −54, −9, 30, $T = 4.48$, $p < 0.0005$; cluster-level: $p = 0.006$ FWE-corrected, $k_E = 559$ voxels, assigned to Brodmann area (BA) 4p/3b, 2nd peak-level: −50, −7, 19, $T = 4.07$, assigned to BA 3a; 3rd peak-level: −57, −1, 12, $T = 4.41$, assigned to BA 3b/44; **Figure 2**, second row]. In right parietal cortex, directly opposite to the former cluster, we identified another cluster with a single peak which spreads from the parietal operculum into postcentral gyrus. This cluster, however, did not reach cluster significance level (peak-level: 60, −7, 9, $T = 4.85$, $p < 0.001$; cluster-level: $p = 0.763$ FWE-corrected, $k_E = 99$ voxels, **Figure 2**, third row). The only region that presented significant increases in GMD was the right lateral OFC (peak-level: 44, 36, −8, $T = 5.24$, $p < 0.0005$; cluster-level: $p = 0.020$ FWE-corrected, $k_E = 438$ voxels; **Figure 2**, bottom row).

After 1 year (pre as compared to 12 months after surgery), we found no GMD decreases surviving corrected FWE-threshold. One cluster in the left caput caudate just missed significance (peak-level: −11, 17, −6, $T = 5.09$, $p < 0.0005$; cluster-level: $p = 0.029$ FWE-corrected, $k_E = 364$ voxels; **Figure 3**, first row). Directly opposite to this cluster, we identified another cluster in right caput caudate. Although peak level was higher as compared to the left cluster, cluster level did not reach significant cluster level (peak-level: 17, 20, −6, $T = 6.36$, $p < 0.0005$; cluster-level: $p = 0.141$ FWE-corrected, $k_E = 236$ voxels; **Figure 3**, first row). We, nevertheless, considered both clusters together as relevant for the discussion due to their symmetry. We also observed significantly increased GMD that overlapped with the right cerebellar lobule VII (peak-level: 32, −58, −53, $T = 5.53$, $p < 0.0005$; cluster-level: $p = 0.009$ FWE-corrected, $k_E = 464$ voxels; **Figure 3**, second row).

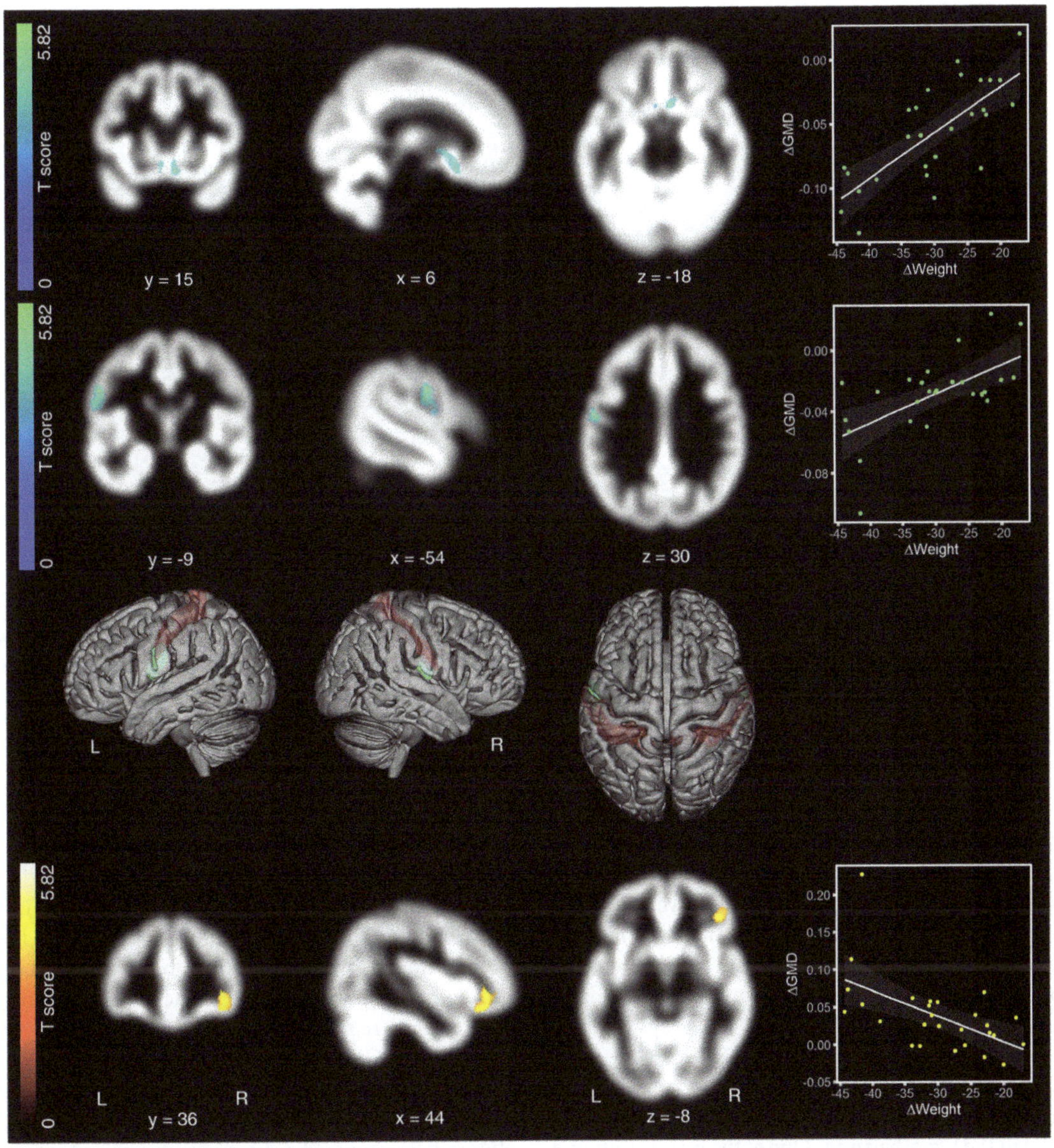

FIGURE 2 | Regression analyses between changes in gray matter density (GMD) maps and weight, 6 months after surgery. The loss of body weight (in kg) from pre to 6 months after surgery was associated with decreased GMD in the hypothalamus (top row) and the left postcentral gyrus (second row). In right postcentral gyrus, directly opposite to the left-sided cluster, we identified another cluster, which did not survive significance threshold. Due to the symmetry of both clusters across both hemispheres, we considered this non-significant cluster, nevertheless, as relevant for the discussion (third row). The only region that presented significantly increased GMD was the right lateral OFC (bottom row). Significant GMD clusters are projected on patients' mean GMD template. Hot colors indicate positive and cold colors negative associations. GMD effects are presented on a coronal, sagittal, and axial brain slice (from left to right). Coordinates below each brain slice indicate clusters' peak coordinates in Montreal Neurological Institute (MNI) space. "L" indicates the left, "R" the right brain hemisphere. The color bar on the left side indicates the T-scores for the cluster presented in that row. In the 3rd row, we superimposed effects on both postcentral gyri on a rendered brain. Postcentral gyri are colored in red. Scatter plots on the right to the brain slices show the relationship between changes in GMD and changes in weight. Changes in GMD, as shown in the scatter plots, were extracted as the 1st Eigenvariate at $p = 0.025$ family-wise error (FWE), cluster-threshold and $p = 0.0005$, uncorrected peak threshold.

DISCUSSION

Here, we applied three MRI methods to investigate surgery-induced voxel-by-voxel structural and functional plasticity of gray and white matter in association to individual improvements in adiposity, metabolism and inflammation [as indexed by changes in body weight (kg), fat mass (%) and the blood levels of cholesterol, HDL, LDL, triglyceride, HbA1c, CrP, TSH]. Only the loss of body weight (in kg) was significantly associated with surgery-induced brain plasticity, and this only for GMD changes. Due to the longitudinal design of our study, body weight (kg) and the BMI (kg/m^2) were redundant measures, since body length (m) did not change over time. Unexpectedly, reductions in fat mass (%) and reductions in body weight (kg) correlated

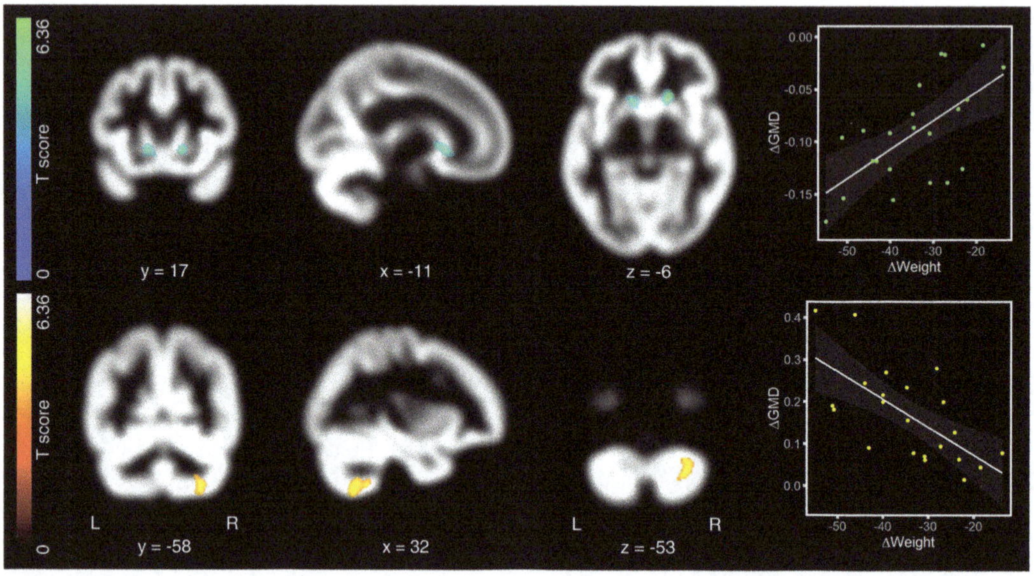

FIGURE 3 | Regression analyses between changes in GMD maps and weight, 12 months after surgery. After 12 months, the loss of body weight was associated with decreased GMD in the left caput caudate. This cluster reached peak significance level, but just missed significant cluster threshold ($p = 0.029$; threshold at $p = 0.025$, FWE-corrected; first row). Directly opposite to this cluster, we also identified the right caput caudate, but below the significant threshold. We, nevertheless, considered both clusters together as relevant for the discussion due to the symmetry of effects. Increased GMD after 12 months was observed in the right cerebellar lobule VII (second row). As in **Figure 2**, hot colors indicate positive and cold colors negative associations. Significant clusters are projected on patients' mean GMD template, presented on a coronal, sagittal, and axial brain slice (from left to right). Coordinates below each slice index coordinates of the clusters' peak in MNI space. "L" indexes the left, "R" the right brain hemisphere. The left-sided color bar shows the T-scores for the respective GMD cluster. Right-sided scatter plots present the association between changes in GMD and changes in body weight. As for **Figure 2**, changes in GMD in the scatter plots were extracted as the 1st Eigenvariate at $p = 0.025$ FWE, cluster-threshold and $p = 0.0005$, uncorrected peak threshold.

only by trend 6 months after surgery ($r = 0.03$), whereas after 12 months we found no correlation between them. Significant brain-associations were only identified for the weight loss, but not for the loss of fat mass suggesting that both markers address different aspects of adiposity.

Six Months After Surgery

Six months after surgery, reduced body weight overlapped with decreased GMD in the hypothalamus. One of the hypothalamus's central functional attribution is to receive metabolic feedback from the digestive tract and fat depots to control hedonic responses to food (Hollmann et al., 2013; Schlogl et al., 2016). We found that the higher the individual BMI loss, the higher the loss of GMD in the hypothalamus was. Previous functional MRI studies in patients after bariatric surgery revealed increases in neural activity in the hypothalamus as a response to standardized glucose load (van de Sande-Lee et al., 2011), suggesting a surgery-induced regain in hypothalamic responsivity to sweet and high-calorie food. Although it is generally difficult to infer the functional relevance of GMD changes, the loss in hypothalamic GMD in our study may reflect structural correlates of surgery-induced improved hypothalamic sensitivity to an altered homeostatic demand.

Besides the hypothalamus, we found weight-loss related decreases in GMD in the left parietal cortex, around the central sulcus, comprising the pre- (i.e., BA 4p) and postcentral gyrus (i.e., BA 3a/b). The postcentral gyrus is known to host the primary somatosensory cortex. Its organization is well described by the so-called homunculus (i.e., the little man in the brain), with different sub-regions being involved in processing somatosensory feedback from distinct body parts (i.e., cortical representations; Pleger and Villringer, 2013). The location of GMD effects in the present study overlapped with the representation of the digestive system, suggesting that the loss of GMD relates to adaptation processes of abdominal organs, like the stomach, with associated influences on the somatosensory feedback to corresponding cortical representations. Neighbored BA 4p (p for posterior) in the precentral gyrus is cytoarchitectonically different from the more anteriorily located primary motor cortex, BA 4a. BA 4p seems to be involved in both, motor and somatosensory processing suggesting close functional-anatomical associations to directly neighboring S1 (i.e., BA 3b; Geyer et al., 1996). On the contralateral hemisphere, we also found a cluster in the same topographic location. This cluster did not reach significance, but its symmetric occurrence across both hemispheres, nevertheless, complicates the discussion about a hemispherical dominance of the observed effects.

The last region that presented changes in GMD related to the surgery-induced weight loss was the right lateral orbitofrontal cortex, well known as a key region of the brain's reward circuity (Noonan et al., 2012). As compared to the hypothalamus and postcentral gyri, lateral OFC presented not decreased but increased GMD. In previous studies, activity in lateral OFC was found to positively correlate with the subjective appeal of high-calorie food in the fasting state, suggesting that fasting biases regions of the brain reward circuitry, such as the lateral OFC, towards high-calorie food (Goldstone et al., 2009). Besides its role in food reward, studies in the late 90th suggest its contribution to taste and smell processing (Small et al., 1997; Zald et al., 1998), suggesting that the lateral OFC, especially in the right hemisphere, plays a role in gustatory processes, too (Small et al., 1997, 1999; Zald et al., 1998; Rolls, 2005). Thus, elevated GMD in lateral OFC may not only reflect altered food reward but also gustatory processing.

Twelve Months After Surgery

Twelve months after surgery, we also found decreased GMD, not in the hypothalamus as after the first 6 months, but in the caput caudate. The caput caudate belongs to the dorsal striatum. It is a dopamine-rich reward region involved in guiding food consumption and its devaluation when eating beyond satiety (Small et al., 2001). Its activity during the consumption of chocolate milkshake seems to correspond to future gains in body weight in young adolescence females (Stice et al., 2008). Obese individuals, like drug addicts, present attenuated reward responses in the dorsal striatum during the ingestion of food, probably promoting compensatory overconsumption (Wang et al., 2001; Stice et al., 2008; Johnson and Kenny, 2010). The dorsal striatum is permanently exchanging information with the hypothalamus to sustain energy homeostasis. The weight loss related decrease of GMD in the hypothalamus 6 months after surgery, together with the GMD decrease in caput caudate 6 months later, may thus indicate a progressively improving hedonic-homeostatic crosstalk over the 1-year observation period.

Besides weight-loss related decreased GMD, 12 months after surgery, we also found significantly increased GMD that comprised the right cerebellar lobule VII. The higher the BMI-loss, the more GMD increased. The functional attribution of this cerebellar effect is difficult since this region remains less well investigated as the other regions we found. A series of studies investigated the attribution of the cerebellar lobule VII to phonological storage, which is assumed to depend on projections between parietal regions and right caudo-lateral lobule VIIb (Desmond et al., 1997; Chen and Desmond, 2005), specifically during late memory encoding, when encoding and the transfer of verbal items to phonological storage run in parallel (Macher et al., 2014). Whether an increased GMD relates to improved verbal memory capacities or other cognitive gains remains unanswered. These speculations clearly warrant further longitudinal studies combining brain imaging with cognitive tests.

Limitations

Some important limitations of our study must be taken into consideration. First, our study does not contain control persons, neither lean nor comparably obese, that were investigated over the same observation period with the same clinical or imaging methods. Furthermore, our study does not address how the amelioration of obesity-related comorbidities may relate to differences in neural plasticity. This is due to the small sample size that limits generalization of brain-adiposity associations and analyses of sub-populations, such as those patients that recovered from diabetes after surgery (see the drop of HbA1c levels into normal range in three patients in **Table 1**). Not only the sample size *per se*, but also the imbalance between male and female patients should be considered as a further limitation. Our sample mainly consisted of female patients. That is why we accounted for gender effects during data analyses to minimize potential confounding influences. Gender-related differences in neural plasticity, however, remain unaddressed by our study. The small sample size may also explain why we found statistical evidence for adiposity-related neural plasticity only for GMD and not for any other plasticity marker or any other clinical parameter.

Outlook

Future studies should include a larger sample size that allows sub-population analyses. These studies should furthermore combine cognitive tests and metabolic/inflammatory markers with measurements of structural and functional brain plasticity to assess brain representations of integrative cognitive-metabolic/inflammatory improvements induced by bariatric surgery. An understanding of such relationships may support the development of new therapeutic strategies against obesity.

ETHICS STATEMENT

The study was carried out in accordance with the recommendation of the ethics guideline, ethics committee of the medical faculty, University of Leipzig. The protocol was approved by the same ethics committee. All patients gave written informed consent in accordance with the Declaration of Helsinki.

AUTHOR CONTRIBUTIONS

MR, SvP, SH, TS, and BP designed the study. MR, SvP, SiP, SH, JH, TS, and AD performed the experiments. MR, KG, KM, and MH analyzed the data. MR and BP prepared figures, tables and wrote the article. All authors approved the final version of this manuscript.

FUNDING

This study is supported by the IFB AdiposityDiseases, Federal Ministry of Education and Research Bundesministerium für Bildung und Forschung (Bundesministerium für Bildung und Forschung, BMBF), Germany, FKZ: 01E01001 (http://www.bmbf.de). The study was also supported by the Deutsche Forschungsgemeinschaft (DFG)—project number 209933838—SFB 1052 to BP and MR.

REFERENCES

Amlung, M., Petker, T., Jackson, J., Balodis, I., and MacKillop, J. (2016). Steep discounting of delayed monetary and food rewards in obesity: a meta-analysis. *Psychol. Med.* 46, 2423–2434. doi: 10.1017/s0033291716000866

Ashburner, J. (2007). A fast diffeomorphic image registration algorithm. *Neuroimage* 38, 95–113. doi: 10.1016/j.neuroimage.2007.07.007

Bryant, E. J., King, N. A., and Blundell, J. E. (2008). Disinhibition: its effects on appetite and weight regulation. *Obes. Rev.* 9, 409–419. doi: 10.1111/j.1467-789x.2007.00426.x

Chen, S. H., and Desmond, J. E. (2005). Cerebrocerebellar networks during articulatory rehearsal and verbal working memory tasks. *Neuroimage* 24, 332–338. doi: 10.1016/j.neuroimage.2004.08.032

Davis, C., Patte, K., Levitan, R., Reid, C., Tweed, S., and Curtis, C. (2007). From motivation to behaviour: a model of reward sensitivity, overeating and food preferences in the risk profile for obesity. *Appetite* 48, 12–19. doi: 10.1016/j.appet.2006.05.016

Debette, S., Beiser, A., Hoffmann, U., Decarli, C., O'Donnell, C. J., Massaro, J. M., et al. (2010). Visceral fat is associated with lower brain volume in healthy middle-aged adults. *Ann. Neurol.* 68, 136–144. doi: 10.1002/ana.22062

Debette, S., Seshadri, S., Beiser, A., Au, R., Himali, J. J., Palumbo, C., et al. (2011). Midlife vascular risk factor exposure accelerates structural brain aging and cognitive decline. *Neurology* 77, 461–468. doi: 10.1212/WNL.0b013e318227b227

Desmond, J. E., Gabrieli, J. D., Wagner, A. D., Ginier, B. L., and Glover, G. H. (1997). Lobular patterns of cerebellar activation in verbal working-memory and finger-tapping tasks as revealed by functional MRI. *J. Neurosci.* 17, 9675–9685. doi: 10.1523/JNEUROSCI.17-24-09675.1997

Dixon, J. B. (2010). The effect of obesity on health outcomes. *Mol. Cell. Endocrinol.* 316, 104–108. doi: 10.1016/j.mce.2009.07.008

Ebbert, J. O., Elrashidi, M. Y., and Jensen, M. D. (2014). Managing overweight and obesity in adults to reduce cardiovascular disease risk. *Curr. Atheroscler. Rep.* 16:445. doi: 10.1007/s11883-014-0445-x

Eickhoff, S. B., Stephan, K. E., Mohlberg, H., Grefkes, C., Fink, G. R., Amunts, K., et al. (2005). A new SPM toolbox for combining probabilistic cytoarchitectonic maps and functional imaging data. *Neuroimage* 25, 1325–1335. doi: 10.1016/j.neuroimage.2004.12.034

Geiger, B. M., Behr, G. G., Frank, L. E., Caldera-Siu, A. D., Beinfeld, M. C., Kokkotou, E. G., et al. (2008). Evidence for defective mesolimbic dopamine exocytosis in obesity-prone rats. *FASEB J.* 22, 2740–2746. doi: 10.1096/fj.08-110759

Geiger, B. M., Haburcak, M., Avena, N. M., Moyer, M. C., Hoebel, B. G., and Pothos, E. N. (2009). Deficits of mesolimbic dopamine neurotransmission in rat dietary obesity. *Neuroscience* 159, 1193–1199. doi: 10.1016/j.neuroscience.2009.02.007

Geyer, S., Ledberg, A., Schleicher, A., Kinomura, S., Schormann, T., Bürgel, U., et al. (1996). Two different areas within the primary motor cortex of man. *Nature* 382, 805–807. doi: 10.1038/382805a0

Gianos, M., Abdemur, A., Fendrich, I., Gari, V., Szomstein, S., and Rosenthal, R. J. (2012). Outcomes of bariatric surgery in patients with body mass index <35 kg/m2. *Surg. Obes. Relat. Dis.* 8, 25–30. doi: 10.1016/j.soard.2011.08.012

Goldstone, A. P., Prechtl De Hernandez, C. G., Beaver, J. D., Muhammed, K., Croese, C., Bell, G., et al. (2009). Fasting biases brain reward systems towards high-calorie foods. *Eur. J. Neurosci.* 30, 1625–1635. doi: 10.1111/j.1460-9568.2009.06949.x

Gurka, M. J., Filipp, S. L., Musani, S. K., Sims, M., and Deboer, M. D. (2018). Use of BMI as the marker of adiposity in a metabolic syndrome severity score: derivation and validation in predicting long-term disease outcomes. *Metabolism* 83, 68–74. doi: 10.1016/j.metabol.2018.01.015

Ho, A. J., Raji, C. A., Becker, J. T., Lopez, O. L., Kuller, L. H., Hua, X., et al. (2010). Obesity is linked with lower brain volume in 700 AD and MCI patients. *Neurobiol. Aging* 31, 1326–1339. doi: 10.1016/j.neurobiolaging.2010.04.006

Hollmann, M., Pleger, B., Villringer, A., and Horstmann, A. (2013). Brain imaging in the context of food perception and eating. *Curr. Opin. Lipidol.* 24, 18–24. doi: 10.1097/mol.0b013e32835b61a4

Horstmann, A., Busse, F. P., Mathar, D., Müller, K., Lepsien, J., Schlogl, H., et al. (2011). Obesity-related differences between women and men in brain structure and goal-directed behavior. *Front. Hum. Neurosci.* 5:58. doi: 10.3389/fnhum.2011.00058

Jagust, W., Harvey, D., Mungas, D., and Haan, M. (2005). Central obesity and the aging brain. *Arch. Neurol.* 62, 1545–1548. doi: 10.1001/archneur.62.10.1545

Jenkinson, M., Bannister, P., Brady, M., and Smith, S. (2002). Improved optimization for the robust and accurate linear registration and motion correction of brain images. *Neuroimage* 17, 825–841. doi: 10.1016/s1053-8119(02)91132-8

Johnson, P. M., and Kenny, P. J. (2010). Dopamine D2 receptors in addiction-like reward dysfunction and compulsive eating in obese rats. *Nat. Neurosci.* 13, 635–641. doi: 10.1038/nn.2519

Knopman, D. S., Petersen, R. C., Rocca, W. A., Larson, E. B., and Ganguli, M. (2011). Passive case-finding for Alzheimer's disease and dementia in two U.S. communities. *Alzheimers Dement.* 7, 53–60. doi: 10.1016/j.jalz.2010.11.001

Lohmann, G., Müller, K., Bosch, V., Mentzel, H., Hessler, S., Chen, L., et al. (2001). LIPSIA—a new software system for the evaluation of functional magnetic resonance images of the human brain. *Comput. Med. Imaging Graph.* 25, 449–457. doi: 10.1016/s0895-6111(01)00008-8

Macher, K., Bohringer, A., Villringer, A., and Pleger, B. (2014). Cerebellar-parietal connections underpin phonological storage. *J. Neurosci.* 34, 5029–5037. doi: 10.1523/JNEUROSCI.0106-14.2014

Mueller, K., Horstmann, A., Möller, H. E., Anwander, A., Lepsien, J., Schroeter, M. L., et al. (2014). Obesity associated cerebral gray and white matter alterations are interrelated in the female brain. *PLoS One* 9:e114206. doi: 10.1371/journal.pone.0114206

Mugler, J. P. III., and Brookeman, J. R. (1990). Three-dimensional magnetization-prepared rapid gradient-echo imaging (3D MP RAGE). *Magn. Reson. Med.* 15, 152–157. doi: 10.1002/mrm.1910150117

Noonan, M. P., Kolling, N., Walton, M. E., and Rushworth, M. F. (2012). Re-evaluating the role of the orbitofrontal cortex in reward and reinforcement. *Eur. J. Neurosci.* 35, 997–1010. doi: 10.1111/j.1460-9568.2012.08023.x

Oguz, I., Farzinfar, M., Matsui, J., Budin, F., Liu, Z., Gerig, G., et al. (2014). DTIPrep: quality control of diffusion-weighted images. *Front. Neuroinform.* 8:4. doi: 10.3389/fninf.2014.00004

Pleger, B., and Villringer, A. (2013). The human somatosensory system: from perception to decision making. *Prog. Neurobiol.* 103, 76–97. doi: 10.1016/j.pneurobio.2012.10.002

Reese, T. G., Heid, O., Weisskoff, R. M., and Wedeen, V. J. (2003). Reduction of eddy-current-induced distortion in diffusion MRI using a twice-refocused spin echo. *Magn. Reson. Med.* 49, 177–182. doi: 10.1002/mrm.10308

Robinson, M. K. (2009). Surgical treatment of obesity—weighing the facts. *N. Engl. J. Med.* 361, 520–521. doi: 10.1056/nejme0904837

Rolls, E. T. (2005). Taste, olfactory, and food texture processing in the brain and the control of food intake. *Physiol. Behav.* 85, 45–56. doi: 10.1016/j.physbeh.2005.04.012

Rullmann, M., Preusser, S., Poppitz, S., Heba, S., Hoyer, J., Schütz, T., et al. (2018). Gastric-bypass surgery induced widespread neural plasticity of the obese human brain. *Neuroimage* 172, 853–863. doi: 10.1016/j.neuroimage.2017.10.062

Schlogl, H., Horstmann, A., Villringer, A., and Stumvoll, M. (2016). Functional neuroimaging in obesity and the potential for development of novel treatments. *Lancet Diabetes Endocrinol.* 4, 695–705. doi: 10.1016/s2213-8587(15)00475-1

Sjöström, L. (2013). Review of the key results from the Swedish Obese Subjects (SOS) trial—a prospective controlled intervention study of bariatric surgery. *J. Intern. Med.* 273, 219–234. doi: 10.1111/joim.12012

Sjöström, L., Lindroos, A. K., Peltonen, M., Torgerson, J., Bouchard, C., Carlsson, B., et al. (2004). Lifestyle, diabetes, and cardiovascular risk factors 10 years after bariatric surgery. *N. Engl. J. Med.* 351, 2683–2693. doi: 10.1056/NEJMoa035622

Small, D. M., Jones-Gotman, M., Zatorre, R. J., Petrides, M., and Evans, A. C. (1997). Flavor processing: more than the sum of its parts. *Neuroreport* 8, 3913–3917. doi: 10.1097/00001756-199712220-00014

Small, D. M., Zald, D. H., Jones-Gotman, M., Zatorre, R. J., Pardo, J. V., Frey, S., et al. (1999). Human cortical gustatory areas: a review of functional neuroimaging data. *Neuroreport* 10, 7–14. doi: 10.1097/00001756-199901180-00002

Small, D. M., Zatorre, R. J., Dagher, A., Evans, A. C., and Jones-Gotman, M. (2001). Changes in brain activity related to eating chocolate: from pleasure to aversion. *Brain* 124, 1720–1733. doi: 10.1093/brain/124.9.1720

Smith, S. M., Jenkinson, M., Johansen-Berg, H., Rueckert, D., Nichols, T. E., MacKay, C. E., et al. (2006). Tract-based spatial statistics: voxelwise analysis of multi-subject diffusion data. *Neuroimage* 31, 1487–1505. doi: 10.1016/j.neuroimage.2006.02.024

Smith, S. M., Jenkinson, M., Woolrich, M. W., Beckmann, C. F., Behrens, T. E., Johansen-Berg, H., et al. (2004). Advances in functional and structural MR image analysis and implementation as FSL. *Neuroimage* 23, S208–S219. doi: 10.1016/j.neuroimage.2004.07.051

Stice, E., Spoor, S., Bohon, C., and Small, D. M. (2008). Relation between obesity and blunted striatal response to food is moderated by TaqIA A1 allele. *Science* 322, 449–452. doi: 10.1126/science.1161550

Stice, E., Yokum, S., Bohon, C., Marti, N., and Smolen, A. (2010). Reward circuitry responsivity to food predicts future increases in body mass: moderating effects of DRD2 and DRD4. *Neuroimage* 50, 1618–1625. doi: 10.1016/j.neuroimage.2010.01.081

Stoeckel, L. E., Weller, R. E., Cook, E. W. III., Twieg, D. B., Knowlton, R. C., and Cox, J. E. (2008). Widespread reward-system activation in obese women in response to pictures of high-calorie foods. *Neuroimage* 41, 636–647. doi: 10.1016/j.neuroimage.2008.02.031

Tosto, G., and Reitz, C. (2013). Genome-wide association studies in Alzheimer's disease: a review. *Curr. Neurol. Neurosci. Rep.* 13:381. doi: 10.1007/s11910-013-0381-0

Tuulari, J. J., Karlsson, H. K., Antikainen, O., Hirvonen, J., Pham, T., Salminen, P., et al. (2016). Bariatric surgery induces white and grey matter density recovery in the morbidly obese: a voxel-based morphometric study. *Hum. Brain Mapp.* 37, 3745–3756. doi: 10.1002/hbm.23272

van de Sande-Lee, S., Pereira, F. R., Cintra, D. E., Fernandes, P. T., Cardoso, A. R., Garlipp, C. R., et al. (2011). Partial reversibility of hypothalamic dysfunction and changes in brain activity after body mass reduction in obese subjects. *Diabetes* 60, 1699–1704. doi: 10.2337/db10-1614

Walther, K., Birdsill, A. C., Glisky, E. L., and Ryan, L. (2010). Structural brain differences and cognitive functioning related to body mass index in older females. *Hum. Brain Mapp.* 31, 1052–1064. doi: 10.1002/hbm.20916

Wang, G. J., Volkow, N. D., Logan, J., Pappas, N. R., Wong, C. T., Zhu, W., et al. (2001). Brain dopamine and obesity. *Lancet* 357, 354–357. doi: 10.1016/S0140-6736(00)03643-6

Zald, D. H., Lee, J. T., Fluegel, K. W., and Pardo, J. V. (1998). Aversive gustatory stimulation activates limbic circuits in humans. *Brain* 121, 1143–1154. doi: 10.1093/brain/121.6.1143

Zang, Y., Jiang, T., Lu, Y., He, Y., and Tian, L. (2004). Regional homogeneity approach to fMRI data analysis. *Neuroimage* 22, 394–400. doi: 10.1016/j.neuroimage.2003.12.030

Zhang, C., Wei, N. L., Wang, Y., Wang, X., Zhang, J. G., and Zhang, K. (2015). Deep brain stimulation of the nucleus accumbens shell induces anti-obesity effects in obese rats with alteration of dopamine neurotransmission. *Neurosci. Lett.* 589, 1–6. doi: 10.1016/j.neulet.2015.01.019

Zou, Q. H., Zhu, C. Z., Yang, Y., Zuo, X. N., Long, X. Y., Cao, Q. J., et al. (2008). An improved approach to detection of amplitude of low-frequency fluctuation (ALFF) for resting-state fMRI: fractional ALFF. *J. Neurosci. Methods* 172, 137–141. doi: 10.1016/j.jneumeth.2008.04.012

17

A Randomized Controlled ERP Study on the Effects of Multi-Domain Cognitive Training and Task Difficulty on Task Switching Performance in Older Adults

*Kristina Küper *, Patrick D. Gajewski, Claudia Frieg and Michael Falkenstein*

Aging Research Group, Leibniz Research Centre for Working Environment and Human Factors, Dortmund, Germany

Edited by:
Louis Bherer,
Université de Montréal, Canada

Reviewed by:
Tilo Strobach,
Medical School Hamburg, Germany
Bruno Kopp,
Hannover Medical School, Germany

***Correspondence:**
Kristina Küper
kueper@ifado.de

Executive functions are subject to a marked age-related decline, but have been shown to benefit from cognitive training interventions. As of yet, it is, however, still relatively unclear which neural mechanism can mediate training-related performance gains. In the present electrophysiological study, we examined the effects of multi-domain cognitive training on performance in an untrained cue-based task switch paradigm featuring Stroop color words: participants either had to indicate the word meaning of Stroop stimuli (word task) or perform the more difficult task of color naming (color task). One-hundred and three older adults (>65 years old) were randomly assigned to a training group receiving a 4-month multi-domain cognitive training, a passive no-contact control group or an active (social) control group receiving a 4-month relaxation training. For all groups, we recorded performance and EEG measures before and after the intervention. For the cognitive training group, but not for the two control groups, we observed an increase in response accuracy at posttest, irrespective of task and trial type. No training-related effects on reaction times were found. Cognitive training was also associated with an overall increase in N2 amplitude and a decrease of P2 latency on single trials. Training-related performance gains were thus likely mediated by an enhancement of response selection and improved access to relevant stimulus-response mappings. Additionally, cognitive training was associated with an amplitude decrease in the time window of the target-locked P3 at fronto-central electrodes. An increase in the switch positivity during advance task preparation emerged after both cognitive and relaxation training. Training-related behavioral and event-related potential (ERP) effects were not modulated by task difficulty. The data suggest that cognitive training increased slow negative potentials during target processing which enhanced the N2 and reduced a subsequent P3-like component on both switch and non-switch trials and irrespective of task difficulty. Our findings further corroborate the effectiveness of multi-domain cognitive training in older adults and indicate that ERPs can be instrumental in uncovering the neural processes underlying training-related performance gains.

Keywords: cognitive training, task difficulty, aging, Stroop switch task, switch positivity, P3, P2, N2

INTRODUCTION

All planned goal-directed behavior is mediated by executive control functions, such as selective attention, working memory, the inhibition of irrelevant information or the selection and coordination of relevant task sets. Previous research has indicated that these functions are subject to a marked age-related decline beginning as early as in midlife (Li et al., 2004; Sander et al., 2012). Given the crucial role of executive control functions for activities of daily living, age-related deficits in this domain can be particularly detrimental to the well-being and autonomy of older adults (Burgess et al., 1998; Jonides et al., 2008). Cognitive functions show a remarkable degree of plasticity across the lifespan, however, and can hence benefit from different types of training interventions up to a very old age (Hertzog et al., 2008; Karbach and Schubert, 2013; for reviews see Kueider et al., 2012; Ballesteros et al., 2015).

Cognitive training regimen which focus on a single domain or task, such as working memory or task switching, have been shown to consistently improve performance in the trained task (for meta-analyses, see Karbach and Verhaeghen, 2014; Lampit et al., 2014b; Au et al., 2015). Transfer of such training gains to untrained tasks or everyday functioning appears to be more limited, however, and has been reported only in some cases (Karbach and Verhaeghen, 2014; Au et al., 2015), but not in others (Ball et al., 2002; Melby-Lervåg and Hulme, 2013; Melby-Lervåg et al., 2016).

It has been hypothesized that a substantial overlap between the processes underlying performance in the training task and those underlying performance in the transfer task is necessary for successful transfer to occur (Jonides, 2004; Dahlin et al., 2008; Lustig et al., 2009; Buschkuehl et al., 2012). In light of this, cognitive training interventions which focus not only on a single function but on multiple cognitive functions have recently been discussed as a more effective training measure which may potentially yield broader transfer effects (Gates and Valenzuela, 2010; Karbach, 2014). In keeping with this, cognitive training programs integrating multiple tasks have shown both near and far transfer effects to measures of perceptual processing, working memory updating, memory accuracy and reasoning (Mahncke et al., 2006; Wild-Wall et al., 2012; Walton et al., 2014; Baniqued et al., 2015). Moreover, Lampit et al. (2014a) reported transfer gains from a multi-domain training aimed at reasoning, memory, attention and visuo-spatial abilities to a bookkeeping task closely mirroring a real-world work scenario. In direct comparisons to single-domain interventions, multi-domain cognitive training has additionally been associated with more pronounced benefits in far transfer tasks measuring executive attentional control (Binder et al., 2016) and increased longevity of training-related performance benefits (Cheng et al., 2012).

Recent resting-state fMRI studies have been able to offer some insights into the neural processes which may mediate performance gains associated with multi-domain cognitive training: older adults who have undergone multi-domain cognitive training show increased neural lateralization and functional connectivity (Cao et al., 2016; Li et al., 2016; Luo et al., 2016; see also Binder et al., 2017, for similar electrophysiological data). Such brain activation patterns are commonly found in much younger adults suggesting that multi-domain cognitive training may be able to compensate age-related changes to neural connectivity at least to some degree. In keeping with this, multi-domain cognitive training has also been associated with a reduction in age-related cortical thinning in fronto-temporal areas (Kim et al., 2015; Jiang et al., 2016).

A drawback of these imaging studies is that they employed predominantly passive control groups. It is thus possible that the structural differences observed between training and control groups reflect differences in general activity rather than training-specific benefits (see Redick et al., 2013). Moreover, it is still relatively unclear what functional consequences the observed structural changes may have, especially for the crucial domain of executive control. In two previous studies, we thus compared middle-aged and older adults who had undergone multi-domain cognitive training to both active and passive control groups and examined event-related potential (ERP) indices of performance in a task switching paradigm (Gajewski and Falkenstein, 2012; Gajewski et al., 2017).

Task switching paradigms have the advantage of yielding indices of multiple distinct subcomponents of executive control. The paradigm requires participants to attend to two or more different tasks in distinct experimental blocks. In single blocks, participants always have to perform only one of the tasks whereas they have to flexibly switch between different tasks on a trial-by-trial basis in the mixed block. Mixed blocks thus feature stay trials on which the same task as in the preceding trial has to be performed and switch trials on which a different task has to be performed. In memory-based switch tasks, participants have to memorize a fixed task order for these mixed blocks. In cue-based paradigms, the task order is instead random and a cue preceding each target stimulus indicates which task is to be performed.

Despite the fact that both single and stay trials constitute task repetitions, performance on trials in the single block is usually better than on stay trials in the mixed block. These general switch costs or mixing costs have been interpreted as indexing the ability to maintain a task set in the context of a different, interfering task set. The ability to flexibly switch between tasks on a trial-by trial basis is instead reflected in specific or local switch costs, i.e., performance decrements in switch trials relative to stay trials (Allport et al., 1994; Rogers and Monsell, 1995; Meiran, 1996; see Kiesel et al., 2010, for a review). Age-comparative research has indicated that older adults show increased general switch costs relative to younger adults, but similar specific switch costs (Kramer et al., 1999; Kray and Lindenberger, 2000; Mayr, 2001). It thus appears that aging negatively affects the ability to simultaneously maintain and coordinate distinct task sets, but leaves task switching abilities relatively intact.

Our previous training studies have indicated that multi-domain cognitive training has the potential to compensate at least some of this age-related deficit and can lead to a reduction in general switch costs (Gajewski and Falkenstein, 2012; Gajewski et al., 2017). In our studies, these performance gains were accompanied by amplitude increases in three ERPs, the N2, the P3 and the error negativity (Ne). The target-locked N2 is a negative deflection with a fronto-central maximum, which has been linked to both the detection of stimulus novelty and cognitive control, in terms of response inhibition and the resolution of response conflict during responding (Folstein and Van Petten, 2008). It is thus thought to reflect the implementation of stimulus-response associations, i.e., response selection, which is hampered on interference or conflict trials (Gajewski et al., 2008). In the context of task switching paradigms, the N2 has been found to be decreased in latency and amplitude for task repetitions (Gajewski et al., 2010a). A training-related increase in N2 amplitude may thus reflect improved response selection. The subsequent target-P3, a positive deflection with a parietal focus, has been associated with the allocation of processing resources, specifically memory operations (e.g., Polich, 2007). As such, its amplitude is largest for single trials, intermediate for stay trials and lowest for switch trials (Kieffaber and Hetrick, 2005; Jost et al., 2008; Gajewski et al., 2010b; Gajewski and Falkenstein, 2012). A training-related increase in P3 amplitude can thus be interpreted in terms of improved resource allocation. Finally, the error negativity (Ne or error-related negativity, ERN) is an early negative deflection which is elicited by the detection of a response error (Falkenstein et al., 1991). A training-related increase in Ne amplitude thus reflects improvements in error monitoring.

In the present study, we wanted to corroborate and extend our previous findings on the functional neural processes mediating gains in executive functioning associated with multi-domain cognitive training in older adults. To this end, we employed a different task-switching transfer task than in our earlier study which featured two rather than three distinct tasks and introduced different levels of task difficulty. In order to gain more thorough insights into neural processes involved in task preparation and response selection we examined not only the ERP components described in our earlier study, but also the switch positivity during advance task preparation (Karayanidis et al., 2010) and the target-locked P2 (Kieffaber and Hetrick, 2005).

One-hundred and three healthy older adults were randomly assigned to either a multi-domain cognitive training group, an active control group receiving relaxation training or a passive no-contact control group. At pretest and posttest, we used a binary cue-based switch paradigm featuring two tasks with asymmetric difficulty levels as transfer task. Participants had to indicate either the font color or the word meaning of Stroop stimuli, that is color words which were printed in colored fonts which could either be congruent to the word meaning (i.e., the word "yellow" presented in yellow font) or incongruent to it (i.e., the word "red" presented in yellow font). Word reading is the dominant behavior in this context, rendering the color task much more difficult than the word task (Stroop, 1935). Previous research has indicated that age-related cognitive deficits can be exacerbated with increasing task difficulty (e.g., Bierre et al., 2016). As of yet, relatively little is known, however, about the impact of task difficulty on training and transfer gains in older adults. An fMRI study by Brehmer et al. (2011) has indicated that training-related benefits to neural efficiency may come to bear mainly under more difficult task conditions for this age group. The present study aimed to further examine this issue and pinpoint the specific neural processes which may benefit from multi-domain cognitive training under difficult as compared to easy task conditions. In order to do this, we examined two additional ERP components which were omitted in our earlier study on older adults (Gajewski and Falkenstein, 2012), the switch positivity and the target-locked P2. The cue-locked switch positivity has been linked to anticipatory processes associated with task-set reconfiguration. Its amplitude is thus highest for switch trials, intermediate for stay trials and lowest for single trials (Eppinger et al., 2007; Wylie et al., 2009; Jamadar et al., 2010; Karayanidis et al., 2010, 2011). The target-locked P2, an early positive deflection with a fronto-central focus, is reduced on switch compared to stay trials and has thus been related to the retrieval of stimulus-response bindings (Kieffaber and Hetrick, 2005; Schapkin et al., 2014).

Irrespective of task difficulty, we expected to observe performance gains from pretest to posttest in the multi-domain cognitive training group but not in the two control groups. In keeping with our earlier study (Gajewski and Falkenstein, 2012), we further expected that these performance gains would be accompanied by modulations of ERP components indexing the resolution of response conflict during response selection (N2) and the allocation of cognitive resources (target-locked P3) as well as the retrieval of stimulus-response bindings (P2) and anticipatory task-set reconfiguration (switch positivity). Based on previous research (Brehmer et al., 2011), we expected between-group differences to be more pronounced under difficult task conditions.

MATERIALS AND METHODS

Participants

Participants were independently living, healthy older adults which were screened for sufficient visual and auditory acuity. Other exclusion criteria were a history of cardio-vascular, motor, oncological, psychiatric or neurological diseases. Participants were also excluded from the study if their self-reported cognitive training activity exceeded 1.5 h per week. As a result of this screening procedure, 32.5% of applicants were included in the study. After completing the pretest, the 114 participants were randomly assigned to a training group receiving a 4-month multi-domain cognitive training (remaining $N = 32$; 20 female, 65–82 years old, mean age: 70.5 years, seven drop-outs due to illness, relocation, technical malfunctions), a passive no-contact control group (remaining $N = 37$; 21 female, 65–88 years old, mean age: 70 years, two drop-outs due to technical malfunctions) and an active (social) control group receiving a 4-month relaxation training (remaining $N = 34$; 21 female, 65–87 years old, mean age: 70.9 years, two drop-outs due to illness). All groups were comparable with respect to age, education and cognitive status as assessed by Mini Mental State

Examination (MMSE German version, Kessler et al., 2000), verbal IQ (MWT-B, Lehrl, 2005), forward and backward digit span and versions A and B of the Trail-Making Test (see, Wild-Wall et al., 2012, for details). All participants were included in the behavioral data analyses. Due to malfunctions of the EEG equipment, data from six participans (one of the cognitive control group, one of the active control group and three of the passive control group) could not be included in the ERP analyses. The study was carried out in accordance with the Declaration of Helsinki and with the recommendations of the local ethics committee of the Leibniz association. All participants gave written informed consent and received 100 Euro to recompense them for travel expenses.

Multi-Domain Cognitive Training and Relaxation Training

Participants in the cognitive training and the active (social) control group completed two 90-min training sessions per week across a period of 4 months. Both trainings were conducted by payed professional trainers in small groups of no more than 12 participants. Participants who had missed regular sessions had the opportunity to take part in two additional sessions after the regular training had been completed. Participants were otherwise not encouraged to train outside of the regular training sessions.

Participants in the cognitive training group were first given basic information on cognitive functions, their relevance for activities of daily living and the impact of aging on these functions. Participants additionally learned memory strategies, such as the method of loci. Subsequently, participants completed 4 weeks of paper-pencil-based exercises focused on improving processing speed, selective attention, short-term memory span, verbal fluency and arithmetic and reasoning skills (sudokus; MAT, Lehrl et al., 1994; Klauer, 2008). Simultaneously, participants without prior computer experience were familiarized with the use of a computer mouse and keyboard. In the final cognitive training phase, participants completed computer-based cognitive exercises focused on perceptual speed, selective attention and memory (peds Braintrainer[1]; mentaga GYM[2]; Mental Aktiv[3]). This multi-domain cognitive training regimen did not include a task-switching task, a Stroop task or a combination thereof. A more thorough description of the multi-domain cognitive training has already been published elsewhere (see appendix of Gajewski and Falkenstein, 2012).

The relaxation training of the active (social) control group was comprised of gymnastic, back therapy, muscle relaxation and stretching exercises as well as techniques from autogenous training, progressive muscle relaxation, Qigong and massage therapy. The training also included elements of health education, giving basic information about healthy nutrition, the negative effects of addictive substances, such as alcohol and nicotine and the benefits of physical exercise.

[1] www.ahano.de
[2] www.mentage.com
[3] www.mental-aktiv.de

Pre- and Posttest Procedure

Before and after the interventions, participants completed pretest and posttest sessions, respectively. These included socio-demographic questionnaires (pretest only), paper-and-pencil-based neuropsychological tests and computer-based cognitive tests with concurrent EEG-recording. While the present study focuses on the Stroop switch task, data from other cognitive tasks has been reported elsewhere (Gajewski and Falkenstein, 2012; Wild-Wall et al., 2012). Cognitive testing and EEG-recording were conducted in a dimly lit, electrically-shielded and sound-attenuated room. All participants were tested individually and were seated 90 cm from a 15 inch CRT monitor with a resolution of 640 × 480. Stimulus presentation and response acquisition were controlled by an IBM-compatible computer running MS-DOS.

In the Stroop switch task, participants had to indicate either the font color or the word meaning of Stroop stimuli. Stroop stimuli (10 × 5–7 mm) were the German words "rot", "grün", "blau" and "gelb" (red, green, blue and yellow, respectively) which were presented on a black background in one of four colored fonts (red, green, blue and yellow). Fonts could either be congruent to the word meaning (i.e., the word "yellow" presented in yellow font) or incongruent to it (i.e., the word "red" presented in yellow font). Prior to the Stroop stimulus, participants were presented with a cue which indicated which task had to be performed in the current trial. A white square (37 × 37 mm) indicated that font color was the relevant stimulus dimension, whereas a white diamond (37 × 37 mm) indicated that participants had to respond to the word meaning. Responses were given by pressing one of four response keys which were mounted in a response box and each corresponded to a specific color.

A given trial thus began with the presentation of a fixation cross for 300 ms, followed by the presentation of the cue (diamond/square). After 1000 ms, the Stroop stimulus appeared within the cue and remained onscreen until the participant had responded by pressing one of the four response keys. Five-hundred milliseconds after the participant's response a positive (plus sign) or negative (minus sign) feedback appeared. When the reaction time exceeded 2500 ms, the word "schneller" (faster) was presented in addition to the feedback in order to encourage participants to respond more quickly on subsequent trials.

Participants completed a total of 250 trials (50% congruent and 50% incongruent) in three distinct experimental blocks. The first two blocks were single blocks in which participants always had to perform either the word (52 trials) or the color task (52 trials). In the subsequent mixed block (146 trials), participants instead had to perform the color task (73 trials) or the word task (73 trials) in random order, as signaled by the cue. Thirty-six trials of each task type were stay trials in which the same task as in the preceding trial had to be performed. The other 37 trials were switch trials in which a different task than in the preceding trial had to be completed. Across all conditions, half of the trials featured congruent Stroop stimuli whereas the other half featured incongruent Stroop stimuli.

Electrophysiological Recording and Analyses

EEG activity was recorded continuously from 32 active BioSemi Pin-Type electrodes arranged according to the extended 10–20 system in a preconfigured cap (Easy Cap, Easycap GmbH, Herrsching-Breitbrunn, Germany). Electrodes were placed at positions Fp1, Fpz, Fp2, F7, F3, Fz, F4, F8, FC3, FCz, FC4, T7, C3, Cz, C4, T8, CP3, CPz, CP4, P7, P3, Pz, P4, P8, PO3, POz, PO4, O1, Oz and O2. Eight additional electrodes were used to record the EOG and activity at the left and right mastoids. In the Bio-Semi system, ground and reference electrodes are replaced by a feedback loop between an active and a passive electrode at positions C1 and C2, respectively. Impedances for all electrodes were kept below 10 kΩ. Signals were digitized with a BioSemi Active Two amplifier at a sampling rate of 2048 Hz and a bandpass of 0.01–140 Hz.

For off-line analysis, data were downscaled to a sampling rate of 1000 Hz and digitally bandpass filtered at 0.05–17 Hz. The first trial of each experimental block and trials with an incorrect, very fast (<100 ms) or very slow (>2500 ms) response were excluded from further analyses. The EEG was segmented into cue-locked and target-locked epochs and baseline-corrected with respect to the 100 ms pre-stimulus interval. Vertical and horizontal ocular artifacts were corrected off-line (Gratton et al., 1983), while trials with other artifacts (maximum amplitude in the segment, ±150 μV; maximum voltage step between two successive sampling points, 50 μV; maximum difference between two sampling points within the segment, ±300 μV, lowest activity in a 100 ms interval, 0.5 μV) were excluded from averaging. Electrodes were re-referenced to linked mastoids. ERPs were averaged separately for each of the two tasks (color, word) and the three trial types (single, switch, stay).

The switch positivity and the target-locked P3 were quantified as mean amplitudes between 300 ms and 600 ms post-cue and post-stimulus, respectively, at electrode positions Fz, Cz and Pz. The target-locked P2 was quantified as the most positive local amplitude between 150 ms and 300 ms after stimulus onset at FCz. The subsequent target-locked N2 was measured as the most negative local amplitude between 200 ms and 400 ms post-stimulus at Cz. Electrode positions and time windows were selected on the basis of previous research (e.g., Polich, 2007; Folstein and Van Petten, 2008; Gajewski and Falkenstein, 2012; Schapkin et al., 2014).

RESULTS

Behavioral Data

The first trial of each experimental block was excluded from further analyses. Trials with an incorrect, very fast (<100 ms) or very slow (>2500 ms) response were not included in the reaction time analyses. Mean accuracy and reaction times as well as the linear integrated speed-accuracy score (LISAS = mean reaction $\text{times}_{\text{condition}}$ + standard deviation of reaction $\text{times}_{\text{total}}$/standard deviation of proportion of $\text{errors}_{\text{total}}$ × proportion of $\text{errors}_{\text{condition}}$; Vandierendonck, 2016) were computed (see **Figure 1**). Due to lack of errors, LISAS could not be computed for one participant from the cognitive training group. All behavioral parameters were analyzed in separate analysis of variances (ANOVAs) with the within-subject factors Test Time (pretest, posttest), Trial Type (single, switch, stay) and Task (color task, word task) and the between-subject factor Group (cognitive training, active control, passive control). For all parameters, we additionally computed mixing/general switch costs (stay trials – single trials) and specific/local switch costs (switch trials – stay trials) which were submitted to separate ANOVAs with the within-subject factors Test Time and Task and the between-subject factor Group. Results were Greenhouse-Geisser corrected, where appropriate. For the sake of brevity, we only list significant effects involving the factor Test Time. In order to specify training-related changes, these effects were further analyzed with Bonferroni *post hoc* tests.

In the reaction time data, we observed a significant main effect of Test Time ($F_{(1,100)} = 8.21, p < 0.01, \eta_p^2 = 0.08$) and a significant interaction of Test Time × Trial Type × Task ($F_{(2,200)} = 5.48$, $p < 0.01$, $\eta_p^2 = 0.05$). *Post hoc* tests indicated that for the color task, reaction times decreased from pretest to posttest on single and stay trials (both $ps < 0.01$), but not on switch trials ($p = 0.18$). In the word task, reaction time benefits were limited to switch trials ($p < 0.01$) and stay trials ($p < 0.05$), but did not emerge on single trials ($p = 0.68$). None of the effects involving interactions of the factors Test Time and Group were significant.

The accuracy data yielded a significant main effect of Test Time ($F_{(1,100)} = 4.1$, $p < 0.05$, $\eta_p^2 = 0.04$) and a significant interaction of Test Time × Group ($F_{(2,100)} = 3.4$, $p < 0.05$, $\eta_p^2 = 0.06$). Bonferroni *post hoc* tests showed reduced error rates at posttest compared to pretest only in the cognitive training group ($p < 0.01$), but not in the two control groups (both $ps > 0.84$). Baseline accuracy at pretest was equivalent for the three groups (all $ps > 0.99$).

For the LISAS data, we similarly found a significant main effect of Test Time ($F_{(1,99)} = 12.21$, $p < 0.01$, $\eta_p^2 = 0.11$) as well as a significant interaction of Test Time × Group ($F_{(2,99)} = 3$, $p = 0.05$, $\eta_p^2 = 0.06$). In keeping with the accuracy data, only the cognitive control group showed decreased LISAS, i.e., better performance, at posttest compared to pretest ($p < 0.001$, both control groups, $ps > 0.18$). At pretest, we observed no significant differences in baseline performance between the three groups (all $ps > 0.89$). The interaction of Test Time × Task ($F_{(1,99)} = 6.01$, $p < 0.05$, $\eta_p^2 = 0.06$) was also significant. *Post hoc* tests nevertheless showed significant performance benefits from pretest to posttest in both the color task ($p < 0.001$) and in the word task ($p < 0.05$).

Our analysis of mixing/general switch costs (stay trials – single trials) and specific/local switch costs (switch trials – stay trials) yielded no significant effects involving the factor Test Time for either accuracy, reaction times or LISAS.

Behavioral Data Summary

Error rates and LISAS indicated performance gains from pretest to posttest only for the cognitive training group, but not for the two control groups. Training-related performance gains emerged for all trial types and could thus not be attributed

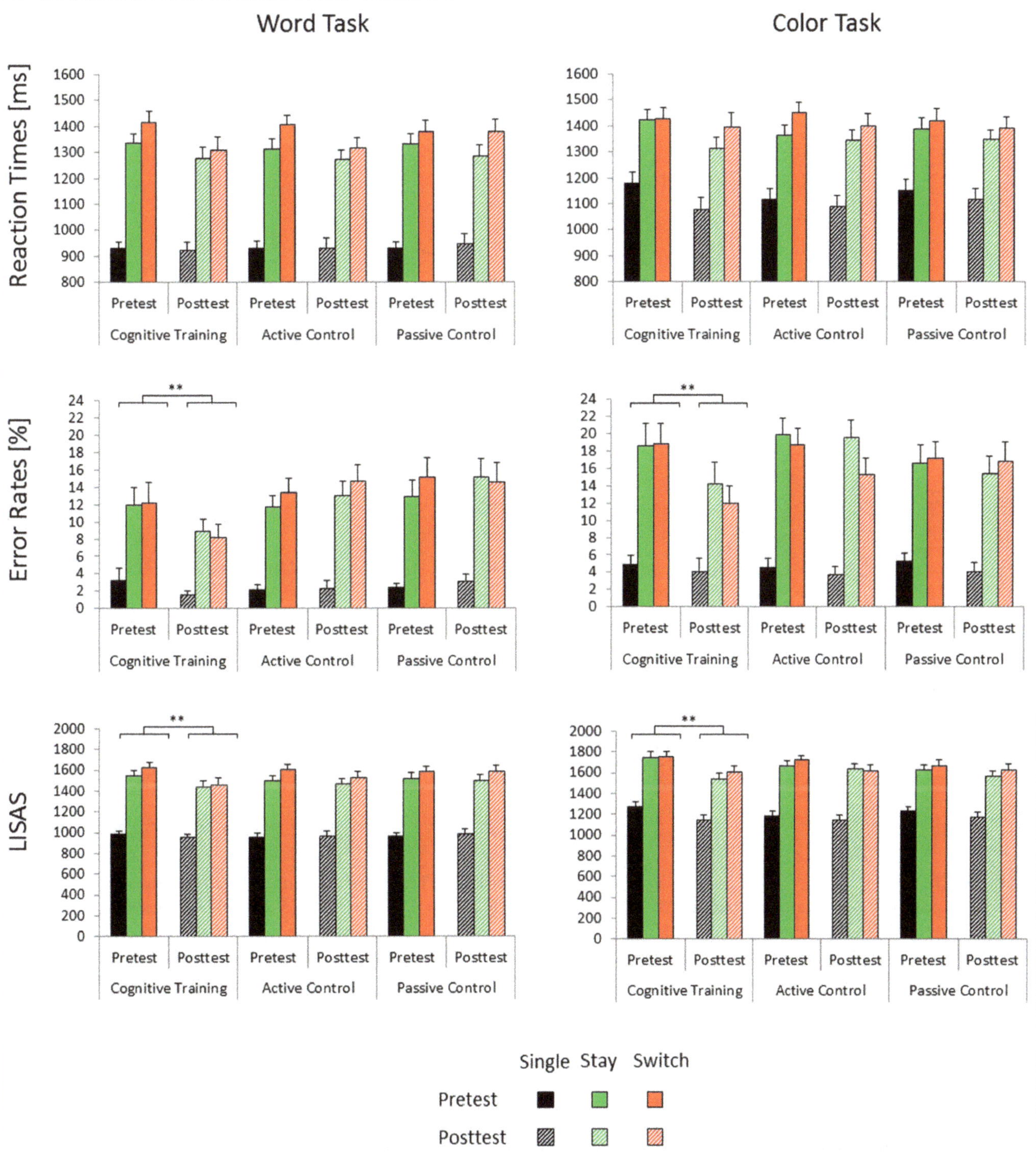

FIGURE 1 | Mean reaction times, error rates and linear integrated speed-accuracy score (LISAS) for the three groups (cognitive training, active control, passive control) as a function of session (pretest, posttest), trial type (single, switch, stay) and task (word task, color task). Error bars indicate the standard error of the mean. Posttest reaction time gains associated with cognitive training are highlighted (**significant at $p < 0.001$).

to reductions of mixing/general switch costs or specific/local switch costs. All groups showed decreased reaction times at posttest compared to pretest. These unspecific practice effects were subject to the task participants had to perform: for the easier word task, reaction time benefits emerged under mixing conditions. For the more difficult color task, they were instead limited to single and stay trials which did not require a task set reconfiguration.

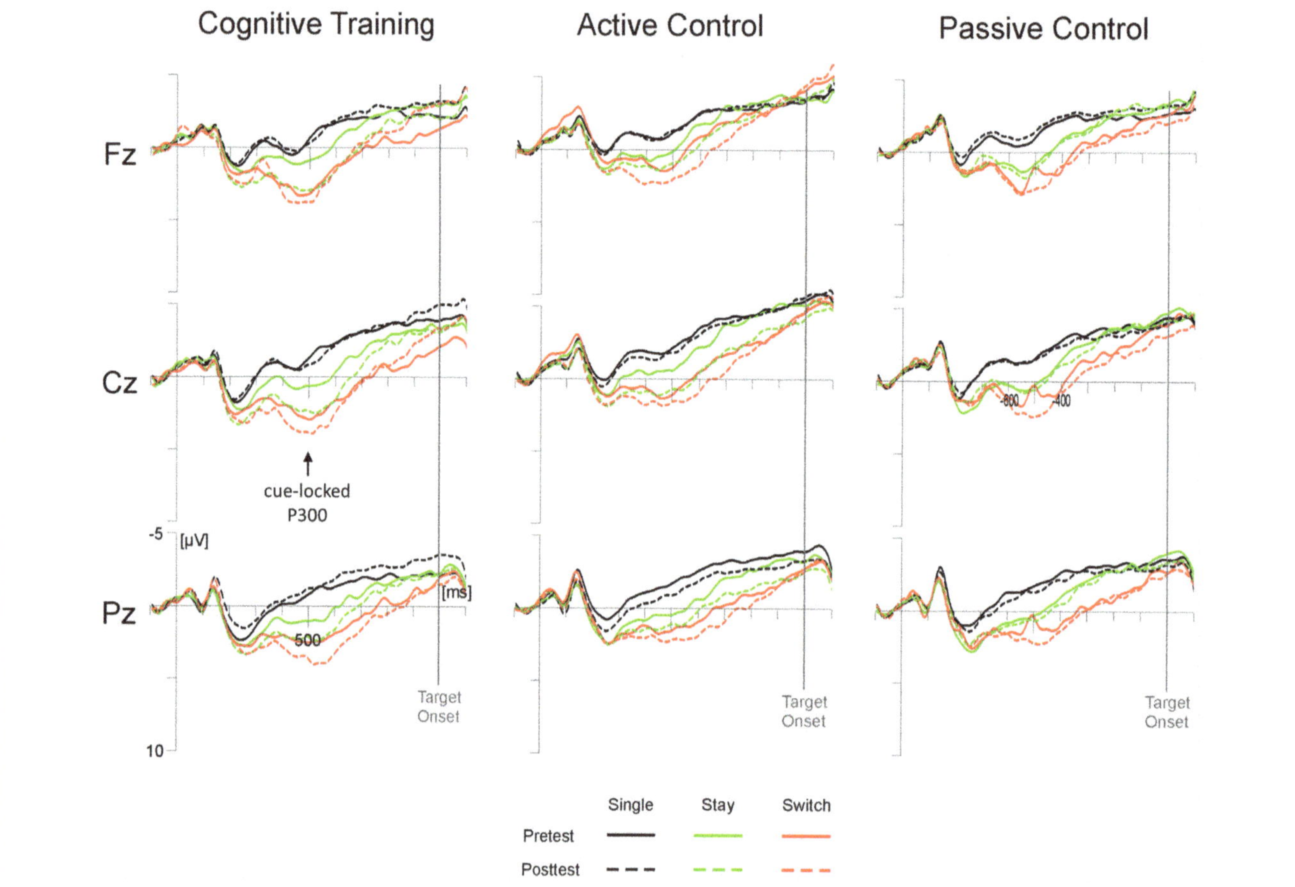

FIGURE 2 | Cue-locked grand average event-related potentials (ERPs) for the three groups (cognitive training, active control, passive control) at Fz, Cz and Pz as a function of session (pretest, posttest) and trial type (single, switch, stay). Time scaling ranges from −100 ms to 1100 ms around cue onset and positive deflections are displayed downward. Cognitive training was associated with increased posttest amplitudes of the highlighted cue-locked P3 on stay trials (green lines).

ERP Data

The switch positivity and the target-locked P3 were analyzed in separate ANOVAs with the within-subject factors Electrode Position (Fz, Cz, Pz), Test Time (pretest, posttest), Trial Type (single, switch, stay) and Task (color task, word task) and the between-subject factor Group (cognitive training, active control, passive control). Target-locked P2 amplitude at FCz and N2 amplitude at Cz were analyzed in separate ANOVAs with the within-subject factors Test Time (pretest, posttest), Trial Type (switch, stay) and Task (color task, word task) and the between-subject factor Group (cognitive training, active control, passive control). Results were Greenhouse-Geisser corrected, where appropriate. Significant effects involving the crucial factor Test Time are listed and were further analyzed with Bonferroni *post hoc* tests.

Cue-Locked Switch Positivity Amplitude

Analyses of the switch positivity amplitude yielded a significant main effect of Test Time ($F_{(1,98)} = 5.79$, $p < 0.05$, $\eta_p^2 = 0.06$) as well as interactions of Test Time × Electrode Position × Trial Type × Task ($F_{(4,392)} = 3.96$, $p < 0.01$, $\eta_p^2 = 0.04$) and, crucially, Test Time × Group × Electrode Position × Trial Type ($F_{(8,392)} = 4.83$, $p = 0.05$, $\eta_p^2 = 0.04$). As illustrated in **Figure 2**, *post hoc* tests indicated that in the cognitive training group, stay trials elicited higher switch positivities at posttest compared to pretest at all sites (Fz and Cz, *ps* < 0.05; Pz, $p = 0.05$; all other *ps* > 0.14). In the active control group, higher posttest amplitudes emerged at Cz for stay trials ($p < 0.05$) and Pz showed a trend towards pre-post differences for single trials ($p = 0.07$; all other *ps* > 0.15). For the passive control group, on the other hand, we found no reliable pre-post differences at any electrode position (all *ps* > 0.29).

Target-Locked P2 Amplitude and Latency

For P2 amplitudes at FCz, we observed a significant interaction of Test Time × Task ($F_{(1,98)} = 4.93$, $p < 0.05$, $\eta_p^2 = 0.05$), yet *post hoc* tests indicated no significant changes from pretest to posttest for either the color or the word task (both *ps* > 0.11). None of the effects involving the factor Group reached significance. The P2 latency analysis yielded a significant main effect of Test Time ($F_{(2,196)} = 4.6$, $p < 0.05$, $\eta_p^2 = 0.05$) and a significant interaction of Test Time × Group × Trial Type ($F_{(4,196)} = 2.42$,

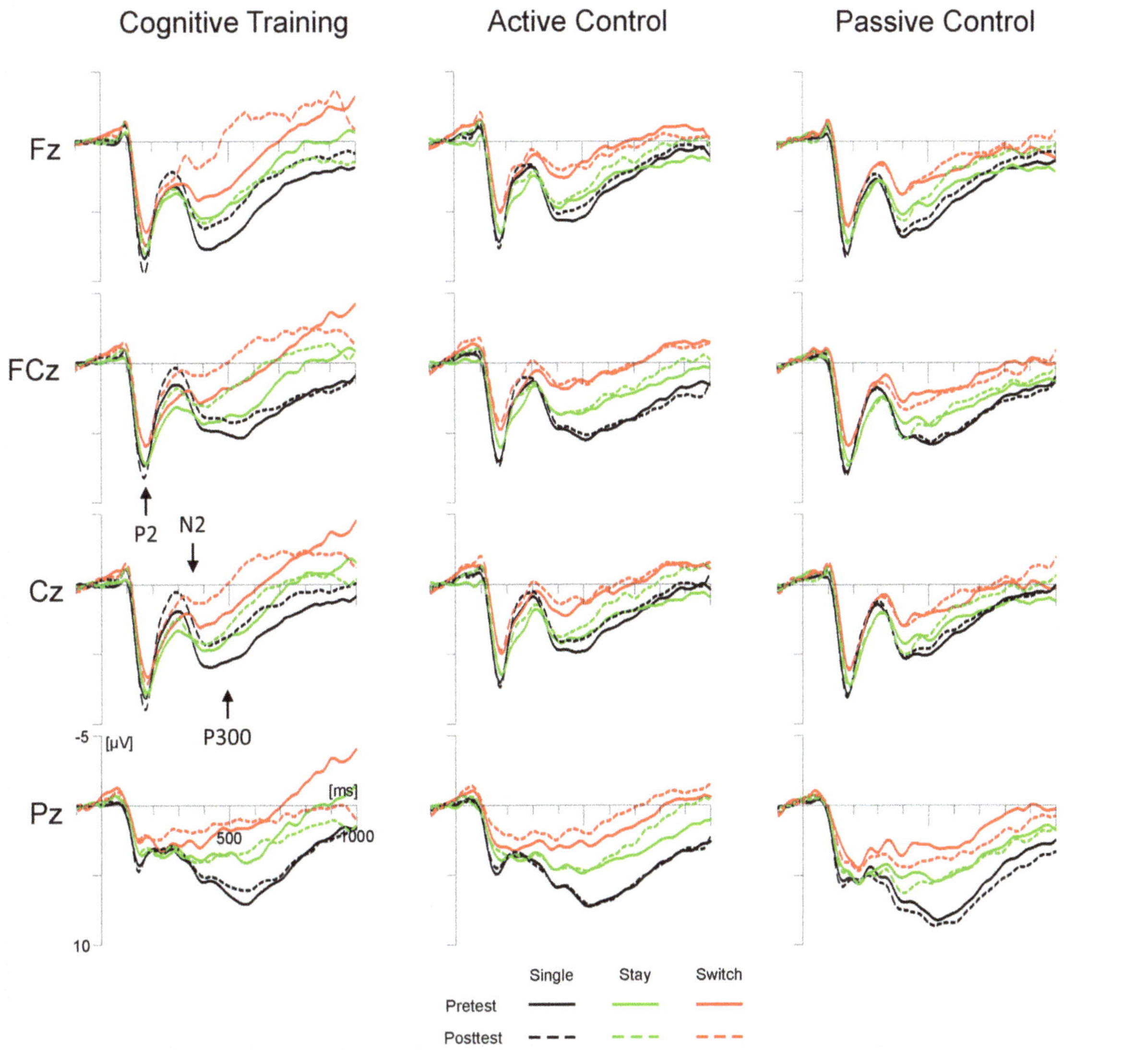

FIGURE 3 | Target-locked grand average ERPs for the three groups (cognitive training, active control, passive control) at Fz, FCz, Cz and Pz as a function of session (pretest, posttest) and trial type (single, switch, stay). Time scaling ranges from −100 ms to 1000 ms around cue onset and positive deflections are displayed downward. Cognitive training was associated with increased posttest amplitudes of the highlighted N2 and decreased amplitudes of the highlighted P3 for all trial types. Single trials (black lines) additionally showed reduced latencies of the highlighted P2 at posttest.

$p = 0.05$, $\eta_p^2 = 0.05$). *Post hoc* tests showed reduced P2 latencies at posttest compared to pretest, but only on single trials of the cognitive training group ($p < 0.01$; all other *ps* > 0.14, see **Figure 3**).

Target-Locked N2 Amplitude and Latency

The analysis of N2 amplitudes at Cz, yielded a significant interaction of Test Time × Group ($F_{(2,98)} = 3.36$, $p < 0.05$, $\eta_p^2 = 0.06$). *Post hoc* tests showed an increase in N2 amplitude from pretest to posttest for the cognitive training group ($p < 0.01$), but not for the two control groups (both *ps* > 0.34, see **Figure 3**). The N2 latency analysis showed a significant interaction of Test Time × Trial Type × Task ($F_{(2,196)} = 6.25$, $p < 0.01$, $\eta_p^2 = 0.06$). According to *post hoc* tests, N2 latencies were shortened from pretest to posttest only on stay trials of the color task ($p < 0.01$; all other *ps* > 0.13).

Target-Locked P3 Amplitude

For the target-locked mean P3 amplitude, we observed significant interactions of Test Time × Electrode Position ($F_{(2,196)} = 4.67$, $p < 0.05$, $\eta_p^2 = 0.05$), and, importantly, Test Time × Group × Electrode Position × Trial Type ($F_{(8,392)} = 2.72$, $p < 0.01$, $\eta_p^2 = 0.05$). For both control groups, *post hoc* tests showed no significant amplitude differences between pre- and posttest, irrespective of trial type and electrode position (all *ps* > 0.21; see **Figure 3**). For the cognitive training group, on the other hand, P3 amplitudes decreased from pretest to posttest: at Fz, amplitude decreases were significant for single and switch trials (both $ps < 0.01$). At Cz, we observed significant decreases for switch and stay trials (both $ps < 0.05$) and a trend towards a decrease for single trials ($p = 0.07$; Pz, all $ps > 0.39$).

ERP Data Summary

For all trial types, cognitive training was associated with an increase of the target-locked N2 and a subsequent amplitude decrease at fronto-central locations in the time range of the target-locked P3. On single trials, we additionally observed a training-related reduction of target-locked P2 latencies. In the cue-target interval, the switch positivity on stay trials was increased at posttest for both the cognitive training group and the active control group. The passive control showed no significant ERP differences between pretest and posttest.

DISCUSSION

The present study was aimed at examining the effects of multi-domain cognitive training and task difficulty on executive functions in older adults. To this end, healthy older adults were randomly assigned to a passive control group, an active control group receiving 4 months of relaxation training and a cognitive training group who completed 4 months of multi-domain cognitive training. In pre- and posttest sessions, we recorded behavioral and ERP indices of performance in an untrained task switching paradigm featuring Stroop stimuli. Participants had to attend two tasks with different difficulty levels, an easier word reading task and a more difficult color naming task (see Stroop, 1935).

At the behavioral level, we observed reduced reaction times at posttest compared to pretest. Although this effect appeared to be driven mainly by reaction time reductions in the cognitive training group and the active control group, it was not significantly modulated by the factor Group. It thus should be considered a practice effect induced by repeated testing rather than a performance gain related to the increased activity associated with training regimen. Interestingly, this practice effect was modulated by task difficulty: in the easier word-task, reaction time benefits emerged on stay and switch trials, but not in single task blocks. In the more difficult color task, reaction times instead decreased for single and stay trials, but not for switch trials. In light of the low difficulty level of the word task, it is feasible that only the more complex mixed block offered room for improvement because performance for the less demanding single trials was already at ceiling at pretest. For the more difficult color task, on the other hand, the task set configuration associated with switch trials may have further elevated the difficulty level to such a degree that practice was not sufficient to generate reliable reaction time benefits.

In the context of the present study, accuracy and LISAS results were more noteworthy than the reaction time data as they indicated performance benefits associated exclusively with multi-domain cognitive training: both parameters were reduced at posttest compared to pretest only for the cognitive training group, but not for the two control groups. This result pattern corroborates and extends previous research on multi-domain cognitive training which could show beneficial transfer effects to executive functions in younger, middle-aged and older adults (e.g., Gajewski and Falkenstein, 2012; Baniqued et al., 2015; Gajewski et al., 2017). In keeping with these studies, training-related performance gains became manifest in increased response accuracy. In contrast to our initial hypothesis, however, these accuracy improvements were equivalent in the color and in the word task.

Cognitive training was not only associated with gains in response accuracy, but also with modulations of cue- and target-locked ERPs from pretest to posttest. Whereas the switch positivity in the task preparation period was larger at posttest both in the cognitive training group and the active control group, changes in target-N2 and target-P3 amplitude as well as target-P2 latency were limited to the cognitive training group. Like the training-related benefits in accuracy, these ERP modulations were not subject to the task participants had to perform.

ERPs in the cue-target interval showed modulations from pretest to posttest after either type of training regimen: on posttest stay trials, we observed an increase in switch positivity which was widespread for the cognitive training group and limited to central sites for the active control group, but absent in the passive control group. Modulations of the switch positivity are thought to reflect the degree of task set updating necessary to prepare for the upcoming task (for a review see Karayanidis et al., 2010). An enhancement of switch positivity amplitude from pretest to posttest, notably in stay trials, may thus indicate a training-related boost to the efficiency of maintaining a task set from one trial to the next under mixing conditions. As both the cognitive training group and the active control group showed an increase in switch positivity amplitude, this efficiency gain may be due to unspecific vitalization associated with training regimen in general (see Gajewski and Falkenstein, 2015a).

Regarding the target-locked ERPs, the present target-P2 data indicate that multi-domain cognitive training has the potential to accelerate the processing operations underlying the P2, at least under single task conditions. Previous research has linked the P2 to the retrieval of stimulus-response bindings (Kieffaber and Hetrick, 2005; Gajewski et al., 2008; Schapkin et al., 2014). The subsequent target-locked N2 has been associated with cognitive control processes, such as response inhibition, the resolution of response conflict and response selection (for a review see Folstein and Van Petten, 2008). The training-related enhancement of the target-locked N2 we observed in the present study is consistent with our previous reports (Gajewski and Falkenstein, 2012; Gajewski et al., 2017): multi-domain cognitive training, was previously associated with an increase in target-locked N2 amplitude in cue-based and memory-based versions of a task switching paradigm featuring three tasks with comparable difficulty levels. Whereas the earlier study showed reliable N2 enhancements mainly for switch trials, the present N2 data as well as data from the later study indicate that cognitive training can also lead to amplitude increases on single and stay trials (see Gajewski and Falkenstein, 2015a,b, for similar N2 enhancements due to habitual physical activity).

Taken together with our previous findings (Gajewski and Falkenstein, 2012; Gajewski et al., 2017), the present ERP data thus corroborate the idea that multi-domain cognitive training can benefit processes involved in response selection, especially in older adults. At the behavioral level, such a training-related improvement of response selection consistently appears to translate into an improvement of response accuracy not only in older adults (the present study, Gajewski and Falkenstein, 2012) but also in younger participants (Gajewski et al., 2017). To be more specific, the present and previous data suggest that target-P2 and target-N2 are related to the retrieval or activation of stimulus-response mappings or task sets (target-P2) and the implementation of these sets (target-N2). The mechanisms reflected in these ERP components are thus essential for successfully executing a task-appropriate reaction, i.e., for pressing the correct response key. When this process is enhanced as indicated, for example, by a negative shift in the target-locked N2, participants are less likely to make an error. In other words, cognitive training enhances the ability to make a correct decision. For the present study, this was the case irrespective of task difficulty and on both switch and non-switch trials.

In contrast to our earlier report on older adults (Gajewski and Falkenstein, 2012), the present data show an amplitude decrease in the time window of the target-locked P3 at fronto-central electrodes following cognitive training. In the earlier study, participants had instead shown a training-related increase in target-locked P3 amplitudes at posterior sites which we interpreted in terms of improved cognitive resource allocation. In younger adults, the P3 usually has a clear-cut parietal focus (for a review see Polich, 2007). For the present older participants, we instead observed cue-locked and target-locked P3s with a more widespread distribution featuring parietal and frontal foci. This is in line with previous age-comparative research which has indicated that older adults may show a broader distribution of the P3 which extends to anterior sites as well and which likely reflects the compensatory increased recruitment of prefrontal brain areas involved in cognitive control (Kray et al., 2005; Eppinger et al., 2007; Adrover-Roig and Barceló, 2010; Kopp et al., 2014). As the target-P3 amplitude decrease observed in the present study was limited to fronto-central electrodes, it could potentially reflect a training-related reduction in this compensatory over-recruitment of frontal areas. Alternatively, the target-P3 amplitude decrease could be related to the enhancement of the preceding fronto-central target-N2 which extends into the P3 peak latency range, or to an even broader negative shift in the time range of both target-locked N2 and P3 (see Gajewski and Falkenstein, 2015a,b). Further ERP research on cognitive training in older adults is needed to clarify this issue.

Previous research on the impact of transfer task difficulty on training-related performance gains is scarce. In one of the few studies on the subject, Brehmer et al. (2011) examined the performance of a cognitive training group and an active control group in a working memory transfer task featuring high and low load conditions. They found that neither group showed performance gains from pretest to posttest in either condition suggesting that performance was already at ceiling at pretest. The present study instead featured a more difficult transfer task which offered room for improvement from pretest to posttest. Under these conditions, practice effects which were not directly associated with cognitive training were subject to task difficulty whereas genuine training-related performance benefits were not. Likewise, cognitive training benefited performance on single, stay and switch trials to a similar degree. As a result, we were unable to link training-related performance gains to reductions of mixing/general switch costs or specific/local switch costs as previous studies have done (e.g., Gajewski and Falkenstein, 2012). Note, however, that particularly specific/local switch costs were minimal at baseline in the cognitive training group. Any potential impact of multi-domain cognitive training on these costs thus would have been difficult to detect, in the present study.

Conclusions

The present study corroborates and extends our understanding of the neural underpinnings of performance gains associated with multi-domain cognitive training in older adults. A 4 month multi-domain cognitive training had beneficial effects on response accuracy in an untrained binary switch paradigm featuring two tasks with distinct difficulty levels. These training-related performance gains were likely mediated by an increase in target-locked N2 amplitude, an amplitude reduction in the time range of the target-locked P3 and a decrease in target-P2 latency. These ERP modulations indicate benefits to neural processes involved in response selection which resulted in reduced error rates on both switch and non-switch trials. Our findings suggest that multi-domain cognitive training increases slow negative potentials during target processing which enhance the N2 and may additionally reduce the amplitude of a subsequent P3-like component on both switch and non-switch trials and irrespective of task difficulty.

AUTHOR CONTRIBUTIONS

KK conducted the data analysis and wrote the manuscript. PDG and MF were involved in study conception and data acquisition and revised and approved the manuscript. CF was involved in study conception as well as the acquisition and analysis of the data and revised and approved the manuscript.

ACKNOWLEDGMENTS

This work was funded by a grant from the German Insurance Association (Gesamtverband der Deutschen Versicherungswirtschaft, GDV). We thank Ludger Blanke for programming the task and technical support and Christiane Westedt, Brita Rietdorf and Pia Deltenre for their help in organizing and conducting the study. This article is based on a reanalysis of data which were first analyzed by CF as part of her dissertation project. The publication of this article was supported by the Open Access Fund of the Leibniz Association and by the Open Access Fund of the Technical University of Dortmund.

REFERENCES

Adrover-Roig, D., and Barceló, F. (2010). Individual differences in aging and cognitive control modulate the neural indexes of context updating and maintenance during task switching. *Cortex* 46, 434–450. doi: 10.1016/j.cortex.2009.09.012

Allport, D. A., Styles, E. A., and Hsieh, S. (1994). "Shifting intentional set: exploring the dynamic control of tasks," in *Attention and Performance XV: Conscious and Nonconscious Information Processing*, eds C. Umiltà and M. Moscovitch (Cambridge, MA: MIT Press), 421–452.

Au, J., Sheehan, E., Tsai, N., Duncan, G. J., Buschkuehl, M., and Jaeggi, S. M. (2015). Improving fluid intelligence with training on working memory: a meta-analysis. *Psychon. Bull. Rev.* 22, 366–377. doi: 10.3758/s13423-014-0699-x

Ball, K., Berch, D. B., Helmers, K. F., Jobe, J. B., Leveck, M. D., Marsiske, M., et al. (2002). Effects of cognitive training interventions with older adults: a randomized controlled trial. *JAMA* 288, 2271–2281. doi: 10.1001/jama.288.18.2271

Ballesteros, S., Kraft, E., Santana, S., and Tziraki, C. (2015). Maintaining older brain functionality: a targeted review. *Neurosci. Biobehav. Rev.* 55, 453–477. doi: 10.1016/j.neubiorev.2015.06.008

Baniqued, P. L., Allen, C. M., Kranz, M. B., Johnson, K., Sipolins, A., Dickens, C., et al. (2015). Working memory, reasoning, and task switching training: transfer effects, limitations, and great expectations? *PLoS One* 10:e0142169. doi: 10.1371/journal.pone.0142169

Bierre, K. L., Lucas, S. J., Guiney, H., Cotter, J. D., and Machado, L. (2016). Cognitive difficulty intensifies age-related changes in anterior frontal hemodynamics: novel evidence from near-infrared spectroscopy. *J. Gerontol. A Biol. Sci. Med. Sci.* 72, 181–188. doi: 10.1093/gerona/glw061

Binder, J. C., Bezzola, L., Haueter, A. I., Klein, C., Kühnis, J., Baetschmann, H., et al. (2017). Expertise-related functional brain network efficiency in healthy older adults. *BMC Neurosci.* 18:2. doi: 10.1186/s12868-016-0324-1

Binder, J. C., Marin, M., Zöllig, J., Röcke, C., Mérillat, S., Eschen, A., et al. (2016). Multi-domain training enhances attentional control. *Psychol. Aging* 31, 390–408. doi: 10.1037/pag0000081

Brehmer, Y., Rieckmann, A., Bellander, M., Westerberg, H., Fischer, H., and Bäckman, L. (2011). Neural correlates of training-related working-memory gains in old age. *Neuroimage* 58, 1110–1120. doi: 10.1016/j.neuroimage.2011.06.079

Burgess, P. W., Alderman, N., Evans, J., Emslie, H., and Wilson, B. A. (1998). The ecological validity of tests of executive function. *J. Int. Neuropsychol. Soc.* 4, 547–558. doi: 10.1017/s1355617798466037

Buschkuehl, M., Jaeggi, S. M., and Jonides, J. (2012). Neuronal effects following working memory training. *Dev. Cogn. Neurosci.* 2, S167–S179. doi: 10.1016/j.dcn.2011.10.001

Cao, W., Cao, X., Hou, C., Li, T., Cheng, Y., Jiang, L., et al. (2016). Effects of cognitive training on resting-state functional connectivity of default mode, salience, and central executive networks. *Front. Aging Neurosci.* 8:70. doi: 10.3389/fnagi.2016.00070

Cheng, Y., Wu, W., Feng, W., Wang, J., Chen, Y., Shen, Y., et al. (2012). The effects of multi-domain versus single-domain cognitive training in non-demented older people: a randomized controlled trial. *BMC Med.* 10:30. doi: 10.1186/1741-7015-10-30

Dahlin, E., Nyberg, L., Bäckman, L., and Neely, A. S. (2008). Plasticity of executive functioning in young and older adults: immediate training gains, transfer, and long-term maintenance. *Psychol. Aging* 23, 720–730. doi: 10.1037/a0014296

Eppinger, B., Kray, J., Mecklinger, A., and John, O. (2007). Age differences in task switching and response monitoring: evidence from ERPs. *Biol. Psychol.* 75, 52–67. doi: 10.1016/j.biopsycho.2006.12.001

Falkenstein, M., Hohnsbein, J., Hoormann, J., and Blanke, L. (1991). Effects of crossmodal divided attention on late ERP components. II. Error processing in choice reaction tasks. *Electroencephalogr. Clin. Neurophysiol.* 78, 447–455. doi: 10.1016/0013-4694(91)90062-9

Folstein, J. R., and Van Petten, C. (2008). Influence of cognitive control and mismatch on the N2 component of the ERP: a review. *Psychophysiology* 45, 152–170. doi: 10.1111/j.1469-8986.2007.00602.x

Gajewski, P. D., and Falkenstein, M. (2012). Training-induced improvement of response selection and error detection in aging assessed by task switching: effects of cognitive, physical, and relaxation training. *Front. Hum. Neurosci.* 6:130. doi: 10.3389/fnhum.2012.00130

Gajewski, P. D., and Falkenstein, M. (2015a). Lifelong physical activity and executive functions in older age assessed by memory based task switching. *Neuropsychologia* 73, 195–207. doi: 10.1016/j.neuropsychologia.2015.04.031

Gajewski, P. D., and Falkenstein, M. (2015b). Long-term habitual physical activity is associated with lower distractibility in a Stroop interference task in aging: behavioral and ERP evidence. *Brain Cogn.* 98, 87–101. doi: 10.1016/j.bandc.2015.06.004

Gajewski, P. D., Freude, G., and Falkenstein, M. (2017). Cognitive training sustainably improves executive functioning in middle aged industry workers assessed by task switching: a randomized controlled ERP study. *Front. Hum. Neurosci.* 11:81. doi: 10.3389/fnhum.2017.00081

Gajewski, P. D., Kleinsorge, T., and Falkenstein, M. (2010a). Electrophysiological correlates of residual switch costs. *Cortex* 46, 1138–1148. doi: 10.1016/j.cortex.2009.07.014

Gajewski, P. D., Wild-Wall, N., Schapkin, S. A., Erdmann, U., Freude, G., and Falkenstein, M. (2010b). Effects of aging and job demands on cognitive flexibility assessed by task switching. *Biol. Psychol.* 85, 187–199. doi: 10.1016/j.biopsycho.2010.06.009

Gajewski, P. D., Stoerig, P., and Falkenstein, M. (2008). ERP—correlates of response selection in a response conflict paradigm. *Brain Res.* 1189, 127–134. doi: 10.1016/j.brainres.2007.10.076

Gates, N., and Valenzuela, M. (2010). Cognitive exercise and its role in cognitive function in older adults. *Curr. Psychiatry Rep.* 12, 20–27. doi: 10.1007/s11920-009-0085-y

Gratton, G., Coles, M. G. H., and Donchin, E. (1983). A new method for off-line removal of ocular artifact. *Electroencephalogr. Clin. Neurophysiol.* 55, 468–484. doi: 10.1016/0013-4694(83)90135-9

Hertzog, C., Kramer, A. F., Wilson, R. S., and Lindenberger, U. (2008). Enrichment effects on adult cognitive development can the functional capacity of older adults be preserved and enhanced? *Psychol. Sci. Public Interest* 9, 1–65. doi: 10.1111/j.1539-6053.2009.01034.x

Jamadar, S., Hughes, M., Fulham, W. R., Michie, P. T., and Karayanidis, F. (2010). The spatial and temporal dynamics of anticipatory preparation and response inhibition in task-switching. *Neuroimage* 51, 432–449. doi: 10.1016/j.neuroimage.2010.01.090

Jiang, L., Cao, X., Li, T., Tang, Y., Li, W., Wang, J., et al. (2016). Cortical thickness changes correlate with cognition changes after cognitive training: evidence from a chinese community study. *Front. Aging Neurosci.* 8:118. doi: 10.3389/fnagi.2016.00118

Jonides, J. (2004). How does practice makes perfect? *Nat. Neurosci.* 7, 10–11. doi: 10.1038/nn0104-10

Jonides, J., Lewis, R. L., Nee, D. E., Lustig, C. A., Berman, M. G., and Moore, K. S. (2008). The mind and brain of short-term memory. *Annu. Rev. Psychol.* 59, 193–224. doi: 10.1146/annurev.psych.59.103006.093615

Jost, K., Mayr, U., and Rösler, F. (2008). Is task switching nothing but cue priming? Evidence from ERPs. *Cogn. Affect. Behav. Neurosci.* 8, 74–84. doi: 10.3758/cabn.8.1.74

Karayanidis, F., Jamadar, S., Ruge, H., Phillips, N., Heathcote, A., and Forstmann, B. U. (2010). Advance preparation in task-switching: converging evidence from behavioral, brain activation and model-based approaches. *Front. Psychol.* 1:25. doi: 10.3389/fpsyg.2010.00025

Karayanidis, F., Provost, A., Brown, S., Paton, B., and Heathcote, A. (2011). Switch-specific and general preparation map onto different ERP components in a task-switching paradigm. *Psychophysiology* 48, 559–568. doi: 10.1111/j.1469-8986.2010.01115.x

Karbach, J. (2014). Game-based cognitive training for the aging brain. *Front. Psychol.* 5:1100. doi: 10.3389/fpsyg.2014.01100

Karbach, J., and Schubert, T. (2013). Training-induced cognitive and neural plasticity. *Front. Hum. Neurosci.* 7:48. doi: 10.3389/fnhum.2013.00048

Karbach, J., and Verhaeghen, P. (2014). Making working memory work: a meta-analysis of executive-control and working memory training in older adults. *Psychol. Sci.* 25, 2027–2037. doi: 10.1177/0956797614548725

Kessler, J., Markowitsch, H. J., and Denzler, P. (2000). *Mini-Mental-Status-Test (MMST).* Göttingen: Beltz Test GmbH.

Kieffaber, P. D., and Hetrick, W. P. (2005). Event-related potential correlates of task switching and switch costs. *Psychophysiology* 42, 56–71. doi: 10.1111/j.1469-8986.2005.00262.x

Kiesel, A., Steinhauser, M., Wendt, M., Falkenstein, M., Jost, K., Philipp, A. M., et al. (2010). Control and interference in task switching—a review. *Psychol. Bull.* 136, 849–874. doi: 10.1037/a0019842

Kim, G. H., Jeon, S., Im, K., Kwon, H., Lee, B. H., Kim, G. Y., et al. (2015). Structural brain changes after traditional and robot-assisted multi-domain cognitive training in community-dwelling healthy elderly. *PLoS One* 10:e0123251. doi: 10.1371/journal.pone.0123251

Klauer, K. J. (2008). *Denksport Für Ältere—Geistig Fit Bleiben.* Bern: Hans Huber.

Kopp, B., Lange, F., Howe, J., and Wessel, K. (2014). Age-related changes in neural recruitment for cognitive control. *Brain Cogn.* 85, 209–219. doi: 10.1016/j.bandc.2013.12.008

Kramer, A. F., Hahn, S., and Gopher, D. (1999). Task coordination and aging: explorations of executive control processes in the task switching paradigm. *Acta Psychol. (Amst)* 101, 339–378. doi: 10.1016/s0001-6918(99)00011-6

Kray, J., Eppinger, B., and Mecklinger, A. (2005). Age differences in attentional control: an event-related potential approach. *Psychophysiology* 42, 407–416. doi: 10.1111/j.1469-8986.2005.00298.x

Kray, J., and Lindenberger, U. (2000). Adult age differences in task switching. *Psychol. Aging* 15, 126–147. doi: 10.1037/0882-7974.15.1.126

Kueider, A. M., Parisi, J. M., Gross, A. L., and Rebok, G. W. (2012). Computerized cognitive training with older adults: a systematic review. *PLoS One* 7:e40588. doi: 10.1371/journal.pone.0040588

Lampit, A., Ebster, C., and Valenzuela, M. (2014a). Multi-domain computerized cognitive training program improves performance of bookkeeping tasks: a matched-sampling active-controlled trial. *Front. Psychol.* 5:794. doi: 10.3389/fpsyg.2014.00794

Lampit, A., Hallock, H., and Valenzuela, M. (2014b). Computerized cognitive training in cognitively healthy older adults: a systematic review and meta-analysis of effect modifiers. *PLoS Med.* 11:e1001756. doi: 10.1371/journal.pmed.1001756

Lehrl, S. (2005). *Mehrfachwahl-Wortschatz-Intelligenztest (MWT-B).* Göttingen: Hogrefe.

Lehrl, S., Lehrl, M., and Weickmann, E. (1994). *MAT Gehirnjogging: Einführung in Das Mentale Aktivierungs Training.* Ebersberg: Vless.

Li, S. C., Lindenberger, U., Hommel, B., Aschersleben, G., Prinz, W., and Baltes, P. B. (2004). Transformations in the couplings among intellectual abilities and constituent cognitive processes across the life span. *Psychol. Sci.* 15, 155–163. doi: 10.1111/j.0956-7976.2004.01503003.x

Li, T., Yao, Y., Cheng, Y., Xu, B., Cao, X., Waxman, D., et al. (2016). Cognitive training can reduce the rate of cognitive aging: a neuroimaging cohort study. *BMC Geriatr.* 16:12. doi: 10.1186/s12877-016-0194-5

Luo, C., Zhang, X., Cao, X., Gan, Y., Li, T., Cheng, Y., et al. (2016). The lateralization of intrinsic networks in the aging brain implicates the effects of cognitive training. *Front. Aging Neurosci.* 8:32. doi: 10.3389/fnagi.2016.00032

Lustig, C., Shah, P., Seidler, R., and Reuter-Lorenz, P. A. (2009). Aging, training, and the brain: a review and future directions. *Neuropsychol. Rev.* 19, 504–522. doi: 10.1007/s11065-009-9119-9

Mahncke, H. W., Connor, B. B., Appelman, J., Ahsanuddin, O. N., Hardy, J. L., Wood, R. A., et al. (2006). Memory enhancement in healthy older adults using a brain plasticity-based training program: a randomized, controlled study. *Proc. Natl. Acad. Sci. U S A* 103, 12523–12528. doi: 10.1073/pnas.0605194103

Mayr, U. (2001). Age differences in the selection of mental sets: the role of inhibition, stimulus ambiguity and response-set overlap. *Psychol. Aging* 16, 96–109. doi: 10.1037//0882-7974.16.1.96

Meiran, N. (1996). Reconfiguration of processing mode prior to task performance. *J. Exp. Psychol. Learn. Mem. Cogn.* 22, 1423–1442. doi: 10.1037/0278-7393.22.6.1423

Melby-Lervåg, M., and Hulme, C. (2013). Is working memory training effective? A meta-analytic review. *Dev. Psychol.* 49, 270–291. doi: 10.1037/a0028228

Melby-Lervåg, M., Redick, T. S., and Hulme, C. (2016). Working memory training does not improve performance on measures of intelligence or other measures of "Far Transfer": evidence from a meta-analytic review. *Perspect. Psychol. Sci.* 11, 512–534. doi: 10.1177/1745691616635612

Polich, J. (2007). Updating P300: an integrative theory of P3a and P3b. *Clin. Neurophysiol.* 118, 2128–2148. doi: 10.1016/j.clinph.2007.04.019

Redick, T. S., Shipstead, Z., Harrison, T. L., Hicks, K. L., Fried, D. E., Hambrick, D. Z., et al. (2013). No evidence of intelligence improvement after working memory training: a randomized, placebo-controlled study. *J. Exp. Psychol. Gen.* 142, 359–379. doi: 10.1037/a0029082

Rogers, R. D., and Monsell, S. (1995). Costs of a predictible switch between simple cognitive tasks. *J. Exp. Psychol. Gen.* 124, 207–231. doi: 10.1037//0096-3445.124.2.207

Sander, M. C., Lindenberger, U., and Werkle-Bergner, M. (2012). Lifespan age differences in working memory: a two-component framework. *Neurosci. Biobehav. Rev.* 36, 2007–2033. doi: 10.1016/j.neubiorev.2012.06.004

Schapkin, S. A., Gajewski, P. D., and Freude, G. (2014). Age differences in memory-based task switching with and without cues: an ERP study. *J. Psychophysiol.* 28, 187–201. doi: 10.1027/0269-8803/a000125

Stroop, J. R. (1935). Studies of interference in serial verbal reactions. *J. Exp. Psychol.* 18, 643–662. doi: 10.1037/h0054651

Vandierendonck, A. (2016). A comparison of methods to combine speed and accuracy measures of performance: a rejoinder on the binning procedure. *Behav. Res. Methods* doi: 10.3758/s13428-016-0721-5 [Epub ahead of print].

Walton, C. C., Kavanagh, A., Downey, L. A., Lomas, J., Camfield, D. A., and Stough, C. (2014). Online cognitive training in healthy older adults: a preliminary study on the effects of single versus multi-domain training. *Transl. Neurosci.* 6, 13–19. doi: 10.1515/tnsci-2015-0003

Wild-Wall, N., Falkenstein, M., and Gajewski, P. D. (2012). Neural correlates of changes in a visual search task due to cognitive training in seniors. *Neural Plast.* 2012:529057. doi: 10.1155/2012/529057

Wylie, G. R., Murray, M. M., Javitt, D. C., and Foxe, J. J. (2009). Distinct neurophysiological mechanisms mediate mixing costs and switch costs. *J. Cogn. Neurosci.* 21, 105–118. doi: 10.1162/jocn.2009.21009

18

The Toll Route to Structural Brain Plasticity

*Guiyi Li and Alicia Hidalgo**

Plasticity and Regeneration Lab, School of Biosciences, University of Birmingham, Birmingham, United Kingdom

Edited by:
Gaia Tavosanis, German Center for Neurodegeneratives, Helmholtz Association of German Research Centers (HZ), Germany

Reviewed by:
Daewoo Lee, Ohio University, United States
Bruno Van Swinderen, The University of Queensland, Australia

***Correspondence:**
Alicia Hidalgo
a.hidalgo@bham.ac.uk

The human brain can change throughout life as we learn, adapt and age. A balance between structural brain plasticity and homeostasis characterizes the healthy brain, and the breakdown of this balance accompanies brain tumors, psychiatric disorders, and neurodegenerative diseases. However, the link between circuit modifications, brain function, and behavior remains unclear. Importantly, the underlying molecular mechanisms are starting to be uncovered. The fruit-fly *Drosophila* is a very powerful model organism to discover molecular mechanisms and test them *in vivo*. There is abundant evidence that the *Drosophila* brain is plastic, and here we travel from the pioneering discoveries to recent findings and progress on molecular mechanisms. We pause on the recent discovery that, in the *Drosophila* central nervous system, Toll receptors—which bind neurotrophin ligands—regulate structural plasticity during development and in the adult brain. Through their topographic distribution across distinct brain modules and their ability to switch between alternative signaling outcomes, Tolls can enable the brain to translate experience into structural change. Intriguing similarities between Toll and mammalian Toll-like receptor function could reveal a further involvement in structural plasticity, degeneration, and disease in the human brain.

Keywords: *Drosophila*, structural brain plasticity, neurodegeneration, adult neurogenesis, neurotrophin, Toll, TLR, homeostasis

INTRODUCTION

The brain can change throughout life. Cells, neurites (axons and dendrites), and synapses are generated with experience and learning as we adapt to the environment. They are also eliminated, maintaining neural circuit stability and normal behavior. The balance between the former, known as structural plasticity, and the latter, known as structural homeostasis, characterizes brain health, and its breakdown accompanies a brain disease—such as brain tumors, psychiatric disorders, and neurodegenerative diseases (e.g., Alzheimer's and Parkinson's diseases). Structural plasticity and homeostasis may reveal how the brain works, as brain function relies on structural changes to cells.

Structural plasticity is often understood to be "hebbian," whereby co-active synapses are stabilized, reinforcing connections. Structural homeostasis is also known as "non-hebbian plasticity" and includes elimination and "compensatory plasticity," such as increases in synapse number as arborizations decrease, to deliver normal function. Synapses can also manifest physiological plasticity such as synaptic potentiation, depression, or homeostatic plasticity (e.g., involving regulatory adjustments in neurotransmitter release or post-synaptic excitability to maintain a normal function). Here we will deal only with structural changes.

Mammalian cortical plasticity has long been known (Feldman and Brecht, 2005). Classical experiments by Wiesel and Hubel showed that synapses and neurites are modified in response to neuronal activity and experience (Wiesel and Hubel, 1965). When kittens were deprived of light in one eye, arborizations from active neurons originating from the open eye outcompeted the silent ones from the closed eye, altering the pattern of innervation in the cortex. Importantly, recurrent cycles of light deprivation and exposure did not cause spine elimination to restore original spine profiles but instead maintained and built on newly formed synapses (Hofer et al., 2009). This suggests that structural changes in neurons may store information from the past, enabling the brain to adapt and respond in the future. However, plasticity may not necessarily be adaptive nor beneficial, but just a consequence of available connectivity opportunities for neurons (Feldman and Brecht, 2005).

Structural plasticity can also involve neurogenesis. Enriched environments, exercise, voluntary running, and learning can induce neurogenesis in the adult mammalian brain (Gage, 2004, 2019; Deng et al., 2010). In mammals, neurogenesis occurs in restricted brain areas, including the dentate gyrus of the hippocampus and the subventricular zone generating olfactory bulb neurons (Eriksson et al., 1998; Spalding et al., 2013; Goncalves et al., 2016; Simoes and Rhiner, 2017). Hippocampal neurogenesis may be required for spatial navigation and learning and memory to encode time into memory and prevent interference with old memories (Deng et al., 2010). However, this remains to be established.

The molecular mechanisms underlying structural brain plasticity and homeostasis remain virtually unknown. The neurotrophin BDNF and its receptor TrkB are currently the key factors known to be involved, and there is evidence that Toll-like receptors (TLRs) could also be involved (Lu et al., 2005, 2013; Okun et al., 2011; Park and Poo, 2013). Progress in understanding the link between molecular mechanisms, circuits, structural brain plasticity, homeostasis, and brain health in mammals has long been challenging.

The fruit-fly *Drosophila* is a powerful model organism to discover molecular mechanisms and link genes to neurons, circuits, and behavior. Here we review pioneering work on structural brain plasticity and homeostasis in *Drosophila*, current evidence of underlying molecular mechanisms, and how they could relate to the mammalian brain.

STRUCTURAL PLASTICITY AND HOMEOSTASIS IN THE ADULT *DROSOPHILA* BRAIN

Structural Plasticity: Brain Size Is Variable and Regulated by Experience

Pioneering work by Martin Heisenberg's lab started the structural plasticity journey through the *Drosophila* brain. Gerhard Technau showed that, in *Drosophila*, fiber number in the adult mushroom body peduncle can increase by 15% at 1 week after adult fly eclosion, and this was influenced by environmental stimuli (Technau, 1984). Flies reared in isolation, constant darkness, or olfactory deprivation had a significantly reduced fiber number (Technau, 1984). In fact, Kenyon cell number in wild-type flies is variable and can change depending on larval growth conditions and experience in the first week of adult fly life (Balling et al., 1987; Heisenberg et al., 1995). Brain size also changed with experience. Eclosed adult flies were kept either in isolation or single sex populations (i.e., deprived environment) or in large population cages or mixed sexes (i.e., enriched) for 19 days, and then the brain volume was measured. The volume of various brain structures increased in enriched vs. deprived flies, including the mushroom bodies, calyces, and the visual system lamina, medulla, and lobula (Heisenberg et al., 1995). Furthermore, compared to flies reared in constant darkness, stimulation of the visual system by breeding flies in constant light during a critical period spanning the first 5 days after eclosion increased the volume of the lamina and lobula plate, the size of photoreceptors and glial cells, the mushroom body calyces, and the central complex (Barth and Heisenberg, 1997; Barth et al., 1997). These pioneering studies did not resolve the cellular bases of structural brain plasticity. Some limited proliferation was detected in adult brains, but it was deemed to be insufficient to explain the extent of structural brain change (Technau, 2007). This work altogether showed that brain size can be modified by experience and that different experiences can affect brain regions differentially.

Findings from the olfactory system provided independent evidence for structural plasticity during the critical period in other brain regions (Devaud et al., 2003). The olfactory glomeruli continue to grow between days 1 and 12 of adult fly life, and the volume of particular glomeruli was influenced by experience—i.e., exposure to odorant—concomitantly with the maturation of odorant-induced behavior (Devaud et al., 2003). Similarly, when flies were exposed to a high concentration of carbon dioxide (CO_2) during the critical period, the volume of the CO_2-specific V glomerulus in the antennal lobe significantly increased (Sachse et al., 2007). This structural change was reversible after recovering at normal air exposure for another 5 days. By contrast, CO_2 exposure after the critical period did not cause a significant structural alteration in the V glomerulus (Sachse et al., 2007). The microglomeruli that form as projection neurons from the antennal lobe connecting to the Kenyon cell dendrites at the calyx are also modified by experience. After conditioning young flies with an odorant (11-*cis*-vaccenylacetate) to form long-term memory, the size of the microglomeruli responding to this odorant decreased, but the number of such microglomeruli increased (Baltruschat et al., 2021). This demonstrated that new synaptic boutons are formed during learning and for long-term memory and that structural change is linked to brain function.

To conclude, multiple regions within the adult brain—visual and olfactory systems and central complex—can be modified by experience (**Figure 1**). Whether this is restricted to a critical period within the first week of adult fly life or continues throughout the life course remains to be tested further and established. Most studies show that plasticity takes place within a critical period in the first week of adult life but do not carry out test beyond. Heisenberg showed that, at least under some

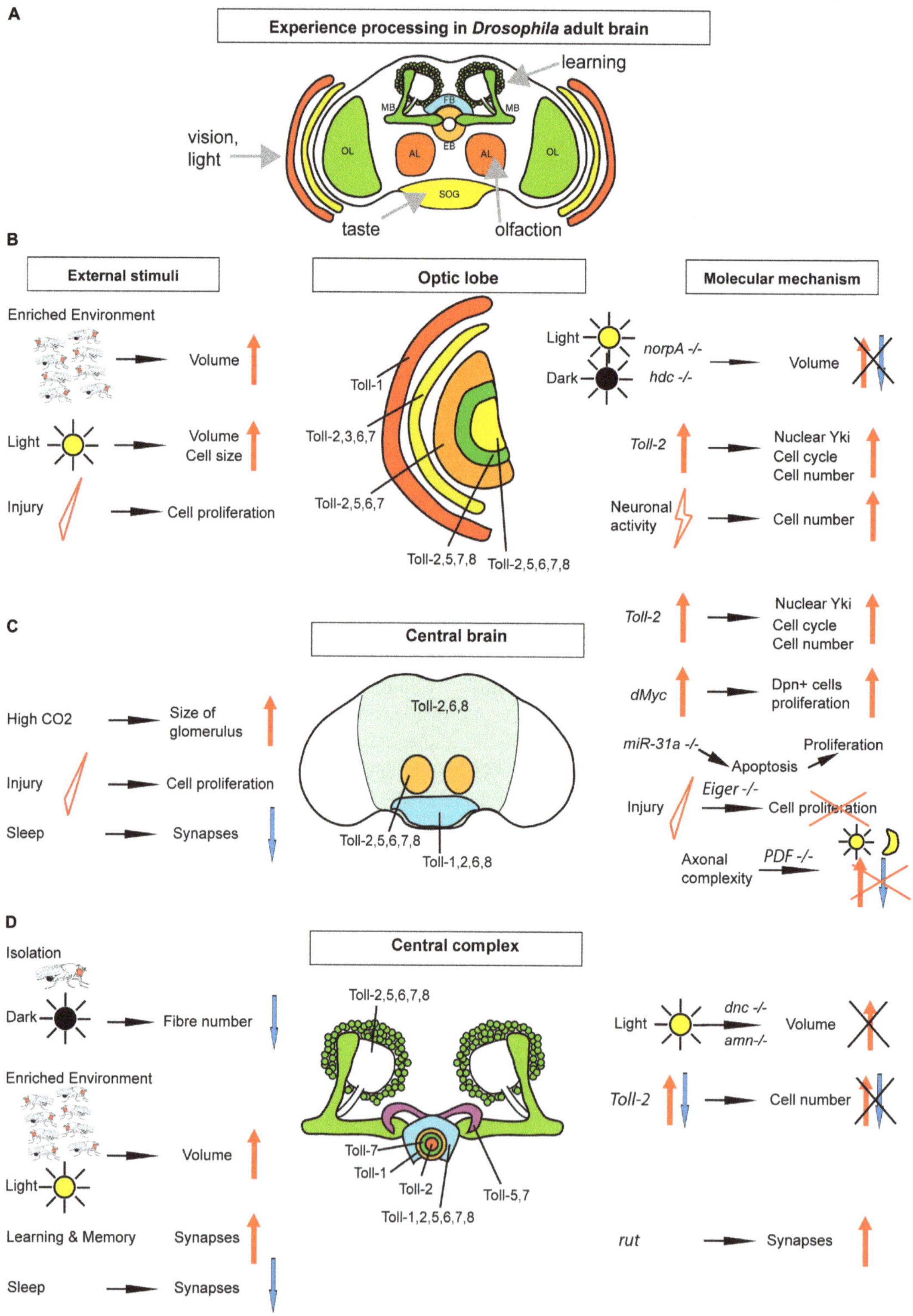

FIGURE 1 | Map of Toll receptors in a *Drosophila* adult brain. **(A)** *Drosophila* adult brain illustrating some modules receiving sensory input and involved in learning. **(B)** Optic lobe (including retina, lamina, medulla, lobula, and lobula plate from outer to inner layers). **(C)** Central brain [including neuropiles (pale green), antennal lobes (orange), and sub-esophageal ganglion (bright blue)]. **(D)** Central complex: mushroom bodies (green) ellipsoid body in rings, fan-shaped body (bright blue), and protocerebral bridge (purple). Each brain module expresses different Tolls or a combination of Tolls; thus, they could be regulated differentially in distinct brain modules. From **(B–D)**, the key findings involved in structural brain plasticity are summarized with external stimuli on the left and molecular manipulations and mechanisms on the right. OL, optic lobe; MB, mushroom body; FB, fan-shaped body; EB, ellipsoid body; AL, antennal lobe; SOG, sub-esophageal ganglion.

conditions, the brain remains plastic beyond this period and into at least the second week (Heisenberg et al., 1995). This varies across brain regions, suggesting that different mechanisms with distinct dynamics regulate plasticity in the different brain domains (Heisenberg et al., 1995).

Structural Homeostasis: Elimination and Compensation

Structural homeostasis was initially reported in the adult brain of *Musca domestica* (Kral and Meinertzhagen, 1989). Eclosed adult flies were subjected for 2 days to two regimens: they were either kept in constant darkness or stimulated by flickering green light (Kral and Meinertzhagen, 1989). As a result, the synapse number in lamina neurons that connect to photoreceptors decreased with light exposure and increased in flies reared in the dark (Kral and Meinertzhagen, 1989). Thus, neuronal stimulation provoked synapse elimination, and the lack of stimulation increased synapse formation. Subjecting adult flies to cold-shock also decreased the synapse number, and synapses could be recovered by transferring the flies to warmer temperatures (Brandstatter and Meinertzhagen, 1995). These findings provided evidence for structural homeostasis in the lamina of the visual system of the house fly. Structural homeostasis was also revealed in the context of olfaction in *Drosophila*. Exposure of adult fruit-flies to a high concentration of an odorant for 4 days resulted in behavioral adaptation to the odorant, normal olfactory transduction, and a reduction in olfactory glomeruli size in the antennal lobes (Devaud et al., 2001).

A subcellular evidence of structural homeostasis in the *Drosophila* brain was found in the mushroom body calyx and photoreceptor terminals in the lamina (Kremer et al., 2010; Sugie et al., 2015). Inhibiting action potential firing in antennal lobe projection neurons that connect to mushroom body Kenyon cells increased the size of microglomeruli in the mushroom body calyx (Kremer et al., 2010). Pre-synaptic active zone density also increased, which means that, upon a reduction in neuronal activity, the neurons increase in synapse number to restore function (Kremer et al., 2010). This is evidence of compensatory plasticity. On the other hand, exposing flies to constant light for the first 1–3 days after eclosion decreased the number of synaptic active zones and T-bars from photoreceptors in the lamina (Sugie et al., 2015). Thus, neuronal stimulation induced the disassembly of presynaptic active zones.

The adult fly brain altogether manifests activity-dependent structural homeostasis, as neuronal activity decreased the olfactory glomeruli size and caused synapse elimination, and compensatory plasticity, as the microglomeruli size and synapse number increased in the absence of stimulation (**Figure 1**).

Circadian Plasticity and Sleep

Structural changes in the brain have long been known to occur with circadian rhythms. Neurotransmitters were first shown to affect cell size with circadian periodicity (Pyza and Meinertzhagen, 1996). The size of the nuclei of lamina L2 neurons changes with the circadian rhythm, larger in the morning and smaller at night (Gorska-Andrzejak et al., 2005). L2 neuron dendrites are also largest in the morning and smallest in the middle of the night (Weber et al., 2009). However, whether this reflects changes directly controlled by the circadian clock or changes in response to the environment is less clear. For instance, lamina neuron dendritic changes were eliminated when flies were kept in constant light (Weber et al., 2009). Axonal arborizations of clock neurons, such as pigment-dispensing factor (PDF) neurons, are also more complex during the day than at night (Herrero et al., 2020), but activating PDF neurons with TrpA1 increased axonal complexity in the night to the same level as in the morning (Herrero et al., 2020). Thus, changes induced in daytime, by light, could reflect activity-dependent plasticity in clock neurons as well as other neuron types.

Sleep is linked to the circadian clock, and fruit-flies also sleep during night-time. The synapse number and size increase in the brain during waking time, synapse accumulation during the day drives sleep need, and synapse number decreases with sleep (Bushey et al., 2011; Huang et al., 2020). Thus, sleep is required for the homeostatic re-normalization in synapse number (Bushey et al., 2011; Huang et al., 2020). Whether sleep or the lack of it can have further structural consequences in circuits is an interesting question.

Cell Number Plasticity in the Adult Brain

Cell number plasticity reflects changes in cell proliferation, survival, or death. Apoptosis in the adult fruit-fly brain is limited to the critical period. Dying cells were detected in multiple brain areas, but by the fifth day of adult life, apoptosis was no longer detected (Ito and Hotta, 1992; Kato et al., 2009). In the intact, normal, young brain, glial proliferation was observed adjacently to apoptotic cells, suggesting that apoptosis in the adult brain induces compensatory proliferation in the nearby glia (Kato et al., 2009).

Evidence of adult neurogenesis in adult *Drosophila* was recently reviewed in Li and Hidalgo (2020) and will not be dealt with in detail here. In brief, [^{3}H]-thymidine and BrdU experiments labeling cells going through S-phase had suggested that cell proliferation might take place (Technau, 1984, see also Li and Hidalgo, 2020), but this could reflect polyploidy instead (Nandakumar et al., 2020). Importantly, the developmental neuroblasts that make the adult brain are eliminated through either apoptosis or cell cycle exit in the larva or pupa, before the adult ecloses (Siegrist et al., 2010; Li and Hidalgo, 2020). Thus, in the absence of neuroblasts, it was unclear how neurogenesis could proceed. A careful temporal profile of BrdU pulses applied to the adult brain showed that not only there are cells in S-phase in the adult brain but also the number of labeled cells critically increased over time (Kato et al., 2009). This was robust evidence of cell division in the adult brain. Cell proliferation was also reported using clonal analyses (Kato et al., 2009; Fernandez-Hernandez et al., 2013; Foo et al., 2017) and cell cycle markers (Li et al., 2020). The incidence of cell proliferation increased with genetic manipulations and injury (Kato et al., 2009; Fernandez-Hernandez et al., 2013). Injury in the optic lobe or central brain by stabbing with a needle and antennal ablation induced the proliferation of glial cells (Kato et al., 2009; Fernandez-Hernandez et al., 2013). Injury-induced cell proliferation seemed to be restricted to a critical period in the first 10 days of young flies, although this remains to be confirmed. The dividing cells were shown to be, in some cases, glia but could also include progenitor cells, as in the normal, intact, adult brain, there are cells that express the common neural stem cell marker *deadpan* (Fernandez-Hernandez et al., 2013; Li et al., 2020).

These findings altogether mean that cell number plasticity in the adult *Drosophila* brain includes both loss and generation of new cells (**Figure 1**). There is suggestive evidence for a critical period in cell number plasticity in the young fly, but this remains to be confirmed.

STRUCTURAL BRAIN PLASTICITY IS COMMON IN INSECTS

Structural brain plasticity occurs in other insects and could be widespread. In moths, pre-exposure to bat sound increased the volume of some glomeruli in antennal lobes and mushroom body calyces (Anton et al., 2016). In bumblebees kept in complete darkness for 7 days, lack of visual stimulation increased the relative volume of antennal lobes, mushroom body calyces, and neuropils (Jones et al., 2013). In honeybees, the synaptic bouton number in the calyx of the lip—one of the mushroom body compartments—increased when the bees were reared in impoverished conditions with reduced social interactions and olfactory and visual stimuli compared to bees reared in the hive (Cabirol et al., 2017). The structure of both the lip and dense collar (also mushroom body compartments) were also affected by foraging behavior. The volume and bouton number of the lip and dense collar correlated positively with the time spent foraging (Cabirol et al., 2018). These and further findings (Hourcade et al., 2009) showed that, in honeybees, the volume and synapse number of both antennal lobes and mushroom bodies can be modified by environmental stimuli, which, in turn, modified the behavior.

Thus, like in the mammalian brain, environmental stimuli induce structural brain plasticity in multiple insect species, including fruit-flies, bumblebees, honeybees, and moths. This suggests that structural brain plasticity is a fundamental property of how brains work and are modified through experience. In both insects and humans, the brain modules involved in olfaction and learning and memory were found to be plastic. Remarkably, contrary to the limited neurogenic sites of the human brain but similar to its cortical brain plasticity, plasticity appears to be widespread throughout the insect brain.

MOLECULAR MECHANISMS OF STRUCTURAL BRAIN PLASTICITY

The molecular mechanisms underlying structural brain plasticity are beginning to be uncovered (**Table 1** and **Figure 1**). Pioneering work first addressed this question by testing genes involved in phototransduction and learning and memory. Mutations in genes required for phototransduction such as *norpA* (causing loss of phospholipase-C) and hdc^{jk910} (deficient in histamine, the main neurotransmitter in the retina) obliterated the differences in brain volume observed when rearing fruit-flies in constant light vs. darkness (Barth and Heisenberg, 1997). This meant that visual experience is required for light-induced structural brain plasticity in the optic lobes. By contrast, mutations in genes involved in cAMP signaling *dunce* (*dnc*), *rutabaga* (*rut*), and *amnesiac* (*amn*), involved in learning, did not cause volume changes in the optic lobe with light rearing, but *dnc* and *amn* did cause volume changes in the mushroom body calyx (Barth and Heisenberg, 1997). Furthermore, when kept in the dark, wild-type flies in large social groups had larger calyces than flies housed in smaller groups, but this effect was lost in all three mutants (Barth and Heisenberg, 1997). It was recently shown that rut, which encodes Ca^{2+}/CaM-dependent adenyl cyclase, is also required for structural plasticity at the calyx. In fact, long-term memory modifies the size and number of microglomeruli in the calyx, but this effect was abolished in *rut* mutants or by blocking protein synthesis (Baltruschat et al., 2021). Thus, cAMP regulates plasticity in calyx but not the visual system, which means that distinct molecular pathways may underlie structural plasticity in distinct brain regions (Barth and Heisenberg, 1997).

Several genes promoting cell proliferation in the adult *Drosophila* brain were identified. The TNF homolog Eiger is required for cell proliferation in response to injury in the adult brain, as cell proliferation was not induced in injured *eiger* mutants (Kato et al., 2009). Over-expression of the oncogene *dMyc* in the adult brain increased the proliferation of Dpn^{+} progenitor cells (Fernandez-Hernandez et al., 2013). Mutant microRNA miR-31a induced the apoptosis of glia in young adult flies, which was followed by compensatory proliferation (Foo et al., 2017). So, these data altogether suggested that, in the adult brain, common fundamental cellular processes can also drive cell number adjustments, at least upon cell death or injury.

In clock neurons, the expression of PDF increases during the day, positively correlating with an increase in axonal complexity of PDF neurons (Herrero et al., 2020). Conversely, conditional PDF knock-down in the adult prevents structural plasticity. These findings altogether demonstrate that PDF regulates structural plasticity in clock neurons (Herrero et al., 2020).

Drosophila neurotrophins are encoded by the *spätzle* (*spz*) paralog gene family, which includes *Drosophila* neurotrophin-1 (DNT1, also called spz-2), DNT2/spz-5, and Spz-1 (Zhu et al., 2008; Sutcliffe et al., 2013; Foldi et al., 2017). During nervous system development, DNTs promote neuronal survival, cell death, connectivity, structural synaptic plasticity, and compensatory plasticity (Zhu et al., 2008; Sutcliffe et al., 2013; Foldi et al., 2017; Ulian-Benitez et al., 2017). Mammalian neurotrophins bind Trk and p75 receptors, but DNTs bind kinase-free Trk homolog encoded by the *kekkon* genes and Toll receptors (Mandai et al., 2009; Ulian-Benitez et al., 2017). Toll-1 in *Drosophila* is responsible for dorso-ventral body axis in embryogenesis and for innate immunity (Hashimoto et al., 1988; Lemaitre et al., 1996), and it led to the discovery of TLRs throughout most organisms. Tolls and TLRs not only have universal, evolutionarily conserved functions controlling innate immunity, but they also have non-immune functions

TABLE 1 | Genes involved in structural brain plasticity in *Drosophila*.

	Gene	What does it encode?	What does it do in structural brain plasticity?	References
Classical pathways Involved in neuro-transmission or learning	norpA	Phospholipase C Regulates phototransduction	Regulate volume of lamina.	Barth and Heisenberg, 1997
	hdc	Histidine decarboxylase catalyses the decarboxylation of histidine to form histamine that is involved in neurotransmission	Regulate volume of lobula plate.	Barth and Heisenberg, 1997
	Dunce (dnc)	cAMP phosphodiesterase	Regulates volume of the mushroom body calyx.	Barth and Heisenberg, 1997
	Rutabaga (rut)	Homolog of adenylate cyclase generates cAMP	Regulates volume of MB calyx and synapse formation during learning.	Barth and Heisenberg, 1997; Baltruschat et al., 2021
	Amnesiac (amn)	Suppressor of dunce	Regulates the volume of the MB calyx	Barth and Heisenberg, 1997
Neuro- and glio-genesis	Eiger	Type II transmembrane protein, homolog of tumo r necrosis factor (TNF).	Required for cell proliferation in response to stubbing injury in adult brain.	Kato et al., 2009
	dMyc	homolog of vertebrate MYC, a transcription factor	Promote proliferation of Dpn^+ cells.	Fernandez-Hernandez et al., 2013
	miR-31a	microRNA-31a	Induces cell apoptosis of glia in young adult flies.	Foo et al., 2017
Circadian	Pigment dispersing factor (PDF)	Neuropeptide	Transmits circadian information from ventrolateral neurons (LNvs).	Herrero et al., 2020
	Bruchpilot (Brp)	Active zone scaffold protein	Promotes synapse formation and sleep need	Huang et al., 2020
Toll signaling	Toll-2 (also known as 18 wheeler)	Toll-2 of the family of *Drosophila* Toll receptors (Toll-1 to Toll-9)	Regulates cell survival, and proliferation. Toll-2 loss causes axon and dendrite degeneration.	Li et al., 2020.
	MyD88	Canonical downstream adaptor of Tolls	Promotes cell survival and keep progenitors quiescent	Li et al., 2020
	Weckle (Wek)	Downstream adaptor of Tolls	Promotes cell death and cell proliferation	Li et al., 2020
	Yorkie (Yki)	Transcriptional coactivator, ortholog of mammalian yes-associated protein (YAP)	Promotes cell proliferation	Li et al., 2020

(Anthoney et al., 2018). There are nine Tolls in the *Drosophila* genome, and during embryonic and larval nervous system development, at least some Tolls have been shown to be involved in connectivity, cell number plasticity, and structural synaptic plasticity (Zhu et al., 2008; McIlroy et al., 2013; Ballard et al., 2014; Ward et al., 2015; McLaughlin et al., 2016; Foldi et al., 2017; Ulian-Benitez et al., 2017; Li et al., 2020). At least seven Tolls are expressed in the adult brain (Toll-1, −2, −3, −5, −6, −7, and −8), in overlapping but distinct expression patterns that coincide with brain anatomical domains (Li et al., 2020; **Figure 1**).

Tolls can promote either cell quiescence, proliferation, neuronal survival, or death, depending on time, cell type, and cell context, in the CNS (McIlroy et al., 2013; Foldi et al., 2017; Li et al., 2020; **Figure 2**). Canonical Toll signaling proceeds *via* the MyD88 adaptor, leading to the activation of NF-κB homologs Dorsal and Dif downstream, which in the CNS promote cell survival (Foldi et al., 2017; Anthoney et al., 2018). Tolls can also function *via* Weckle (Wek) and Sarm to promote cell death (Foldi et al., 2017). Sarm is an evolutionarily conserved inhibitor of MyD88, and it induces apoptosis *via* JNK downstream (Foldi et al., 2017). Tolls bind Wek, which binds Sarm facilitating its inhibition of MyD88 (Foldi et al., 2017). Sarm also has NAD-ase activity which drives axonal degeneration (Carty and Bowie, 2019). Toll-2 also regulates cell proliferation during development, *via* Wek and Yorkie (Yki) (Li et al., 2020). Concerted knock-down of multiple *Tolls* throughout development causes dramatic reductions in brain size, most likely due to combined increased cell death and reduced cell proliferation (Li et al., 2020). Although Tolls can have redundant functions, they are not equal, and they can lead to distinct cellular outcomes. For example, in the pupal CNS, Toll-1 and Toll-6 can induce both cell survival and cell death, but Toll-1 has a stronger pro-apoptotic effect, whereas Toll-2 does not induce cell death (Foldi et al., 2017; Li et al., 2020).

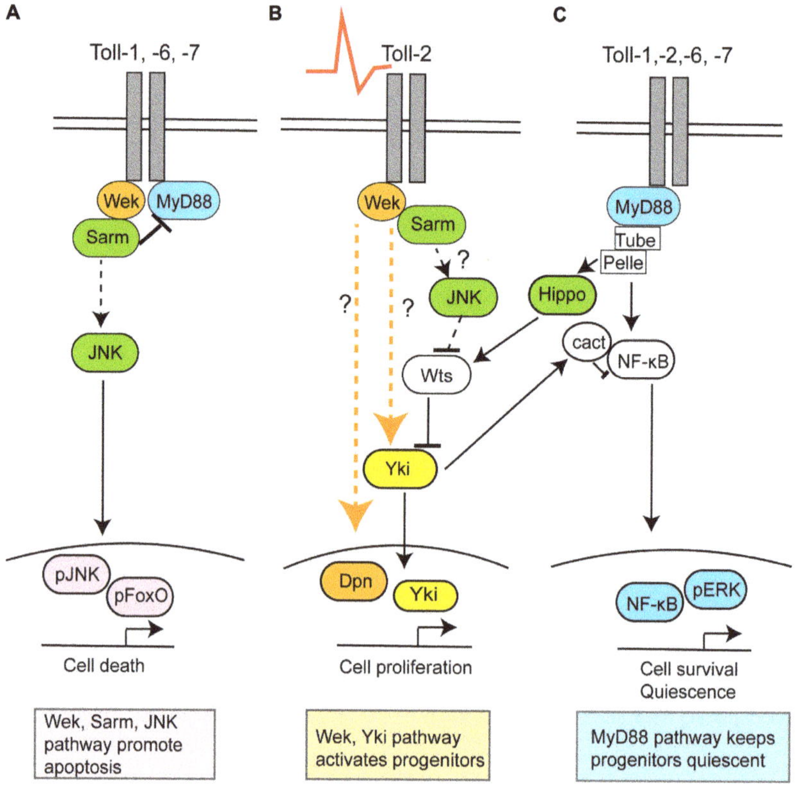

FIGURE 2 | Toll receptors can regulate cell survival, death, quiescence, or proliferation *via* alternative signaling pathways. Toll receptors share common functions, but they can also each elicit distinct cellular outcomes. This is a summary of data evidence on signaling by Toll-1, −2, −6, and −7 in the central nervous system in embryonic, larval, and/or pupal development and Toll-2 in the adult brain. **(A)** During development, Toll receptors can promote cell apoptosis *via* Wek, Sarm, and JNK, **(B)** but in the adult brain, Toll-2 receptors can also function *via* Wek and Yki to promote cell proliferation. Question marks denote how or whether Wek signals remain unknown. **(C)** Toll receptors can promote cell survival *via* MyD88-NFkB signaling both throughout development and in the adult. Moreover, adult progenitor cells are normally kept quiescent *via* MyD88. In other contexts, the activation of Toll by gram-positive bacteria prevents proliferation by activating the Hippo pathway, thus inhibiting Yki, although whether this is also the case in the brain is unknown.

Toll-2, at least, is responsible for generative processes underlying structural brain plasticity in the adult (Li et al., 2020). It is neuroprotective, and *Toll-2* knock-down causes axonal misrouting, loss of axons and dendrites, and loss of neurons and impairs behavior (Li et al., 2020). Toll-2 promotes neurogenesis in the adult brain, as the conditional over-expression of *Toll-2* restricted to the adult promotes cell proliferation *via* Yki, and increases cell number and brain size (Li et al., 2020). Neuronal activation with TrpA1 also increases cell number, and this depends on Toll-2 (42). There are Dpn^{+} progenitors in the adult *Drosophila* brain (Li et al., 2020), which express MyD88. Toll signaling *via* MyD88 inhibits the proliferation of progenitor cells, whereas signaling *via wek* promotes cell proliferation (Li et al., 2020). Similarly, in immunity, Toll signaling *via* MyD88 activates Hippo signaling, inhibiting Yki and cell proliferation (Liu et al., 2016). Thus, Toll signaling *via* MyD88 keeps progenitor cells quiescent, and neuronal activity or Toll-2 signaling can activate an alternative Wek downstream pathway that promotes cell proliferation *via* Yki (Li et al., 2020; **Figure 2**). Thus, depending on the availability of downstream adaptors, Toll receptors can function *via* alternative signaling pathways, with distinct cellular outcomes (Foldi et al., 2017). What enables Tolls to switch between signaling *via* MyD88, Sarm, or Wek to promote cell survival and quiescence, apoptosis, or cell proliferation, respectively, is not known.

The topographic expression of Tolls together with the multiple possible outcomes downstream (**Figures 1, 2**) contributes to the formation of the distinct brain modules in development and could have driven the formation and diversification of distinct brain types in the course of evolution. Importantly, it enables them to regulate structural plasticity independently in different brain domains. In fact, the cell number in the optic lobe medulla and central brain was found to be more plastic than mushroom body Kenyon cells (Li et al., 2020). By regulating the cell number independently in distinct brain domains (e.g., visual, olfactory), Tolls can match a sensory experience (e.g., vision and olfaction) to a structural change. In contrast to the limited neurogenic niches of the mammalian brain, cell cycling markers and changes in cell number were found spread out through the *Drosophila* brain, reminiscent of widespread adult neurogenesis in zebrafish. These findings meant that the cell number in the adult fruit-fly brain is plastic, and experience can elicit structural changes in the brain *via* Toll receptor signaling.

Sleep need can be driven by increasing the levels of the active zone scaffold protein Bruchpilot (Brp) (Huang et al., 2020). Increasing the levels of Brp led to a dose-dependent increase in synapse formation, and this was sufficient to quantitatively tune sleep patterns reminiscent of sleep deprivation (Huang et al., 2020). When knocking down sleep-regulating genes, such as *wide awake*, *insomniac*, or *fumin*, the expression level of the active zone scaffold protein Bruchpilot significantly increased in a brain-wide manner (Huang et al., 2020). Moreover, knocking down brp expression in R2 neurons in flies that otherwise over-expressed Brp was sufficient to partially rescue a sleepless behavior and a deficient short-term memory, thus demonstrating the importance of these neurons and Brp in the regulation of sleep (Huang et al., 2020).

Toll and Spz are also involved in regulating sleep homeostasis. Astroglial calcium increases with sleep need and is required for sleep rebound after sleep deprivation (Blum et al., 2021). It has been proposed that astrocytes secrete Spz, which signals *via* Toll-1 in R5 neurons to promote a sleep rebound (Blum et al., 2021). The intracellular Ca^{2+} level in R5 neurons significantly increased after sleep deprivation, and knocking down Toll suppressed this increase (Blum et al., 2021). Moreover, knocking down *Spz* in astroglia or *Toll* in R5 neurons reduced the homeostatic sleep rebound (Blum et al., 2021). However, whether Spz and Toll-1 can also cause structural modifications in R5 neurons and whether this is linked to sleep homeostasis was not investigated.

To conclude, evidence indicates that these and other yet-to-be-discovered molecular mechanisms underlie structural changes in the fly brain, modifying neural circuits in response to experience to deliver appropriate behavior, learning, and sleep and to adapt to the environment.

SIMILARITIES BETWEEN TOLLS AND MAMMALIAN TLRS IN STRUCTURAL BRAIN PLASTICITY

There are 10 TLRs in the human brain. Investigation of TLR function in the mammalian brain has mostly focused on their immune-like functions in microglia and astrocytes (Okun et al., 2009, #76; Okun et al., 2011, #87; Shmueli et al., 2018, #308; Anthoney et al., 2018, #35; Chen et al., 2019, #312; Donnelly et al., 2020, #311), but TLRs are also expressed in neural stem cells, NG2 glia, and neurons throughout development and in the adult. TLRs also have non-immune functions in the mammalian nervous system (Rolls et al., 2007, #78; Okun et al., 2010, #221; Chen et al., 2019, #312; Donnelly et al., 2020, #311). They are required to either promote or prevent neural stem cell proliferation and differentiation into neurons or glia and to regulate cell survival or death, neurite growth or retraction, synaptogenesis, and the compensation of spine density and size. In neurons, they can regulate slow cellular processes through the canonical MyD88 and ERK signaling pathways and gene expression (Rolls et al., 2007; Okun et al., 2010) and also fast neuronal action (e.g., < 1 min) in interaction with channels (e.g., TrpA1 and TrpV1), enabling fast responses to sensory stimuli, such as heat, pain, and itch (Donnelly et al., 2020, #311). This repertoire of functions reveals that TLRs could be involved in regulating brain function and plasticity independently of immunity.

Drosophila Tolls can carry out overlapping yet distinct functions (Foldi et al., 2017). Similarly, in mammals, TLR-2, −3, and -4 regulate neurogenesis and cell differentiation; TLR-7, −8, and -9 can induce apoptosis; and TLR-3, −7, and -8 regulate arborizations through neurite growth and retraction, spine density, and size (Ma et al., 2006; Cameron et al., 2007; Rolls et al., 2007; Okun et al., 2010; Chen et al., 2019). Thus, not all Tolls and TLRs are equal, and they may each elicit distinct cellular outcomes.

Whether *TLRs* are expressed topographically in the brain, like *Drosophila* Tolls, is not yet known. There is evidence that *TLRs* are expressed with distinct temporal profiles from brain development to the adult brain (Ma et al., 2006; Kaul et al., 2012; Barak et al., 2014; Arnaboldi et al., 2020). They might be expressed in partly overlapping and at least partly distinct cell types in the brain, as their loss of function causes region-specific behavioral phenotypes. For instance, TLR4 regulates the levels of neuromodulators in the frontal cortex and hippocampus (Femenia et al., 2018). Mice with altered TLR-3 or -4 function have altered spatial navigation, learning and memory, anxiety, and social interactions (Okun et al., 2012). However, these observations were made in mutant mice, and it is compelling to find out whether conditional alterations in TLR function restricted to the adult would also influence behavior and in a spatially dependent manner. Finding out whether TLRs are distributed topographically like in *Drosophila* would explain the experience-dependent regulation of brain plasticity and the consequences in behavior.

The endogenous ligands that could regulate non-immune neuronal TLR functions in the sterile, undamaged brain are unknown. Neurotrophins are ligands for Tolls in *Drosophila*, but whether they can also bind mammalian TLRs remains unexplored. Interestingly, *TLR4* knock-out mice with anxiety behavior also had an altered expression of BDNF in the frontal cortex and hippocampus (Femenia et al., 2018). Intriguingly, in cell culture, human neurotrophins BDNF and NGF can modify human TLR signaling in response to their endogenous ligands and induce TLR-4 signaling in the absence of any other ligand (McIlroy et al., 2013; Foldi et al., 2017; Li et al., 2020). This means either that binding of NGF and BDNF to Trk or p75 receptors modifies TLR signaling or that NGF and BDNF can directly bind at least TLR4 (Foldi et al., 2017). It is compelling to find out whether TLRs could also respond to NGF or BDNF *in vivo* in the mammalian brain.

Understanding TLR function in the brain is important, as alterations result in brain diseases, including anxiety, neuropsychiatric disorders, schizophrenia, autism, Alzheimer's disease, autoimmune diseases (e.g., multiple sclerosis), and stroke (Okun et al., 2011).

CONCLUSION

There is abundant evidence of structural brain plasticity in the *Drosophila* brain, involving modifications to regional volumes, cell number, cell shape, and synapses, altogether modifying neural circuits. In *Drosophila*, Toll receptors regulate structural brain plasticity topographically, activating alternative signaling pathways downstream that can promote cell proliferation, quiescence, survival, or death. In this way, Tolls enable the link between sensory experience and structural brain change. There are striking similarities in the way *Drosophila* Tolls and mammalian TLRs function in the brain, including through distinct Toll-specific functions, cellular outcomes, and consequences in behavior. Although mammalian TLRs have been investigated mostly in the context of immunity, they also have non-immune functions in the sterile, undamaged brain, and these functions could be crucial to understanding brain diseases. Communication between *Drosophila* and mammalian findings can expedite the understanding of structural change in the human brain—in health and disease.

AUTHOR CONTRIBUTIONS

GL and AH wrote and revised the manuscript. Both authors contributed to the article and approved the submitted version.

FUNDING

This work was funded by the BBSRC project grants BB/R017034/1 and BB/R00871X/1.

ACKNOWLEDGMENTS

We thank our lab members for the discussions and comments on the manuscript.

REFERENCES

Anthoney, N., Foldi, I., and Hidalgo, A. (2018). Toll and Toll-like receptor signalling in development. *Development* 145:dev156018.

Anton, S., Chabaud, M. A., Schmidt-Busser, D., Gadenne, B., Iqbal, J., Juchaux, M., et al. (2016). Brief sensory experience differentially affects the volume of olfactory brain centres in a moth. *Cell Tissue Res.* 364, 59–65. doi: 10.1007/s00441-015-2299-0

Arnaboldi, F., Sommariva, M., Opizzi, E., Rasile, M., Camelliti, S., Busnelli, M., et al. (2020). Expression of Toll-like receptors 4 and 7 in murine peripheral nervous system development. *Ann Anat.* 231:151526. doi: 10.1016/j.aanat.2020.151526

Ballard, S. L., Miller, D. L., and Ganetzky, B. (2014). Retrograde neurotrophin signaling through Tollo regulates synaptic growth in Drosophila. *J. Cell Biol.* 204, 1157–1172. doi: 10.1083/jcb.201308115

Balling, A., Technau, G. M., and Heisenberg, M. (1987). Are the structural changes in adult Drosophila mushroom bodies memory traces? Studies on biochemical learning mutants. *J. Neurogenet.* 4, 65–73. doi: 10.3109/01677068709102334

Baltruschat, L., Prisco, L., Ranft, P., Lauritzen, J. S., Fiala, A., Bock, D. D., et al. (2021). Circuit reorganization in the Drosophila mushroom body calyx accompanies memory consolidation. *Cell Rep.* 34:08871.

Barak, B., Feldman, N., and Okun, E. (2014). Toll-like receptors as developmental tools that regulate neurogenesis during development: an update. *Front. Neurosci.* 8:272. doi: 10.3389/fnins.2014.00272

Barth, M., and Heisenberg, M. (1997). Vision affects mushroom bodies and central complex in Drosophila melanogaster. *Learn. Mem.* 4, 219–229. doi: 10.1101/lm.4.2.219

Barth, M., Hirsch, H. V., Meinertzhagen, I. A., and Heisenberg, M. (1997). Experience-dependent developmental plasticity in the optic lobe of Drosophila melanogaster. *J. Neurosci.* 17, 1493–1504. doi: 10.1523/jneurosci.17-04-01493.1997

Blum, I. D., Keles, M. F., Baz, E. S., Han, E., Park, K., Luu, S., et al. (2021). Astroglial Calcium Signaling Encodes Sleep Need in Drosophila. *Curr. Biol.* 31, 150–162.e7.

Brandstatter, J. H., and Meinertzhagen, I. A. (1995). The rapid assembly of synaptic sites in photoreceptor terminals of the fly's optic lobe recovering from cold shock. *Proc. Natl. Acad. Sci. U. S. A.* 92, 2677–2681. doi: 10.1073/pnas.92.7.2677

Bushey, D., Tononi, G., and Cirelli, C. (2011). Sleep and synaptic homeostasis: structural evidence in Drosophila. *Science* 332, 1576–1581. doi: 10.1126/science.1202839

Cabirol, A., Brooks, R., Groh, C., Barron, A. B., and Devaud, J. M. (2017). Experience during early adulthood shapes the learning capacities and the number of synaptic boutons in the mushroom bodies of honey bees (Apis mellifera). *Learn. Mem.* 24, 557–562. doi: 10.1101/lm.045492.117

Cabirol, A., Cope, A. J., Barron, A. B., and Devaud, J. M. (2018). Relationship between brain plasticity, learning and foraging performance in honey bees. *PLoS One.* 13:e0196749. doi: 10.1371/journal.pone.0196749

Cameron, J. S., Alexopoulou, L., Sloane, J. A., DiBernardo, A. B., Ma, Y., Kosaras, B., et al. (2007). Toll-like receptor 3 is a potent negative regulator of axonal growth in mammals. *J. Neurosci.* 27, 13033–13041. doi: 10.1523/jneurosci.4290-06.2007

Carty, M., and Bowie, A. G. S. A. R. M. (2019). From immune regulator to cell executioner. *Biochem. Pharmacol.* 161, 52–62. doi: 10.1016/j.bcp.2019.01.005

Chen, C. Y., Shih, Y. C., Hung, Y. F., and Hsueh, Y. P. (2019). Beyond defense: regulation of neuronal morphogenesis and brain functions via Toll-like receptors. *J. Biomed. Sci.* 26:90.

Deng, W., Aimone, J. B., and Gage, F. H. (2010). New neurons and new memories: how does adult hippocampal neurogenesis affect learning and memory? *Nat. Rev. Neurosci.* 11, 339–350. doi: 10.1038/nrn2822

Devaud, J. M., Acebes, A., and Ferrus, A. (2001). Odor exposure causes central adaptation and morphological changes in selected olfactory glomeruli in Drosophila. *J. Neurosci.* 21, 6274–6282. doi: 10.1523/jneurosci.21-16-06274.2001

Devaud, J. M., Acebes, A., Ramaswami, M., and Ferrus, A. (2003). Structural and functional changes in the olfactory pathway of adult Drosophila take place at a critical age. *J. Neurobiol.* 56, 13–23. doi: 10.1002/neu.10215

Donnelly, C. R., Chen, O., and Ji, R. R. (2020). How do sensory neurons sense danger signals? *Trends Neurosci.* 43, 822–838. doi: 10.1016/j.tins.2020.07.008

Eriksson, P. S., Perfilieva, E., Bjork-Eriksson, T., Alborn, A. M., Nordborg, C., Peterson, D. A., et al. (1998). Neurogenesis in the adult human hippocampus. *Nat. Med.* 4, 1313–1317.

Feldman, D. E., and Brecht, M. (2005). Map plasticity in somatosensory cortex. *Science* 310, 810–815. doi: 10.1126/science.1115807

Femenia, T., Qian, Y., Arentsen, T., Forssberg, H., and Diaz Heijtz, R. (2018). Toll-like receptor-4 regulates anxiety-like behavior and DARPP-32 phosphorylation. *Brain Behav. Immun.* 69, 273–282. doi: 10.1016/j.bbi.2017.11.022

Fernandez-Hernandez, I., Rhiner, C., and Moreno, E. (2013). Adult neurogenesis in Drosophila. *Cell Rep.* 3, 1857–1865. doi: 10.1016/j.celrep.2013.05.034

Foldi, I., Anthoney, N., Harrison, N., Gangloff, M., Verstak, B., Nallasivan, M. P., et al. (2017). Three-tier regulation of cell number plasticity by neurotrophins and Tolls in Drosophila. *J. Cell Biol.* 216, 1421–1438. doi: 10.1083/jcb.201607098

Foo, L. C., Song, S., and Cohen, S. M. (2017). miR-31 mutants reveal continuous glial homeostasis in the adult Drosophila brain. *EMBO J.* 36, 1215–1226. doi: 10.15252/embj.201695861

Gage, F. H. (2004). Structural plasticity of the adult brain. *Dialogues Clin. Neurosci.* 6, 135–141. doi: 10.31887/dcns.2004.6.2/fgage

Gage, F. H. (2019). Adult neurogenesis in mammals. *Science* 364, 827–828. doi: 10.1126/science.aav6885

Goncalves, J. T., Schafer, S. T., and Gage, F. H. (2016). Adult Neurogenesis in the Hippocampus: from Stem Cells to Behavior. *Cell* 167, 897–914. doi: 10.1016/j.cell.2016.10.021

Gorska-Andrzejak, J., Keller, A., Raabe, T., Kilianek, L., and Pyza, E. (2005). Structural daily rhythms in GFP-labelled neurons in the visual system of Drosophila melanogaster. *Photochem. Photobiol. Sci.* 4, 721–726. doi: 10.1039/b417023g

Hashimoto, C., Hudson, K. L., and Anderson, K. V. (1988). The Toll gene of Drosophila, required for dorsal-ventral embryonic polarity, appears to encode a transmembrane protein. *Cell* 52, 269–279. doi: 10.1016/0092-8674(88)90516-8

Heisenberg, M., Heusipp, M., and Wanke, C. (1995). Structural plasticity in the Drosophila brain. *J. Neurosci.* 15, 1951–1960.

Herrero, A., Yoshii, T., Ispizua, J. I., Colque, C., Veenstra, J. A., Muraro, N. I., et al. (2020). Coupling Neuropeptide Levels to Structural Plasticity in Drosophila Clock Neurons. *Curr. Biol.* 30, 3154–3166.e4.

Hofer, S. B., Mrsic-Flogel, T. D., Bonhoeffer, T., and Hubener, M. (2009). Experience leaves a lasting structural trace in cortical circuits. *Nature* 457, 313–317. doi: 10.1038/nature07487

Hourcade, B., Perisse, E., Devaud, J. M., and Sandoz, J. C. (2009). Long-term memory shapes the primary olfactory center of an insect brain. *Learn. Mem.* 16, 607–615. doi: 10.1101/lm.1445609

Huang, S., Piao, C., Beuschel, C. B., Gotz, T., and Sigrist, S. J. (2020). Presynaptic Active Zone Plasticity Encodes Sleep Need in Drosophila. *Curr. Biol.* 30, 1077–1091.e5.

Ito, K., and Hotta, Y. (1992). Proliferation pattern of postembryonic neuroblasts in the brain of Drosophila melanogaster. *Dev. Biol.* 149, 134–148. doi: 10.1016/0012-1606(92)90270-q

Jones, B. M., Leonard, A. S., Papaj, D. R., and Gronenberg, W. (2013). Plasticity of the worker bumblebee brain in relation to age and rearing environment. *Brain Behav. Evol.* 82, 250–261. doi: 10.1159/000355845

Kato, K., Awasaki, T., and Ito, K. (2009). Neuronal programmed cell death induces glial cell division in the adult Drosophila brain. *Development* 136, 51–59. doi: 10.1242/dev.023366

Kaul, D., Habbel, P., Derkow, K., Kruger, C., Franzoni, E., Wulczyn, F. G., et al. (2012). Expression of Toll-like receptors in the developing brain. *PLoS One.* 7:e37767. doi: 10.1371/journal.pone.0037767

Kral, K., and Meinertzhagen, I. A. (1989). Anatomical plasticity of synapses in the lamina of the optic lobe of the fly. *Philos. Trans. R. Soc. Lond. B Biol. Sci.* 323, 155–183. doi: 10.1098/rstb.1989.0004

Kremer, M. C., Christiansen, F., Leiss, F., Paehler, M., Knapek, S., Andlauer, T. F., et al. (2010). Structural long-term changes at mushroom body input synapses. *Curr. Biol.* 20, 1938–1944. doi: 10.1016/j.cub.2010.09.060

Lemaitre, B., Nicolas, E., Michaut, L., Reichhart, J. M., and Hoffmann, J. A. (1996). The dorsoventral regulatory gene cassette spatzle/Toll/cactus controls the potent antifungal response in Drosophila adults. *Cell* 86, 973–983. doi: 10.1016/s0092-8674(00)80172-5

Li, G., Forero, M. G., Wentzell, J. S., Durmus, I., Wolf, R., Anthoney, N. C., et al. (2020). A Toll-receptor map underlies structural brain plasticity. *Elife* 9:e52743.

Li, G., and Hidalgo, A. (2020). Adult Neurogenesis in the Drosophila Brain: the Evidence and the Void. *Int. J. Mol. Sci.* 21:6653. doi: 10.3390/ijms21186653

Liu, B., Zheng, Y., Yin, F., Yu, J., Silverman, N., and Pan, D. (2016). Toll Receptor-Mediated Hippo Signaling Controls Innate Immunity in Drosophila. *Cell* 164, 406–419. doi: 10.1016/j.cell.2015.12.029

Lu, B., Nagappan, G., Guan, X., Nathan, P. J., and Wren, P. (2013). BDNF-based synaptic repair as a disease-modifying strategy for neurodegenerative diseases. *Nat. Rev. Neurosci.* 14, 401–416. doi: 10.1038/nrn3505

Lu, B., Pang, P. T., and Woo, N. H. (2005). The yin and yang of neurotrophin action. *Nat. Rev. Neurosci.* 6, 603–614. doi: 10.1038/nrn1726

Ma, Y., Li, J., Chiu, I., Wang, Y., Sloane, J. A., Lu, J., et al. (2006). Toll-like receptor 8 functions as a negative regulator of neurite outgrowth and inducer of neuronal apoptosis. *J. Cell Biol.* 175, 209–215. doi: 10.1083/jcb.200606016

Mandai, K., Guo, T., St Hillaire, C., Meabon, J. S., Kanning, K. C., Bothwell, M., et al. (2009). LIG family receptor tyrosine kinase-associated proteins modulate growth factor signals during neural development. *Neuron* 63, 614–627. doi: 10.1016/j.neuron.2009.07.031

McIlroy, G., Foldi, I., Aurikko, J., Wentzell, J. S., Lim, M. A., Fenton, J. C., et al. (2013). Toll-6 and Toll-7 function as neurotrophin receptors in the Drosophila melanogaster CNS. *Nat. Neurosci.* 16, 1248–1256. doi: 10.1038/nn.3474

McLaughlin, C. N., Nechipurenko, I. V., Liu, N., and Broihier, H. T. A. (2016). Toll receptor-FoxO pathway represses Pavarotti/MKLP1 to promote microtubule dynamics in motoneurons. *J. Cell Biol.* 214, 459–474. doi: 10.1083/jcb.201601014

Nandakumar, S., Grushko, O., and Buttitta, L. A. (2020). Polyploidy in the adult Drosophila brain. *Elife* 9:e54385.

Okun, E., Barak, B., Saada-Madar, R., Rothman, S. M., Griffioen, K. J., Roberts, N., et al. (2012). Evidence for a developmental role for TLR4 in learning and memory. *PLoS One.* 7:e47522. doi: 10.1371/journal.pone.0047522

Okun, E., Griffioen, K., Barak, B., Roberts, N. J., Castro, K., Pita, M. A., et al. (2010). Toll-like receptor 3 inhibits memory retention and constrains adult hippocampal neurogenesis. *Proc. Natl. Acad. Sci. U. S. A.* 107, 15625–15630. doi: 10.1073/pnas.1005807107

Okun, E., Griffioen, K. J., Lathia, J. D., Tang, S.-C., Mattson, M. P., and Arumugam, T. V. (2009). Toll-like receptors in neurodegeneration. *Brain Res. Rev.* 59, 278–292. doi: 10.1016/j.brainresrev.2008.09.001

Okun, E., Griffioen, K. J., and Mattson, M. P. (2011). Toll-like receptor signaling in neural plasticity and disease. *Trends Neurosci.* 34, 269–281. doi: 10.1016/j.tins.2011.02.005

Park, H., and Poo, M. M. (2013). Neurotrophin regulation of neural circuit development and function. *Nat. Rev. Neurosci.* 14, 7–23. doi: 10.1038/nrn3379

Pyza, E., and Meinertzhagen, I. A. (1996). Neurotransmitters regulate rhythmic size changes amongst cells in the fly's optic lobe. *J. Comp. Physiol. A* 178, 33–45.

Rolls, A., Shechter, R., London, A., Ziv, Y., Ronen, A., Levy, R., et al. (2007). Toll-like receptors modulate adult hippocampal neurogenesis. *Nat. Cell Biol.* 9, 1081–1088. doi: 10.1038/ncb1629

Sachse, S., Rueckert, E., Keller, A., Okada, R., Tanaka, N. K., Ito, K., et al. (2007). Activity-dependent plasticity in an olfactory circuit. *Neuron* 56, 838–850. doi: 10.1016/j.neuron.2007.10.035

Shmueli, A., Shalit, T., Okun, E., and Shohat-Ophir, G. (2018). The toll pathway in the central nervous system of flies and mammals. *Neuromolecular Med.* 20, 419–436. doi: 10.1007/s12017-018-8515-9

Siegrist, S. E., Haque, N. S., Chen, C. H., Hay, B. A., and Hariharan, I. K. (2010). Inactivation of both Foxo and reaper promotes long-term adult neurogenesis in Drosophila. *Curr. Biol.* 20, 643–648. doi: 10.1016/j.cub.2010.01.060

Simoes, A. R., and Rhiner, C. A. (2017). Cold-Blooded View on Adult Neurogenesis. *Front. Neurosci.* 11:327. doi: 10.3389/fnins.2017.00327

Spalding, K. L., Bergmann, O., Alkass, K., Bernard, S., Salehpour, M., Huttner, H. B., et al. (2013). Dynamics of hippocampal neurogenesis in adult humans. *Cell* 153, 1219–1227.

Sugie, A., Hakeda-Suzuki, S., Suzuki, E., Silies, M., Shimozono, M., Mohl, C., et al. (2015). Molecular Remodeling of the Presynaptic Active Zone of Drosophila Photoreceptors via Activity-Dependent Feedback. *Neuron* 86, 711–725. doi: 10.1016/j.neuron.2015.03.046

Sutcliffe, B., Forero, M. G., Zhu, B., Robinson, I. M., and Hidalgo, A. (2013). Neuron-type specific functions of DNT1, DNT2 and Spz at the Drosophila neuromuscular junction. *PLoS One.* 8:e75902. doi: 10.1371/journal.pone.0075902

Technau, G. M. (1984). Fiber number in the mushroom bodies of adult Drosophila melanogaster depends on age, sex and experience. *J. Neurogenet.* 1, 113–126. doi: 10.3109/01677068409107077

Technau, G. M. (2007). Fiber number in the mushroom bodies of adult Drosophila melanogaster depends on age, sex and experience. *J. Neurogenet.* 21, 183–196. doi: 10.1080/01677060701695359

Ulian-Benitez, S., Bishop, S., Foldi, I., Wentzell, J., Okenwa, C., Forero, M. G., et al. (2017). Kek-6: a truncated-Trk-like receptor for Drosophila neurotrophin 2 regulates structural synaptic plasticity. *PLoS Genet.* 13:e1006968. doi: 10.1371/journal.pgen.1006968

Ward, A., Hong, W., Favaloro, V., and Luo, L. (2015). Toll receptors instruct axon and dendrite targeting and participate in synaptic partner matching in a Drosophila olfactory circuit. *Neuron* 85, 1013–1028. doi: 10.1016/j.neuron.2015.02.003

Weber, P., Kula-Eversole, E., and Pyza, E. (2009). Circadian control of dendrite morphology in the visual system of Drosophila melanogaster. *PLoS One.* 4:e4290. doi: 10.1371/journal.pone.0004290

Wiesel, T. N., and Hubel, D. H. (1965). Comparison of the effects of unilateral and bilateral eye closure on cortical unit responses in kittens. *J. Neurophysiol.* 28, 1029–1040. doi: 10.1152/jn.1965.28.6.1029

Zhu, B., Pennack, J. A., McQuilton, P., Forero, M. G., Mizuguchi, K., Sutcliffe, B., et al. (2008). Drosophila neurotrophins reveal a common mechanism for nervous system formation. *PLoS Biol.* 6:e284. doi: 10.1371/journal.pbio.0060284

19

Transfer Effects to a Multimodal Dual-Task after Working Memory Training and Associated Neural Correlates in Older Adults

Stephan Heinzel[1,2,3], Jérôme Rimpel[4], Christine Stelzel[2,5,6] and Michael A. Rapp[2*]

[1] Clinical Psychology and Psychotherapy, Freie Universität Berlin, Berlin, Germany, [2] Social and Preventive Medicine, University of Potsdam, Potsdam, Germany, [3] Department of Psychology, Humboldt-Universität zu Berlin, Berlin, Germany, [4] Clinical Psychology and Neuropsychology, Johannes Gutenberg University Mainz, Mainz, Germany, [5] International Psychoanalytic University, Berlin, Germany, [6] Berlin School of Mind and Brain, Berlin, Germany

Edited by:
Claudia Voelcker-Rehage, Chemnitz University of Technology, Germany

Reviewed by:
Mario Bonato, Ghent University, Belgium
Daniel Barulli, Columbia University, USA

***Correspondence:**
Michael A. Rapp
michael.rapp@uni-potsdam.de

Working memory (WM) performance declines with age. However, several studies have shown that WM training may lead to performance increases not only in the trained task, but also in untrained cognitive transfer tasks. It has been suggested that transfer effects occur if training task and transfer task share specific processing components that are supposedly processed in the same brain areas. In the current study, we investigated whether single-task WM training and training-related alterations in neural activity might support performance in a dual-task setting, thus assessing transfer effects to higher-order control processes in the context of dual-task coordination. A sample of older adults (age 60–72) was assigned to either a training or control group. The training group participated in 12 sessions of an adaptive n-back training. At pre and post-measurement, a multimodal dual-task was performed in all participants to assess transfer effects. This task consisted of two simultaneous delayed match to sample WM tasks using two different stimulus modalities (visual and auditory) that were performed either in isolation (single-task) or in conjunction (dual-task). A subgroup also participated in functional magnetic resonance imaging (fMRI) during the performance of the n-back task before and after training. While no transfer to single-task performance was found, dual-task costs in both the visual modality ($p < 0.05$) and the auditory modality ($p < 0.05$) decreased at post-measurement in the training but not in the control group. In the fMRI subgroup of the training participants, neural activity changes in left dorsolateral prefrontal cortex (DLPFC) during one-back predicted post-training auditory dual-task costs, while neural activity changes in right DLPFC during three-back predicted visual dual-task costs. Results might indicate an improvement in central executive processing that could facilitate both WM and dual-task coordination.

Keywords: working memory, cognitive training, modality, dual-task, aging, transfer, fMRI, neuroimaging

INTRODUCTION

Aging is associated with neurochemical, structural, and functional brain changes (Grady, 2012) that affect various cognitive functions. One central cognitive function which is affected by these changes and known to be declined in older age is working memory (WM) (Bopp and Verhaeghen, 2005). Neuroimaging studies have identified brain areas that play a key role in WM processing including lateral prefrontal cortex, inferior parietal lobule, as well as medial frontal regions (Miller and Cohen, 2001; Owen et al., 2005; D'Esposito, 2007). It has been suggested that efficient functioning of such a fronto-parietal WM network is reduced in older adults, as indicated by relatively higher activation at low WM load and relatively lower activation at high WM load when compared to younger adults (Schneider-Garces et al., 2010; Nagel et al., 2011; Heinzel et al., 2014a). These age-related changes in WM load-dependent activation patterns have been described within the framework of the compensation-related utilization of neural circuits hypothesis (CRUNCH, Reuter-Lorenz and Cappell, 2008). Specifically, an over-recruitment of neural resources at low WM load has been associated with inefficient neural processing (Barulli and Stern, 2013).

With respect to training effects, several studies have indicated that WM training leads to an increase in WM performance (Klingberg et al., 2002, 2005; Westerberg et al., 2007; Holmes et al., 2009, 2010; Thorell et al., 2009; Strobach et al., 2014). More importantly, WM training has been shown to improve performance in a broad range of other cognitive domains, such as executive control (Olesen et al., 2004; Klingberg et al., 2005; Westerberg et al., 2007; Thorell et al., 2009; Chein and Morrison, 2010; Brehmer et al., 2012; Strobach et al., 2014), episodic memory (Dahlin et al., 2008b; Lövdén et al., 2010; Richmond et al., 2011), and fluid intelligence (Klingberg et al., 2002; Olesen et al., 2004; Jaeggi et al., 2008, 2010; Rudebeck et al., 2012; Stephenson and Halpern, 2013; Au et al., 2015). Moreover, WM training is effective in older adults and has the potential to reduce age-related WM decline (Li et al., 2008; Schmiedek et al., 2010; Richmond et al., 2011; Brehmer et al., 2012; Buschkuehl et al., 2012; Heinzel et al., 2014b, 2016). Likewise, training of specific executive control processes, so-called process-based interventions, show similar beneficial effects in young and older adults (e.g., Li et al., 2008; Karbach and Kray, 2009; Brehmer et al., 2012; Zinke et al., 2012, see Karbach and Verhaeghen, 2014 for a review). Research on dual-task training is an important field in this research domain with promising effects on both training and transfer tasks (Liepelt et al., 2011; Strobach et al., 2012, 2015). Cognitive training research assumes similar mechanisms underlying training and transfer effects. Most WM training studies suppose that training improves executive control processes that are involved in the transformation and coordination of WM contents (Baddeley, 2003; Curtis and D'Esposito, 2003; Fuster, 2004). Likewise, many dual-task training studies assume that executive control processes involved in the coordination of the two component tasks (Meyer and Kieras, 1997; Szameitat et al., 2002; Stelzel et al., 2007) is optimized via training (Liepelt et al., 2011; Strobach et al., 2012, 2015) and that learning such stimulus-independent processes forms the basis for transfer effects rather than the mere improvement in the specific component tasks.

Importantly, it has been suggested that age-related deficits in dual-task performance (Lindenberger et al., 2000; Hartley, 2001; Verhaeghen and Cerella, 2002; Dubost et al., 2006; Göthe et al., 2007; Granacher et al., 2011) and corresponding changes in neural activation (Hartley et al., 2011; Chmielewski et al., 2014) may result from an underlying WM dysfunction (Awh et al., 2006; Gazzaley and Nobre, 2012).

Considering the effectiveness of WM and dual-task training programs to achieve both training and transfer effects in older adults as well as the overlapping constructs of WM and dual-task (Sala et al., 1995; Baddeley, 1996; Hegarty et al., 2000), we assume that improvements in dual-task performance reflected by a decrease in dual-task costs can be obtained by a WM training. According to notions of "neural transfer" (Dahlin et al., 2008a; Buschkuehl et al., 2012; Heinzel et al., 2014a), a training-related increase in neural efficiency of WM processing may facilitate executively demanding dual-task coordination due to an increased availability of neural resources related to dual-task coordination over and above modality-specific improvements in the component single-tasks.

To our knowledge, it has not been studied systematically if dual-task costs can be reduced by the training of a single n-back WM task in older adults. Thus, the present study aimed to contribute by answering the question whether this WM training leads to a transfer effect to dual-task performance. We trained older adults in a single n-back task with visually presented numerical stimuli (Cohen et al., 1997). The transfer dual-task consisted of a novel multimodal delayed match-to-sample paradigm that includes visual and auditory stimulus modalities. We hypothesized that the transfer from WM training effects to executive dual-task processes would improve performance in both stimulus modalities in the dual-task context, as measured by reduced dual-task costs for both tasks.

The results of the current study included older participants from a previously published training group that performed the n-back task during functional magnetic resonance imaging (fMRI) measurement pre and post-training (Heinzel et al., 2014a, 2016) as well as an unpublished control group. As reported in (Heinzel et al., 2014a, 2016), blood-oxygen-level-dependent (BOLD) signal in WM-related fronto-parietal regions was found to decrease in lower WM load after training in the training group, thus indicating a training-related increase in processing efficiency in WM (Lustig et al., 2009).

We investigated the hypothesis that training-related changes of BOLD response in literature-based WM-related regions of interest (ROIs) during one-back (low WM load) predict dual-task costs after training. According to previous research on neural correlates of both central executive components of WM (D'Esposito et al., 2000; Collette and Van der Linden, 2002; Baddeley, 2003; Mohr et al., 2006) and dual-task coordination (Goldberg et al., 1998; Herath, 2001; Loose et al., 2003; Schubert and Szameitat, 2003; Nebel et al., 2005; Yildiz and Beste, 2015), we expect that changes in BOLD response in dorsolateral prefrontal cortex (DLPFC) will be related to behavioral transfer effects to a dual-task.

MATERIALS AND METHODS

Participants

Altogether, 38 older adults (range: 60–72 years) were recruited by announcements in local newspaper and the internet. In four participants the dual-task data was not correctly recorded due to technical failures during data acquisition. Therefore, the total sample consisted of 34 participants (see **Table 1**). Eighteen participants (11 females; mean ± SD age = 65.78 ± 3.04) were included in the training group and 16 participants (11 females, mean ± SD age = 65.00 ± 3.67) in a no-contact control group that was matched one by one to the training group according to age, sex, and education to ensure parallelization of the two groups. Thirteen participants of the training group in the current study also participated in fMRI sessions before and after the training program. Detailed fMRI results have been previously reported (Heinzel et al., 2014a, 2016). FMRI-analyses presented in the current paper specifically test the hypothesis that pre–post activation changes in a DLPFC ROI may predict results in a behavioral dual-task at T2. All participants were native German speakers, right-handed (Oldfield, 1971), had normal or corrected-to-normal vision, no psychopharmacological medication or history of any psychiatric disease, and achieved 27 or more points in the Mini Mental Status Examination (MMSE, Folstein et al., 1975). Written informed consent was obtained from each participant after the procedures had been explained. The study was approved by the local Ethics Committee of the Charité Universitätsmedizin Berlin, Germany and was conducted in accordance with the Declaration of Helsinki.

Design and Procedure

At the beginning and the end of the training/waiting period, all participants completed both an n-back and a dual-task. Note that other results from the training group including neuropsychological tests and a Sternberg transfer task are reported elsewhere (Heinzel et al., 2016). The WM training was accomplished over a period of 4 weeks and contained 12 training session of an adaptive n-back training (approximately 45 min each). Training sessions took place on Mondays, Wednesdays, and Fridays in a quiet room at St Hedwig Hospital, Berlin, Germany. The control group was not contacted during this time. All tasks were presented with the software Presentation (Version 14.9; Neurobehavioral Systems).

n-Back Task and Adaptive Training

The n-back task comprised two runs, each consisted of 16 blocks which were counterbalanced across subjects and presented in four pseudorandomized orders. Between the blocks, a white fixation cross was presented for 12 s. During the n-back paradigm a randomly assigned sequence of 16 numerical stimuli (0–9) was presented (Cohen et al., 1997) (**Figure 1**). The stimuli were presented separately in the center of a black screen for 500 ms. Two difficulty levels are induced by two different interstimulus intervals (ISIs) of 500 or 1500 ms (pseudorandomized between blocks). The subjects were required to indicate the re-occurrence of a number which has previously presented one, two, or three trials before (1-, 2-, 3-back) by a button press. During a zero-back condition, the participants were obliged to detect the number ‘0.’ The respective WM load condition (0-, 1-, 2-, and 3-back) was indicated by a cue 2 s before a block began. The n-back task lasted approximately 22 min.

The training group participated in an n-back training program over a period of 4 weeks with three sessions per week, resulting in 12 training sessions. Participants accomplished three runs of the n-back task in each training session, lasting approximately 45 min. Each run consisted of 12 blocks. At run 1 in session 1, all participants began the training with the difficulty level 1 (four blocks of zero-back, four-blocks of one-back, and four-blocks of two-back, at an ISI of 1500 ms). Difficulty level was individually adapted throughout all 12 training sessions in

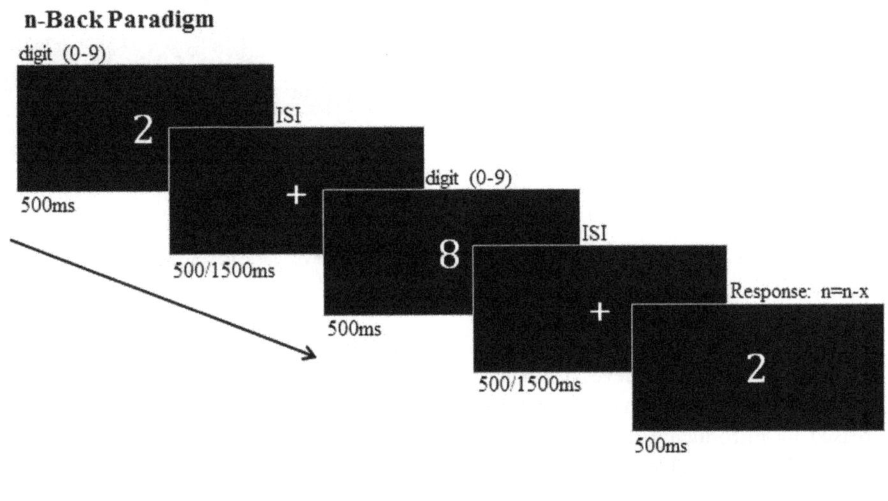

FIGURE 1 | n-back paradigm (example: two-back target).

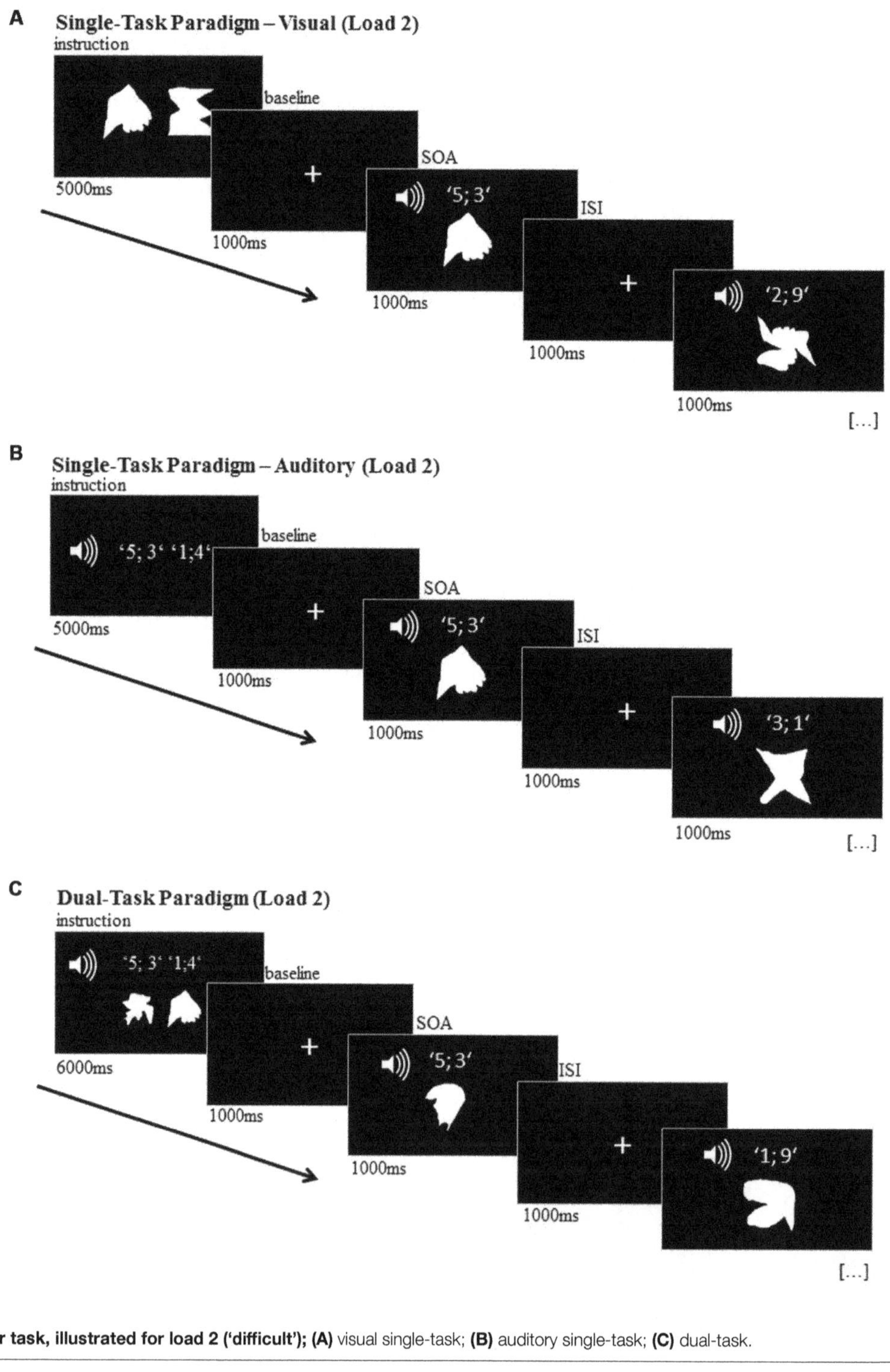

FIGURE 2 | Transfer task, illustrated for load 2 ('difficult'); (A) visual single-task; **(B)** auditory single-task; **(C)** dual-task.

order to keep the task challenging during the entire training program (Doumas et al., 2009). The difficulty level of the task varied across training runs according to individual performance. Task difficulty was increased by introducing higher WM load levels and by shortening the ISI (Heinzel et al., 2014c). If a participant successfully completed one run with a hit rate of 80% or above within each block and with a false alarm rate below 15%, the next difficulty level was introduced in the following run. From level 1 to level 3, ISI was gradually decreased from 1500 to 500 ms in steps of 500 ms. At level 4, the next n-level was introduced (three-back), and zero-back was removed, i.e., participants completed 1-, 2-, and 3-back tasks. In addition, ISI was set back to 1500 ms. At level 7, four-back was introduced and one-back was removed.

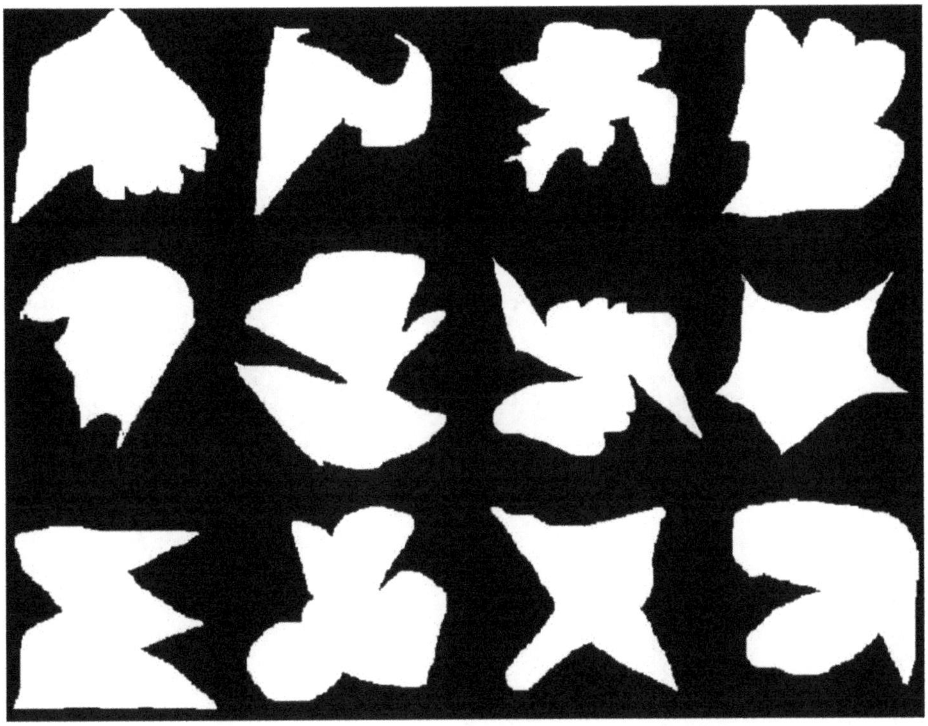

FIGURE 3 | Visual stimulus set: 12 meaningless shapes.

Transfer Task

The transfer dual-task consisted of a delayed match-to-sample paradigm in which the participants had to remember previously presented visual and/or auditory target stimuli. During the probe phase of the experiment, 16 visual and 16 auditory stimuli were presented successively, while one visual and one auditory stimulus was always presented simultaneously. In the single-task conditions, participants were instructed to attend to either the visual stimuli in the visual task (**Figure 2A**) and to auditory stimuli in the auditory task (**Figure 2B**). In the dual-task condition, participants had to attend to both visual and auditory stimuli (**Figure 2C**). There were two difficulty conditions for each task (memory load 1 and memory load 2) and each condition was presented twice in a pseudo-randomized order.

Visual and auditory single-tasks

The visual stimulus set consisted of 12 meaningless white shapes (**Figure 3**) and the auditory stimulus set consisted of 12 different pairs of digits, ranging from 0 to 9 (e.g., '4; 1') and were presented by a female voice via speakers. In the encoding phase at the beginning of each block of the visual single-tasks, 1 (load 1: 'easy') or 2 (load 2: 'difficult') visual target stimuli were presented for 4000 ms (load 1) or 5000 ms (load 2), respectively. In the auditory single-task blocks, 1 (load 1) or 2 (load 2) number pairs were presented vocally as target stimuli. During this encoding phase, subjects were required to encode the target(s). Subsequently, in the probe phase of all conditions of the experiment, 16 visual and 16 auditory stimuli were presented randomly for 1000 ms each with ISIs of 1000 ms, while one visual and one auditory stimulus was always presented simultaneously. Each block included six target stimuli. Participants were requested to press the right mouse key on the laptop with the right index finger each time a target stimulus appeared. Thus, response modality was a motor response for all types of targets.

Dual-task

In the dual-task condition, 1 (load 1) or 2 (load 2) visual target stimuli and 1 or 2 auditory target stimuli were presented during the encoding phase of each block for 5000 ms (load 1) or 6000 ms (load 2). The probe phase in the dual-task conditions was identical to the single-task conditions, however, participants were required to attend to both visual and auditory stimuli at the same time. Each time one of the memorized targets matched a presented stimulus, the participant had to indicate the match by a button press.

Performance and Dual-Task-Costs

The absolute task performance (percent correct) was calculated as the difference of the mean of hits minus false alarms (Eq. 1):

$$\text{hits} - \text{false alarms} = \text{absolute performance} \qquad (1)$$

The dual-task costs (relative dual-task performance) were calculated as the difference of the mean of single-task performance minus the mean of dual-task performance divided

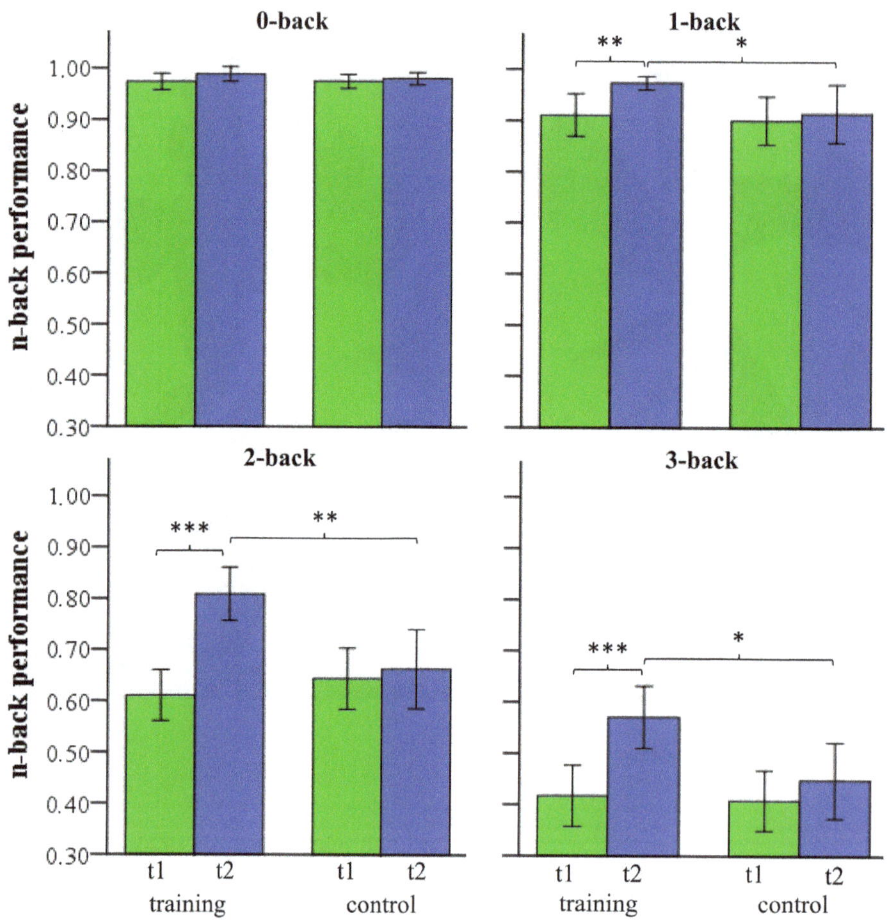

FIGURE 4 | n-back performance of the training and control group at pre-test (T1) and post-test (T2) for 0-, 1-, 2-, and 3-back (*$p < 0.05$; **$p < 0.01$; ***$p < 0.001$).

by the mean of single-task performance (Eq. 2):

$$\frac{\text{Performance Single Task} - \text{Performance Dual Task}}{\text{Performance Single Task}} \cdot 100 = \text{DualTaskCosts} \quad (2)$$

Analyses of transfer effects to the dual-task were focused on dual-task costs because this measure defines dual-task performance in relation to and controlling for individual differences in single task performances. Therefore, dual-task costs are a more specific measure of executive control functions that are required to simultaneously perform two tasks and might be specifically sensitive for detecting age-related changes (Göthe et al., 2007).

Analyses in fMRI Subgroup

MR Image Acquisition and Processing

A detailed description of the MR image acquisition and processing can be derived from (Heinzel et al., 2014a). 13 participants of the older training group of the current dual-task study also participated in pre- and post- fMRI-measurements during n-back as reported in (Heinzel et al., 2014a, 2016). In the beginning of each scanning procedure, one T1-weighted 3D pulse sequence was obtained. Functional data were obtained using a gradient echo echo-planar imaging (GE-EPI) pulse sequence (TR = 2000 ms, TE = 35 ms, flip angle = 80°, matrix size = 64 × 64, voxel size = 3.1 mm × 3.1 mm × 3.8 mm). 31 slices were acquired approximately axial to the bicommissural plane.

TABLE 1 | Demographic variables.

	Training group *M (SD)*	Control group	Training vs. Control group *t*(32) (*p*)
Sex	7 males/ 11 females	5 males/ 11 females	$\chi^2(34,1) = 0.216$, $p = 0.729$
Age (years)	65.78 (3.04)	65.00 (3.67)	0.676 (0.504)
Education (years)	15.53 (2.76)	16.34 (3.63)	0.743 (0.463)
MMSE (points)	29.22 (1.17)	29.07 (0.99)	0.426 (0.673)

MMSE, Mini Mental Status Examination.

TABLE 2 | Working memory performance.

Task	Training group			Control group			t-test (between-subject)	
	T1	T2	t-test (T1 to T2)	T1	T2	t-test (T1 to T2)	T1	T2
Zero-back	0.97 (0.04)	0.99 (0.03)	$t_{(15)} = 1.515, p = 0.148$	0.97 (0.03)	0.98 (0.03)	$t_{(17)} = 0.794, p = 0.440$	$t_{(32)} = 0.003, p = 0.998$	$t_{(32)} = 0.810, p = 0.424$
One-back	0.91 (0.09)	0.97 (0.03)	$t_{(15)} = 3.400, p = 0.003$	0.91 (0.09)	0.91 (0.11)	$t_{(17)} = 0.131, p = 0.898$	$t_{(32)} = 0.022, p = 0.983$	$t_{(32)} = 2.159, p = 0.038$
Two-back	0.61 (0.11)	0.81 (0.11)	$t_{(15)} = 7.368, p < 0.001$	0.65 (0.12)	0.66 (0.16)	$t_{(17)} = 0.448, p = 0.661$	$t_{(32)} = -1.135, p = 0.265$	$t_{(32)} = 3.203, p = 0.003$
Three-back	0.42 (0.13)	0.57 (0.13)	$t_{(15)} = 4.568, p < 0.001$	0.42 (0.12)	0.45 (0.15)	$t_{(17)} = 1.670, p = 0.116$	$t_{(32)} = 0.048, p = 0.962$	$t_{(32)} = 2.578, p = 0.015$

Mean (SD); T1, pre-test; T2, post-test.

Estimation of BOLD Effect Sizes in n-Back

The WM experiment was analyzed within the framework of the general linear model (GLM). To this end, at the single subject level, we created design matrices comprising the experimental conditions of 0-, 1-, 2-, and 3-back as separate regressors of interest and all other experimental conditions (cue, button presses, and the six rigid body realignment parameters) as regressors of no interest. The GLM was fitted voxel-wise into the filtered time series using the restricted maximum likelihood algorithm as implemented in SPM8. We computed differential contrasts 1-back vs. 0-back, 2-back vs. 0-back, and 3-back vs. 0-back. Parameter estimates of BOLD response were extracted for seven literature-based ROIs (see Heinzel et al., 2014a for the procedure) which comprised the bilateral DLPFC, rostrate cingulate zone (RCZ), lateral premotor cortex (LPMC), and intraparietal sulcus (IPS). All ROIs combined define the WM network here. Change scores of n-back activity were calculated by subtracting parameter estimates at T2 from T1.

RESULTS

WM Training

In order to assess WM training success a 2 (group) by 2 (time) by 4 (WM load) repeated-measures ANOVA was conducted (**Figure 4**). The ANOVA revealed significant interactions of the factors group by time by WM load ($F_{(3,30)} = 7.309$, $p = 0.001$, $\eta_p^2 = 0.422$) and group by time ($F_{(1,32)} = 25.602$, $p < 0.001$, $\eta_p^2 = 0.444$), as well as a significant main effect of time ($F_{(1,32)} = 41.431$, $p < 0.001$, $\eta_p^2 = 0.564$) and a non-significant main effect of group ($F_{(1,32)} = 3.158$, $p = 0.085$, $\eta_p^2 = 0.090$). *Post hoc* two-sample *t*-test revealed that both groups did not differ in any condition (0-, 1-, 2-, 3-back) at time T1 (**Table 2**). At time T2 both groups did not differ in the zero-back condition ($t_{(32)} = 0.810$, $p = 0.424$). Both groups differed significantly in the one-back ($t_{(32)} = 2.159$, $p = 0.038$), two-back ($t_{(32)} = 3.203$, $p = 0.003$), and three-back conditions ($t_{(32)} = 2.578$, $p = 0.015$). The control group did not show an improvement from T1 to T2 (all p's > 0.11), whereas the training group improved significantly in WM performance from T1 to T2 for one-back ($t_{(15)} = 3.400$, $p = 0.003$), two-back ($t_{(15)} = 7.368$, $p < 0.001$), and three-back ($t_{(15)} = 4.568$, $p < 0.001$, see **Table 2**).

Single-Task Performance (Percent Correct)

Single-task performance of visual and auditory single-tasks are reported in **Table 3**.

Visual Single-Task Performance (Percent Correct)

A 2 (group) by 2 (time) by 2 (load) repeated-measures ANOVA showed no significant group by time by load interaction ($F_{(1,32)} = 0.600$, $p = 0.444$, $\eta_p^2 = 0.018$). Also, the group by time interaction ($F_{(1,32)} = 0.500$, $p = 0.485$, $\eta_p^2 = 0.015$) as well as all other interactions were not significant (all p's > 0.32). A significant main effect of load ($F_{(1,32)} = 69.595$, $p < 0.001$, $\eta_p^2 = 0.685$) shows that performance decreased with increasing load. A significant main effect of time ($F_{(1,32)} = 5.537$, $p = 0.025$, $\eta_p^2 = 0.147$) indicates general improvement in visual task performance from T1 to T2. There was no significant effect of group ($F_{(1,32)} = 0.030$, $p = 0.864$, $\eta_p^2 = 0.001$).

Auditory Single-Task Performance (Percent Correct)

Comparable to the findings in visual single-task performance, a 2 (group) by 2 (time) by 2 (load) repeated-measures ANOVA in auditory task performance showed no significant group by time by load interaction ($F_{(1,32)} = 0.196$, $p = 0.661$, $\eta_p^2 = 0.006$). The group by time interaction ($F_{(1,32)} = 0.508$, $p = 0.481$, $\eta_p^2 = 0.016$) as well as all other interactions were not significant (all p's > 0.44). A significant main effect of load ($F_{(1,32)} = 42.558$, $p < 0.001$, $\eta_p^2 = 0.571$) shows that performance decreased with increasing load. The main effect of time ($F_{(1,32)} = 3.938$, $p = 0.056$, $\eta_p^2 = 0.110$) was not significant. On a trend-level, this result may suggest a general improvement in auditory task performance from T1 to T2. There was no significant effect of group ($F_{(1,32)} = 0.250$, $p = 0.620$, $\eta_p^2 = 0.008$).

Taken together, the results of single-task analyses show that there is no transfer effect to any measure of single-task performance indicated by non-significant group by time interactions. This is also reflected by non-significant *post hoc* two-sample *t*-test (all p's > 0.19).

Absolute Dual-Task Performance (Percent Correct)

Mean values and standard deviations of absolute dual-task performance are reported in **Table 3**. A 2 (group) by 2 (time) by 2 (load) by 2 (modality) repeated-measures ANOVA showed no significant four-way interaction ($F_{(1,32)} = 2.435$, $p = 0.129$, $\eta_p^2 = 0.071$) and none of the three-way interactions was significant (all p's > 22). A significant group by time interaction ($F_{(1,32)} = 4.686$, $p = 0.038$, $\eta_p^2 = 0.128$), indicated a training-related improvement in dual-task performance in the training group but not in the control group independently of load or modality. A significant main effect of time ($F_{(1,32)} = 14.507$, $p = 0.001$, $\eta_p^2 = 0.312$) shows a general improvement in dual-task performance from pre- to post-test. A significant main effect of load ($F_{(1,32)} = 262.019$, $p < 0.001$, $\eta_p^2 = 0.891$) reflects a generally lower performance at high load. No main effect of group was found ($F_{(1,32)} = 0.031$, $p = 0.861$, $\eta_p^2 = 0.001$). *Post hoc* two-sample *t*-test showed lower performance in the training group for visual targets during dual-task in the high load condition at T1 ($t_{(32)} = 2.163$, $p = 0.038$) and higher performance in the training group for auditory targets during dual-task in the low load condition at T2 ($t_{(32)} = 2.074$, $p = 0.046$). All other two-sample *t*-test were non-significant (all p's > 0.46).

Relative Dual-Task Performance (Dual-Task Costs)

Mean dual-task costs and standard deviations as well as the results of the *post hoc* analyses are reported in **Table 4**. A 2 (group) by 2 (time) by 2 (load) by 2 (modality) repeated-measures ANOVA revealed a significant interaction of group by time by load by modality ($F_{(1,32)} = 4.559$, $p = 0.041$, $\eta_p^2 = 0.125$) and non-significant interactions of the factors group by time by modality ($F_{(1,32)} = 0.587$, $p = 0.449$, $\eta_p^2 = 0.018$) and group by time by load ($F_{(1,32)} = 1.000$, $p = 0.325$, $\eta_p^2 = 0.030$) and group by time ($F_{(1,32)} = 3.066$, $p = 0.090$, $\eta_p^2 = 0.087$). A significant main effect of time ($F_{(1,32)} = 5.648$, $p = 0.024$, $\eta_p^2 = 0.150$) indicates changes of dual-task cost from time T1 to T2. There was no significant effect of group ($F_{(1,32)} = 0.007$, $p = 0.937$, $\eta_p^2 < 0.001$). For the visual modality, *post hoc* two-sample *t*-test show that both groups differed significantly at T1 for load 2 ($t_{(32)} = 2.564$, $p = 0.015$). From T1 to T2, dual-task costs in the training group decreased from 83 to 54% ($t_{(17)} = 3.531$, $p = 0.003$) but did not change significantly in the control group (T1: 50%; T2: 59%, $t_{(15)} = -0.541$, $p = 0.596$, see **Figure 5A**). Both groups did not differ at T2 for load 2 ($t_{(32)} = -0.302$, $p = 0.764$). Within the auditory condition, *post hoc t*-test revealed that dual-task costs decreased in the training group from T1 (20%) to T2 (5%, $t_{(17)} = 3.324$, $p = 0.004$) but did not change in the control group (T1: 20%; T2: 17%, $t_{(17)} = 0.405$, $p = 0.691$) for load 1 (see **Figure 5B**). Both groups did not differ in load 1 at T1 ($t_{(32)} = -0.035$, $p = 0.972$) but at T2 ($t_{(32)} = -2.415$, $p = 0.022$). Within-subject comparisons can be found in **Table 4**. Dual-task costs for each condition are illustrated in **Figure 5**.

Analyses in fMRI Subgroup

As reported in Heinzel et al. (2014a), there was a training-related reduction in BOLD-response during n-back in the WM network. This reduction was found to be specifically strong in the low

TABLE 3 | Single- and dual-task performance (in %).

Modality	Load	Training group				Control group			
		Single task		Dual task		Single task		Dual task	
		T1	T2	T1	T2	T1	T2	T1	T2
Visual	1	0.91 (0.15)	0.98 (0.04)	0.76 (0.22)	0.88 (0.18)	0.96 (0.05)	0.96 (0.06)	0.75 (0.34)	0.84 (0.21)
Visual	2	0.70 (0.23)	0.78 (0.17)	0.12 (0.26)	0.36 (0.27)	0.67 (0.20)	0.75 (0.23)	0.32 (0.28)	0.32 (0.31)
Auditory	1	0.96 (0.07)	0.98 (0.07)	0.77 (0.22)	0.93 (0.07)	0.97 (0.06)	0.99 (0.03)	0.77 (0.25)	0.82 (0.21)
Auditory	2	0.79 (0.17)	0.85 (0.17)	0.36 (0.28)	0.40 (0.24)	0.83 (0.16)	0.85 (0.19)	0.33 (0.29)	0.34 (0.23)

Mean (SD); T1, pre-test; T2, post-test.

TABLE 4 | Dual-task costs (relative performance in %).

Modality	Load	Training group			Control group			t-test (between subject)	
		T1	T2	t-test (T1 to T2)	T1	T2	t-test (T1 to T2)	T1	T2
Visual	1	16.55 (21.13)	10.67 (19.71)	$t(17) = 0.897, p = 0.382$	23.60 (35.11)	12.63 (22.24)	$t(15) = 1.458, p = 0.166$	$t(32) = -0.719, p = 0.478$	$t(32) = -0.272, p = 0.787$
Visual	2	83.37 (31.24)	54.33 (34.03)	$t(17) = 3.531, p = 0.003$	49.94 (44.34)	58.50 (46.07)	$t(15) = -0.541, p = 0.596$	$t(32) = 2.564, p = 0.015$	$t(32) = -0.302, p = 0.764$
Auditory	1	19.89 (21.52)	4.60 (8.00)	$t(17) = 3.324, p = 0.004$	20.19 (27.54)	17.20 (20.49)	$t(15) = 0.405, p = 0.691$	$t(32) = -0.035, p = 0.972$	$t(32) = -2.415, p = 0.022$
Auditory	2	53.39 (36.72)	52.33 (25.84)	$t(17) = 0.098, p = 0.923$	59.50 (37.32)	57.13 (30.65)	$t(15) = 0.191, p = 0.851$	$t(32) = -0.481, p = 0.634$	$t(32) = -0.495, p = 0.624$

Mean (SD); T1, pre-test; T2, post-test.

WM load condition one-back, indicating an increase in neural efficiency. Here, we tested the hypothesis whether this training-related reduction in BOLD-response in the WM network and more specifically in DLPFC, can predict dual-task costs at post-test.

Individual Differences in the Training Group: Correlations with Dual-Task Costs

While no correlations between the entire WM network ROI (see **Figure 6C**) and dual-task costs were found (p's > 0.24), analysis in left DLPFC revealed a significant correlation between training-related reduction in one-back activity and auditory dual-task costs at post-test ($r = 0.625$, $p = 0.022$), indicating lower dual-task costs in participants that showed a stronger reduction in one-back activity (**Figure 6A**). No correlations were found between right DLPFC and auditory dual-task costs ($r = 0.297$, $p = 0.325$). No significant correlations were found between DLPFC activation changes during one-back and visual dual-task costs (p's > 0.35). However, exploratory analyses in 2- and 3-back revealed a significant negative correlation between changes in right DLPFC activity during three-back and visual dual-task costs at post-test ($r = -0.711$, $p = 0.006$, see **Figure 6B**), indicating an increase in three-back activity could have been beneficial for visual dual-task performance.

DISCUSSION

In the present study, we aimed to investigate the influence of WM training on dual-task costs in a novel delayed match-to-sample dual-task. The results indicate that 12 sessions of numerical n-back training can improve the performance in the trained task. Moreover, we found a transfer to the performance in a dual-task. The transfer was reflected by a reduction of dual-task costs in the 'easy' auditory condition in the training but not the control group. Further, we found a reduction of dual-task costs in the 'difficult' visual condition. No training-associated changes in single task performance were found. This is in line with previous research (e.g., Liepelt et al., 2011; Bonato et al., 2013), indicating that measures of dual-task coordination seem to be more sensitive to both subtle cognitive deficits and training-related changes. An additional analysis of a subsample within the training group of this dual-task study that also participated in a previously published fMRI study (Heinzel et al., 2014a, 2016), revealed that a reduction in one-back activity from pre- to post-test in the left DLPFC predicted dual-task costs in the auditory task at post-test. Additional exploratory analyses indicated that changes in three-back activity in right DLPFC were associated with dual-task costs in the visual task at post-test. Thus, taken together, fMRI results may suggest that a training-related reduction in DLPFC activity during low WM load as well as an increase during high WM load might support dual-task performance.

Transfer Effects

The assumption that numerical n-back training can reduce dual-task costs in an untrained transfer task has been partly confirmed. Unexpectedly, modality-specific transfer effects were found to be dependent on the task demand. While transfer to the auditory task occurred in the 'easy' condition, transfer to the visual task was found in the 'difficult' condition. Especially in the training group, performance in the high load condition of the visual task was lower compared to the auditory task at T1, possibly indicating a task-prioritization (Stelzel et al., 2009) biased toward the auditory task. A diminished difference between visual and auditory performance during dual task after training, supports the notion of a shift toward a more efficient dual-task coordination, accompanied by the ability to focus on both component tasks.

Since a transfer effect to both modalities of the dual-task and no transfer to the single-tasks was found, the WM training in this study might have led to an improved modality-independent executive control that was not restricted to the modality of the internal stimulus representation of the trained n-back task (verbal representation of numbers). Therefore, n-back training may facilitate the coordination of two simultaneous tasks as suggested by models and empirical work on central executive processes (Morris and Jones, 1990; Baddeley, 2000; Collette and Van der Linden, 2002). These central executive processes are thought to comprise an attentional control system that governs other WM subsystems including information storage and rehearsal (Baddeley, 2000), and can be divided into separate subfunctions [e.g., updating, inhibition, shifting, dual task coordination (Miyake et al., 2000; Collette and Van der Linden, 2002)].

The results of the current study add an important piece of information to the current cognitive training literature, as we could show that improvements in dual-task performance do not necessarily require an explicit dual-task training if the applied single task training includes executive control processes that are continuously demanding on the WM system. This notion may be derived from studies comparing different training and transfer paradigms including single choice reaction tasks (Strobach et al., 2012, 2015) and studies comparing adaptive to non-adaptive training regimes (Brehmer et al., 2011, 2012). In fact, improvements in dual-task performance in older adults may be enlarged if crucial components are specifically trained (Strobach et al., 2012) and task demand of the training task is adaptively increased according to individual performance (Brehmer et al., 2012).

Please note that the term "transfer effects" that is used in the current study refers to a relatively narrow concept of transfer ["near transfer," see taxonomy by Noack et al. (2009)], as training and transfer tasks share several process components. On the other

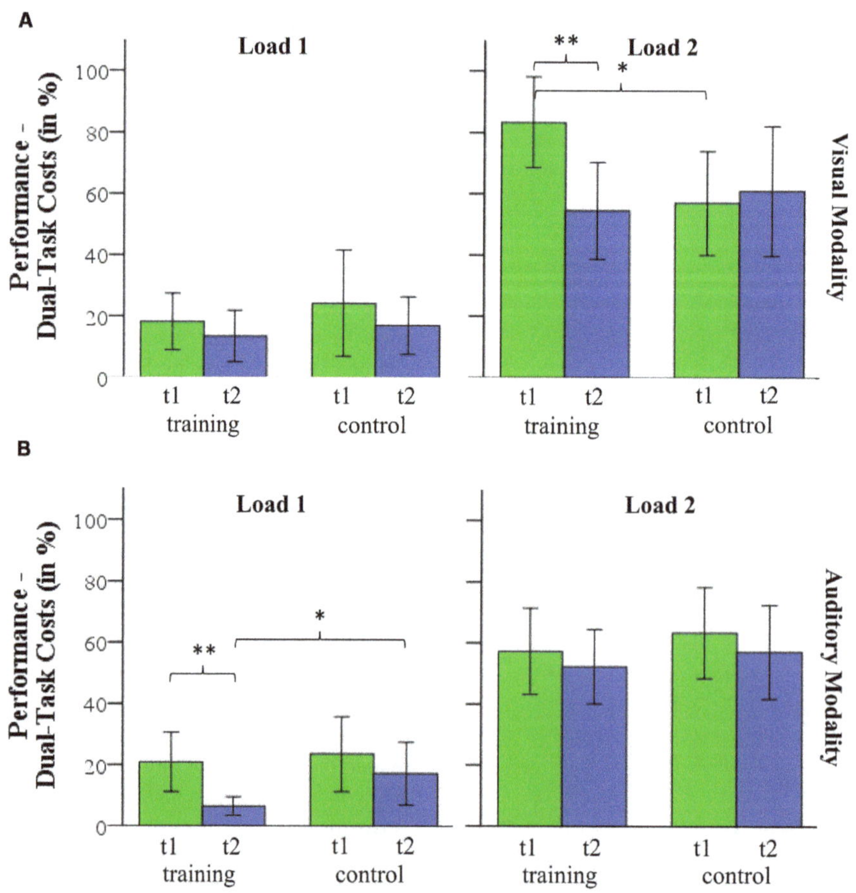

FIGURE 5 | Dual-task costs for load 1 and load 2 for (A) visual and **(B)** auditory modality. *$p < 0.05$; **$p < 0.01$.

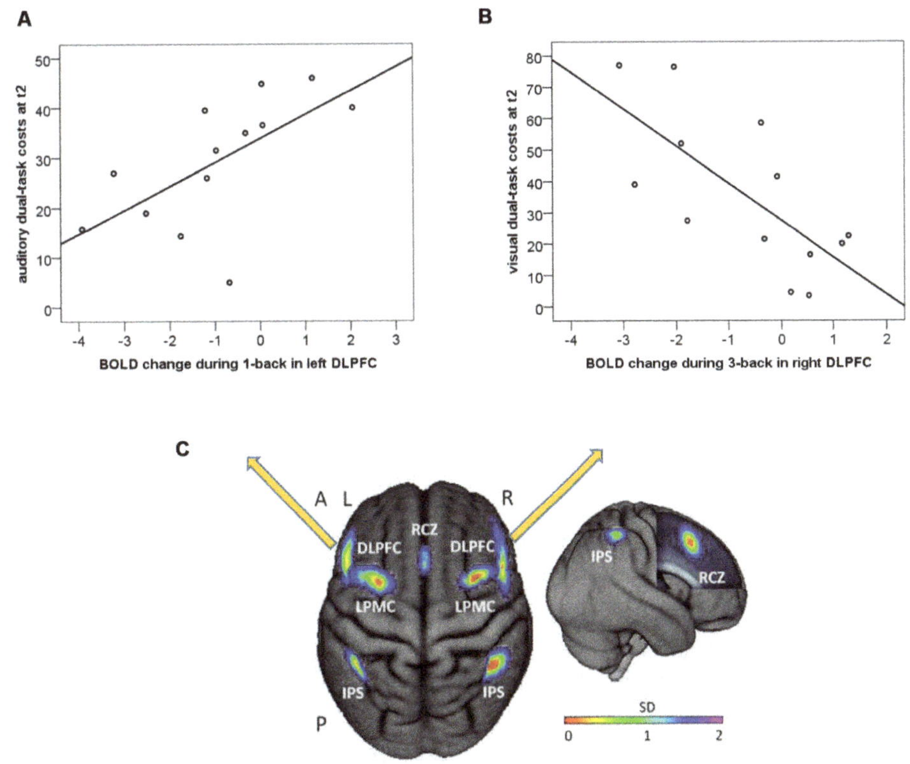

FIGURE 6 | Correlation of one-back BOLD change from T1 to T2 (arbitrary units) and auditory dual-task costs at post-test (T2) for (A) left dorsolateral prefrontal cortex (DLPFC); and **(B)** right dorsolateral prefrontal cortex (DLPFC); **(C)** Location of literature-based probabilistic ROIs of the WM network. Left item: dorsal view of the ROIs overlaid onto the surface of the sample mean brain. Right item: right lateral view. The frontal lobe was cut to display the mid-sagittal ROI. RCZ, rostral cingulate zone; DLPFC, dorsolateral prefrontal cortex; LPMC, lateral premotor cortex; IPS, intraparietal sulcus; A, anterior; P, posterior; L, left; R, right; SD, standard deviation.

hand, the transfer task (dual-task) also differed in crucial aspects from the training task (e.g., attending to two modalities instead of one, use of different stimuli, complex delayed match to sample instead of updating task). Furthermore, no improvements were found in the control group, neither in the training nor in the transfer task. Thus, we are confident that improvements in the transfer task were not just due to familiarity effects in the training task. Since we only used a no-contact control group in the current study, however, we cannot rule out an additional influence of familiarity effects.

The investigation of neural mechanisms underlying "far transfer," e.g., transfer to tasks that include motor coordination such as postural control tasks could be an interesting focus for future research in older adults. In fact, recent work on cognitive-motor dual-tasking in older adults (for review see Boisgontier et al., 2013) has indicated that training-related cognitive improvements might also facilitate postural control performance, a strong predictor for risk of falls (Beauchet et al., 2009).

Analyses within the fMRI Subgroup

As an additional analysis in a subsample ($N = 13$ training participants), we investigated whether a WM training-related increase in neural efficiency in n-back can predict dual-task costs at post-test. Our hypothesis of a DLPFC-modulated transfer to auditory dual-task costs was confirmed by the current data. A reduction in left DLPFC activation during one-back from pre- to post-test in the training group may indicate an increase in neural efficiency in WM, which could have facilitated auditory task performance in a multimodal dual-task. However, as re-test effects cannot be excluded, this cannot be directly derived from the current investigation and requires confirmation in further studies.

Against our hypothesis, the magnitude of visual dual-task costs was not predicted by a DLPFC activity reduction during one-back. However, exploratory analyses revealed that those participants showing a training-related increase in three-back activity in right DLPFC also showed the lowest visual dual-task costs at post-test. Previous research on DLPFC functions suggests its role in higher order executive control such as chunking (Bor et al., 2003, 2004; Owen et al., 2005), maintaining (Courtney, 1998; Nee et al., 2013), updating, and manipulating of information (Owen, 1997; Roth et al., 2006; Barbey et al., 2013). Thus, a more efficient processing in, e.g., chunking may have been beneficial for dual-task performance in the present study in terms of a reduction in auditory dual-task demands by an improvement in the conjunction of stimulus information. Potentially, an overlapping internal stimulus representation (a verbal "code," Wickens, 2002) of the training task and the auditory transfer task may have additionally supported transfer effects within this modality domain.

Hypothetically, the modality-specific findings in DLPFC may relate to a predominantly left lateralized processing of verbal information in WM as compared to predominantly right lateralized processing of visuospatial information (Smith and Jonides, 1999). More specifically, previous research indicates that right hemispheric DLPFC might be predominantly involved in controlling visuospatial WM, whereas left hemispheric DLPFC would mainly control verbal WM (Baddeley, 2003). The association between right-hemispheric DLPFC activity changes during three-back and transfer to visual dual-task could relate to a training-related improvement in neural capacity (Barulli and Stern, 2013) in some subjects as discussed in the model of training-related neural adaptations by Lustig et al. (2009). This potential capacity adaptation may have facilitated the visuospatial task performance within the dual-task condition. However, due to the small sample size of the current pilot study and limitations in study design, these interpretations are only preliminary.

General Limitations and Perspectives

There are several limitations that need to be taken into account when interpreting the results of this study. First, we did not measure fMRI during the dual-task. Thus, we cannot make reliable statements about neuronal effects during dual-task processing in this study. The pre–post fMRI results reported here are based on a relatively small sample and no pre–post fMRI data from the dual-task control group was available. Therefore, any kind of conclusion should be made with restraints as re-test effects cannot be excluded. Further limitations are the lower dual-task performance for visual targets in the high load condition of the training compared to the control group at pre-test and very high performance in both groups in single tasks at low load. Thus, the possibility for further improvement was restricted in the easy conditions of the single tasks. Future studies should include larger samples and compare different age groups such as children and young adults. This would increase the significance in terms of allowing extensive assumptions about cognitive plasticity across the life span. Also, for reasons of feasibility, we only included a no-contact control group. Therefore, social interaction or other unspecific effects associated with the training procedure might have influenced results in the training group and the influence familiarity/practice effects cannot be ruled out. In future studies, an active control group should be included in the study design. Another limitation is related to the sustainability of the results. The current experimental design does not allow any assumptions about long-lasting training or transfer effects. Future studies should take account of implementing follow-up measures.

CONCLUSION

In the current study, a 4-week WM training intervention (single n-back task) in a sample of older adults was associated with an increase in WM performance in the training group but not in an untrained control group. Furthermore, a transfer effect from single-task n-back training to dual-task performance was reported in older adults for the first time. Additional analyses of training-related changes of BOLD response during WM processing in relation to post-training dual-task performance provide preliminary evidence for neural underpinnings of this transfer effect. The findings support the notion of a training-related increase in neural efficiency, as indicated by a reduced activity in DLPFC during one-back performance that may have facilitated the reduction of auditory dual-task costs at post-test after training. Additional analyses in right DLPFC during performance of three-back suggest that increased WM capacity might support performance in a visuospatial dual-task condition. Findings may indicate a training-related improvement of central executive functioning.

AUTHOR CONTRIBUTIONS

SH and MR designed the study. SH programmed the experiments. SH and JR supervised and conducted the experiments. SH, JR, CS, and MR analyzed the data. SH, JR, CS, and MR wrote the paper.

FUNDING

This work was supported by a German National Academic Foundation scholarship to SH, in part by the German Ministry for Education and Research (BMBF 01QG87164 and 01GS08195 and 01GQ0914) and in part by the German Research Foundation (Deutsche Forschungsgemeinschaft, DFG, FOR 1617: grant RA1047/2-1; DFG SPP 1772 "Human performance under multiple cognitive task requirements": grants RA1047/4-1 and HE7464/1-1), and by a MaxNetAging award to MR.

ACKNOWLEDGMENTS

The authors would like to acknowledge the Open Access Publishing Fund of the University of Potsdam supported publication of this work. Fractions of the current work are part of an unpublished thesis. We thank Laura Oliveras Puig, Wolf-Rüdiger Brockhaus, Sabrina Saase, and Sven Breitmeyer for assistance during data acquisition and Robert Lorenz for support during fMRI analyses.

REFERENCES

Au, J., Sheehan, E., Tsai, N., Duncan, G. J., Buschkuehl, M., and Jaeggi, S. M. (2015). Improving fluid intelligence with training on working memory: a meta-analysis. *Psychon. Bull. Rev.* 22, 366–377. doi: 10.3758/s13423-014-0699-x

Awh, E., Vogel, E. K., and Oh, S.-H. (2006). Interactions between attention and working memory. *Neuroscience* 139, 201–208. doi: 10.1016/j.neuroscience.2005.08.023

Baddeley, A. (1996). Exploring the central executive. *Q. J. Exp. Psychol. A* 49, 5–28. doi: 10.1080/713755608

Baddeley, A. (2000). The episodic buffer: a new component of working memory? *Trends Cogn. Sci.* 4, 417–423. doi: 10.1016/S1364-6613(00)01538-2

Baddeley, A. (2003). Working memory: looking back and looking forward. *Nat. Rev. Neurosci.* 4, 829–839. doi: 10.1038/nrn1201

Barbey, A. K., Koenigs, M., and Grafman, J. (2013). Dorsolateral prefrontal contributions to human working memory. *Cortex* 49, 1195–1205. doi: 10.1016/j.cortex.2012.05.022

Barulli, D., and Stern, Y. (2013). Efficiency, capacity, compensation, maintenance, plasticity: emerging concepts in cognitive reserve. *Trends Cogn. Sci.* 17, 502–509. doi: 10.1016/j.tics.2013.08.012

Beauchet, O., Annweiler, C., Dubost, V., Allali, G., Kressig, R. W., Bridenbaugh, S., et al. (2009). Stops walking when talking: a predictor of falls in older adults? *Eur. J. Neurol.* 16, 786–795. doi: 10.1111/j.1468-1331.2009.02612.x

Boisgontier, M. P., Beets, I. A. M., Duysens, J., Nieuwboer, A., Krampe, R. T., and Swinnen, S. P. (2013). Age-related differences in attentional cost associated with postural dual tasks: increased recruitment of generic cognitive resources in older adults. *Neurosci. Biobehav. Rev.* 37, 1824–1837. doi: 10.1016/j.neubiorev.2013.07.014

Bonato, M., Priftis, K., Umiltà, C., and Zorzi, M. (2013). Computer-based attention-demanding testing unveils severe neglect in apparently intact patients. *Behav. Neurol.* 26, 179–181. doi: 10.3233/BEN-2012-129005

Bopp, K. L., and Verhaeghen, P. (2005). Aging and verbal memory span: a meta-analysis. *J. Gerontol. B. Psychol. Sci. Soc. Sci.* 60, 223–233. doi: 10.1093/geronb/60.5.P223

Bor, D., Cumming, N., Scott, C. E. L., and Owen, A. M. (2004). Prefrontal cortical involvement in verbal encoding strategies: modality independent PFC involvement in strategies. *Eur. J. Neurosci.* 19, 3365–3370. doi: 10.1111/j.1460-9568.2004.03438.x

Bor, D., Duncan, J., Wiseman, R. J., and Owen, A. M. (2003). Encoding strategies dissociate prefrontal activity from working memory demand. *Neuron* 37, 361–367. doi: 10.1016/S0896-6273(02)01171-6

Brehmer, Y., Rieckmann, A., Bellander, M., Westerberg, H., Fischer, H., and Bäckman, L. (2011). Neural correlates of training-related working-memory gains in old age. *Neuroimage* 58, 1110–1120. doi: 10.1016/j.neuroimage.2011.06.079

Brehmer, Y., Westerberg, H., and Bäckman, L. (2012). Working-memory training in younger and older adults: training gains, transfer, and maintenance. *Front. Hum. Neurosci.* 6:63. doi: 10.3389/fnhum.2012.00063

Buschkuehl, M., Jaeggi, S. M., and Jonides, J. (2012). Neuronal effects following working memory training. *Dev. Cogn. Neurosci.* 2(Suppl. 1), S167–S179. doi: 10.1016/j.dcn.2011.10.001

Chein, J. M., and Morrison, A. B. (2010). Expanding the mind's workspace: training and transfer effects with a complex working memory span task. *Psychon. Bull. Rev.* 17, 193–199. doi: 10.3758/PBR.17.2.193

Chmielewski, W. X., Yildiz, A., and Beste, C. (2014). The neural architecture of age-related dual-task interferences. *Front. Aging Neurosci.* 6:193. doi: 10.3389/fnagi.2014.00193

Cohen, J. D., Perlstein, W. M., Braver, T. S., Nystrom, L. E., Noll, D. C., Jonides, J., et al. (1997). Temporal dynamics of brain activation during a working memory task. *Nature* 386, 604–608. doi: 10.1038/386604a0

Collette, F., and Van der Linden, M. (2002). Brain imaging of the central executive component of working memory. *Neurosci. Biobehav. Rev.* 26, 105–125.

Courtney, S. M. (1998). An area specialized for spatial working memory in human frontal cortex. *Science* 279, 1347–1351. doi: 10.1126/science.279.5355.1347

Curtis, C. E., and D'Esposito, M. (2003). Persistent activity in the prefrontal cortex during working memory. *Trends Cogn. Sci.* 7, 415–423.

Dahlin, E., Neely, A. S., Larsson, A., Bäckman, L., and Nyberg, L. (2008a). Transfer of learning after updating training mediated by the striatum. *Science* 320, 1510–1512. doi: 10.1126/science.1155466

Dahlin, E., Nyberg, L., Bäckman, L., and Neely, A. S. (2008b). Plasticity of executive functioning in young and older adults: immediate training gains, transfer, and long-term maintenance. *Psychol. Aging* 23, 720–730. doi: 10.1037/a0014296

D'Esposito, M. (2007). From cognitive to neural models of working memory. *Philos. Trans. R. Soc. B Biol. Sci.* 362, 761–772. doi: 10.1098/rstb.2007.2086

D'Esposito, M., Postle, B. R., and Rypma, B. (2000). Prefrontal cortical contributions to working memory: evidence from event-related fMRI studies. *Exp. Brain Res.* 133, 3–11.

Doumas, M., Rapp, M. A., and Krampe, R. T. (2009). Working memory and postural control: adult age differences in potential for improvement, task priority, and dual tasking. *J. Gerontol. B Psychol. Sci. Soc. Sci.* 64, 193–201. doi: 10.1093/geronb/gbp009

Dubost, V., Kressig, R. W., Gonthier, R., Herrmann, F. R., Aminian, K., Najafi, B., et al. (2006). Relationships between dual-task related changes in stride velocity and stride time variability in healthy older adults. *Hum. Mov. Sci.* 25, 372–382. doi: 10.1016/j.humov.2006.03.004

Folstein, M. F., Folstein, S. E., and McHugh, P. R. (1975). "Mini-mental state": a practical method for grading the cognitive state of patients for the clinician. *J. Psychiatr. Res.* 12, 189–198.

Fuster, J. M. (2004). Upper processing stages of the perception-action cycle. *Trends Cogn. Sci.* 8, 143–145.

Gazzaley, A., and Nobre, A. C. (2012). Top-down modulation: bridging selective attention and working memory. *Trends Cogn. Sci.* 16, 129–135. doi: 10.1016/j.tics.2011.11.014

Goldberg, T. E., Berman, K. F., Fleming, K., Ostrem, J., Van Horn, J. D., Esposito, G., et al. (1998). Uncoupling cognitive workload and prefrontal cortical physiology: a PET rCBF study. *Neuroimage* 7, 296–303. doi: 10.1006/nimg.1998.0338

Göthe, K., Oberauer, K., and Kliegl, R. (2007). Age differences in dual-task performance after practice. *Psychol. Aging* 22, 596–606. doi: 10.1037/0882-7974.22.3.596

Grady, C. (2012). The cognitive neuroscience of ageing. *Nat. Rev. Neurosci.* 13, 491–505. doi: 10.1038/nrn3256

Granacher, U., Bridenbaugh, S. A., Muehlbauer, T., Wehrle, A., and Kressig, R. W. (2011). Age-related effects on postural control under multi-task conditions. *Gerontology* 57, 247–255. doi: 10.1159/000322196

Hartley, A. A. (2001). Age differences in dual-task interference are localized to response-generation processes. *Psychol. Aging* 16, 47–54. doi: 10.1037/0882-7974.16.1.47

Hartley, A. A., Jonides, J., and Sylvester, C.-Y. C. (2011). Dual-task processing in younger and older adults: similarities and differences revealed by fMRI. *Brain Cogn.* 75, 281–291. doi: 10.1016/j.bandc.2011.01.004

Hegarty, M., Shah, P., and Miyake, A. (2000). Constraints on using the dual-task methodology to specify the degree of central executive involvement in cognitive tasks. *Mem. Cogn.* 28, 376–385. doi: 10.3758/BF03198553

Heinzel, S., Lorenz, R. C., Brockhaus, W.-R., Wüstenberg, T., Kathmann, N., Heinz, A., et al. (2014a). Working memory load-dependent brain response predicts behavioral training gains in older adults. *J. Neurosci.* 34, 1224–1233. doi: 10.1523/JNEUROSCI.2463-13.2014

Heinzel, S., Lorenz, R. C., Pelz, P., Heinz, A., Walter, H., Kathmann, N., et al. (2016). Neural correlates of training and transfer effects in working memory in older adults. *Neuroimage* 134, 236–249. doi: 10.1016/j.neuroimage.2016.03.068

Heinzel, S., Riemer, T. G., Schulte, S., Onken, J., Heinz, A., and Rapp, M. A. (2014b). Catechol-O-methyltransferase (COMT) genotype affects age-related changes in plasticity in working memory: a pilot study. *BioMed Res. Int.* 2014:414351. doi: 10.1155/2014/414351

Heinzel, S., Schulte, S., Onken, J., Duong, Q.-L., Riemer, T. G., Heinz, A., et al. (2014c). Working memory training improvements and gains in non-trained cognitive tasks in young and older adults. *Neuropsychol. Dev. Cogn. B Aging Neuropsychol. Cogn.* 21, 146–173. doi: 10.1080/13825585.2013.790338

Herath, P. (2001). Neural correlates of dual task interference can be dissociated from those of divided attention: an fMRI study. *Cereb. Cortex* 11, 796–805. doi: 10.1093/cercor/11.9.796

Holmes, J., Gathercole, S. E., and Dunning, D. L. (2009). Adaptive training leads to sustained enhancement of poor working memory in children. *Dev. Sci.* 12, F9–F15. doi: 10.1111/j.1467-7687.2009.00848.x

Holmes, J., Gathercole, S. E., Place, M., Dunning, D. L., Hilton, K. A., and Elliott, J. G. (2010). Working memory deficits can be overcome: impacts of training and medication on working memory in children with ADHD. *Appl. Cogn. Psychol.* 24, 827–836. doi: 10.1002/acp.1589

Jaeggi, S. M., Buschkuehl, M., Jonides, J., and Perrig, W. J. (2008). Improving fluid intelligence with training on working memory. *Proc. Natl. Acad. Sci. U.S.A.* 105, 6829–6833. doi: 10.1073/pnas.0801268105

Jaeggi, S. M., Buschkuehl, M., Perrig, W. J., and Meier, B. (2010). The concurrent validity of the N -back task as a working memory measure. *Memory* 18, 394–412. doi: 10.1080/09658211003702171

Karbach, J., and Kray, J. (2009). How useful is executive control training? Age differences in near and far transfer of task-switching training. *Dev. Sci.* 12, 978–990. doi: 10.1111/j.1467-7687.2009.00846.x

Karbach, J., and Verhaeghen, P. (2014). Making working memory work: a meta-analysis of executive-control and working memory training in older adults. *Psychol. Sci.* 25, 2027–2037. doi: 10.1177/0956797614548725

Klingberg, T., Fernell, E., Olesen, P. J., Johnson, M., Gustafsson, P., Dahlström, K., et al. (2005). Computerized training of working memory in children with ADHD–a randomized, controlled trial. *J. Am. Acad. Child Adolesc. Psychiatry* 44, 177–186. doi: 10.1097/00004583-200502000-00010

Klingberg, T., Forssberg, H., and Westerberg, H. (2002). Training of working memory in children with ADHD. *J. Clin. Exp. Neuropsychol.* 24, 781–791.

Li, S.-C., Schmiedek, F., Huxhold, O., Röcke, C., Smith, J., and Lindenberger, U. (2008). Working memory plasticity in old age: practice gain, transfer, and maintenance. *Psychol. Aging* 23, 731–742. doi: 10.1037/a0014343

Liepelt, R., Strobach, T., Frensch, P., and Schubert, T. (2011). Improved intertask coordination after extensive dual-task practice. *Q. J. Exp. Psychol.* 64, 1251–1272. doi: 10.1080/17470218.2010.543284

Lindenberger, U., Marsiske, M., and Baltes, P. B. (2000). Memorizing while walking: increase in dual-task costs from young adulthood to old age. *Psychol. Aging* 15, 417–436. doi: 10.1037/0882-7974.15.3.417

Loose, R., Kaufmann, C., Auer, D. P., and Lange, K. W. (2003). Human prefrontal and sensory cortical activity during divided attention tasks. *Hum. Brain Mapp.* 18, 249–259. doi: 10.1002/hbm.10082

Lövdén, M., Bäckman, L., Lindenberger, U., Schaefer, S., and Schmiedek, F. (2010). A theoretical framework for the study of adult cognitive plasticity. *Psychol. Bull.* 136, 659–676. doi: 10.1037/a0020080

Lustig, C., Shah, P., Seidler, R., and Reuter-Lorenz, P. A. (2009). Aging, training, and the brain: a review and future directions. *Neuropsychol. Rev.* 19, 504–522. doi: 10.1007/s11065-009-9119-9

Meyer, D. E., and Kieras, D. E. (1997). A computational theory of executive cognitive processes and multiple-task performance: part I. Basic mechanisms. *Psychol. Rev.* 104, 3–65. doi: 10.1037/0033-295X.104.1.3

Miller, E. K., and Cohen, J. D. (2001). An integrative theory of prefrontal cortex function. *Annu. Rev. Neurosci.* 24, 167–202. doi: 10.1146/annurev.neuro.24.1.167

Miyake, A., Friedman, N. P., Emerson, M. J., Witzki, A. H., Howerter, A., and Wager, T. D. (2000). The unity and diversity of executive functions and their contributions to complex "Frontal Lobe" tasks: a latent variable analysis. *Cogn. Psychol.* 41, 49–100. doi: 10.1006/cogp.1999.0734

Mohr, H. M., Goebel, R., and Linden, D. E. J. (2006). Content- and task-specific dissociations of frontal activity during maintenance and manipulation in visual working memory. *J. Neurosci. Off. J. Soc. Neurosci.* 26, 4465–4471. doi: 10.1523/JNEUROSCI.5232-05.2006

Morris, N., and Jones, D. M. (1990). Memory updating in working memory: the role of the central executive. *Br. J. Psychol.* 81, 111–121. doi: 10.1111/j.2044-8295.1990.tb02349.x

Nagel, I. E., Preuschhof, C., Li, S.-C., Nyberg, L., Bäckman, L., Lindenberger, U., et al. (2011). Load modulation of BOLD response and connectivity predicts working memory performance in younger and older adults. *J. Cogn. Neurosci.* 23, 2030–2045. doi: 10.1162/jocn.2010.21560

Nebel, K., Wiese, H., Stude, P., de Greiff, A., Diener, H.-C., and Keidel, M. (2005). On the neural basis of focused and divided attention. *Cogn. Brain Res.* 25, 760–776. doi: 10.1016/j.cogbrainres.2005.09.011

Nee, D. E., Brown, J. W., Askren, M. K., Berman, M. G., Demiralp, E., Krawitz, A., et al. (2013). A meta-analysis of executive components of working memory. *Cereb. Cortex* 23, 264–282. doi: 10.1093/cercor/bhs007

Noack, H., Lövdén, M., Schmiedek, F., and Lindenberger, U. (2009). Cognitive plasticity in adulthood and old age: gauging the generality of cognitive intervention effects. *Restor. Neurol. Neurosci.* 27, 435–453. doi: 10.3233/RNN-2009-0496

Oldfield, R. C. (1971). The assessment and analysis of handedness: the Edinburgh inventory. *Neuropsychologia* 9, 97–113. doi: 10.1016/0028-3932(71)90067-4

Olesen, P. J., Westerberg, H., and Klingberg, T. (2004). Increased prefrontal and parietal activity after training of working memory. *Nat. Neurosci.* 7, 75–79. doi: 10.1038/nn1165

Owen, A. M. (1997). The functional organization of working memory processes within human lateral frontal cortex: the contribution of functional neuroimaging. *Eur. J. Neurosci.* 9, 1329–1339. doi: 10.1111/j.1460-9568.1997.tb01487.x

Owen, A. M., McMillan, K. M., Laird, A. R., and Bullmore, E. (2005). N-back working memory paradigm: a meta-analysis of normative functional neuroimaging studies. *Hum. Brain Mapp.* 25, 46–59. doi: 10.1002/hbm.20131

Reuter-Lorenz, P. A., and Cappell, K. A. (2008). Neurocognitive aging and the compensation hypothesis. *Curr. Dir. Psychol. Sci.* 17, 177–182. doi: 10.1111/j.1467-8721.2008.00570.x

Richmond, L. L., Morrison, A. B., Chein, J. M., and Olson, I. R. (2011). Working memory training and transfer in older adults. *Psychol. Aging* 26, 813–822. doi: 10.1037/a0023631

Roth, J. K., Serences, J. T., and Courtney, S. M. (2006). Neural system for controlling the contents of object working memory in humans. *Cereb. Cortex* 1991, 1595–1603. doi: 10.1093/cercor/bhj096

Rudebeck, S. R., Bor, D., Ormond, A., O'Reilly, J. X., and Lee, A. C. H. (2012). A potential spatial working memory training task to improve both episodic memory and fluid intelligence. *PLoS ONE* 7:e50431. doi: 10.1371/journal.pone.0050431

Sala, S. D., Baddeley, A., Papagno, C., and Spinnler, H. (1995). Dual-task paradigm: a means to examine the central executive. *Ann. N. Y. Acad. Sci.* 769, 161–172. doi: 10.1111/j.1749-6632.1995.tb38137.x

Schmiedek, F., Lövdén, M., and Lindenberger, U. (2010). Hundred days of cognitive training enhance broad cognitive abilities in adulthood: findings from the COGITO study. *Front. Aging Neurosci.* 2:27. doi: 10.3389/fnagi.2010.00027

Schneider-Garces, N. J., Gordon, B. A., Brumback-Peltz, C. R., Shin, E., Lee, Y., Sutton, B. P., et al. (2010). Span, CRUNCH, and beyond: working memory capacity and the aging brain. *J. Cogn. Neurosci.* 22, 655–669. doi: 10.1162/jocn.2009.21230

Schubert, T., and Szameitat, A. J. (2003). Functional neuroanatomy of interference in overlapping dual tasks: an fMRI study. *Cogn. Brain Res.* 17, 733–746. doi: 10.1016/S0926-6410(03)00198-8

Smith, E. E., and Jonides, J. (1999). Storage and executive processes in the frontal lobes. *Science* 283, 1657–1661. doi: 10.1126/science.283.5408.1657

Stelzel, C., Brandt, S. A., and Schubert, T. (2009). Neural mechanisms of concurrent stimulus processing in dual tasks. *Neuroimage* 48, 237–248. doi: 10.1016/j.neuroimage.2009.06.064

Stelzel, C., Kraft, A., Brandt, S. A., and Schubert, T. (2007). Dissociable neural effects of task order control and task set maintenance during dual-task processing. *J. Cogn. Neurosci.* 20, 613–628. doi: 10.1162/jocn.2008.20053

Stephenson, C. L., and Halpern, D. F. (2013). Improved matrix reasoning is limited to training on tasks with a visuospatial component. *Intelligence* 41, 341–357. doi: 10.1016/j.intell.2013.05.006

Strobach, T., Frensch, P., Mueller, H. J., and Schubert, T. (2012). Testing the limits of optimizing dual-task performance in younger and older adults. *Front. Hum. Neurosci.* 6:39. doi: 10.3389/fnhum.2012.00039

Strobach, T., Frensch, P., Müller, H., and Schubert, T. (2015). Evidence for the acquisition of dual-task coordination skills in older adults. *Acta Psychol.* 160, 104–116. doi: 10.1016/j.actpsy.2015.07.006

Strobach, T., Salminen, T., Karbach, J., and Schubert, T. (2014). Practice-related optimization and transfer of executive functions: a general review and a specific realization of their mechanisms in dual tasks. *Psychol. Res.* 78, 836–851. doi: 10.1007/s00426-014-0563-7

Szameitat, A. J., Schubert, T., Müller, K., and von Cramon, D. Y. (2002). Localization of executive functions in dual-task performance with fMRI. *J. Cogn. Neurosci.* 14, 1184–1199. doi: 10.1162/089892902760807195

Thorell, L. B., Lindqvist, S., Bergman Nutley, S., Bohlin, G., and Klingberg, T. (2009). Training and transfer effects of executive functions in preschool children. *Dev. Sci.* 12, 106–113. doi: 10.1111/j.1467-7687.2008.00745.x

Verhaeghen, P., and Cerella, J. (2002). Aging, executive control, and attention: a review of meta-analyses. *Neurosci. Biobehav. Rev.* 26, 849–857.

Westerberg, H., Jacobaeus, H., Hirvikoski, T., Clevberger, P., Ostensson, M.-L., Bartfai, A., et al. (2007). Computerized working memory training after stroke–a pilot study. *Brain Inj.* 21, 21–29. doi: 10.1080/02699050601148726

Wickens, C. D. (2002). Multiple resources and performance prediction. *Theor. Issues Ergon. Sci.* 3, 159–177. doi: 10.1080/14639220210123806

Yildiz, A., and Beste, C. (2015). Parallel and serial processing in dual-tasking differentially involves mechanisms in the striatum and the lateral prefrontal cortex. *Brain Struct. Funct.* 220, 3131–3142. doi: 10.1007/s00429-014-0847-0

Zinke, K., Zeintl, M., Eschen, A., Herzog, C., and Kliegel, M. (2012). Potentials and limits of plasticity induced by working memory training in old-old age. *Gerontology* 58, 79–87. doi: 10.1159/000324240

20

Dynamic Brains and the Changing Rules of Neuroplasticity: Implications for Learning and Recovery

Patrice Voss†, Maryse E. Thomas†, J. Miguel Cisneros-Franco and Étienne de Villers-Sidani**

Department of Neurology and Neurosurgery, Montreal Neurological Institute, McGill University, Montreal, QC, Canada

Edited by:
Claude Alain,
Rotman Research Institute, Canada

Reviewed by:
Samira Anderson,
University of Maryland, College Park, United States
Vesa Putkinen,
University of Jyväskylä, Finland

***Correspondence:**
Étienne de Villers-Sidani
etienne.de-villers-sidani@mcgill.ca
Patrice Voss
patrice.voss@gmail.com

†These authors have contributed equally to this work.

A growing number of research publications have illustrated the remarkable ability of the brain to reorganize itself in response to various sensory experiences. A traditional view of this plastic nature of the brain is that it is predominantly limited to short epochs during early development. Although examples showing that neuroplasticity exists outside of these finite time-windows have existed for some time, it is only recently that we have started to develop a fuller understanding of the different regulators that modulate and underlie plasticity. In this article, we will provide several lines of evidence indicating that mechanisms of neuroplasticity are extremely variable across individuals and throughout the lifetime. This variability is attributable to several factors including inhibitory network function, neuromodulator systems, age, sex, brain disease, and psychological traits. We will also provide evidence of how neuroplasticity can be manipulated in both the healthy and diseased brain, including recent data in both young and aged rats demonstrating how plasticity within auditory cortex can be manipulated pharmacologically and by varying the quality of sensory inputs. We propose that a better understanding of the individual differences that exist within the various mechanisms that govern experience-dependent neuroplasticity will improve our ability to harness brain plasticity for the development of personalized translational strategies for learning and recovery following brain injury or disease.

Keywords: neuroscience, plasticity regulators, brain, plasticity, learning, recovery, regulators, neuromodulatory systems

INTRODUCTION

Neuroplasticity can be viewed as a general umbrella term that refers to the brain's ability to modify, change, and adapt both structure and function throughout life and in response to experience. Just as individual differences contribute to variability observed in brain structure and function (see Gu and Kanai, 2014, for a review), mechanisms of neuroplasticity also show significant variability across individuals. Indeed, a growing number of recent studies suggest that the rules and mechanisms that govern cortical plasticity are more variable than previously thought. The purpose of this article is to shed light on the various factors that contribute to neuroplastic variability observed within cortical sensory systems, with a special focus on the auditory system as a model. We will establish the role played by critical periods, plasticity inhibitors, and neuromodulator systems and highlight how these factors interact with other elements such as age, sex, and sensory experience to produce a broad variability of plastic processes. We propose that developing a more robust comprehension of the individual differences that exist within neuroplastic mechanisms can have a significant impact on how clinicians and researchers approach a wide range of neurological and neurodevelopmental disorders. The first section of this paper will introduce the concepts of experience dependent plasticity, critical periods, and plasticity inhibitors. The second portion will provide evidence of how the quality and quantity of sensory inputs reaching the brain influence the rules of plasticity within cortical sensory areas. The third part will illustrate how individual differences in neuromodulator tone can differentially affect brain plasticity within sensory cortices throughout the lifetime.

EXPERIENCE-DEPENDENT PLASTICITY IN THE DEVELOPING AND MATURE BRAIN

Critical Periods for Experience-Dependent Plasticity

Age is a key determinant of experience-dependent cortical plasticity. Important structural and functional changes tend to predominantly occur early in life during time-limited epochs of stimulus-driven plasticity known as *critical periods* (Knudsen, 2004). A well-known example of this limited time-window was provided by the classic monocular visual deprivation studies of Wiesel and Hubel (1963). CPs have since been described in all major sensory systems and in a variety of animal species and their identification has been instrumental in the discovery of the cortical machinery involved in their regulation (see Hensch, 2005 for a review). Many studies of CP plasticity have focused on the rat primary auditory cortex (A1) model, which displays a succession of partially overlapping CPs for various stimulus parameters during development (de Villers-Sidani and Merzenich, 2011). For example, frequency tuning has the earliest and shortest CP in the auditory system (around days 11–14 of life), whereas CPs for more complex sound representations, such as frequency modulation tuning, tend to occur slightly later during early infancy (around days 25–33) (Insanally et al., 2009). Several sensitive periods have also been identified in humans, particularly as they relate to hearing restoration following prelingual deafness and language acquisition. Current evidence suggests that the optimal time for cochlear implantation is before 4 years of life and that implantations performed after 7 years are unlikely to produce satisfactory results (see Kral and Sharma, 2012). Although typically associated with early developmental stages, there is a growing body of evidence demonstrating that CPs can be reopened later in life due to a variety of factors that are still being uncovered. These include damage to peripheral sensory organs (Chino et al., 1992; Diamond et al., 1993; Van Brussel et al., 2011) and changes in the sensory environment (He et al., 2006; Zhou et al., 2011). Recent work has shown that plastic changes in auditory cortex that normally occur within early CPs can even be observed in aging humans and rodents (de Villers-Sidani et al., 2010; Mishra et al., 2014). This suggests that the elements that regulate plasticity change throughout the lifespan and do not only operate around developmental CPs.

Plasticity Inhibitors and Cellular Brakes

With CP closure, sensory representations are stabilized (Rice and Van der Loos, 1977; Fagiolini et al., 1994; Zhang et al., 2002; de Villers-Sidani et al., 2007). This process requires the maturation of inhibitory (GABAergic) cellular networks and the maintenance of sufficient GABAergic tone in the cortex (Hensch, 2005; Fritschy and Panzanelli, 2014). Any further modification of these networks and associated cortical plasticity is regulated by a series of plasticity inhibitors and molecular brakes, so-called because of their role in limiting plasticity in the mature brain (see Hensch, 2005; Bavelier et al., 2010, for reviews). Functional and structural elements that promote and constrain plasticity include the inhibitory activity of GABAergic interneurons such as parvalbumin positive (PV+) cells (Kuhlman et al., 2013), extracellular matrix components including perineuronal nets (PNNs) (Wang and Fawcett, 2012), and myelin associated proteins (McGee et al., 2005). For a summary of these elements, see **Figure 1**.

Throughout life, the proportion of GABAergic interneurons in the cortex remains relatively stable. However, the number of PV+ and somatostatin positive (SOM+) interneurons decreases with age, indicating that different interneuron subtypes are differentially affected by aging (Stanley et al., 2012; Ouellet and de Villers-Sidani, 2014). Furthermore, PV staining intensity has been shown to be positively correlated with the degree of experience-dependent plasticity (de Villers-Sidani et al., 2008; Zhou et al., 2011). Adult brain CP-like plastic remodeling can be induced by down-regulating cortical inhibition (Fagiolini and Hensch, 2000) or disrupting PNNs (Pizzorusso et al., 2002; McRae et al., 2007; Wang and Fawcett, 2012) or myelin (Kartje et al., 1999; McGee et al., 2005), which form structural barriers to limit plasticity and stabilize cortical representations.

Loss of inhibition during aging could lead to a state of cortical instability where sensory representations are easily distorted by non-specific passive experiences as is the case during CPs (Zhou et al., 2011) (**Figures 1A,B**). Indeed, we recently observed that experience-dependent plasticity is not only paradoxically enhanced, it is also unstable (i.e., producing plastic changes that decayed rapidly in time) in old rats compared to young controls, and was paralleled by a reduction in PV+ cell density, GABA concentration, and PNNs (Cisneros-Franco et al., unpublished). We also found that passive distortions of the auditory map decayed rapidly, indicating an ongoing instability of A1 tuning in the aging cortex. These observations led us to propose that the inhibitory regulation of plasticity, rather than plasticity *per se*, is reduced in the aged brain. This finding has important repercussions for the development of rehabilitation strategies targeted toward aging and opposes the traditional view that aging is a period of limited plasticity.

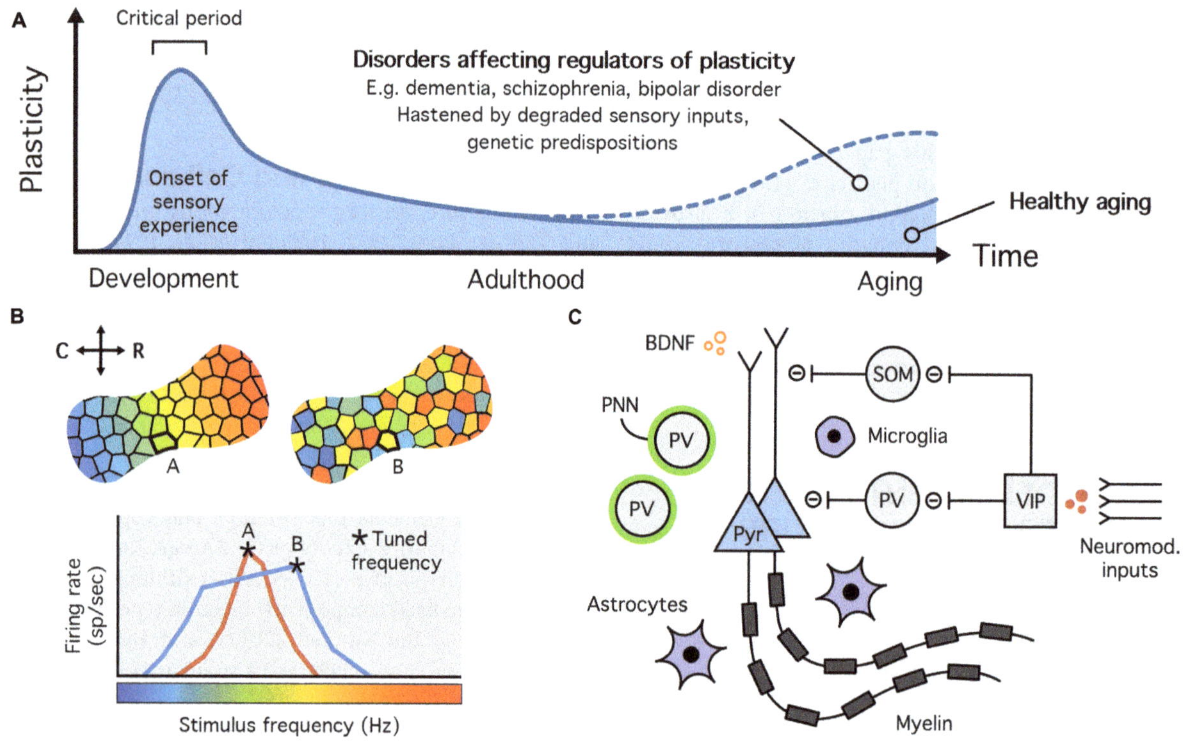

D

Regulators of plasticity and examples of associated disorders

GABAergic interneurons including those expressing parvalbumin (**PV**), somatostatin (**SOM**), and vasoactive intestinal peptide (**VIP**) drive cortical oscillations, maintain excitatory-inhibitory balance in cortical circuits, and regulate activity-dependent plasticity through inhibition. Inhibitory deficits have been strongly linked to schizophrenia through post-mortem analyses, mouse model studies, and surveys of susceptibility genes. PV+ cell function in particular has been shown to be disrupted in schizophrenia, leading to defective inhibition of pyramidal cells and irregular neuronal rhythms. More general inhibitory deficits such as excitatory-inhibitory imbalance and reductions in GABA transmission and receptors have also been linked to a variety of neurodevelopmental disorders including autism, Down's syndrome, and fragile X syndrome[1].

Peri-neuronal nets (**PNN**) are components of the extracellular matrix that densely surround neurons, particularly PV+ cells, and provide a physical barrier to plasticity by stabilizing synapses. PNN disruption has been implicated in schizophrenia, bipolar disorder, major depression, autism, and addiction[2].

Neuromodulatory inputs and **neuromodulators** are critical for many forms of cortical plasticity in the mature brain and mediate plasticity through the recruitment of neural pathways associated with states of cognition including motivation, attention, and emotion. Neurological conditions are typically associated with deficits in one or more neuromodulatory systems. For instance, Parkinson's arises from the cell death of dopaminergic cells in the substantia nigra, however deficiencies of the serotonergic, noradrenergic, and cholinergic systems have also been identified in the progression of the disease.[3,4].

Myelin and **myelin associated proteins** play an important role in neuronal connectivity and inhibit large-scale plasticity by limiting axonal growth and regeneration, especially after injury in adult animals. Diffusion tensor and magnetization transfer imaging studies have shown alterations in white matter associated with illnesses including multiple sclerosis, schizophrenia, bipolar disorder, and depression[5,6,7,8].

Glial cells including **astrocytes** and **microglia** are being increasingly understood to contribute to synaptic plasticity through monitoring the extracellular milieu and absorbing and releasing synaptically active molecules. Astrocytes are known to communicate with neurons by releasing gliotransmitters, especially glutamate. Microglia are involved in neuroimmune responses following brain injury and are capable of physically remodeling synapses. Altered astrocyte and microglia function has been linked to neurodegenerative diseases including Alzheimer's, Parkinson's, Huntington's, and amyotrophic lateral sclerosis[9,10].

Neurotrophins such as **BDNF** promote plasticity during adulthood through mediating local protein synthesis, dendritic arborization and synaptic growth. Deficient neurotrophin levels may lead to some of the deficits in synaptic transmission observed in various dementias[11].

FIGURE 1 | Continued

FIGURE 1 | Regulation of experience dependent plasticity. **(A)** Trajectory of experience dependent plasticity during the lifetime. The onset of sensory experience triggers the opening of critical period windows during which the sensory cortex is rapidly organized in response to passive stimulation from the external environment. With maturation, the critical period closes and sensory representations are stabilized. Plasticity continues to take place during adulthood but is tightly regulated by a variety of cellular and molecular processes. These mechanisms tend to decrease with age allowing for non-specific passive experience to elicit plasticity during aging. Disorders that affect regulators of plasticity increase the likelihood for maladaptive plastic changes to take place in the brain. **(B)** Auditory tonotopic map plasticity. Example of a mature tonotopic map from the rat primary auditory cortex (top left) and that of a rat demonstrating irregular plasticity (top right). The tonotopic map typically exhibits a smooth gradient with neurons in the most caudal (C) part of the cortex firing preferentially (or tuned to) low frequencies and neurons in the most rostral (R) part tuned to high frequencies. In unusual plastic states, such as aging and after long-term exposure to white noise, this functional gradient becomes disrupted as tuning of individual neurons becomes less selective (bottom). For example, a neuron's tuning may shift from being narrow and selective (site A – red line) to broad and flat peaked (site B – blue line), sometimes altering its tuning frequency (**A,B** based on Cisneros-Franco et al., unpublished and Thomas et al., unpublished). **(C)** Some of the major regulators of plasticity in the auditory cortex. Plasticity regulators limit plasticity in the mature brain by controlling the activity of excitatory cells, primarily pyramidal (Pyr) neurons. They include cells such as inhibitory interneurons and glia, structural molecules like peri-neuronal nets and myelin associated proteins, neuromodulatory control from other brain regions, and neurotrophic factors. **(D)** Table of regulators of plasticity and associated disorders. Altered neuroplasticity has been implicated in a variety of neurological disorders including psychiatric, neurodevelopmental, and neurodegenerative disorders. This table highlights just a few examples of disorders associated with specific regulators of plasticity. References: (1) Marín, 2012 (Review); (2) Sorg et al., 2016; (3) Brichta et al., 2013 (Review); (4) Higley and Picciotto, 2014; (5) Wen et al., 2014; (6) Bellani et al., 2016; (7) Mighdoll et al., 2015; (8) Mandl et al., 2015; (9) Singh and Abraham, 2017 (Review); (10) Morris et al., 2013; (11) Arancio and Chao, 2007.

SENSORY INPUTS REACHING THE BRAIN INFLUENCE THE RULES OF PLASTICITY

The Quality and Quantity of Sensory Inputs Affect the Timing of Critical Period Windows

Studies of CPs have demonstrated the importance of sensory experience for normal neurodevelopment and sensory map acquisition. The quality and quantity of sensory experience, however, can have diverse effects on CP duration and outcome. Enriched sensory environments, for example, can prolong CP plasticity (Greifzu et al., 2014), stimulate dendritic growth (Leggio et al., 2005; Bose et al., 2010), and improve neuronal response properties (Engineer et al., 2004; Feldman, 2005), whereas deprived or unstructured noisy environments postpone CP onset and maintain cortical neurons in an immature state (Cynader and Mitchell, 1980; Mower, 1991; Fagiolini et al., 1994). In general, the excess presence of a specific stimulus during the CP appears to result in its exaggerated incorporation into the sensory map. For instance, altering the visual environment of the kitten through striped surroundings (Sengpiel et al., 1999) or goggles (Tanaka et al., 2009) shifts the orientation selectivity of visual cortical neurons to prefer the dominant orientation of their environment. In auditory cortex, pure tone pips of a chosen frequency played continuously result in the overrepresentation of that frequency within the tonotopic map (Zhang et al., 2001; de Villers-Sidani et al., 2007). However, there is evidence for hardwired preferences for ethologically relevant stimuli such as tone pips played at a temporal modulation rate similar to that of communication (Kim and Bao, 2009) and vocalizations from members of the same species (Soha and Marler, 2001). The quantity of salient stimuli present during development can also affect the timing of CP closure. Exposure to temporally modulated white noise produces a shorter than usual CP for spectral tuning in auditory cortex, whereas the masking of normal auditory inputs with continuous white noise keeps it open indefinitely (Chang and Merzenich, 2003). Similarly, exposure to bandlimited noise results only in the selective functional and inhibitory maturation of sectors of the tonotopic map outside of the noise band (de Villers-Sidani et al., 2008).

Sensory Inputs with Low Signal-to-Noise Ratio Can Trigger Plasticity in the Mature Cortex

While the fidelity of sensory inputs has long been known to affect perceptual development, the potential effects of weak, absent, or noisy sensory inputs on mature brain function are only beginning to be understood. Sensory information reaching the brain can be degraded due to exogenous or endogenous factors. Exogenous factors are environmental noise that reduce the discriminability of a stimulus, such as listening to a voice in a crowded room, whereas endogenous factors refer to limits of the peripheral sensory organs or central processing disorders that affect the perception of sensory inputs. In all cases, plastic processes determine how the brain responds and adapts to these challenging perceptual situations and a major goal of neuroscience research should be to understand and integrate our knowledge of these different contexts. We previously demonstrated the similarity between auditory impairments that arise with natural aging in old rats and young adult rats exposed to continuous white noise for 8 weeks (Kamal et al., 2013). Aged rats displayed poor tuning selectivity, neuronal desynchronization, and reduced sensitivity to low-probability sounds, which was nearly indistinguishable from the young adult rats that had been housed in a noisy auditory environment. Furthermore, these impairments were associated with reduced inhibitory interneuron expression and decreased cortical myelin density in both groups of animals. More recently, we observed that exposure to amplitude-modulated noise did not produce the same plastic changes as continuous noise in young adult rats (Thomas et al., unpublished). We concluded that auditory inputs with a high temporal signal-to-noise ratio are protective for auditory function well into adulthood. Together, these findings strongly suggest that noisy sensory inputs, whether originating from the environment or endogenous processes associated with aging could manifest similar functional and structural deficits. Other studies have also demonstrated the ability of noisy environments to induce plastic changes in the mature auditory cortex resulting in impaired function (Pienkowski and Eggermont, 2010; Zheng, 2012; Gourévitch et al., 2014). When returned to normal environments, however, most of these changes appear to be completely or partially reversible indicating ongoing mechanisms of homeostatic plasticity. This in turn suggests that interventions that target plasticity such as enriched environments (e.g., musical training and experience) and discrimination training could be used to counteract or prevent the effects of degraded sensory inputs on mature brains (White-Schwoch et al., 2013; Alain et al., 2014; Mishra et al., 2014).

BRAIN PLASTICITY IS MEDIATED BY NEUROMODULATOR SYSTEMS

Neuromodulator Systems As Drivers of Plasticity

In addition to sensory experience, various neuromodulator systems can affect both CPs and adult cortical plasticity by increasing neuronal excitability, improving signal to noise ratio, and controlling the propagation of activity through the cortex (Kirkwood, 2007). Early studies indicated that norepinephrine, a key neurotransmitter of the noradrenergic system, is necessary for ocular dominance column plasticity during the critical period (Kasamatsu and Pettigrew, 1976; Kasamatsu et al., 1979). Subsequent work, however, suggested that both noradrenergic and cholinergic networks need to be impaired to affect cortical plasticity, suggesting a functional redundancy between the two systems (Bear and Daniels, 1983; Bear and Singer, 1986). More recent studies have demonstrated that the cholinergic system is a potent neuromodulator of attention, learning and memory, in both humans (Rokem and Silver, 2010; Beer et al., 2013; Moran et al., 2013; Chamoun et al., 2017) and animal models (Herrero et al., 2008; Hasselmo and Sarter, 2011). Furthermore, Shepard et al. (2015) has provided evidence that mice lacking norepinephrine failed to reorganize auditory cortex frequency representation in response to prolonged sound exposure, suggesting that norepinephrine is a necessary driver of CP plasticity within auditory cortex. The dopaminergic and the noradrenalinergic systems have also been shown to significantly modulate and shape cortical plasticity. For instance, dopamine upregulation has been linked with increases in the auditory cortical representation of paired tones (Bao et al., 2001) and increases in noradrenaline have been shown to increase the threshold of acoustic excitatory responses in auditory neurons (Manunta and Edeline, 1998).

Taken together, these findings highlight the critical role of neuromodulator systems as the main gating mechanisms of plasticity in adult sensory cortex, as well as their important role in shaping cortical function and cognitive abilities. Indeed, both neurochemically boosting cholinergic transmission (Greuel et al., 1988; Voss et al., 2016) and stimulating the basal forebrain — from which the cholinergic neurons project to the cortex — (Kilgard and Merzenich, 1998; Froemke et al., 2007; Kang and Vaucher, 2009; Kang et al., 2014) have been shown to have a significant effect on learning rates and the cortical processing of stimuli. Stimulating the dopaminergic system has also been shown to improve cortical signal-to-noise ratio (Winterer and Weinberger, 2004; Kroener et al., 2009), to enhance visual perceptual performance (Müller et al., 1998; Noudoost and Moore, 2011) and to modulate plasticity within sensory cortex (Bao et al., 2001; Hui et al., 2009). These data provide interesting research avenues worth exploring to develop methods to promote neuroplasticity in situations of learning difficulties or of recovery following brain injury.

Inter-individual Variability of Neuromodulator Tone Affects Brain Plasticity and Cognition

One of the hallmarks of cognitive processes is the inter-individual variability that exists among healthy individuals. Indeed, a growing body of evidence suggests that this variability is intrinsically linked to variability within the neuromodulator systems. In particular, the potency of the dopaminergic and cholinergic systems changes across the lifespan and cognitive abilities tend to correlate with the maturation of these systems. For instance, the inverted u-shaped function of dopamine signaling (Arnsten, 1998; Goldman-Rakic et al., 2000), where an optimal dopamine level results in improved neuronal function while both insufficient or excessive dopamine levels impair function, is well-suited to model the link between changes in cognitive performance across the lifespan and age-related changes in dopamine signaling, both which also follow an inverted u-shaped function (Störmer et al., 2012). Similarly, cholinergic functions have also been shown to decline during the course of healthy aging (Gibson et al., 1981; McGeer et al., 1984; Voss et al., 2016) and are linked to age-related cognitive and perceptual decline (Everitt and Robbins, 1997; Schliebs and Arendt, 2011). The degeneration of neuromodulatory function with normal aging is likely to contribute to both the diminished and enhanced plasticity observed in aging individuals because neuromodulatory control is weakened overall. While older adults have poorer learning outcomes traditionally perceived as a reduction in plasticity, they are also more vulnerable to maladaptive plastic changes (Mahncke et al., 2006; Oberman and Pascual-Leone, 2013).

There is also an increasing number of studies demonstrating important sex differences regarding neuromodulator levels and how they affect cognition. Research with both animal models and humans have reported that nicotine — a receptor agonist of the cholinergic system—, for instance, can increase learning rates in a sexually dimorphic manner (Levin et al., 1993; Algan et al., 1997). Similarly, animal studies have found that dopaminergic neurotransmission is modulated by sex steroids (Becker, 1990; Booze et al., 1999). In particular, estrogen considerably enhances striatal dopamine synthesis, baseline dopamine release, and the behavioral and neurochemical response to d-amphetamines (Becker, 1990, 1999). It is generally agreed that estrogen has an overall facilitating effect on dopaminergic neurotransmission (Jacobs and D'Esposito, 2011; Uban et al., 2012) and that

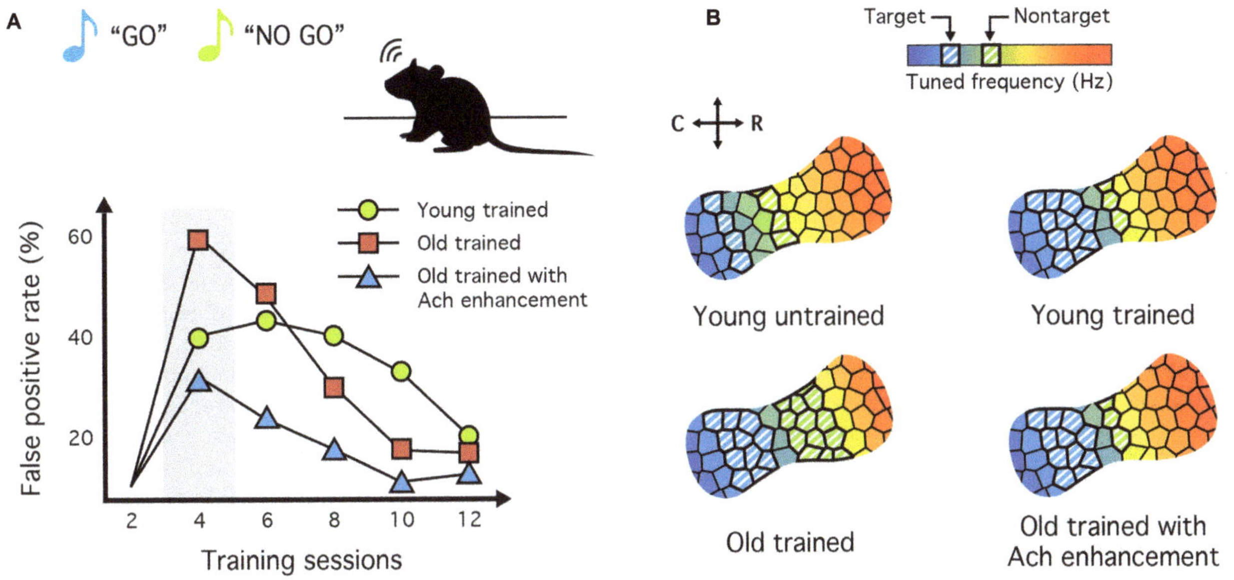

C

Interventions targeting regulators of plasticity

Cognitive training encompasses a broad range of exercises usually performed on a computer that may train attention, working memory, problem solving, low-level sensory processing, and/or executive functioning. The benefit of cognitive training exercises are their versatility and ease of implementation in multiple settings however the extent to which training in one domain generalizes to others remains a pertinent concern. If individual differences in plasticity are taken into consideration, then cognitive training exercises designed to recruit specific plasticity regulators are most likely to result in meaningful changes. For example, exercises that train sustained attention are best suited to recruit the cholinergic system and bring about changes in clinical populations that exhibit cholinergic deficits[1,2].

Neuropharmaceuticals have the potential to target any of the vast number of cellular and molecular processes that contribute to plasticity. In particular, drugs that influence neuromodulatory systems are well positioned to affect plasticity in neuronal circuits. L-DOPA, the dopamine precursor, has been successfully used to treat movement deficits in Parkinson's disease for decades and cholinergic enhancers are often employed in the treatment of dementias. The effects of certain drugs on plasticity are not always taken into account when medications are prescribed for certain conditions, however. Both positive and negative effects of L-DOPA on cognitive performance have been described in Parkinson's patients and cholinergic blockers used in the treatment of psychosis have also been suggested to have negative effects on cognition[3,4,5].

Physical exercise has been shown to increase levels of BDNF in the periphery and brain, which in turn has been suggested to improve mood and cognitive abilities. Given this, exercise is a potential strategy to boost mood and cognition in older adults and in conditions characterized by low BDNF levels such as dementia and Alzheimer's[6,7].

Enriched environments have been shown to increase neurotrophic factors that promote cell survival, dendritic branching, and synaptogenesis at all stages of life in animal studies. To this end, environments that encourage sensory, motor, cognitive, and social behaviors are proposed to promote recovery from neurodegenerative conditions and acute brain injuries, however the difficulties of implementing standard enrichment programs in clinical settings make them difficult to study in humans[8,9,10].

A **combination** of neurotherapeutics is most likely to have the largest effect on plasticity. Effects of cognitive training, for example, may be enhanced through neuropharmacology. Valproate, a histone-deacetylase inhibitor, was shown to facilitate learning of absolute pitch during adulthood, presumably through lifting epigenetic restraints on plasticity[10]. Tinnitus, a plasticity syndrome in which individuals experience ringing in the ears, is often treated with a combination of music, noise generators and perceptual training[11,12].

FIGURE 2 | Neurotherapeutic interventions targeting regulators of plasticity. **(A)** Cholinergic enhancement paired with training reduces the probability of false positives (FP) in aged rats. Young adult and old (>24-month-old) rats were trained on a "Go (target frequency)/No-Go (non-target frequency)" auditory perceptual learning task. The FP rate can be used as an indicator of distractibility, and aged humans and rodents tend to have particularly high FP rates during early stages of training. When aged rats were given the cholinesterase inhibitor rivastigmine before each training session their FP rate was halved. This suggests that boosting the cholinergic system can enhance perception and behavioral performance in the elderly by reducing distractibility. **(B)** The tonotopic map of trained aged rats resembles young rats when training is paired with cholinergic enhancement. Compared to a naive, young adult rat (top left), the map of a trained rat (top right) will have a greater proportion of sites tuned to the target stimulus frequency and a smaller proportion tuned to the non-target frequency. This differential representation is believed to help the rat assign more importance to the target tone and ignore the non-target. In old rats (bottom left), however, training results in an equal enlargement of both the target and non-target frequency regions. While these rats are capable of learning the discrimination task, this alternative learning mechanism

(Continued)

FIGURE 2 | Continued
may result in their elevated FP rate. Indeed, old rats trained with rivastigmine (bottom right), which exhibit less distractibility exhibit map plasticity like young adult rats (**A,B** modified from Voss et al., 2016). **(C)** Table of neurotherapeutic interventions aimed at mechanisms of plasticity. By targeting the various regulators of plasticity, the goal of neurotherapeutics is to utilize the brain's innate capacity to change to improve learning, memory, and recovery from neurological injury or disease. This brief selection demonstrates a broad range of behavioral, pharmaceutical, and environmental interventions either currently available or under exploration today. References: (1) Vinogradov et al., 2012; (2) Cramer et al., 2011; (3) Cools, 2006; (4) Suraweera et al., 2015; (5) Grinevich et al., 2009; (6) Coelho et al., 2013; (7) Szuhany et al., 2015; (8) Mora et al., 2007; (9) Nithianantharajah and Hannan, 2006; (10) Alwis and Rajan, 2014; (11) Gervain et al., 2013; (12) Zenner et al., 2017.

interactions between estrogen and dopamine significantly affect memory functions (Jacobs and D'Esposito, 2011; Quinlan et al., 2013).

Finally, psychological traits have also been shown to covary with neuromodulator levels. Previous research has identified a relatively strong relationship between dopamine receptors and individual differences in self-reported novelty-seeking personality (Norbury and Husain, 2015) and individual differences in sensation-seeking behaviors have been linked to brain dopamine function (Hamidovic et al., 2009; Derringer et al., 2010). Furthermore, risk-taking behavior in humans can be directly manipulated with dopaminergic drugs, but the effectiveness of such a manipulation depends on baseline sensation-seeking traits (Norbury et al., 2013).

Taken together, these findings provide multiple lines of evidence demonstrating that important inter-individual differences exist within the various neuromodulator systems, and that, therefore, these individual differences are likely also reflected, to a certain extent, in measures of cortical plasticity. Future studies would benefit from taking these individual differences into account when investigating the relationship between neuromodulator tone and cortical plasticity.

Neuropathological Condition and Drug Treatments Can Alter Neuromodulator Balance

Several neuropathological conditions present with significant neuromodulator imbalances. For instance, hallmark pathophysiological features of schizophrenia and Parkinson's disease include the disruption of dopaminergic networks, whereas Alzheimer's disease and multiple forms of dementia are associated with disturbances in the cholinergic and noradrenergic systems. These neuropathological conditions are also often associated with perceptual impairments, which could be caused or exacerbated by neuromodulatory imbalances. In schizophrenia, for instance, in addition to deficits in higher-order processes, deficits can be found throughout the cortex at the level of early sensory processing (Javitt, 2015; Javitt and Freedman, 2015). In particular, schizophrenia has been recently associated with a variety of low-level auditory dysfunctions evidenced by behavioral, electrophysiological, and structural metrics (Javitt and Sweet, 2015), and although more limited, there is also evidence that visual cortex plasticity may also be compromised in the disease (Cavuş et al., 2012). Central auditory dysfunction, in the absence of severe peripheral hearing loss, is also associated with high incidences of cognitive decline and Alzheimer's disease (Gates et al., 2008; Albers et al., 2015). In transgenic mice overexpressing amyloid precursor protein, the presence of Alzheimer's disease pathology is associated with loss of GABAergic inhibition (Huang and Mucke, 2012) and significant changes in auditory evoked responses within the primary auditory cortex (Wang et al., 2003).

Several medications have been developed to specifically target the neuromodulator systems involved in neuropathological disorders, and therefore, also affect brain plasticity and sensory processes. In theory, these drugs could be used to target mechanisms of sensory plasticity in healthy adults and be paired with training to ward off perceptual deficits associated with natural aging. For instance, cholinergic antagonists have been shown to significantly improve occipital cortical responsiveness in rats (Kang et al., 2015) and visual perceptual learning in humans (Rokem and Silver, 2010), and recent evidence suggests that these learning effects can last several months after ceasing cholinergic enhancement (Rokem and Silver, 2013). Cholinergic function can also be enhanced through the use of cholinesterase inhibitors such as rivastigmine or donepezil (Colović et al., 2013), which are currently used to treat Alzheimer's disease and diverse dementia (Ellis, 2005; Birks, 2006). We recently showed in the aged rat that a daily administration of rivastigmine paired with training on an auditory discrimination task led to profound plastic changes within auditory cortex compared with age-matched controls who only underwent perceptual training (Voss et al., 2016) (**Figures 2A,B**). Not only did boosting cholinergic function produce robust frequency map and tuning bandwidth changes within auditory cortex, it also significantly improved the speed with which rats learned to perform the task. Furthermore, the magnitude of the functional changes was found to correlate with each rat's individual discrimination performance. These results demonstrate that combining perceptual training with neuromodulation of the cholinergic system can restore cortical functional deficits observed as a result of normal aging. Taken together, these findings highlight the therapeutic potential and the powerful potentiating effect of neuromodulator systems for improving the recovery or prevention of age-related and disease-related deficits. See **Figure 2C** for a selection of current and proposed therapeutic interventions targeting various modulators of plasticity.

FUTURE DIRECTIONS

The research described here demonstrates that the propensity for experience dependent plasticity throughout life can be more or less potentiated by diverse factors including individual genetic, cellular, molecular, and environmental differences. These findings have lead us to understand that the rules that regulate plasticity are not only more intrinsically variable than were previously thought, but can also be shaped in mature brains. Although plasticity within sensory systems is greatest during time-limited epochs during early development, plasticity regulators in the adult brain can be manipulated by acting on various neuromodulators and by precisely regulating sensory input. Indeed, our lab and others have shown that degraded sensory inputs can trigger plasticity within primary sensory cortex, possibly the result of an adaptive mechanism to facilitate cortical rewiring in cases of neurological injury or trauma to peripheral sensory systems. The idea that plasticity mechanisms can operate throughout the lifespan suggests that many functional properties of sensory neurons can be altered, and even reversed in some cases. This is particularly relevant for neurodegenerative and neuropsychiatric conditions where plasticity mechanisms appear to be dysregulated. Additional research will be required to more completely model age and disease-related plastic changes within sensory cortex, which will then allow us to better tailor stimulus-exposure or behavioral training paradigms to produce the desired functional and behavioral outcome measures. Indeed, without properly establishing a link with behavior, the nature of the reorganization, whether adaptive or maladaptive, will remain difficult to establish. Studies focusing on this goal will be important, with procedures allowing functional perturbation of particular relevance to establish causality.

Moving forward, it will also be necessary to take into account individual differences including age, sex, drug use, and pathological conditions in order to advance personalized treatments that aid learning, memory, and recovery from brain injury and disease. Neuromodulator systems, in particular, display immense variability between individuals. This is particularly evident when considering the huge range of interindividual variability in the effects of cholinergic, dopaminergic and noradrenergic drugs, regardless of the desired outcome measure (Keers and Aitchison, 2010; Tang et al., 2014; Turner et al., 2015). Individual differences in baseline perceptual abilities (Wong and Perrachione, 2007; Perrachione et al., 2011) and in brain connectivity (Lee et al., 2014; Voss and Zatorre, 2015) are also likely to affect learning and recovery rates. As with many medical and health-related fields where personalized and precision medicine are increasingly becoming mainstream, neurotherapeutic interventions targeting mechanisms of plasticity and cognition should also follow an individualized approach by harnessing individual differences to best utilize the brain's innate capacity to change.

AUTHOR CONTRIBUTIONS

PV, MT, JC-F, and EdV-S conceived and wrote the manuscript. MT conceived and designed the figures.

FUNDING

This work was supported by the Canadian Institutes for Health Research, the Natural Sciences and Engineering Research Council of Canada, the Canadian Foundation for Innovation and the Fonds de Recherche du Quebec.

ACKNOWLEDGMENT

The authors would like to thank Lydia Ouellet for her technical support during various experiments described in this paper.

REFERENCES

Alain, C., Zendel, B. R., Hutka, S., and Bidelman, G. M. (2014). Turning down the noise: the benefit of musical training on the aging auditory brain. *Hear. Res.* 308, 162–173. doi: 10.1016/j.heares.2013.06.008

Albers, M. W., Gilmore, G. C., Kaye, J., Murphy, C., Wingfield, A., Bennett, D. A., et al. (2015). At the interface of sensory and motor dysfunctions and Alzheimer's disease. *Alzheimer's Dement.* 11, 70–98. doi: 10.1016/j.jalz.2014.04.514

Algan, O., Furedy, J. J., Demirgören, S., Vincent, A., and Pöğün, Ş (1997). Effects of tobacco smoking and gender on interhemispheric cognitive function: performance and confidence measures. *Behav. Pharmacol* 8, 416–428. doi: 10.1097/00008877-199710000-00006

Alwis, D. S., and Rajan, R. (2014). Environmental enrichment and the sensory brain: the role of enrichment in remediating brain injury. *Front. Syst. Neurosci.* 8:156. doi: 10.3389/fnsys.2014.00156

Arancio, O., and Chao, M. V. (2007). Neurotrophins, synaptic plasticity and dementia. *Curr. Opin. Neurobiol.* 17, 325–330. doi: 10.1016/j.conb.2007.03.013

Arnsten, A. F. (1998). Catecholamine modulation of prefrontal cortical cognitive function. *Trends Cogn. Sci.* 2, 436–447. doi: 10.1016/S1364-6613(98)01240-6

Bao, S., Chan, V. T., and Merzenich, M. M. (2001). Cortical remodelling induced by activity of ventral tegmental dopamine neurons. *Nature* 412, 79–83. doi: 10.1038/35083586

Bavelier, D., Levi, D. M., Li, R. W., Dan, Y., and Hensch, T. K. (2010). Removing brakes on adult brain plasticity: from molecular to behavioral interventions. *J. Neurosci.* 30, 14964–14971. doi: 10.1523/JNEUROSCI.4812-10.2010

Bear, M., and Daniels, J. (1983). The plastic response to monocular deprivation persists in kitten visual cortex after chronic depletion of norepinephrine. *J. Neurosci.* 3, 407–416.

Bear, M. F., and Singer, W. (1986). Modulation of visual cortical plasticity by acetylcholine and noradrenaline. *Nature* 320, 172–176. doi: 10.1038/320172a0

Becker, J. B. (1990). Estrogen rapidly potentiates amphetamine-induced striatal dopamine release and rotational behavior during microdialysis. *Neurosci. Lett.* 118, 169–171. doi: 10.1016/0304-3940(90)90618-J

Becker, J. B. (1999). Gender differences in dopaminergic function in striatum and nucleus accumbens. *Pharmacol. Biochem. Behav.* 64, 803–812. doi: 10.1016/S0091-3057(99)00168-9

Beer, A. L., Vartak, D., and Greenlee, M. W. (2013). Nicotine facilitates memory consolidation in perceptual learning. *Neuropharmacology* 64, 443–451. doi: 10.1016/j.neuropharm.2012.06.019

Bellani, M., Boschello, F., Delvecchio, G., Dusi, N., Altamura, C. A., Ruggeri, M., et al. (2016). DTI and myelin plasticity in bipolar disorder: integrating neuroimaging and neuropathological findings. *Front. Psychiatry* 7:21. doi: 10.3389/fpsyt.2016.00021

Birks, J. S. (2006). "Cholinesterase inhibitors for Alzheimer's disease," in *Cochrane Database of Systematic Reviews*, ed. J. S. Birks (Chichester: John Wiley & Sons, Ltd).

Booze, R. M., Welch, M. A., Wood, M. L., Billings, K. A., Apple, S. R., and Mactutus, C. F. (1999). Behavioral sensitization following repeated intravenous nicotine administration: gender differences and gonadal hormones. *Pharmacol. Biochem. Behav.* 64, 827–839. doi: 10.1016/S0091-3057(99)00169-0

Bose, M., Muñoz-Llancao, P., Roychowdhury, S., Nichols, J. A., Jakkamsetti, V., Porter, B., et al. (2010). Effect of the environment on the dendritic morphology of the rat auditory cortex. *Synapse* 64, 97–110. doi: 10.1002/syn.20710

Brichta, L., Greengard, P., and Flajolet, M. (2013). Advances in the pharmacological treatment of Parkinson's disease: targeting neurotransmitter systems. *Trends Neurosci.* 36, 543–554. doi: 10.1016/j.tins.2013.06.003

Cavuş, I., Reinhart, R. M. G., Roach, B. J., Gueorguieva, R., Teyler, T. J., Clapp, W. C., et al. (2012). Impaired visual cortical plasticity in schizophrenia. *Biol. Psychiatry* 71, 512–520. doi: 10.1016/j.biopsych.2012.01.013

Chamoun, M., Huppé-Gourgues, F., Legault, I., Rosa-Neto, P., Dumbrava, D., Faubert, J., et al. (2017). Cholinergic potentiation improves perceptual-cognitive training of healthy young adults in three dimensional multiple object tracking. *Front. Hum. Neurosci.* 11:128. doi: 10.3389/fnhum.2017.00128

Chang, E. F., and Merzenich, M. M. (2003). Environmental noise retards auditory cortical development. *Science* 300, 498–502. doi: 10.1126/science.1082163

Chino, Y. M., Kaas, J. H., Smith, E. L., Langston, A. L., and Cheng, H. (1992). Rapid reorganization of cortical maps in adult cats following restricted deafferentation in retina. *Vis. Res.* 32, 789–796. doi: 10.1016/0042-6989(92)90021-A

Coelho, F. G., de, M., Gobbi, S., Andreatto, C. A. A., Corazza, D. I., Pedroso, R. V., et al. (2013). Physical exercise modulates peripheral levels of brain-derived neurotrophic factor (BDNF): a systematic review of experimental studies in the elderly. *Arch. Gerontol. Geriatr.* 56, 10–15. doi: 10.1016/j.archger.2012.06.003

Colović, M. B., Krstić, D. Z., Lazarević-Pašti, T. D., Bondžić, A. M., and Vasić, V. M. (2013). Acetylcholinesterase inhibitors: pharmacology and toxicology. *Curr Neuropharmacol.* 11, 315–335. doi: 10.2174/1570159X11311030006

Cools, R. (2006). Dopaminergic modulation of cognitive function-implications for l-DOPA treatment in Parkinson's disease. *Neurosci. Biobehav. Rev.* 30, 1–23. doi: 10.1016/j.neubiorev.2005.03.024

Cramer, S. C., Sur, M., Dobkin, B. H., O'Brien, C., Sanger, T. D., Trojanowski, J. Q., et al. (2011). Harnessing neuroplasticity for clinical applications. *Brain* 134, 1591–1609. doi: 10.1093/brain/awr039

Cynader, M., and Mitchell, D. E. (1980). Prolonged sensitivity to monocular deprivation in dark-reared cats. *J. Neurophys.* 43, 1026–1040.

de Villers-Sidani, E., Alzghoul, L., Zhou, X., Simpson, K. L., Lin, R. C., and Merzenich, M. M. (2010). Recovery of functional and structural age-related changes in the rat primary auditory cortex with operant training. *Proc. Natl. Acad. Sci. U.S.A.* 107, 13900–13905. doi: 10.1073/pnas.1007885107

de Villers-Sidani, E., Chang, E. F., Bao, S., and Merzenich, M. M. (2007). Critical period window for spectral tuning defined in the primary auditory cortex (A1) in the rat. *J. Neurosci.* 27, 180–189. doi: 10.1523/JNEUROSCI.3227-06.2007

de Villers-Sidani, E., and Merzenich, M. M. (2011). Lifelong plasticity in the rat auditory cortex: basic mechanisms and role of sensory experience. *Prog. Brain Res.* 191, 119–131. doi: 10.1016/B978-0-444-53752-2.00009-6

de Villers-Sidani, E., Simpson, K. L., Lu, Y. F., Lin, R. C., and Merzenich, M. M. (2008). Manipulating critical period closure across different sectors of the primary auditory cortex. *Nat. Neurosci.* 11, 957–965. doi: 10.1038/nn.2144

Derringer, J., Krueger, R. F., Dick, D. M., Saccone, S., Grucza, R. A., Agrawal, A., et al. (2010). Predicting sensation seeking from dopamine genes. *Psychol. Sci.* 21, 1282–1290. doi: 10.1177/0956797610380699

Diamond, M. E., Armstrong-James, M., and Ebner, F. F. (1993). Experience-dependent plasticity in adult rat barrel cortex. *Proc. Natl. Acad. Sci. U.S.A.* 90, 2082–2086. doi: 10.1073/pnas.90.5.2082

Ellis, J. M. (2005). Cholinesterase inhibitors in the treatment of dementia. *J. Am. Osteopath. Assoc.* 105, 145–158.

Engineer, N. D., Percaccio, C. R., Pandya, P. K., Moucha, R., Rathbun, D. L., and Kilgard, M. P. (2004). Environmental enrichment improves response strength, threshold, selectivity, and latency of auditory cortex neurons. *J. Neurophys.* 92, 73–82. doi: 10.1152/jn.00059.2004

Everitt, B. J., and Robbins, T. W. (1997). Central cholinergic systems and cognition. *Annu. Rev. Psychol.* 48, 649–684. doi: 10.1146/annurev.psych.48.1.649

Fagiolini, M., and Hensch, T. K. (2000). Inhibitory threshold for critical-period activation in primary visual cortex. *Nature* 404, 183–186. doi: 10.1038/35004582

Fagiolini, M., Pizzorusso, T., Berardi, N., Domenici, L., and Maffei, L. (1994). Functional postnatal development of the rat primary visual cortex and the role of visual experience: dark rearing and monocular deprivation. *Vis. Res.* 34, 709–720. doi: 10.1016/0042-6989(94)90210-0

Feldman, D. E. (2005). Map plasticity in somatosensory cortex. *Science* 310, 810–815. doi: 10.1126/science.1115807

Fritschy, J. M., and Panzanelli, P. (2014). GABAA receptors and plasticity of inhibitory neurotransmission in the central nervous system. *Eur. J. Neurosci.* 39, 1845–1865. doi: 10.1111/ejn.12534

Froemke, R. C., Merzenich, M. M., and Schreiner, C. E. (2007). A synaptic memory trace for cortical receptive field plasticity. *Nature* 450, 425–429. doi: 10.1038/nature06289

Gates, G. A., Anderson, M. L., Feeney, M. P., McCurry, S. M., and Larson, E. B. (2008). Central auditory dysfunction in older persons with memory impairment or Alzheimer dementia. *Arch. Otolaryngol. Neck Surg.* 134, 771–777. doi: 10.1001/archotol.134.7.771

Gervain, J., Vines, B. W., Chen, L. M., Seo, R. J., Hensch, T. K., Werker, J. F., et al. (2013). Valproate reopens critical-period learning of absolute pitch. *Front. Syst. Neurosci.* 7:102. doi: 10.3389/fnsys.2013.00102

Gibson, G., Peterson, C., and Jenden, D. (1981). Brain acetylcholine synthesis declines with senescence. *Science* 213, 674–676. doi: 10.1126/science.7256270

Goldman-Rakic, P. S., Castner, S., and Williams, G. (2000). Clinical implications of the inverted U-shaped curve relating D1 stimulation and behavior. *Biol. Psychiatry* 47, S62. doi: 10.1016/S0006-3223(00)00296-1

Gourévitch, B., Edeline, J. M., Occelli, F., and Eggermont, J. J. (2014). Is the din really harmless? Long-term effects of non-traumatic noise on the adult auditory system. *Nat. Rev. Neurol.* 15, 483–491. doi: 10.1038/nrn3744

Greifzu, F., Pielecka-Fortuna, J., Kalogeraki, E., Krempler, K., Favaro, P. D., Schlüter, O. M., et al. (2014). Environmental enrichment extends ocular dominance plasticity into adulthood and protects from stroke-induced impairments of plasticity. *Proc. Natl. Acad. Sci. U.S.A.* 111, 1150–1155. doi: 10.1073/pnas.1313385111

Greuel, J. M., Luhmann, H. J., and Singer, W. (1988). Pharmacological induction of use-dependent receptive field modifications in the visual cortex. *Science* 242, 74–77. doi: 10.1126/science.2902687

Grinevich, V. P., Papke, R. L., Lippiello, P. M., and Bencherif, M. (2009). Atypical antipsychotics as noncompetitive inhibitors of $\alpha 4\beta 2$ and $\alpha 7$ neuronal nicotinic receptors. *Neuropharmacology* 57, 183–191. doi: 10.1016/j.neuropharm.2009.05.003

Gu, J., and Kanai, R. (2014). What contributes to individual differences in brain structure? *Front. Hum. Neurosci.* 8:262. doi: 10.3389/fnhum.2014.00262

Hamidovic, A., Dlugos, A., Skol, A., Palmer, A. A., and de Wit, H. (2009). Evaluation of genetic variability in the dopamine receptor D2 in relation to behavioral inhibition and impulsivity/sensation seeking: an exploratory study with d-amphetamine in healthy participants. *Exp. Clin. Psychopharmacol.* 17, 374–383. doi: 10.1037/a0017840

Hasselmo, M. E., and Sarter, M. (2011). Modes and models of forebrain cholinergic neuromodulation of cognition. *Neuropsychopharmacology* 36, 52–73. doi: 10.1038/npp.2010.104

He, H.-Y., Hodos, W., and Quinlan, E. M. (2006). Visual deprivation reactivates rapid ocular dominance plasticity in adult visual cortex. *J. Neurosci.* 26, 2951–2955. doi: 10.1523/JNEUROSCI.5554-05.2006

Hensch, T. K. (2005). Critical period plasticity in local cortical circuits. *Nat. Rev. Neurosci.* 6, 877–888. doi: 10.1038/nrn1787

Herrero, J. L., Roberts, M. J., Delicato, L. S., Gieselmann, M. A., Dayan, P., and Thiele, A. (2008). Acetylcholine contributes through muscarinic receptors to attentional modulation in V1. *Nature* 454, 1110–1114. doi: 10.1038/nature07141

Higley, M. J., and Picciotto, M. R. (2014). Neuromodulation by acetylcholine: examples from schizophrenia and depression. *Curr. Opin. Neurobiol.* 29, 88–95. doi: 10.1016/j.conb.2014.06.004

Huang, Y., and Mucke, L. (2012). Alzheimer mechanisms and therapeutic strategies. *Cell* 148, 1204–1222. doi: 10.1016/j.cell.2012.02.040

Hui, G. K., Wong, K. L., Chavez, C. M., Leon, M. I., Robin, K. M., and Weinberger, N. M. (2009). Conditioned tone control of brain reward behavior produces highly specific representational gain in the primary auditory cortex. *Neurobiol. Learn. Mem.* 92, 27–34. doi: 10.1016/j.nlm.2009.02.008

Insanally, M. N., Köver, H., Kim, H., and Bao, S. (2009). Feature-dependent sensitive periods in the development of complex sound representation. *J. Neurosci.* 29, 5456–5462. doi: 10.1523/JNEUROSCI.5311-08.2009

Jacobs, E., and D'Esposito, M. (2011). Estrogen shapes dopamine-dependent cognitive processes: implications for Women's health. *J. Neurosci.* 31, 5286–5293. doi: 10.1523/JNEUROSCI.6394-10.2011

Javitt, D. C. (2015). Neurophysiological models for new treatment development in schizophrenia: early sensory approaches. *Ann. N. Y. Acad. Sci.* 1344, 92–104. doi: 10.1111/nyas.12689

Javitt, D. C., and Freedman, R. (2015). Sensory processing dysfunction in the personal experience and neuronal machinery of schizophrenia. *Am. J. Psychiatry* 172, 17–31. doi: 10.1176/appi.ajp.2014.13121691

Javitt, D. C., and Sweet, R. A. (2015). Auditory dysfunction in schizophrenia: integrating clinical and basic features. *Nat. Rev. Neurosci.* 16, 535–550. doi: 10.1038/nrn4002

Kamal, B., Holman, C., and de Villers-Sidani, E. (2013). Shaping the aging brain: role of auditory input patterns in the emergence of auditory cortical impairments. *Front. Syst. Neurosci.* 7:52. doi: 10.3389/fnsys.2013.00052

Kang, J.-I., Huppé-Gourgues, F., and Vaucher, E. (2015). Pharmacological mechanisms of cortical enhancement induced by the repetitive pairing of visual/cholinergic stimulation. *PLOS ONE* 10:e0141663. doi: 10.1371/journal.pone.0141663

Kang, J.I., Groleau, M., Dotigny, F., Giguère, H., and Vaucher, E. (2014). Visual training paired with electrical stimulation of the basal forebrain improves orientation-selective visual acuity in the rat. *Brain Struct. Funct.* 219, 1493–1507. doi: 10.1007/s00429-013-0582-y

Kang, J.I., and Vaucher, E. (2009). Cholinergic pairing with visual activation results in long-term enhancement of visual evoked potentials. *PLOS ONE* 4:e5995. doi: 10.1371/journal.pone.0005995

Kartje, G. L., Schulz, M. K., Lopez-Yunez, A., Schnell, L., and Schwab, M. E. (1999). Corticostriatal plasticity is restricted by myelin-associated neurite growth inhibitors in the adult rat. *Ann. Neurol.* 45, 778–786. doi: 10.1002/1531-8249(199906)45:6<778::AID-ANA12>3.0.CO;2-B

Kasamatsu, T., and Pettigrew, J. (1976). Depletion of brain catecholamines: failure of ocular dominance shift after monocular occlusion in kittens. *Science* 194, 206–209. doi: 10.1126/science.959850

Kasamatsu, T., Pettigrew, J. D., and Ary, M. (1979). Restoration of visual cortical plasticity by local microperfusion of norepinephrine. *J. Comp. Neurol.* 185, 163–181. doi: 10.1002/cne.901850110

Keers, R., and Aitchison, K. J. (2010). Gender differences in antidepressant drug response. *Int. Rev. Psychiatry* 22, 485–500. doi: 10.3109/09540261.2010.496448

Kilgard, M. P., and Merzenich, M. M. (1998). Cortical map reorganization enabled by nucleus basalis activity. *Science* 279, 1714–1718. doi: 10.1126/science.279.5357.1714

Kim, H., and Bao, S. (2009). Selective increase in representations of sounds repeated at an ethological rate. *J. Neurosci.* 29, 5163–5169. doi: 10.1523/JNEUROSCI.0365-09.2009

Kirkwood, A. (2007). "Neuromodulation of cortical synaptic plasticity," in *Monoaminergic Modulation of Cortical Excitability*, eds K. Y. Tseng and M. Atzori (Boston, MA: Springer), 209–216. doi: 10.1007/978-0-387-72256-6_14

Knudsen, E. I. (2004). Sensitive periods in the development of the brain and behavior. *J. Cogn. Neurosci.* 16, 1412–1425. doi: 10.1162/0898929042304796

Kral, A., and Sharma, A. (2012). Developmental neuroplasticity after cochlear implantation. *Trends Neurosci.* 35, 111–122. doi: 10.1016/j.tins.2011.09.004

Kroener, S., Chandler, L. J., Phillips, P. E. M., and Seamans, J. K. (2009). Dopamine modulates persistent synaptic activity and enhances the signal-to-noise ratio in the prefrontal cortex. *PLOS ONE.* 4:e6507. doi: 10.1371/journal.pone.0006507

Kuhlman, S. J., Olivas, N. D., Tring, E., Ikrar, T., Xu, X., and Trachtenberg, J. T. (2013). A disinhibitory microcircuit initiates critical-period plasticity in the visual cortex. *Nature* 501, 543–546. doi: 10.1038/nature12485

Lee, N. R., Raznahan, A., Wallace, G. L., Alexander-Bloch, A., Clasen, L. S., Lerch, J. P., et al. (2014). Anatomical coupling among distributed cortical regions in youth varies as a function of individual differences in vocabulary abilities. *Hum. Brain Mapp.* 35, 1885–1895. doi: 10.1002/hbm.22299

Leggio, M. G., Mandolesi, L., Federico, F., Spirito, F., Ricci, B., Gelfo, F., et al. (2005). Environmental enrichment promotes improved spatial abilities and enhanced dendritic growth in the rat. *Behav. Brain Res.* 163, 78–90. doi: 10.1016/j.bbr.2005.04.009

Levin, E. D., Briggs, S. J., Christopher, N. C., and Rose, J. E. (1993). Chronic nicotinic stimulation and blockade effects on working memory. *Behav. Pharmacol.* 4, 179–182. doi: 10.1097/00008877-199304000-00010

Mahncke, H. W., Bronstone, A., and Merzenich, M. M. (2006). Brain plasticity and functional losses in the aged: scientific bases for a novel intervention. *Prog. Brain Res.* 157, 81–109. doi: 10.1016/S0079-6123(06)57006-2

Mandl, R. C. W., Pasternak, O., Cahn, W., Kahn, R. S., and Hulshoff Pol, H. E. (2015). Comparing free water imaging and magnetization transfer measurements in schizophrenia. *Schizophr. Res.* 161, 126–132. doi: 10.1016/j.schres.2014.09.046

Manunta, Y., and Edeline, J. M. (1998). Effects of noradrenaline on rate-level function of auditory cortex neurons: is there a "gating" effect of noradrenaline? *Exp. Brain Res.* 118, 361–372. doi: 10.1007/s002210050290

Marín, O. (2012). Interneuron dysfunction in psychiatric disorders. *Nat. Rev. Neurosci.* 13, 107–120. doi: 10.1038/nrn3155

McGee, A. W., Yang, Y., Fischer, Q. S., Daw, N. W., and Strittmatter, S. M. (2005). Experience-driven plasticity of visual cortex limited by myelin and Nogo receptor. *Science* 309, 2222–2226. doi: 10.1126/science.1114362

McGeer, P. L., McGeer, E. G., Suzuki, J., Dolman, C. E., and Nagai, T. (1984). Aging, Alzheimer's disease, and the cholinergic system of the basal forebrain. *Neurology* 34, 741–745. doi: 10.1212/WNL.34.6.741

McRae, P. A., Rocco, M. M., Kelly, G., Brumberg, J. C., and Matthews, R. T. (2007). Sensory deprivation alters aggrecan and perineuronal net expression in the mouse barrel cortex. *J. Neurosci.* 27, 5405–5413. doi: 10.1523/JNEUROSCI.5425-06.2007

Mighdoll, M. I., Tao, R., Kleinman, J. E., and Hyde, T. M. (2015). Myelin, myelin-related disorders, and psychosis. *Schizophr. Res.* 161, 85–93. doi: 10.1016/j.schres.2014.09.040

Mishra, J., de Villers-Sidani, E., Merzenich, M., and Gazzaley, A. (2014). Adaptive training diminishes distractibility in aging across species. *Neuron* 84, 1091–1103. doi: 10.1016/j.neuron.2014.10.034

Mora, F., Segovia, G., and del Arco, A. (2007). Aging, plasticity and environmental enrichment: Structural changes and neurotransmitter dynamics in several areas of the brain. *Brain Res. Rev.* 55, 78–88. doi: 10.1016/j.brainresrev.2007.03.011

Moran, R. J., Campo, P., Symmonds, M., Stephan, K. E., Dolan, R. J., and Friston, K. J. (2013). Free energy, precision and learning: the role of cholinergic neuromodulation. *J. Neurosci.* 33, 8227–8236. doi: 10.1523/JNEUROSCI.4255-12.2013

Morris, G. P., Clark, I. A., Zinn, R., and Vissel, B. (2013). Microglia: a new frontier for synaptic plasticity, learning and memory, and neurodegenerative disease research. *Neurobiol. Learn. Mem.* 105, 40–53. doi: 10.1016/j.nlm.2013.07.002

Mower, G. D. (1991). The effect of dark rearing on the time course of the critical period in cat visual cortex. *Brain Res. Dev. Brain Res.* 58, 151–158. doi: 10.1016/0165-3806(91)90001-Y

Müller, U., von Cramon, D. Y., and Pollmann, S. (1998). D1- Versus D2-receptor modulation of visuospatial working memory in humans. *J. Neurosci.* 18, 2720–2728.

Nithianantharajah, J., and Hannan, A. J. (2006). Enriched environments, experience-dependent plasticity and disorders of the nervous system. *Nat. Rev. Neurosci.* 7, 697–709. doi: 10.1038/nrn1970

Norbury, A., and Husain, M. (2015). Sensation-seeking: dopaminergic modulation and risk for psychopathology. *Behav. Brain Res.* 288, 79–93. doi: 10.1016/j.bbr.2015.04.015

Norbury, A., Manohar, S., Rogers, R. D., and Husain, M. (2013). Dopamine modulates risk-taking as a function of baseline sensation-seeking trait. *J. Neurosci.* 33, 12982–12986. doi: 10.1523/JNEUROSCI.5587-12.2013

Noudoost, B., and Moore, T. (2011). Control of visual cortical signals by prefrontal dopamine. *Nature* 474, 372–375. doi: 10.1038/nature09995

Oberman, L., and Pascual-Leone, A. (2013). Changes in plasticity across the lifespan: cause of disease and target for intervention. *Prog. Brain Res.* 207, 91–120. doi: 10.1016/B978-0-444-63327-9.00016-3

Ouellet, L., and de Villers-Sidani, E. (2014). Trajectory of the main GABAergic interneuron populations from early development to old age in the rat primary auditory cortex. *Front. Neuroanat.* 8:40. doi: 10.3389/fnana.2014.00040

Perrachione, T. K., Lee, J., Ha, L. Y., and Wong, P. C. (2011). Learning a novel phonological contrast depends on interactions between individual differences and training paradigm design. *J. Acoust. Soc. Am.* 130, 461–472. doi: 10.1121/1.3593366

Pienkowski, M., and Eggermont, J. J. (2010). Intermittent exposure with moderate-level sound impairs central auditory function of mature animals without concomitant hearing loss. *Hear. Res.* 261, 30–35. doi: 10.1016/j.heares.2009.12.025

Pizzorusso, T., Medini, P., Berardi, N., Chierzi, S., Fawcett, J. W., and Maffei, L. (2002). Reactivation of ocular dominance plasticity in the adult visual cortex. *Science* 298, 1248–1251. doi: 10.1126/science.1072699

Quinlan, M. G., Almey, A., Caissie, M., LaChappelle, I., Radiotis, G., and Brake, W. G. (2013). Estradiol and striatal dopamine receptor antagonism influence memory system bias in the female rat. *Neurobiol. Learn. Mem.* 106, 221–229. doi: 10.1016/j.nlm.2013.08.018

Rice, F. L., and Van der Loos, H. (1977). Development of the barrels and barrel field in the somatosensory cortex of the mouse. *J. Comp. Neurol.* 171, 545–560. doi: 10.1002/cne.901710408

Rokem, A., and Silver, M. A. (2010). Cholinergic enhancement augments magnitude and specificity of visual perceptual learning in healthy humans. *Curr. Biol.* 20, 1723–1728. doi: 10.1016/j.cub.2010.08.027

Rokem, A., and Silver, M. A. (2013). The benefits of cholinergic enhancement during perceptual learning are long-lasting. *Front. Comput. Neurosci.* 7:66. doi: 10.3389/fncom.2013.00066

Schliebs, R., and Arendt, T. (2011). The cholinergic system in aging and neuronal degeneration. *Behav. Brain Res.* 221, 555–563. doi: 10.1016/j.bbr.2010.11.058

Sengpiel, F., Stawinski, P., and Bonhoeffer, T. (1999). Influence of experience on orientation maps in cat visual cortex. *Nat. Neurosci.* 2, 727–732. doi: 10.1038/11192

Shepard, K. N., Liles, L. C., Weinshenker, D., and Liu, R. C. (2015). Norepinephrine is necessary for experience-dependent plasticity in the developing mouse auditory cortex. *J. Neurosci.* 35, 2432–2437. doi: 10.1523/JNEUROSCI.0532-14.2015

Singh, A., and Abraham, W. C. (2017). Astrocytes and synaptic plasticity in health and disease. *Exp. Brain Res.* 235, 1645–1655. doi: 10.1007/s00221-017-4928-1

Soha, J. A., and Marler, P. (2001). Cues for early discrimination of conspecific song in the white-crowned sparrow (*Zonotrichia leucophrys*). *Ethology* 107, 813–826. doi: 10.1046/j.1439-0310.2001.00713.x

Sorg, B. A., Berretta, S., Blacktop, J. M., Fawcett, J. W., Kitagawa, H., Kwok, J. C. F., et al. (2016). Casting a wide net: role of perineuronal nets in neural plasticity. *J. Neurosci.* 36, 11459–11468. doi: 10.1523/JNEUROSCI.2351-16.2016

Stanley, E. M., Fadel, J. R., and Mott, D. D. (2012). Interneuron loss reduces dendritic inhibition and GABA release in hippocampus of aged rats. *Neurobiol. Aging* 33, 431, e1–13. doi: 10.1016/j.neurobiolaging.2010.12.014

Störmer, V. S., Passow, S., Biesenack, J., and Li, S.-C. (2012). Dopaminergic and cholinergic modulations of visual-spatial attention and working memory: insights from molecular genetic research and implications for adult cognitive development. *Dev. Psychol.* 48, 875–889. doi: 10.1037/a0026198

Suraweera, C., Hanwella, R., and de Silva, V. A. (2015). Medications used in dementia: a review of evidence. *Sri Lanka J. Psychiatry* 6, 3–8. doi: 10.4038/sljpsyc.v6i2.8073

Szuhany, K. L., Bugatti, M., and Otto, M. W. (2015). A meta-analytic review of the effects of exercise on brain-derived neurotrophic factor. *J. Psychiatr. Res.* 60, 56–64. doi: 10.1016/j.jpsychires.2014.10.003

Tanaka, S., Tani, T., Ribot, J., O'Hashi, K., and Imamura, K. (2009). A postnatal critical period for orientation plasticity in the cat visual cortex. *PLOS ONE* 4:e5380. doi: 10.1371/journal.pone.0005380

Tang, H., McGowan, O. O., and Reynolds, G. P. (2014). Polymorphisms of serotonin neurotransmission and their effects on antipsychotic drug action. *Pharmacogenomics* 15, 1599–1609. doi: 10.2217/pgs.14.111

Turner, R. M., Park, B. K., and Pirmohamed, M. (2015). Parsing interindividual drug variability: an emerging role for systems pharmacology. *Wiley Interdiscip. Rev. Syst. Biol. Med.* 7, 221–241. doi: 10.1002/wsbm.1302

Uban, K. A., Rummel, J., Floresco, S. B., and Galea, L. A. M. (2012). Estradiol modulates effort-based decision making in female rats. *Neuropsychopharmacology* 37, 390–401. doi: 10.1038/npp.2011.176

Van Brussel, L., Gerits, A., and Arckens, L. (2011). Evidence for cross-modal plasticity in adult mouse visual cortex following monocular enucleation. *Cereb. Cortex* 21, 2133–2146. doi: 10.1093/cercor/bhq286

Vinogradov, S., Fisher, M., and de Villers-Sidani, E. (2012). Cognitive training for impaired neural systems in neuropsychiatric illness. *Neuropsychopharmacology* 37, 43–76. doi: 10.1038/npp.2011.251

Voss, P., Thomas, M., Chou, Y. C., Cisneros-Franco, J. M., Ouellet, L., and de Villers-Sidani, E. (2016). Pairing cholinergic enhancement with perceptual training promotes recovery of age-related changes in rat primary auditory cortex. *Neural Plast.* 2016, 1–18. doi: 10.1155/2016/1801979

Voss, V., and Zatorre, R. J. (2015). Early visual deprivation changes cortical anatomical covariance in dorsal-stream structures. *Neuroimage* 108, 194–202. doi: 10.1016/j.neuroimage.2014.12.063

Wang, D., and Fawcett, J. (2012). The perineuronal net and the control of CNS plasticity. *Cell Tissue Res.* 349, 147–160. doi: 10.1007/s00441-012-1375-y

Wang, J., Ikonen, S., Gurevicius, K., Van Groen, T., and Tanila, H. (2003). Altered auditory-evoked potentials in mice carrying mutated human amyloid precursor protein and presenilin-1 transgenes. *Neuroscience* 116, 511–517. doi: 10.1016/S0306-4522(02)00714-5

Wen, M. C., Steffens, D. C., Chen, M. K., and Zainal, N. H. (2014). Diffusion tensor imaging studies in late-life depression: systematic review and meta-analysis. *Int. J. Geriatr. Psychiatry* 29, 1173–1184. doi: 10.1002/gps.4129

White-Schwoch, T., Woodruff Carr, K., Anderson, S., Strait, D. L., and Kraus, N. (2013). Older adults benefit from music training early in life: biological evidence for long-term training-driven plasticity. *J. Neurosci.* 33, 7667–7674. doi: 10.1523/JNEUROSCI.2560-13.2013

Wiesel, T. N., and Hubel, D. H. (1963). Effects of visual deprivation on morphology and physiology of cells in the cat's lateral geniculate body. *J. Neurophys.* 26, 978–993.

Winterer, G., and Weinberger, D. R. (2004). Genes, dopamine and cortical signal-to-noise ratio in schizophrenia. *Trends Neurosci.* 27, 683–690. doi: 10.1016/j.tins.2004.08.002

Wong, P. C. M., and Perrachione, T. K. (2007). Learning pitch patterns in lexical identification by native English-speaking adults. *Appl. Psycholinguist.* 28, 565–585. doi: 10.1017/S0142716407070312

Zenner, H.-P., Delb, W., Kröner-Herwig, B., Jäger, B., Peroz, I., Hesse, G., et al. (2017). A multidisciplinary systematic review of the treatment for chronic idiopathic tinnitus. *Eur. Arch. Otorhinolaryngol.* 274, 2079–2091. doi: 10.1007/s00405-016-4401-y

Zhang, L. I., Bao, S., and Merzenich, M. M. (2001). Persistent and specific influences of early acoustic environments on primary auditory cortex. *Nat. Neurosci.* 4, 1123–1130. doi: 10.1038/nn745

Zhang, L. I., Bao, S., and Merzenich, M. M. (2002). Disruption of primary auditory cortex by synchronous auditory inputs during a critical period. *Proc. Natl. Acad. Sci. U.S.A.* 99, 2309–2314. doi: 10.1073/pnas.261707398

Zheng, W. (2012). Auditory map reorganization and pitch discrimination in adult rats chronically exposed to low-level ambient noise. *Front. Syst. Neurosci.* 6:65. doi: 10.3389/fnsys.2012.00065

Zhou, X., Panizzutti, R., de Villers-Sidani, E., Madeira, C., and Merzenich, M. M. (2011). Natural restoration of critical period plasticity in the juvenile and adult primary auditory cortex. *J. Neurosci.* 31, 5625–5634. doi: 10.1523/JNEUROSCI.6470-10.2011

Permissions

All chapters in this book were first published in CBPIPECTVGCI, by Frontiers; hereby published with permission under the Creative Commons Attribution License or equivalent. Every chapter published in this book has been scrutinized by our experts. Their significance has been extensively debated. The topics covered herein carry significant findings which will fuel the growth of the discipline. They may even be implemented as practical applications or may be referred to as a beginning point for another development.

The contributors of this book come from diverse backgrounds, making this book a truly international effort. This book will bring forth new frontiers with its revolutionizing research information and detailed analysis of the nascent developments around the world.

We would like to thank all the contributing authors for lending their expertise to make the book truly unique.

They have played a crucial role in the development of this book. Without their invaluable contributions this book wouldn't have been possible. They have made vital efforts to compile up to date information on the varied aspects of this subject to make this book a valuable addition to the collection of many professionals and students.

This book was conceptualized with the vision of imparting up-to-date information and advanced data in this field. To ensure the same, a matchless editorial board was set up. Every individual on the board went through rigorous rounds of assessment to prove their worth. After which they invested a large part of their time researching and compiling the most relevant data for our readers.

The editorial board has been involved in producing this book since its inception. They have spent rigorous hours researching and exploring the diverse topics which have resulted in the successful publishing of this book. They have passed on their knowledge of decades through this book. To expedite this challenging task, the publisher supported the team at every step. A small team of assistant editors was also appointed to further simplify the editing procedure and attain best results for the readers.

Apart from the editorial board, the designing team has also invested a significant amount of their time inunderstanding the subject and creating the most relevant covers. They scrutinized every image to scout for the most suitable representation of the subject and create an appropriate cover for the book.

The publishing team has been an ardent support to the editorial, designing and production team. Their endless efforts to recruit the best for this project, has resulted in the accomplishment of this book. They are a veteran in the field of academics and their pool of knowledge is as vast as their experience in printing. Their expertise and guidance has proved useful at every step. Their uncompromising quality standards have made this book an exceptional effort. Their encouragement from time to time has been an inspiration for everyone.

The publisher and the editorial board hope that this book will prove to be a valuable piece of knowledge for researchers, students, practitioners and scholars across the globe.

List of Contributors

Kang K. L. Liu
Laboratory for Network Physiology, Department of Physics, Boston University, Boston, MA, USA
Department of Neurology, Beth Israel Deaconess Medical Center, Harvard Medical School, Boston, MA, USA

Ronny P. Bartsch
Department of Physics, Bar-Ilan University, Ramat Gan, Israel

Aijing Lin
Laboratory for Network Physiology, Department of Physics, Boston University, Boston, MA, USA
Department of Mathematics, School of Science, Beijing Jiaotong University, Beijing, China

Rosario N. Mantegna
Dipartimento di Fisica e Chimica, Viale delle Scienze, University of Palermo, Palermo, Italy
Center for Network Science and Department of Economics, Central European University, Budapest, Hungary

Plamen Ch. Ivanov
Laboratory for Network Physiology, Department of Physics, Boston University, Boston, MA, USA
Division of Sleep Medicine, Brigham and Women's Hospital, Harvard Medical School, Boston, MA, USA
Institute of Solid State Physics, Bulgarian Academy of Sciences, Sofia, Bulgaria

Sarah A. Fraser
Interdisciplinary School of Health Sciences, University of Ottawa, Ottawa, ON, Canada

Karen Z.-H. Li and Kiran Vadaga
Department of Psychology, Concordia University, Montréal, QC, Canada

Nicolas Berryman
Sports Studies, Bishop's University, Sherbrooke, QC, Canada
Centre de Recherche de l'Institut Universitaire de Gériatrie de Montréal, Montréal, QC, Canada

Laurence Desjardins-Crépeau
Centre de Recherche de l'Institut Universitaire de Gériatrie de Montréal, Montréal, QC, Canada
Department of Psychology, Université du Québec à Montréal, Montréal, QC, Canada

Maxime Lussier
Centre de Recherche de l'Institut Universitaire de Gériatrie de Montréal, Montréal, QC, Canada

Lora Lehr, Thien Tuong Minh Vu and Louis Bherer
Centre de Recherche de l'Institut Universitaire de Gériatrie de Montréal, Montréal, QC, Canada
Medecine, Université de Montréal, Montréal, QC, Canada

Laurent Bosquet
Laboratoire MOVE (EA6314), Faculté des Sciences du Sport, Université de Poitiers, Poitiers, France

Jessika I. V. Buitenweg, Renate M. van de Ven, Sam Prinssen and Jaap M. J. Murre
Department of Psychology, University of Amsterdam, Amsterdam, Netherlands

K. Richard Ridderinkhof
Department of Psychology, University of Amsterdam, Amsterdam, Netherlands
Amsterdam Brain and Cognition, University of Amsterdam, Amsterdam, Netherlands

Jesper Lundbye-Jensen and Kasper Skriver
Department of Nutrition, Exercise and Sports, University of Copenhagen, Copenhagen, Denmark
Department of Neuroscience and Pharmacology, University of Copenhagen, Copenhagen, Denmark
Copenhagen Centre for Team Sport and Health, University of Copenhagen, Copenhagen, Denmark

Jens B. Nielsen
Department of Neuroscience and Pharmacology, University of Copenhagen, Copenhagen, Denmark

Marc Roig
Memory and Motor Rehabilitation Laboratory (MEMORY-LAB), Feil and Oberfeld Research Centre, Jewish Rehabilitation Hospital, Montreal Center for Interdisciplinary Research in Rehabilitation (CRIR), Laval, QC, Canada
School of Physical and Occupational Therapy, Faculty of Medicine, McGill University, Montreal, QC, Canada

Normand Teasdale and Martin Simoneau
Department of Kinesiology, Faculty of Medicine, Université Laval, Quebec City, QC, Canada
Centre intégré universitaire de santé et de services sociaux de la Capitale-Nationale et Centre d'excellence sur le vieillissement de Québec, Quebec City, QC, Canada

Lisa Hudon Mathieu and Germain Robitaille
Department of Kinesiology, Faculty of Medicine, Université Laval, Quebec City, QC, Canada

Thierry Moszkowicz and Denis Laurendeau
Computer Vision and Systems Laboratory, Department of Electrical Engineering, Université Laval, Quebec City, QC, Canada

Louis Bherer
PERFORM Centre, Concordia University, Montreal, QC, Canada
Department of Medicine, University of Montreal and Montreal Heart Institute, Montreal, QC, Canada

Simon Duchesne
Centre de recherche de l'Institut universitaire en santé mentale de Québec, Quebec City, QC, Canada
Département de Radiologie, Faculté de Médecine, Université Laval, Quebec City, QC, Canada

Carol Hudon
Centre de recherche de l'Institut universitaire en santé mentale de Québec, Quebec City, QC, Canada
École de psychologie, Université Laval, Quebec City, QC, Canada

Jérôme Nicolas Spring and Jérôme Barral
Institute of Sport Sciences, Faculty of Social and Political Sciences, University of Lausanne, Lausanne, Switzerland

Nicolas Place and Bengt Kayser
Institute of Sport Sciences and Department of Physiology, Faculty of Biology and Medicine, University of Lausanne, Lausanne, Switzerland

Fabio Borrani
Institute of Sport Sciences, Faculty of Biology and Medicine, University of Lausanne, Lausanne, Switzerland

Chelsea M. Stillman
Department of Psychiatry, School of Medicine, University of Pittsburgh Medical Center, Pittsburgh, PA, USA
Center for the Neural Basis of Cognition, University of Pittsburgh, Pittsburgh, PA, USA

Jamie Cohen
Center for the Neural Basis of Cognition, University of Pittsburgh, Pittsburgh, PA, USA
Department of Psychology, University of Pittsburgh, Pittsburgh, PA, USA

Morgan E. Lehman
Department of Psychology, University of Pittsburgh, Pittsburgh, PA, USA

Kirk I. Erickson
Department of Psychiatry, School of Medicine, University of Pittsburgh Medical Center, Pittsburgh, PA, USA
Center for the Neural Basis of Cognition, University of Pittsburgh, Pittsburgh, PA, USA
Department of Psychology, University of Pittsburgh, Pittsburgh, PA, USA

Madeleine Ordnung, Maike Hoff and Elisabeth Kaminski
Department of Neurology, Max Planck Institute for Human Cognitive and Brain Sciences, Leipzig, Germany

Arno Villringer
Department of Neurology, Max Planck Institute for Human Cognitive and Brain Sciences, Leipzig, Germany
Mind and Brain Institute, Charité and Humboldt University, Berlin, Germany

Patrick Ragert
Department of Neurology, Max Planck Institute for Human Cognitive and Brain Sciences, Leipzig, Germany
Institute for General Kinesiology and Exercise Science, University of Leipzig, Leipzig, Germany

Ben Godde
Department of Psychology and Methods, Jacobs University Bremen, Bremen, Germany
Jacobs Center on Lifelong Learning and Institutional Development, Jacobs University Bremen, Bremen, Germany
Center for Cognitive Science, Bremen University, Bremen, Germany

Claudia Voelcker-Rehage
Jacobs Center on Lifelong Learning and Institutional Development, Jacobs University Bremen, Bremen, Germany
Center for Cognitive Science, Bremen University, Bremen, Germany
Institute of Human Movement Science and Health, Technische Universität Chemnitz, Chemnitz, Germany

Zahraa Chorghay and Edward S. Ruthazer
Department of Neurology and Neurosurgery, Montreal Neurological Institute, McGill University, Montreal, QC, Canada

Ragnhildur Thóra Káradóttir
Department of Veterinary Medicine, Wellcome Trust - Medical Research Council Stem Cell Institute, University of Cambridge, Cambridge, United Kingdom

Xiao-Ying Tan
School of Physical Education and Coaching, Shanghai University of Sport, Shanghai, China

Yan-Ling Pi
Shanghai Punan Hospital of Pudong New District, Shanghai, China

Jue Wang
Institutes of Psychological Sciences, HangZhou Normal University, Hangzhou, China

Xue-Pei Li, Lan-Lan Zhang, Wen Dai, Hua Zhu and Jian Zhang
School of Kinesiology, Shanghai University of Sport, Shanghai, China

Zhen Ni
Division of Neurology, Krembil Neuroscience Centre and Toronto Western Research Institute, University Health Network, University of Toronto, Toronto, ON, Canada

Yin Wu
School of Economics and Management, Shanghai University of Sport, Shanghai, China

Man-Man Wang, Ya-Shuo Feng, Ying Xing and Jing Zhang
Department of Rehabilitation Medicine, The Third Hospital of Hebei Medical University, Shijiazhuang, China

Si-Dong Yang
Department of Spine Surgery, The Third Hospital of Hebei Medical University, Shijiazhuang, China

Fang Dong
Department of Clinical Laboratory Medicine, The Third Hospital of Hebei Medical University, Shijiazhuang, China

Feng Zhang
Department of Rehabilitation Medicine, The Third Hospital of Hebei Medical University, Shijiazhuang, China
Hebei Provincial Orthopedic Biomechanics Key Laboratory, The Third Hospital of Hebei Medical University, Shijiazhuang, China

Mikkel M. Beck, Rune R. Lind, Svend S. Geertsen, Jesper Lundbye-Jensen and Jacob Wienecke
Department of Nutrition, Exercise and Sports, University of Copenhagen, Copenhagen, Denmark
Department of Neuroscience and Pharmacology, University of Copenhagen, Copenhagen, Denmark

Christian Ritz
Department of Nutrition, Exercise and Sports, University of Copenhagen, Copenhagen, Denmark

Fan Su and Wendong Xu
Department of Hand Surgery Huashan Hospital, Shanghai Medical College, Fudan University, Shanghai, China

Changshen Yu, Wanjun Wang, Shoufeng Liu, Chunlin Gao and Jialing Wu
Department of Neurorehabilitation, Department of Neurology, Tianjin Huanhu Hospital, Tianjin Key Laboratory of Cerebrovascular and Neurodegenerative Diseases, Tianjin, China

Yue Zhang, Yizhao Wang and Weijia Hou
Department of Rehabilitation Medicine, Tianjin Huanhu Hospital, Tianjin Key Laboratory of Cerebrovascular and Neurodegenerative Diseases, Tianjin, China

Chen Wang and Lidong Mo
Neurological Disease Biobank, Tianjin Neurosurgical Institute, Tianjin Huanhu Hospital, Tianjin Key Laboratory of Cerebrovascular and Neurodegenerative Diseases, Tianjin, China

Michael Rullmann
IFB Adiposity Diseases, Leipzig University Medical Centre, Leipzig, Germany
Department of Nuclear Medicine, University Hospital Leipzig, Leipzig, Germany
Department of Neurology, Max Planck Institute for Human Cognitive and Brain Sciences, Leipzig, Germany
Collaborative Research Centre 1052 Obesity Mechanisms, University of Leipzig, Leipzig, Germany

Sven Preusser and Karsten Müller
Department of Neurology, Max Planck Institute for Human Cognitive and Brain Sciences, Leipzig, Germany

Sindy Poppitz
IFB Adiposity Diseases, Leipzig University Medical Centre, Leipzig, Germany
Department of Neurology, Max Planck Institute for Human Cognitive and Brain Sciences, Leipzig, Germany

Stefanie Heba
Department of Neurology, BG University Hospital Bergmannsheil, Ruhr-University Bochum, Bochum, Germany

Konstantinos Gousias
Department of Neurosurgery, BG University Hospital Bergmannsheil, Ruhr-University Bochum, Bochum, Germany

Jana Hoyer
Department of Behavioral Epidemiology, Technische Universität Dresden, Dresden, Germany
Department of Psychology, Technische Universität Dresden, Dresden, Germany

Tatjana Schütz
IFB Adiposity Diseases, Leipzig University Medical Centre, Leipzig, Germany

Arne Dietrich
IFB Adiposity Diseases, Leipzig University Medical Centre, Leipzig, Germany
Department of Bariatric Surgery, University Hospital Leipzig, Leipzig, Germany

Mohammed K. Hankir
Department of Experimental Surgery, University Hospital Würzburg, Würzburg, Germany

Burkhard Pleger
IFB Adiposity Diseases, Leipzig University Medical Centre, Leipzig, Germany
Department of Neurology, Max Planck Institute for Human Cognitive and Brain Sciences, Leipzig, Germany
Collaborative Research Centre 1052 Obesity Mechanisms, University of Leipzig, Leipzig, Germany
Department of Neurology, BG University Hospital Bergmannsheil, Ruhr-University Bochum, Bochum, Germany

Kristina Küper, Patrick D. Gajewski, Claudia Frieg and Michael Falkenstein
Aging Research Group, Leibniz Research Centre for Working Environment and Human Factors, Dortmund, Germany

Guiyi Li and Alicia Hidalgo
Plasticity and Regeneration Lab, School of Biosciences, University of Birmingham, Birmingham, United Kingdom

Stephan Heinzel
Clinical Psychology and Psychotherapy, Freie Universität Berlin, Berlin, Germany
Social and Preventive Medicine, University of Potsdam, Potsdam, Germany
Department of Psychology, Humboldt-Universität zu Berlin, Berlin, Germany

Jérôme Rimpel
Clinical Psychology and Neuropsychology, Johannes Gutenberg University Mainz, Mainz, Germany

Christine Stelzel
Social and Preventive Medicine, University of Potsdam, Potsdam, Germany
International Psychoanalytic University, Berlin, Germany
Berlin School of Mind and Brain, Berlin, Germany

Michael A. Rapp
Social and Preventive Medicine, University of Potsdam, Potsdam, Germany

Patrice Voss, Maryse E. Thomas, J. Miguel Cisneros-Franco and Étienne de Villers-Sidani
Department of Neurology and Neurosurgery, Montreal Neurological Institute, McGill University, Montreal, QC, Canada

Index

CPSIA information can be obtained
at www.ICGtesting.com
Printed in the USA
LVHW060854030122
707669LV00002B/146

9 781639 871179